T0229987

The New Psychology
of Health

Why do people who are more socially connected live longer and have better health than those who are socially isolated?

Why are social ties at least as good for your health as not smoking, having a good diet, and taking regular exercise?

Why is treatment more effective when there is an alliance between therapist and client?

Until now, researchers and practitioners have lacked a strong theoretical foundation for answering such questions. This ground-breaking book fills this gap by showing how social identity processes are key to understanding and effectively managing a broad range of health-related problems.

Integrating a wealth of evidence that the authors and colleagues around the world have built up over the last decade, *The New Psychology of Health* provides a powerful framework for reconceptualising the psychological dimensions of a range of conditions – including stress, trauma, ageing, depression, addiction, eating behaviour, brain injury, and pain.

Alongside reviews of current approaches to these various issues, each chapter provides an in-depth analysis of the ways in which theory and practice can be enriched by attention to social identity processes. Here the authors show not only how an array of social and structural factors shape health outcomes through their impact on group life, but also how this analysis can be harnessed to promote the delivery of 'social cures' in a range of fields.

This is a must-have volume for service providers, practitioners, students, and researchers working in a wide range of disciplines and fields, and will also be essential reading for anyone whose goal it is to improve the health and well-being of people and communities in their care.

Catherine Haslam (PhD, Australian National University) is Professor of Clinical Psychology at The University of Queensland.

Jolanda Jetten (PhD, University of Amsterdam) is a Professor of Social Psychology and former Australian Research Council Future Fellow at The University of Queensland.

Tegan Cruwys (PhD, Australian National University) is an Australian Research Council Developing Early Career Researcher and Senior Lecturer in Psychology at The University of Queensland.

Genevieve Dingle (PhD, University of Queensland) is a Senior Lecturer in Clinical Psychology at The University of Queensland.

S. Alexander Haslam (PhD, Macquarie University) is a Professor of Social and Organisational Psychology and Australian Research Council Laureate Fellow at The University of Queensland.

The New Psychology of Health

Unlocking the Social Cure

Catherine Haslam | Jolanda Jetten
Tegan Cruwys | Genevieve A. Dingle
S. Alexander Haslam

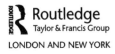

Routledge
Taylor & Francis Group

LONDON AND NEW YORK

First published 2018
by Routledge
2 Park Square, Milton Park, Abingdon, Oxon OX14 4RN

and by Routledge
711 Third Avenue, New York, NY 10017

Routledge is an imprint of the Taylor & Francis Group, an informa business

British Library Cataloguing-in-Publication Data
A catalogue record for this book is available from the British Library

Library of Congress Cataloguing-in-Publication Data
Names: Haslam, Catherine, author.
Title: The new psychology of health : unlocking the social cure / Catherine Haslam,
    Jolanda Jetten, Tegan Cruwys, Genevieve Dingle, and Alexander Haslam.
Description: 1 Edition. | New York : Routledge, 2018.
Identifiers: LCCN 2018015644 (print) | LCCN 2018015909 (ebook) | ISBN 9781315648569
    (Master) | ISBN 9781317301394 (Web PDF) | ISBN 9781317301387 (ePub) |
    ISBN 9781317301370 (Mobipocket) | ISBN 9781138123878 (hb) |
    ISBN 9781138123885 (pb)
Subjects: LCSH: Social service—Psychological aspects. | Health—Psychological aspects.
Classification: LCC HV41 (ebook) | LCC HV41 .H387 2018 (print) | DDC 362.1/0425—dc23
LC record available at https://lccn.loc.gov/2018015644

ISBN: 978-1-138-12387-8
ISBN: 978-1-138-12388-5
ISBN: 978-1-315-64856-9

Typeset in Times New Roman
by Apex CoVantage, LLC

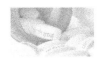

Contents

List of figures   xi
List of tables   xiv
The authors   xv
Foreword   xvii
Preface   xviii
Acknowledgements   xix

1. **Introduction: Why do we need a new psychology of health?**   1
    Current approaches to health   4
        Biomedical approaches   4
        Psychological approaches   5
        Social approaches   7
            Social capital   7
            Social determinants of health   8
    The social identity approach to health   9

2. **The social identity approach to health**   12
    Social identity: definition and origins   14
    Why social identity is important for health   15
    Social identity theory: the psychology of intergroup relations   18
    Self-categorization theory: the psychology of group behaviour   21
        The depersonalisation process   21
        Determinants of social identity salience   22
        Social influence   24
    Applying the social identity approach to health   26
        Social identities are an important health-related resource   26
        Psychological resources that result from shared social identity   27
            Connectedness and positive orientation to others   27
            Meaning, purpose, and worth   29
            Social support   29
            Control, efficacy, and power   30

3. **Social status and disadvantage**   36
    Current approaches to the health effects of social status   39
        Physiological models   39
        Human biological models   41
        Sociological and epidemiological models   42
    The social identity approach to social status and health   45
        Social identities are important determinants of social status   46
        Features of socio-structural context determine responses to group disadvantage   47
            Resisting identification with disadvantaged groups   47
            Leaving disadvantaged groups   48

Social identification is beneficial for well-being even in disadvantaged groups   51
Social identity resources facilitate adjustment to life transitions   52
     The social identity model of identity change (SIMIC)   53
Disadvantage can be a barrier to successful social identity change   56
     Education contexts   56
     Housing contexts   58
     Community contexts   59

4. Stigma   **63**
Stigma and its effects on health   63
     Quantifying the relationship between stigma and health   66
Current approaches to stigmatised group membership   67
     The dispositional model: the role of personality and individual differences   68
     The situational model: concealing stigma   70
The social identity approach to stigma and health   71
     Social identity affects coping with stigma and discrimination   71
     Social identity affects the appraisal of stigma   74
     Features of the broader socio-structural context affect responses to stigma   76
          Pervasiveness of discrimination   76
          Permeability of group boundaries   77
          Cognitive alternatives to the status quo   78
     Social identity affects engagement with health services   79

5. Stress   **84**
Current approaches to understanding stress   84
     The biomedical model: the importance of physiology and adaptation   84
     The dispositional model: the role of personality and individual differences   86
     The situational model: the role of life events   87
     The transactional model: the role of appraisals of threat and support   89
The social identity approach to stress   92
     Social identity is a determinant of primary stress appraisal   92
     Social identity is a basis for effective social support   95
     Social identity can transform the experience of stress   97

6. Trauma and resilience   **104**
Current approaches to trauma and resilience   109
     Biological models   109
     Psychoanalytic models   111
     Cognitive and behavioural models   112
The social identity approach to trauma and resilience   115
     Social identity is central to the experience and appraisal of
     traumatic events   116
     Social identity is central to the experience of posttraumatic stress   120
     Social identity is a basis for resilience and posttraumatic growth   123

7. Ageing   **131**
Current approaches to ageing   133
     Medical and biological approaches   133
     Psychological approaches   135
          The role of individual differences   135

The role of behaviour change 136
Social determinants of healthy ageing 136
The social identity approach to ageing 139
    Older adults' perceptions are shaped by age-based self-categorization
    and internalised age stereotypes 139
    Older adults' performance is shaped by age-based self-categorization
    and internalised age stereotypes 141
    Group memberships are protective in the context of age-related life transition 146
    Meaningful group identification improves health outcomes 149

8. Depression **157**
Current approaches to depression 158
    The biochemical model 158
    The cognitive-behavioural model 160
    The interpersonal stress model 161
The social identity approach to depression 163
    Social relationships counteract depression when they inform the self-concept 163
    Social identities counteract depression because they are a basis for meaning,
    agency, purpose, and support 165
    Social identities structure depression-related thoughts and perception 166
    Depression interventions are effective to the extent that they modify social
    identities or the social realities that inform them 170

9. Addiction **175**
Current approaches to addiction treatment 178
    Biological and pharmacotherapy approaches 178
    Psychotherapeutic approaches 179
    Psychosocial approaches 183
        Couple and family therapies 184
        Residential and community treatment 185
        Mutual support groups 186
The social identity approach to addiction 188
    Addiction trajectories are shaped by social identification, group norms,
    and social influence 188
    Stigma affects intentions to quit 189
    Addiction trajectories are shaped by multiple group memberships 190
    Addiction trajectories centre on processes of social identity change 193
        Social identity pathways are implicated in addiction onset
        and recovery 193
        Therapy groups facilitate social identity change 195
        Recovery involves shifting identification from using to non-using groups 197

10. Eating behaviour **203**
Current models of eating behaviour 204
    Biological models 204
    Individual-difference models 206
    Social cognitive models 207
    Socio-cultural models 211
    Interactionist models 214
The social identity approach to eating 215

Social context provides cues that shape eating norms and invoke eating-relevant
identities   216
Social identity determines attention and conformity to eating norms   218
Eating behaviour reflects and enacts ingroup norms   221
Group-based stigma can fuel an epidemic of unhealthy eating   222

11. Acquired brain injury   **227**
The nature and impact of ABI   227
Current approaches to acquired brain injury   231
   The cognitive behavioural approach   231
   The self-concept approach   232
   The holistic approach   235
The social identity approach to acquired brain injury   236
   Adjustment to acquired brain injury involves processes of social
   identity change   236
   People with ABI can pursue a range of different self-enhancement strategies 240
      People with ABI can pursue a strategy of individual mobility by choosing
      not to disclose their injury   243
      People with ABI can pursue a strategy of social creativity that is a basis
      for posttraumatic growth   244
   Cognitive deficits can interfere with self-categorization processes   247

12. Acute pain   **252**
Defining pain   252
Current approaches to acute pain   254
   Physiological models: the role of sensory pathways   254
   Psychological models: the role of cognitive appraisal and
   individual differences   258
   The hedonic model: pain as a basis for growth   260
The social identity approach to acute pain   263
   Pain is a social glue that binds people to the group   264
   "Our" pain is more real than "their" pain   267
   Social identity affects the appraisal of pain   268
   Social identity can help people cope with physical pain   269
   Social identity can help people cope with social pain   272

13. Chronic mental health conditions   **278**
The nature and impact of CMHC   278
Current approaches to CMHC   283
   Environmental risk factors   283
   Genetic and biomedical approaches   283
   Cognitive behavioural therapy   287
   Interpersonal and social rhythm therapy   288
   Family environment and family-focused therapy   289
   Community approaches to mental health   290
The social identity approach to CMHC   293
   Social identity protects against development of psychosis   294
   Social identity is a basis for recovery from CMHC   297
   Social identification is a basis to manage mental health stigma   302

14. Chronic physical health conditions   **307**
  Current approaches to understanding and managing CPHC   309
    The biomedical approach   309
    The health promotion approach   312
    Psychological approaches   315
    Critical perspectives on health and disability   317
  The social identity approach to CPHC   319
    Social identities affect the way people experience, appraise, and express symptoms   319
    The provision of effective health care services is affected by social
    identity processes   321
    Social identities can motivate both healthy behaviours and health risk behaviours   324
    Social identities provide people with resources to manage threats to
    physical health   326

15. Unlocking the social cure: Groups 4 Health   **332**
  Current strategies to manage social disconnection   332
  The social identity approach to managing social disconnection   334
    Origins and theoretical underpinnings of Groups 4 Health   334
    The Groups 4 Health programme   336
    Proof-of-concept evaluation   339

Appendix: Measures of identity, health, and well-being   **346**
  Social identity measures   346
    Social identification   346
    Multiple identities   348
    Multiple identity compatibility   349
    Multiple group listing   350
    Social identity continuity   351
    Social identity mapping   352
      Stage 1: identifying your groups   353
      Stage 2: thinking about your groups   353
      Stage 3: mapping your groups in relation to each other   354
    Crowd identification   357
    Personal identity strength   358
  Process measures   358
    Group norms   358
    Social support   359
    Unsupportive interactions   361
    Perceived discrimination   362
    Self-stigma   362
    Disclosure and concealment   363
    Perceived personal control   364
  Health and well-being measures   364
    Burnout (chronic stress)   364
    Posttraumatic stress   366
    Depression, anxiety, and stress   367
    Resilience   369
    Affect   370
    Dieting intentions   371

Paranoia   372
Loneliness   373
Personal self-esteem   375
Life satisfaction   376
General health   377

References   380
Author index   447
Subject index   480
Hypotheses associated with the social identity approach to health   489

Figures

P.1 The authors   xvi
1.1 Illustrations from the CSSI report showing engagement in community football
     and a word cloud showing what people feel they would lose if their football
     club disappeared   2
1.2 Perceived and true rankings of the importance of behavioural risk and
     social factors for mortality   3
1.3 A picture of good health: all in the head?   6
1.4 Differences between approaches in their emphasis on psychological and
     social dimensions of health   9
1.5 The rise of 'social cure' research   10
2.1 Unlikely sites of health: Ogliastra, the Magh Mela, and the drought-ridden
     Australian outback   13
2.2 Pathways to self-knowledge   16
2.3 The process of depersonalisation   22
2.4 The principle of comparative fit   23
2.5 The principle of normative fit   24
2.6 The process through which social identity becomes salient   25
2.7 Pilgrims attending the annual Hajj at Mecca   28
2.8 Key resources that flow from shared social identity   32
2.9 The social identity approach to health   32
3.1 The health gradient   37
3.2 Wealth inequality: a cause of ill health for both the poor and the rich   38
3.3 Social support can attenuate the heath-threatening effects of low status   40
3.4 Civil service buildings in Whitehall, London   43
3.5 Prisoners and Guards in the BBC Prison Study   50
3.6 The social identity model of identity change (SIMIC)   54
4.1 The Australian Rules football player Adam Goodes in front of the
     Aboriginal flag   64
4.2 Signs of stigma-related exclusion   65
4.3 Three pathways from stigma and discrimination to ill-health   67
4.4 The rejection-identification model   72
4.5 Dual pathways from group-based discrimination to well-being   73
4.6 Responses to exclusion   74
4.7 Cognitive alternatives have important direct and indirect benefits for health
     and well-being   79
5.1 Stressful experiences? Doing bomb disposal work and undergoing heart surgery   85
5.2 A schematic representation of the transactional model of stress   90
5.3 Perceived and received social support are mediators of the relationship
     between social identification and stress   96
5.4 A schematic representation of the ways in which stress appraisal is moderated
     by self-categorization   98
5.5 The integrated social identity model of stress (ISIS)   100

6.1	Siegfried Sassoon and the commemorative plaque outside his London home	105
6.2	Examples of traumatic events: terrorism, natural disaster, and intergroup conflict	106
6.3	The development of posttraumatic stress disorder (PTSD)	107
6.4	Examples of different trajectories of PTSD symptoms after exposure to trauma	109
6.5	The two cognitive systems implicated in PTSD	113
6.6	Ways in which social identity processes can shape the development of posttraumatic stress disorder (PTSD)	117
6.7	The 1989 Hillsborough disaster	118
6.8	The 2002 Fatboy Slim beach party in Brighton	119
6.9	A sign of everyday social disconnection on the London Underground	124
6.10	The social identity model of collective resilience	125
7.1	Representations of the ageing population in Japan	132
7.2	The distinction between social isolation and loneliness	137
7.3	The negative content of the stereotype of older adults and older adults' responses to that content	140
7.4	Scores on tests of specific memory and general cognitive ability as a function of self-categorization and expectations of the form of ageing decline	143
7.5	The appeal of personal mobility strategies in response to ageing	145
7.6	Challenging age stereotypes through collective action	147
7.7	Square dancing in China	149
7.8	People's cognitive age as a function of their chronological age and the extent of their social group ties	151
7.9	The activity or the group? Identifying the critical ingredient in group interventions	153
8.1	Re-creation of an image from the 1990s Zoloft commercial	159
8.2	A schematic representation of central features of the cognitive-behavioural model of depression	160
8.3	Group memberships predict the likelihood of depression relapse	164
8.4	Social identities as a basis for thoughts, feelings, and actions	167
8.5	Meaningful group activity counteracts depression	171
9.1	Images from Alexander's "Rat Park" study	177
9.2	Some different forms of substance (ab)use commonly treated using behavioural approaches	180
9.3	Practicing meditation	183
9.4	A meeting of Alcoholics Anonymous, with the 'Big Book' in the foreground	186
9.5	Social identity map for "Matt"	192
9.6	Social identity pathways into and out of addiction	194
9.7	The social identity model of cessation maintenance (SIMCM)	196
9.8	The social identity model of recovery (SIMOR)	198
9.9	Identification with substance-using peers and with the therapeutic community as a function of time in treatment	199
10.1	The spectrum of over- and under-eating pathology	205
10.2	Social cognitive models of health behaviour	208
10.3	An example of blatant anti-fat prejudice	210
10.4	Illustrations of the way in which notions of ideal body size change over time	212
10.5	The situated identity enactment model	217
10.6	Popcorn consumption as a function of consumption norms and their source	220
10.7	An example of a body image–related social change strategy	223
11.1	Phineas Gage	228
11.2	The Y-shaped model of rehabilitation	234

11.3	Pathways to successful social identity change in ABI	238
11.4	The importance of maintained group memberships for stroke recovery	239
11.5	Strategies for self-enhancement in the context of ABI	241
11.6	Pursuing social change in ABI management	242
11.7	The stigma and concealment of acquired brain injury	243
11.8	Change processes implicated in successful post-ABI adjustment	246
12.1	Sources of pain: eating a chilli, running a marathon, taking part in a New Year's dive ritual	253
12.2	Descartes' representation of the experience of pain in *Traite de l'homme* [*Treatise of Man*]	255
12.3	Pain on the battlefield	256
12.4	Brain regions involved in registering and processing pain	257
12.5	The expression of pain and suffering	259
12.6	Pain as a vehicle for self-affirmation	262
12.7	Pain as part of group initiation	264
12.8	High-ordeal experiences in the field and the laboratory	266
12.9	Exposure to pain as a function of the number of groups made salient	271
12.10	Aggression as a function of available group memberships following social rejection	274
13.1	Oliver Sacks signing a copy of his book *Musicophilia*	279
13.2	Mood fluctuations in subtypes of bipolar disorder	281
13.3	Living with schizophrenia	282
13.4	Expressed emotion in families	284
13.5	A 1950s advertisement for Thorazine	285
13.6	Addressing the cognitive aspects of schizophrenia	287
13.7	Dr Eric Cunningham Dax AO	291
13.8	Players in a game of Australian Rules Football organised by Reclink	292
13.9	Paranoia in the BBC Prison Study	295
13.10	A social identity model of emergent paranoia	296
13.11	Thematic map of the benefits of choir membership for people with CMHC	298
13.12	Members of the School of Hard Knocks (Queensland) creative writing group and choir	299
13.13	Two pathways through which social identification as a member of a CMHC group has an impact on self-esteem	303
13.14	The Mental Health Australia slogan for the 2016 World Mental Health Day	304
14.1	The worldwide burden of all disease	308
14.2	A person undergoing a full-body computerised topography (CT) scan	310
14.3	Chronic fatigue syndrome	312
14.4	Critical health psychology: questioning assumptions and giving voice	318
14.5	The frequency of older adults reporting symptoms of hearing loss as a function of self-categorization	322
14.6	Frequency of GP appointments before and after an intervention to increase meaningful group membership	324
14.7	Normative influence in health promotion	326
14.8	Groups as an 'active ingredient' in CPHC treatment	328
15.1	Summary of GROUPS 4 HEALTH modules – the 5 S's	336
15.2	An overview of the G4H programme	337
15.3	Social identity maps	338
15.4	Health and well-being outcomes associated with participation in G4H	341
A.1	Overview of measures	347

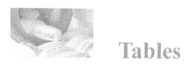

Tables

3.1	Two different lists of top ten tips for health	45
3.2	Examples of alternative self-categorizations in the face of homelessness	48
5.1	Selected events in the Social Readjustment Rating Scale	88
5.2	Social identification and stress in the BBC Prison Study	101
11.1	Mechanisms of injury and common causes of ABI	229
12.1	Three classes of psychological benefit that flow from acute pain	260
13.1	Positive and negative symptoms of chronic mental health conditions	280
13.2	Excerpts from interviews with members of the School of Hard Knocks	300
14.1	RE-AIM guidelines for developing, selecting, and evaluating programmes and policies for health promotion	314
15.1	Change in identification with G4H group and with multiple groups following participation in GROUPS 4 HEALTH programme as a predictor of key outcomes	342
15.2	The top ten social identity tips for better health	343
A.1	Criteria for interpretation of DASS-21 scores	369

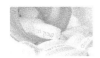

The authors

Catherine Haslam (PhD, Australian National University) is Professor of Clinical Psychology at the University of Queensland. Her research focuses on the social and cognitive consequences of identity-changing life transitions (e.g., trauma, disease, ageing). She was an Associate Fellow of the Canadian Institute for Advanced Research (as part of its Social Interactions, Identity and Well-being Program), is an Associate Editor of the *British Journal of Psychology*, and is on the Editorial Board of *Neuropsychological Rehabilitation*.

Jolanda Jetten (PhD, University of Amsterdam) is a Professor of Social Psychology and former Australian Research Council Future Fellow at the University of Queensland. Her research focuses on social identity, group processes, and intergroup relations. She has published over 150 peer-reviewed articles on these topics, and co-edited *The Social Cure: Identity, Health and Well-Being* (Psychology Press, 2012; with Catherine Haslam and Alex Haslam). She is a former Chief Editor of the *British Journal of Social Psychology* and currently Chief Editor of *Social Issues and Policy Review*.

Tegan Cruwys (PhD, Australian National University) is a Lecturer in the School of psychology at the University of Queensland, a practicing clinical psychologist, and a recipient of the Australian Research Council's Discovery Early Career Research Award. Her research investigates the social-psychological determinants of health, with a particular focus on health behaviours, mental health, and vulnerable populations.

Genevieve Dingle (PhD, University of Queensland) is a Senior Lecturer in Clinical Psychology in the School of Psychology at the University of Queensland. Her research focuses on social factors in addiction, depression, and chronic mental health problems; people experiencing homelessness; and the recovery process. She is on the Editorial Board of the *British Journal of Clinical Psychology*.

S. Alexander Haslam (PhD, Macquarie University) is a Professor of Social and Organisational Psychology and Australian Research Council Laureate Fellow at the University of Queensland. He is a former Chief Editor of the *European Journal of Social Psychology* whose research focuses on the study of group and identity processes in social, organisational, and clinical contexts. Together with colleagues he has written and edited 11 books and over 200 peer-reviewed articles on these topics, including most recently, *The New Psychology of Leadership: Identity, Influence and Power* (Psychology Press, 2011, with Steve Reicher and Michael Platow).

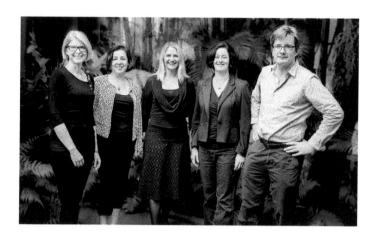

Figure P.1. The authors.

From left to right: Catherine Haslam, Jolanda Jetten, Tegan Cruwys, Genevieve Dingle and Alex Haslam

Source: Jonathan Brazil

Foreword

From the first spark of life and throughout our lives our mental and physical health is profoundly affected by the places we live, the people with whom we spend time and interact, and the communities to which we and they belong. In line with this observation, across the world, governments and policy makers are increasingly recognising the importance of social life for the health of all citizens and turning themselves to the dual task of understanding these processes better and then using that understanding to build healthier societies.

In light of these developments, the bringing together of theory and practice that underpins *The New Psychology of Health* could not have 'come of age' at a more critical point in time. Setting out an analysis that has been meticulously developed and tested over the last decade, this book moves us beyond the stereotyped terms of a debate about whether health is a product of genes, environment, or chance. Instead it argues that what lies at the heart of individuals' health is the nature of the social connections that exist between them and the sense of shared identity that these connections both produce and are produced by.

The result is a masterful text that is a long overdue wake-up call to us all. In my experience, it is rare for a text to successfully combine theory, application, and points for practice into one coherent whole. However, the authors' application of the social identity approach to health does precisely this. In the process, they provide an integrated and essential set of resources for researchers, practitioners, and anyone interested in health promotion.

In the course of expansive treatments of a very broad range of topics, the authors draw on a wealth of expertise pertaining to diverse circumstances, disorders, and diseases. These make the case for a social identity approach to these various topics and point to the ways in which group processes and group psychology are critical to questions of health trajectory and treatment. They then use the approach to address and untangle some of the key dilemmas facing society today. These stretch across issues of disadvantage and depression, of stigma and stress, and of ageing and addiction. In the process, they provide fresh appreciation of, and solutions to, the major 'challenges' faced by health and social care systems today.

This text lays down the foundations of a new way of thinking and learning about how as practitioners – across the spheres of health, social care, education, justice, work, and community – we can truly develop a better 'way of seeing' health. This in turn provides a platform for us to work with others to promote a better 'way of being' in the world. Read on and become part of this revolution.

Professor Dame Sue Bailey, OBE, DBE, FRCPsych
Chair of the Children and Young People's Mental Health Coalition
President, Royal College of Psychiatrists (2011–2014)
Chair, Academy of Medical Royal Colleges (2015–2017)

 Preface

In Siddhartha Mukherjee's magisterial biography of cancer, *The Emperor of All Maladies*, his reflections on the limitations of the medical profession led him to recall Voltaire's observation that "Doctors are men who prescribe medicines of which they know little, to cure diseases of which they know less, in human beings of whom they know nothing" (Mukherjee, 2010, p. 143). In the 300 years since the French social commentator penned these words, much has changed for the better. For a start, doctors are no longer all men. Thankfully too, they also know a lot more about medicines and about disease. But their knowledge of human beings is still limited, and it remains a marginal concern for their profession.

It is here that psychology comes in. Psychology has taught us a lot – especially in the last fifty or so years – about the mental states and processes that make people tick and that are therefore central to their health and well-being. For example, there is now a large literature which explores the role of personality and cognition in shaping health-related attitudes and behaviour. A lot more is also known now about the ways in which these affect individuals' responses to such things as symptoms, stressors, and suffering.

However, we still suspect that this literature would be unlikely to fully satisfy Voltaire's desire for an approach to health that properly appreciates, and engages with, what it means to be a human being. The reason for this is that, writing at a turbulent time in French history, he recognised the powerful ways in which a person's mental state and physical circumstances are shaped by group life and large-scale social forces (e.g., the professions, the church, the aristocracy). A problem that Voltaire might therefore have with prevailing psychologies of health is that while they have a lot to say about people as individuals, until recently, they have had little to say about people as social beings – that is, as members of groups embedded in dynamic social systems.

To date, then, the psychology of health has focused primarily on the personal self of 'I' and 'me'. But health is not all about 'I' and me'. Far from it. It is also about 'we' and 'us' – the social self. This much is evident from the fact that health systems themselves are constituted of people whose primary orientation to those systems is often dictated by relevant group memberships (e.g., as doctors, diabetics, or drug users; as midwives, people with MS, or Medicaid clients). Accordingly, there are grounds for thinking that if we want to get to grips with the richness of the human condition – in ways that Voltaire willed us to – we need *a new psychology of health* that engages with the self as something social and not just personal.

The purpose of this book is to set out this new psychology of health and to demonstrate its explanatory power and practical utility in relation to core topics that define the field. A key point that emerges from these deliberations is that the group-based dimensions of psychology and behaviour on which we focus are not secondary by-products of physical and mental health. Rather, they are *primary drivers* of outcomes. Not only, then, does this new psychology give us a fuller sense of what it means to be human, but it also shows how we can open up new pathways to health by engaging more meaningfully with the social foundations of our humanity.

Acknowledgements

In a book which explores the importance of group life for health, it is appropriate to make clear from the outset that this volume is very much a collective product. Over the four years that it took to produce, the five of us worked very closely together on the various conceptual, structural, and practical tasks that this entailed, and we all had significant input into every chapter (indeed, into almost every sentence). Accordingly, responsibility for the final product is something that we all share equally.

At the same time, though, the book is also a manifestation of collaborations with a large number of other people and groups. For us the most important of these has been the School of Psychology at the University of Queensland, as its members have played a central role in developing our understanding of key issues and in keeping us on the straight and narrow. Katie Greenaway and Nik Steffens deserve special thanks in this regard, but the support and friendship of Tamara Butler, Laura Ferris, Nancy Pachana, Kim Peters, Daniel Skorich, Zoe Walter, and Elyse Williams have also been invaluable. We are also very grateful to Melissa Chang for the painstaking work that she did to check references and permissions and to compile the indices, and to Sarah Bentley for helping to assemble the appendix. Most especially, though, we would like to thank Christine McCoy for the work she did both to help beat the manuscript into shape and to organise our professional lives in ways that allowed us to work productively not only on this book but also on the various projects that have fed into it. Melissa, Sarah, and Christine also had very important roles to play in the development and refinement of GROUPS 4 HEALTH, and their efforts – together with those of all the many other people who have helped and encouraged us as this work has unfolded – are massively appreciated.

Further afield, many other colleagues have also had a pivotal role to play in the book's evolution. Brock Bastian (Melbourne), Nyla Branscombe (Kansas), John Helliwell (British Columbia), Tom Postmes (Gronigen), and Steve Reicher (St Andrews) deserve special mention for the role they have played in shaping our thinking as it has unfolded over the last decade. However, for their generous support and incredibly helpful input – not least in providing detailed feedback on multiple drafts of individual chapters – we would also like to single out Charles Abraham (Exeter), Hymie Anisman (Carleton), Kasia Banas (Edinburgh), Brock Bastian (Melbourne), Janine Baxter (Queensland), Richard Bentall (Liverpool), David Best (Sheffield), Filip Boen (Leuven), Linda Clare (Exeter), Chris Cocking (Brighton), Monique Crane (Macquarie), Mark Daglish (Royal Brisbane and Women's Hospital), John Drury (Sussex), Ilka Gliebs (LSE), Richard Griggs (Florida), Naomi Ellemers (Utrecht), Janelle Jones (Queen Mary), Peter Kay (Exeter), Craig Knight (Exeter), Jason McIntyre (Liverpool), Melissa Johnstone (Macquarie), Niamh McNamara (Nottingham Trent), Kim Matheson (Carleton), Thomas Morton (Exeter), Orla Muldoon (Limerick), David Novelli (Hertfordshire), Heather O'Mahen (Exeter), Tamara Ownsworth (Griffith), Yin Paradies (Deakin), Cameron Parsell (Queensland), Michael Platow (ANU), Kate Reynolds (ANU), Mark Rubin (Newcastle), Fabio Sani (Dundee), Michael Schmitt (Simon Fraser), Mark Tarrant (Exeter), Juliet Wakefield (Nottingham Trent), Richard Williams (Swansea), Barbara Wilson (The Oliver Zangwill Centre for Neuropsychological Rehabilitation and The Raphael Medical Centre), and Renate Ysseldyk (Carleton).

We are also keen to acknowledge the practical support that we received throughout the writing process from friends and the production team at Routledge. Michael Keating, Karlie Keating and Maureen Curtis helped immensely with copy editing. Eleanor Reedy and Tina Cottone did a really great job shepherding us over the finishing line, but we would particularly like to thank Lucy Kennedy who, fortunately for us, had the fortitude to stay with the project from the signing of the contract to the delivery of the bound printed pages.

Finally, we would like to thank the many grant agencies, funding bodies, and charities that have supported our work over the last decade. Over this time we have received generous funding from the Australian Research Council, the Economic and Social Research Council, the British Academy; the Canadian Institute for Advanced Research; and the European Commission for Employment, Social Affairs and Inclusion. Without this many of the studies reported in the pages that follow simply could not have been conducted. We have also been extremely fortunate to collaborate with wonderful people from organisations such as Somerset Care, Cornwall Care, the Housing Associations' Charitable Trust, and the Church Urban Fund in the UK; Lives Lived Well, Reclink, the School of Hard Knocks, and the Salvation Army in Australia; and the Schlegel-University of Waterloo Research Institute for Aging in Canada. We hope that this book does justice to your efforts, and we hope that it helps others to recognise the huge importance of the work that you do.

It is clear, then, that the collective energies of a great many people and a great many groups have gone into bringing this book to fruition. Without these energies not only would the book have languished, but, more importantly for us, the quality of our lives would also have been seriously diminished. So although we are very grateful to our families, colleagues, and communities for helping us to translate the idea for this book into reality, we are yet more grateful for the social cures that they have unlocked along the way. For us, these ensure that the message of this book is not just academic but also deeply personal.

Catherine, Jolanda, Tegan, Genevieve, and Alex
Brisbane, September 2017

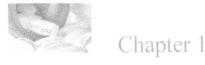

Chapter 1

Introduction: Why do we need a new psychology of health?

Health really matters. Because of this, stories about threats to health and miracle cures feature prominently in newspapers and magazines, and we are inundated with tips about how to stay healthy on a daily basis. So alongside advice to quit smoking, drink less alcohol, and say no to drugs, we are routinely encouraged to engage in regular exercise, to eat more fruit, and to pay attention to our weight.

A large body of empirical evidence suggests that this advice is well grounded. We see this, for example, in research on the benefits of physical activity and sports participation in particular. In one study on this topic the Australian Football League joined forces with researchers at La Trobe University's Centre for Sport and Social Impact (CSSI) to quantify both the health and the economic benefits of physical activity by determining precisely how much participation in sports was worth in financial terms. To do this, they sent a survey to members of 1,677 football clubs asking them not only about football itself, but also about the social connectedness and wider community participation that was associated with their involvement in their club (see Figure 1.1). The findings were striking:

> For every $1 spent to run a club, there is at least a $4.40 return in social value in terms of increased social connectedness, well-being and mental health status; employment outcomes; personal development; physical health; civic pride and support of other community groups.
> (Centre for Sport and Social Impact, 2015)

Interestingly, this return was not dependent on where people lived, the amount of time they had been associated with the club, or their particular role in the club. More strikingly still, the benefits were not restricted to those who actually played football. Instead, they were observed *across the board* – among players, coaches, volunteers, and supporters. This suggests that the health and economic benefits of being involved in sport do not just stem from the physical exercise that this entails. Instead, what also matters for health – but what is often overlooked – is the social connection and sense of community that sport provides.

An investment that increases your financial return by over 400% is nothing to scoff at. This is especially true because many (perhaps most) of the advances that are made in health deliver lower returns than this. For example, a comprehensive review by Luce, Mauskopf, Sloan, Ostermann, and Paramore (2006), which looked at return on investment in U.S. health care between 1980 and 2000, found that every dollar spent on treatment produced benefits of $1.10 for heart attack, $1.49 for stroke, and $1.55 for type 2 diabetes. These are important gains, and they point to the undoubted good sense of investing in medical research and treatment. Nevertheless, alongside data of the form produced by the CSSI, they suggest that it makes very good sense to also invest in social activities that are rather less rarefied and that are typically experienced as part of everyday life by those who engage in them.

This tendency to turn towards physical and medical factors and neglect the importance of everyday social factors when thinking about improving health was confirmed in research that we recently conducted with 500 members of the general public in the United States and the United Kingdom

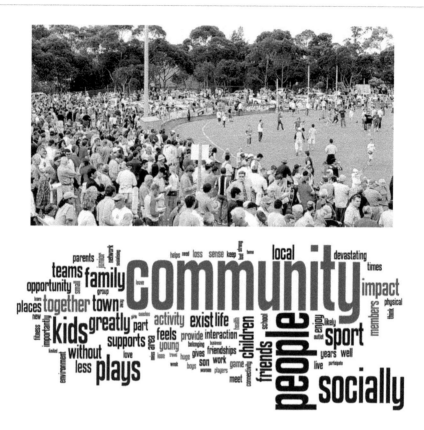

Figure 1.1 Illustrations from the CSSI report showing engagement in community football and a word cloud showing what people feel they would lose if their football club disappeared

Note: We tend to see the health benefits of being involved in sport as resulting from the physical exercise that this involves. However, research suggests that these benefits result not only from playing sport but also from the sense of connection and community that sport provides. Moreover, health economists have put a dollar value to this, showing that for every dollar spent in running a football club, the social return on investment was $4.40.

Source: Centre for Sport and Social Impact (2015)

(Haslam et al., 2018). This involved giving people a survey which asked them to rank 11 factors in terms of their importance for health and mortality. Critically, these were factors whose significance for health had previously been examined by Julianne Holt-Lunstad and her colleagues in an influential meta-analysis of 148 studies involving over 300,000 participants (Holt-Lunstad, Smith, & Layton, 2010; see also Holt-Lunstad, Robles, & Sbarra, 2017). More specifically, this meta-analysis was interested in comparing the impact that social factors, such as social support and social integration, had on mortality to that associated with established physical risks such as smoking, high alcohol consumption, lack of exercise, and obesity – factors which are the traditional focus of medical research.

As the green squares in Figure 1.2 indicate, Holt-Lunstad and colleagues' analysis showed that these social factors were the most important predictors of mortality and that they had an impact that was comparable to (and in fact, slightly higher than) that of the most important behavioural risk

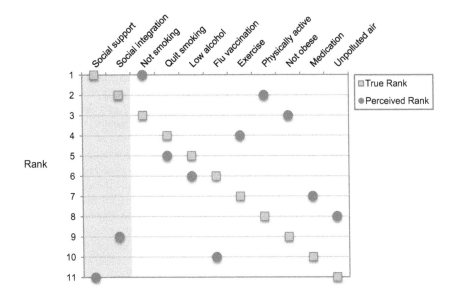

Figure 1.2 Perceived and true rankings of the importance of behavioural risk and social factors for mortality

Note: This figure highlights the degree to which people tend to underestimate the importance of social factors for health relative to that of established behavioural risks that are the traditional focus of medical research. Specifically, whereas Holt-Lunstad et al.'s (2010) meta-analysis found social factors (specifically, social support and social integration) to be most important for health, the general public perceive these to be among the least important.

Source: Haslam, McMahon et al. (2018)

factors. Moreover, as recent research has highlighted, social connectedness makes a contribution to mortality risk that is independent of these other health factors (Holt-Lunstad et al., 2017). Nevertheless, as the red circles in Figure 1.2 indicate, when members of the general public were asked to rank the importance of these same factors, their ordering was strikingly different. In particular, whereas Holt-Lunstad and colleagues found that social support and social integration were the most important predictors of mortality, our respondents ranked these same factors among the *least* important.

So why do people so seriously underestimate the importance of social connectedness and social integration for their health? There is no definitive answer to this question, but it seems likely that multiple factors are at play. One is that the biological mechanisms that impact on health are generally quite well understood theoretically and quite well validated empirically – due in no small part to huge global investment in medical research and technology (Moses et al., 2015; Murphy & Topel, 2010). It is not surprising then, that this has contributed to the dominance of a biomedical model in which the underpinnings of health are understood to be primarily biological or genetic (e.g., see Havelka, Despot Lucanin, & Lucanin, 2009, for a discussion). However, such dominance also appears to be supported by entrenched ideology. This is evident in continued resistance to efforts to expand the medical curriculum beyond the biomedical model (Bowe, Lahey, Kegan, & Armstrong, 2003), and it is also seen in other evidence from our research which suggests that people are more likely to downplay the importance of social factors for health if they have an inclination to follow established authority and convention (Haslam, McMahon et al., 2017).

As a consequence of these and other factors, far less attention has been paid to the role that social processes play in determining health than to biological and medical processes. In part, too, this emphasis reflects the fact that these social processes are harder to pin down. Not least, this is because the ways in which social factors exert their influence on health can vary markedly between individuals – for example, as a function of their living conditions, their culture, their family relationships, their economic circumstances, their work environment, and their social networks. It can also be hard to examine the operation of social factors directly, and so it is often inferred through population-level observations of their impact (e.g., where a lack of social connectedness is found to lead to an increase in depression). We would argue, however, that the existence of this knowledge gap is not a reason to neglect the importance of social factors for health. On the contrary, it is a reason to work harder to try to fill that gap – not only with solid empirical evidence, but also with sound scientific theory.

It is this knowledge gap that the present volume seeks to fill. As we set about this task, we are helped by, and do not want to diminish the significance of, an abundance of previous research which documents the impact and importance of both biological and social factors for health. Nevertheless, what this work is not well placed to provide is an analysis of the *psychological* processes that mediate between societal dynamics and individual health – an analysis for which, we contend, a *new* psychology of health is needed. A key reason for this is that, to date, much of the focus of dominant psychological models has been on understanding the psychology of individuals *as individuals* – the psychology of 'I' and 'me'. What this fails to appreciate is the immense importance of people's psychology *as group members* for their health – the psychology of 'we' and 'us' (Haslam, Jetten, Postmes, & Haslam, 2009; Turner & Oakes, 1986). It is this appreciation that underpins the social identity theorising which informs the novel perspective on health that this book spells out.

In the remainder of this introductory chapter we provide an overview of the biological, psychological, and social approaches that dominate the contemporary health landscape. Rather than explore these in detail (something we will do in later chapters), the goal here is to clarify why a social identity analysis is well placed to provide (1) an overarching framework that integrates and builds upon these existing approaches and (2) a basis from which to develop a new appreciation of the social *and* psychological dimensions of various physical and mental health conditions. This will then provide a platform both for a detailed exposition of the social identity approach in Chapter 2 and for more forensic exploration of these various conditions in the chapters that follow.

Current approaches to health

Biomedical approaches

Of all approaches to health, the biomedical is unquestionably the most influential. This model understands health primarily through the lens of disease, and it attributes the cause of ill health to some breakdown in normal biological and physiological functioning. In so doing, it gives a clear direction in how best to manage health – and this is to focus on repairing or treating the source of breakdown in the body. There are obvious merits to understanding these physiological influences, not least to treat infectious diseases, which were the main cause of ill health and death until early in the 20th century. However, as Engel (1977) recognised, ill health is not reducible to disease processes alone, and if it were, then there should be much greater consistency in how people experience and respond to disease and its treatment than is actually observed. It is also the case that the health landscape has changed dramatically to one in which chronic conditions (e.g., diabetes, depression, cardiovascular disease, arthritis) have become the prevailing cause of ill health. For these conditions, there is generally no simple biomedical fix that can be administered to restore health.

In light of these changing realities, Engel criticized the biomedical approach as overly "physical-istic" (1977, p. 130) and neglectful of both the human condition and the lived experience of disease (see also Deacon, 2013; Hewa & Hetherington, 1995). In this, he led a revolution in medicine to make health more human by supplementing a biological analysis with awareness of the contribution of psy-chological and social factors to the experience of illness. This recognises that a person's health has important cognitive, emotional, and behavioural dimensions and that it is structured by factors such as culture, socio-economic status, family, and religion.

Nevertheless, the challenge has always been to understand how these social and psychological elements present and interact in health contexts to influence outcomes. Engel's solution to this was to advocate for a *biopsychosocial* approach that gives equal weight to the biological, psychological, and social dimensions of health. However, many researchers have argued that the biopsychosocial model is still dominated by the 'bio', even in behavioural medicine where efforts are made to integrate the biological and psychological (Epstein, 1992; Suls, Luger, & Martin, 2010) and that the social elements in particular are not well defined (Havelka et al., 2009). The result is that these elements tend to be 'tacked on' to medical models rather than properly integrated within them. Amongst other things, this means that the model fails to consider the ways in which each of the three elements has the capacity to *restructure* the others – so that, for example, a person's biology is shaped by their psychology, and their psychology is shaped by the groups to which they belong (Caporeal & Brewer, 1995; Ghaemi, 2011).

One consequence of this is that although the biopsychosocial model has proved tremendously appealing, it primarily offers a list of "ingredients" that affect health, rather than a specified theory, and as a consequence it is difficult to test empirically (McLaren, 1998). Moreover, Ghaemi (2009) argues that rather than biological analysis being enriched by a concern for the psychosocial dimensions of health, these limitations have further entrenched the dogma of the traditional biological model. He therefore suggests that if we are to move beyond the limitations of this model and update it in ways that are both theoretically and empirically powerful, we need an approach that is "less eclectic, less generic, less vague" (Ghaemi, 2009, p. 5). As we will see in the chapters that follow, this is a challenge that the new psychology of health takes very seriously and one that it strives to confront head on.

Psychological approaches

Despite the ongoing dominance of the biomedical model (Deacon, 2013), in recent decades psy-chological approaches have proved increasingly influential as a framework for understanding and managing health. This is largely due to the attention they pay to those factors that Engel identified as vital in shaping the manifestation and course of disease. In particular, approaches that attend to the cog-nitive and behavioural dimensions of health now provide a strong and compelling evidence base that informs theory and practice related to a wide range of health conditions (e.g., Beck, 2011; Ehlers & Clark, 2000; Harvey, 2004). This work focuses on understanding the combined influence of a person's thoughts (e.g., their appraisal of symptoms, their sense of personal efficacy) and feelings (e.g., their mood, their sense of loneliness) on their health behaviour (e.g., consuming alcohol, taking medication) and health outcomes (e.g., depression, obesity).

Also prominent is an individual-difference approach that focuses on the way in which health behaviours and outcomes are shaped by psychological traits and personality (e.g., a person's extraver-sion, neuroticism, or conscientiousness; see Figure 1.3). Whereas early models looked at the impact of these factors on their own, latterly more sophisticated models have examined the way in which they interact with a range of situational and environmental factors (Hagger, 2009). At heart, though, such models exemplify a concern with the importance of people's idiosyncratic personal orientations to the world as determinants of their health and well-being.

Although there are a range of other psychological approaches to health (e.g., psychodynamic, sys-temic, critical) and they themselves have many variants, cognitive-behavioural and individual-difference

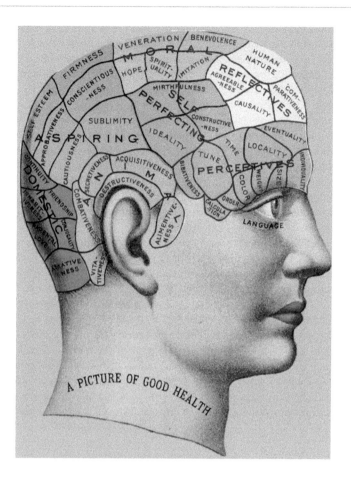

Figure 1.3 A picture of good health: all in the head?

Note: This phrenology chart captures the view that the psychology of health is all about the individual and his or her unique state of mind. Although few people today would subscribe to the idea that personal traits are localised in different areas of the brain as pictured here, the view that individual traits affect health remains very influential.

Source: Pixabay

models are probably the most influential contemporary psychological approaches to health. Despite coming from different theoretical foundations, what all these approaches share is a focus on the psychology of the individual person. For example, when it comes to reflecting on the psychological dimensions of a given health issue (e.g., depression, stress, dysfunctional health behaviour), the individuals' unique personal traits or cognitions are generally seen as the appropriate analytic focus (see Cruwys, Haslam, Fox, & McMahon, 2015, for a discussion). In this way, it is the individual and his or her unique psychology that are seen to lie both at the heart of health problems and at the heart of health solutions.

Interestingly, over time, social factors have come more into the equation. In particular, there has been increased recognition of the importance of group-based elements (e.g., norms, culture) within influential models of behaviour change (e.g., Theory of Planned Behaviour, Ajzen, 1991; Social Cognitive Theory, Bandura, 1986). Practitioners have also increasingly turned to group-based interventions to treat a range of health conditions (e.g., depression, diabetes, coronary heart disease). Here, though, social factors are often seen as secondary and rarely gain theoretical or practical primacy. Moreover, as with the biopsychosocial model, these social elements are *set apart* from psychology and not recognised as having the capacity to fundamentally shape a person (e.g., by (re)structuring cognition and personality; Reynolds et al., 2010) and thereby health. Prevailing conceptualisations of group treatment, for example, still focus almost exclusively on individual-level processes and do not see the group itself either as having higher-order health-relevant properties (because the whole 'us' is irreducible to the constituent 'I's) or as an active ingredient in treatment that makes a distinctive psychological contribution to outcomes (e.g., Farrow, Tarrant, & Khan, 2017; Gleibs, Haslam, Haslam, & Jones, 2011a).

A key limitation here is that by failing to give equal credence to the psychological reality of the group, most psychological approaches to health lack a (meta)theoretical framing for appropriately understanding the power of collectives, and therefore they fail to fully appreciate their influence (whether positive or negative) or to optimally harness their curative potential. And in the absence of this, group processes can be ignored or, worse, treated as something that might be inherently problematic because they could mask an individual's 'true' psychology (Spears, 2010). Accordingly, group interventions where they are embraced tend to be adopted for reasons of efficiency, particularly where there are insufficient funds for individualised treatment. This, again, is a framing that the new psychology of health seeks to challenge, so that, rather than being relegated to the margins, groups and their distinctive psychology can be understood as absolutely central to health.

Social approaches

Social capital

Biomedical and psychological approaches are generally well documented and well understood in health and health psychology literatures. Perhaps less well known are two key frameworks that speak to the ways in which people's health is structured by their social circumstances.

The first of these is the *social capital* approach. This emerged from a large body of research in sociology, political science, and economics which points to the greater prosperity, well-being, and health enjoyed by societies in which people are socially integrated and interconnected. Here, social capital generally refers to the networks, norms of reciprocity, and trust among members of a neighbourhood or community that develop through social interaction and mutual co-operation (though see Szreter & Woolcock, 2004, for a discussion of limitations in conceptualisation of the social capital construct). It is argued that this provides the basis for civic engagement and empowers communities to overcome various challenges that they face through collective action. For example, in his influential book *Making Democracy Work*, Robert Putnam (1993) showed that in regions of Italy where engagement in civic and community activities (e.g., sports clubs, choirs, volunteer groups) was high, government was more economically prosperous and functioned more effectively than it did in those regions where such engagement was low (Putnam, 1993). Putnam (2000) then extended this analysis of 'civic health' in his book *Bowling Alone* to show that these same processes have a bearing on personal health. Indeed, famously, his review of relevant evidence led him to conclude that "As a rough rule of thumb, if you belong to no groups but decide to join one, you cut your risk of dying over the next year in half" (2000, p. 331).

There is considerable discussion within this literature of the mechanisms through which social capital influences health (Kim, Subramanium, & Kawachi, 2006). In particular, it is suggested that such capital can operate by facilitating the sharing of health-related knowledge (e.g., as it relates to facts about health, access to health-related services, and interventions), by promoting healthy norms (e.g., to exercise, to eat well), and by providing access to social support (e.g., Kawachi & Berkman, 2000). However, although these are certainly good examples of the resources that emerge from social capital, research in this tradition offers limited insight into the psychological processes that are involved in these dynamics. How exactly is knowledge created and dispersed? How are norms developed and internalised? How does a person decide who to turn to for social support? Answering such questions is important for a range of reasons – not least because this should help ensure that intervention is as well targeted and effective as possible.

A key way in which social capital research has attempted to address such questions is through concepts of *bonding, bridging*, and *linking* capital (e.g., Kawachi, Subramanian, & Kim, 2008; Putnam & Feldstein, 2004). Bonding capital arises from our relationships with people who are similar to us on some dimension and is often characterised as a horizontal resource because it is typically drawn from within our social networks (e.g., through family, friendship, or neighbourhood ties). Bridging capital tends to be characterised as a vertical resource because it is sourced from people across social and cultural divides (e.g., of ethnicity, class, or religion). Linking capital extends on this construct to identify norms of trust and reciprocity as the mechanisms through which these more vertical relationships and institutional authorities exert their influence on health. The basic argument here is that health can be improved by increasing the quality and quantity of one's 'capital portfolio' in each of these areas.

Yet although these different forms of social capital are descriptively useful in mapping social pathways to health, the underlying mechanisms here are still poorly specified. On what basis do we come to see ourselves as sufficiently similar to others to acquire bonding capital? And what determines when and why the support that flows from these different forms of capital proves effective or ineffective? Here, we would argue that social psychological analysis is needed to explain more precisely *how* social contextual and relational factors structure a person's perceived connection to others and how this then bears upon their health.

Social determinants of health

Despite its clear relevance to a range of health issues, the social capital approach was not developed to target these specifically. This is, however, the primary remit of a second social approach which directly addresses the *social determinants of health*. This approach has its origins in public health and epidemiology and has focused, in particular, on the relationship between social inequality and health. Here, decades of research have shown that the social conditions in which people are born, grow, live, work, and age contribute to unequal health outcomes both within and between societies (Marmot, 2015). This is in large part because social injustice – resulting in poverty, unemployment, inadequate housing, social exclusion, and poor education – reduces opportunities for people to access health services and engage in healthy behaviour.

Importantly, the impact of inequality is felt in both affluent and non-affluent societies. For example, Marmot's studies of British civil servants found that the health of managers was far better than that of their subordinates, despite the fact that the responsibilities associated with senior positions were typically associated with greater stress (Marmot, 2004; see Chapter 3). Clearly, then, people are not immune to the negative health consequences of inequality simply because they are members of an affluent society.

At its heart, work on the social determinants of health focuses primarily on tackling inequality and does so by making a strong case for greater equality in the distribution of the material resources that determine health outcomes through policy interventions (e.g., access to fresh food, recreational facilities, adequate housing, clean air, meaningful employment). Although this has been targeted at the population level – for example, through development of universal health and education policies – it is also intended to build resilience in communities and, through this, enhance individual health.

Yet despite the importance of this message, this approach is less clear about how people's psychology influences their experience of inequality and their health. In this regard, as with other social approaches, it is a challenge to explain individual differences in health outcomes. Why is it that not all people who are exposed to inequality develop disease? And, when they do, why does the impact of disease often vary so much between individuals? One reason that these questions cannot be answered wholly in terms of social factors is that, at a psychological level, there is more involved in the social inequality and social capital stories that needs to be understood (McLeod, Hallett, & Lively, 2015). This, again, is where the social identity approach comes in. In particular, as we will see in the chapters that follow, psychology is structured by higher-order social factors, and this helps us to understand not only when and how inequality has an adverse impact on health, but also when and how those effects might be counteracted.

The social identity approach to health

Each of the above approaches has an important role to play in health. Each also clearly differs in the extent to which it addresses and takes account of the psychological *and* the social dimensions of health. This point can be seen in Figure 1.4 which locates the different approaches in two-dimensional space defined by these two continua. Here, then, we see that in tending to focus on the individual and to neglect issues of psychology, biomedical approaches occupy a position in the bottom-left-hand quadrant of this figure. With their strong focus on the importance of mental state and process, psychological approaches are located in the bottom-right quadrant; and, with their strong emphasis on collective determinants of health, social approaches are located in the top-left quadrant.

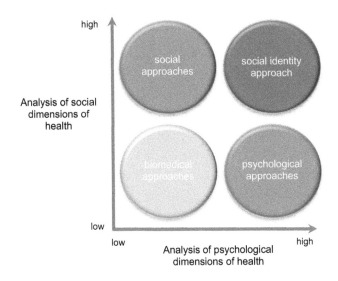

Figure 1.4 Differences between approaches in their emphasis on psychological and social dimensions of health

Note: This figure illustrates the unique contribution that the social identity approach makes to the health literature. In targeting both the social and psychological dimensions of health, it has the capacity to bridge existing approaches to provide an integrated psycho-social analysis of health.

Yet when we map out the ways in which existing approaches fill out this two-dimensional space, it is clear that one key space is left unoccupied: that in the top-right-hand quadrant in which attention is simultaneously paid to *both* the social *and* the psychological dimensions of health. It is this absence, we argue, that creates the demand for a *new* approach to health. This is the gap that the *social identity approach to health* seeks to fill.

Since emerging as a distinct approach to health about a decade ago (Haslam et al., 2009), the goal of the social identity approach to health has been to develop an analysis that integrates concern for both the psychological and the social dimensions of health in ways that give us theoretical, empirical, and practical traction when it comes to understanding and successfully managing a broad range of health conditions and delivering what have come to be known as 'social cures' (after Jetten, Haslam, & Haslam, 2012). There are two distinctive features of the social identity approach that support this goal. The first is an emphasis on *the importance of social groups for health*; the second is an associated appreciation of *the importance of people's psychological identification with those groups*. As we will show in each of the chapters that follow, this means that health is determined in a multitude of ways not only by the groups that people belong to, but also by the extent to which they *internalise* those group memberships *as part of their sense of self* (Turner, 1982). Group identification, for example, plays a key role in how a person understands medical symptoms and potential threats to health, who they turn to for support, how much support they receive, how useful they find it, and how they subsequently behave. And as we will see, such processes have an absolutely critical role to play in the trajectories of a very broad sweep of physical and mental health conditions.

The remainder of this book is primarily concerned with fleshing out and substantiating these ideas. In the process we will see that, despite the fact that the social identity approach to health is new, there is already a large corpus of work – often collectively referred to as *social cure research* – that has tested, and supports, its core hypotheses. Indeed, as the data presented in Figure 1.5 suggest, this

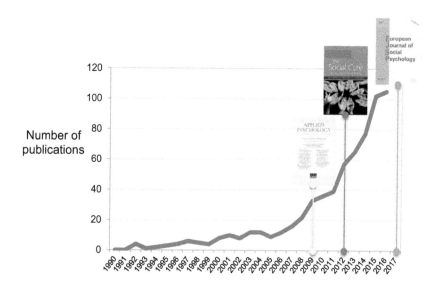

Figure 1.5 The rise of 'social cure' research

Note: This graph plots the number of research papers on "social identity" and "health" published between 1990 and 2016 according to data abstracted from Web of Science in June 2017. A special issue of *Applied Psychology: An International Review* on social identity and health was published in 2009, and another in the *European Journal of Social Psychology* in 2017. The edited volume *The Social Cure: Identity, Health and Well-Being* was published by Psychology Press in 2012.

is an approach that has stimulated rapid and dramatic growth of interest among health researchers and practitioners around the world. As a consequence, there are now well over 400 published studies – with authors from over 20 countries and all six continents – that attest to the fact that people's internalised group memberships have a major bearing on multiple aspects of their health and well-being.

In setting out the case for this approach, Chapter 2 starts by exploring the core hypotheses that define the social identity approach (hypotheses that, for ease of reference, are also listed at the very end of the book and that are also discussed by Jetten et al., 2017). In the remaining chapters we then explore the relevance and explanatory power of social identity processes in relation to a range of specific health-related circumstances and conditions: social disadvantage, stigma, stress, trauma, ageing, depression, chronic mental health conditions, eating behaviour, acquired brain injury, acute pain, addiction, and chronic physical health conditions. In each case we start by reviewing the main existing approaches to the topic in question before going on to show how a social identity analysis enriches our understanding of that topic and provides important new insights for both theory and practice. In our final chapter we then go one important step further by showing how the theoretical insights that we gain from the social identity approach can be translated into a new intervention: GROUPS 4 HEALTH. This seeks to deliver on the second part of this book's title in showing how the approach we have outlined provides a practical framework for mobilising social identities in ways that realise the full potential for social cure.

In all of this, the broad goal of our enterprise is to deliver on Engel's (1977) original vision for a balanced biopsychosocial approach to health in which no single dimension – biological, psychological, or social – is privileged over others. Most importantly, this is an approach in which all three dimensions are understood to be *interdependent* and to have the capacity to structure the other two (e.g., Anisman, 2016; Sapolsky, 2017). Nevertheless, we want to draw particular attention to the importance of social group processes for health because, as we have seen earlier, these have hitherto tended to be neglected. Indeed, as a result, ours is perhaps best thought of as *a sociopsychobio* approach to health. In this reformulation, group psychology is no longer an afterthought. Instead, it assumes a position at the centre of our analytic gaze and is a cornerstone of the social cures that we look to unlock.

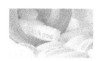

Chapter 2
The social identity approach to health

In the process of doing research for her 2015 book, *The Village Effect*, the journalist and developmental psychologist Susan Pinker travelled to villages in the remote hilltops of central Sardinia to find out more about the people who lived there. The reason she embarked on this journey is that, despite engaging in very hard physical labour for most of their lives, the inhabitants of these villages are some of the healthiest on earth. As a result, men from the region are ten times more likely to live to the age of 100 than is typical elsewhere on the planet (Pinker, 2015).

Seeking to observe larger and more fluid communities, over the last decade a team of intrepid researchers from British and Indian universities has travelled every year to Allahabad in northern India to observe up to 100 million people participating in the Magh Mela. One of the largest religious festivals on earth, amongst other things, this involves many hundreds of thousands of people bathing simultaneously in the water at the confluence of the Ganges and the Yamuna rivers. The site clearly holds abundant potential for the spread of illness, disease, and severe discomfort (e.g., due to pollution of the water and the deafening noise). Yet one of the researchers' key observations is that people return from the event happier and healthier than they set out, and happier and healthier than those who stay at home (Tewari, Khan, Hopkins, Srinivasan, & Reicher, 2012).

Finally, consider the work of various teams of researchers who have studied farming communities in the Australian outback during periods of prolonged drought. At these times there is insufficient water to grow crops or to sustain grazing animals, and farming becomes challenging in the extreme. Yet despite severe financial and physical hardship that are a significant threat to mental health (and that contribute to elevated suicide rates in particular regions; Arnautovska, McPhedran, & De Leo, 2014), farming families prove to be remarkably resilient, and most remain on the land (McLaren & Challis, 2009). Moreover, challenging the image of a group that endures "miseries suffered unvoiced, unknown" (in the words of the poet Henry Lawson), male farmers are *more* likely than urban men to engage in social activities such as chatting to neighbours, attending church services, contacting politicians to discuss local issues, and volunteering time to work on boards or organising committees of clubs, community groups, or other charitable organisations (McPhedran & De Leo, 2013a, 2013b).

As Figure 2.1 suggests, each of these examples is an unlikely site for health. This raises one obvious question: *What is going on here?* In particular, why is it that people who live so far from high-quality medical services, or who are exposed to conditions that are typically considered highly detrimental to health, or who are subjected to extreme physical and psychological challenges are able to withstand their adverse experiences? Indeed, why are they sometimes even made stronger by them?

In each of these cases it is possible to point to specific factors that might be responsible. For example, in Sardinia, the locals attribute their longevity to the superior quality of their genes; in India, religious celebrants point to the analeptic power of their Hindu faith; in rural Australia, communities refer to 'outback spirit'. Each of these factors seems likely to be important in some way or other. However, in this chapter, as in this book as a whole, we want to point to the importance of one critical element that all these examples share and that we suggest is central to the health outcomes that are observed in each of these cases, and in many others besides. That element is *social identity*.

As first defined by Henri Tajfel in the 1970s, social identity refers to the sense of self that people derive from their membership in social groups (Tajfel, 1972). In everyday conversation (and in most psychological literature) when we talk about "the self", we are referring to something unique about a person. So someone who is self-centred thinks only about themselves *as an individual*, someone who

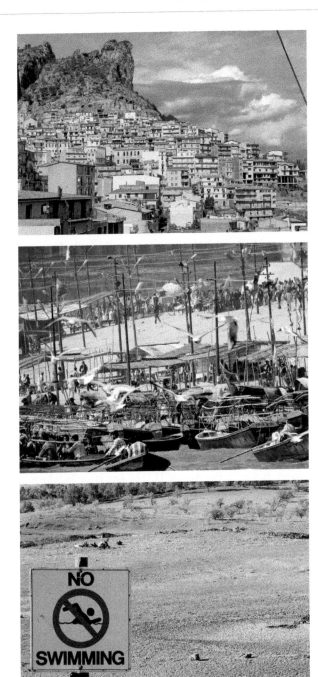

Figure 2.1 Unlikely sites of health: Ogliastra, The Magh Mela, and the drought-ridden Australian outback

Note: These are all places where a strong sense of shared social identity buffers people against significant threats to their health and well-being.

Source: Wikipedia; Adam Jones, Flickr; Wikipedia

has high self-esteem feels good about themselves *as an individual*, someone who has high self-confidence is assured about themselves *as an individual*, and so on. It is also apparent, though, that in everyday conversation when we talk about the self we do not do so only in the first-person singular, as "I" and "me". We also talk about the self in the first-person plural, *in terms of our social identities* as "us" and "we". People do this, for example, when they talk about "us Sardinians", "us Hindus", or "us farmers".

Moreover, rather than being a linguistic artefact or mere figure of speech, social identity theorists argue that our capacity to define the self in terms of group memberships is highly significant. In particular, this is because it speaks to the capacity for the self to be defined not just in terms of our individuality but also by attributes and qualities *that we share with other people*. Amongst other things, this means that all the self-related constructs that psychologists typically approach from the perspective of the individual can also apply to the self as a group member. Sardinians can be self-centred *as group members*, Hindus can have high self-esteem *as group members*, outback farmers can be self-confident *as group members*, and so on.

Looked at in this way, the tendency *not* to think about the self in terms of social identity can be seen to constitute a rather large blind spot in the way we typically think about and understand the self. The significance of this becomes much more marked, however, once we recognise that our capacity to define the self in group-based terms has profound implications for both psychology and behaviour. In this chapter we will spell out what these implications are – with a view to explaining why social identity is such an important concept for human health.

Social identity: definition and origins

The work that first inspired Tajfel to think about social identity ostensibly had very little to do with health. It involved schoolboys from Bristol in England coming into a research laboratory to assign points (signifying small sums of money) to members of two different groups, one to which they apparently belonged and one to which they did not. The whole situation was very contrived, largely because the groups in question were rather meaningless. For example, in one study the groups reflected liking for one of two abstract painters that the boys knew little or nothing about (Klee or Kandinsky); in another, they reflected their supposed tendency to overestimate or underestimate the number of dots on a screen (Tajfel, Flament, Billig, & Bundy, 1971). The key issue in which Tajfel was interested was whether these very stripped-down conditions would be sufficient to induce some form of group behaviour. More particularly, in the absence of factors that had previously been observed to produce prejudice (e.g., a history of conflict or competition for scarce resources; Sherif, 1956, 1966), would the boys still discriminate between the groups in any way?

The answer to Tajfel's question was 'Yes'. Famously, what he and his colleagues found was that even these most minimal conditions were sufficient to encourage the boys to display ingroup favouritism. That is, even though they did not know who the individual beneficiaries would be, and even though they would get nothing themselves, they gave more points to boys who were in their own group (the *ingroup*) than they did to those who were in the other group (the *outgroup*). Indeed, in a later variant of the studies, Marilynn Brewer and Madelyn Silver found that the same pattern of behaviour was observed even when the participants were told that they "were too similar to provide a basis for grouping, so would have to be split into the groups randomly" (1978, pp. 395–396).

These findings proved interesting and important for a wide range of reasons. In the first instance, they challenged theories which suggested that people engage in group behaviour for largely instrumental reasons. A standard economic model, for example, would suggest that people join groups primarily for what they can get out of them, and that, when in those groups, they act in ways that maximise their personal gain and minimise their personal costs. But far from being determined by personal self-interest, behaviour in these minimal group studies (as they became known) instead appeared to reflect something that was *collective*.

It was in attempting to pin down what this 'something' was that Tajfel homed in on the importance of social identity. Through careful analysis of data from a range of minimal group studies, he and his then PhD student, John Turner, came to the conclusion that when participants were assigned to a group (e.g., the group who had supposedly over-estimated dots on a screen), this gave their behaviour a *distinct* meaning. More particularly, they argued that this arose from the process of participants *categorizing themselves* as members of one group (e.g., so that they saw themselves as "Sam the over-estimator" and the group as "us over-estimators" as opposed to the other group "them under-estimators"). Unpacking this further, Tajfel argued:

> Meaning was found by them in the adoption of a strategy for action based on the establishment, through action, of a distinctiveness between their own group and the other, between the two social categories in a truly minimal social system. Distinction from the 'other' category *provided an identity for their own group*, and thus some kind of meaning to an otherwise empty situation.
>
> (Tajfel, 1972, pp. 39–40, emphasis added)

Pinning this down yet further, Tajfel argued that in the minimal group studies the assignment of participants to groups motivated them to develop "a distinct and positively valued *social identity*" (Tajfel, 1972, p. 37, emphasis added). And, in this case, the only way they could achieve a distinct identity was through the differential allocation of points (money) to the two groups.

Tajfel defined social identity as "the individual's knowledge that he [or she] belongs to certain social groups together with some emotional and value significance to him [or her] of this group membership" (p. 31). In other words, social identity refers to *internalised group membership* that serves to define a person's sense of 'who they are' in a given context. This can be formally distinguished from the notion of *personal identity*, which refers to a person's internalised sense of their individuality (e.g., reflecting their unique physical appearance and their idiosyncratic abilities and tastes; Turner, 1982).

As we have already noted, it is the personal definition of self and identity that is the customary focus of psychological analysis and understanding. But it is important to note that in the minimal group studies, knowing about participants' personal identities (e.g., that, as individuals, they were generous and kind or mean and cruel) does not do much to help us understand their behaviour. Instead, it was participants' sense that they were over-estimators (say) that led them to behave as over-estimators and that determined their allocation behaviour (i.e., whether and to whom they were generous and kind or mean and cruel). Similarly, in the world at large, in contexts where people come to define themselves as members of a given group (e.g., as 'us Sardinians', 'us Hindus', or 'us farmers'), then it is these social identities that serve as primary reference points for their behaviour.

Put slightly differently, what the minimal group studies showed very elegantly was that group behaviour does not derive from interdependence, economic exchange, or attraction between individuals. Instead, it flows from the *cognitive process* that enables participants to define the self in terms of group membership. More formally, as Turner (1982) put it, the studies show that "*social identity is the cognitive mechanism which makes group behaviour possible*" (p. 21, emphasis added).

Why social identity is important for health

In the field of social psychology, it is clear that the above analysis goes a long way to helping us understand important forms of social behaviour. In particular, after more than 40 years of research there is a lot of support for the claim that phenomena like prejudice, discrimination, and hatred, as well as cooperation, solidarity, and trust, are more a reflection of people's social identities than of their personal identities (e.g., see Turner, Hogg, Oakes, Reicher, & Wetherell, 1987). In very broad terms, this work can be summarised as showing that how we understand, treat, and engage with other people depends very much on the degree to which we see them as sharing a social identity with us.

Whether we see people as ingroup members or as outgroup members (and the degree to which we do so) thus clearly has very profound implications for our social behaviour, in ways that we will discuss in a lot more detail later. But before we do, it is worth asking why this fact is important for *health*.

As a way of starting to answer this question, consider the experiences of Neil Ansell, a journalist who decided to try to "find himself" by going to live as a hermit in the remote mountains of mid-Wales – something he did for five years (Ansell, 2011a). The idea was simple: with peace and solitude would come insight and self-knowledge. But that wasn't how it turned out. Recounting the experience in his book *Deep Country*, Ansell observes:

> What I found was not what you might expect. You might think that such protracted solitude would lead to introspection, to self-examination, to a growing self-awareness. But not for me. What happened to me was that I began to forget myself, my focus shifted almost entirely outwards to the natural world outside my window. It was as if we gain our sense of self from our interaction with other people; from the reflection of ourselves we see in the eyes of another. Alone, there was no need for identity, for self-definition.
>
> (Ansell, 2011b)

In short, in the absence of interaction with other people, rather than discover his sense of self, Ansell began to lose it. And even though "losing the self" is not necessarily a negative experience in and of itself, as Ansell found, one of the problematic consequences of isolation is that it can lead to a loss of one's bearings (see Figure 2.2). This observation is confirmed in a programme of experimental research led by Namkje Koudenburg which explored the relative impact of introspection and social

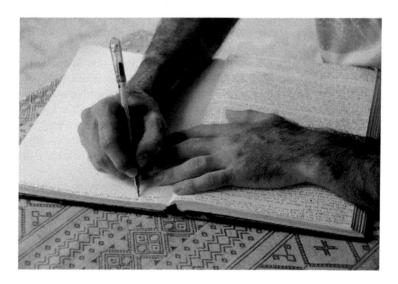

Figure 2.2 Pathways to self-knowledge

Note: Although one might imagine that introspection (e.g., via diary writing) would give us an opportunity to 'find ourselves' and hence be good for our mental health, research by Koudenburg and colleagues (2017) suggests that we are much more likely to gain self-knowledge and a sense of purpose through interaction with others.

Source: Pixabay

interaction on people's sense of personal identity (Koudenburg, Jetten, & Haslam, 2017). This found that, to the extent that they engaged in meaningful social interaction with other people, participants developed a stronger and clearer sense of self (e.g., as measured by items like "I know what I want from life"; see the measure of personal identity strength in the Appendix for details). Importantly, though, this interaction did not have to take the form of face-to-face contact – for example, it could involve writing a letter to a friend or family member. More generally, then, *it is because they make group-based interaction not only possible but also purposeful and meaningful that social identity and social identification are so crucial to health and well-being.*

Fundamentally, this point relates to the fact that, at the core, humans are social animals. In practical terms this means that we live, and have evolved to live, in social groups – the family, the club, the team, the tribe (e.g., Dunbar, 1998, 2013). Group life is therefore central to what we are as humans and it is a key source of meaning, purpose, and direction (see also H13 later). As the metaphysical poet John Donne (1624/1959) observed in a meditation on his own declining health, "No man is an Island, entire of itself" (p. 108). In other words, *groups make us human*, and without them our humanity – and all that goes with it – is diminished. In the most basic sense, *groups make life worth living*, and they are *what we live for*. It therefore follows that because social identity is what makes group behaviour and group life possible, then it, too, must be essential for us to thrive. But by the same token if groups exert a negative influence on our lives (as they sometimes do) or if we lack or lose valuable group memberships, then we can see that social identity processes will tend to be implicated in poor health outcomes.

The previous paragraph is possibly the most important in this book. Indeed, if one had to distil all the work on social identity and health into a summary of less than 200 words, it would probably take something of this form. More formally, though, we can present this as the principal hypothesis of the social identity approach to health:

H1 (the social identity hypothesis): Because it is the basis for meaningful group life, social identity is central to both good and ill health.

This hypothesis is fundamental to the arguments that we advance in this book and that underpin the extensive corpus of social cure research (see Jetten et al., 2017). For this reason the logic that underpins it is worth examining a little more carefully with an example. Imagine that one particular form of group activity that you wanted to take part in was as a member of your local choir. Psychologically, what is it that would allow you to do this? For Turner (1982), the key point was that to behave as a member of the choir, you first have to be able to define yourself as a member of the choir. If you could only ever see yourself and other choir members as individuals (i.e., in terms of *personal identities* as Anne, Bill, Cliff, etc.), this would be impossible.

In short, it is the fact that a choir's members see themselves as singing from the same song sheet (i.e., in terms of a shared social identity) that allows the choir to work as a meaningful entity and that allows its members to contribute to, and benefit from, its collective achievements. Moreover, the more that choir members define themselves in this way – that is, the stronger their *social identification* – the more true this is. To the extent that being in a choir is good for you (and there is plenty of evidence that it is; e.g., see Dingle, Brander, Ballantyne, & Baker, 2013; Stacy, Brittain, & Kerr, 2002; Stewart & Lonsdale, 2016), it therefore follows that social identity and social identification are what allow you to access the benefits (for related evidence, see Dingle, Stark, Cruwys, & Best, 2015). Again, though, if being in a particular group is bad for you (e.g., as might be the case if a group abuses its members; e.g., Temerlin & Temerlin, 1982), then social identity and social identification will serve to compromise your health. This can be summarised in a second hypothesis:

H2 (the identification hypothesis): A person will generally experience the health-related benefits or costs of a given group membership only to the extent that they identify with that group.

These first two hypotheses are both strong and stark. To avoid misunderstanding, we also need to clarify that they (and those that follow) do not suggest that people need to be interacting in meaningful groups all the time in order to be healthy. Speaking to this point, Fabio Sani and his colleagues have shown that what matters for health is not so much the frequency of one's contact with others as the degree of one's identification with the groups of which one is a member (regardless of how much time you spend with them; Sani, Herrera, Wakefield, Boroch, & Gulyas, 2012). Being alone is therefore not necessarily harmful for well-being as long as one has meaningful social identities to fall back on.

Yet if social identities make group life possible and if group life has profound implications for good and bad health, then clearly there is much to be gained from trying to clarify both (1) what leads to social identity and social identification and (2) what their consequences are. Over the last 40 years this has been the primary goal of researchers whose work has been informed by the *social identity approach* and the two theories of which this is comprised: *social identity theory* (Tajfel & Turner, 1979) and *self-categorization theory* (Turner, 1982, 1991; Turner et al., 1987; Turner, Oakes, Haslam, & McGarty, 1994). Moreover, because these theories are central to the ideas that will be explored in the chapters that follow, it is worth discussing each – together with their core implications for health and well-being – in some depth.

Social identity theory: the psychology of intergroup relations

After the minimal group studies had led Tajfel to flesh out the concept of social identity, his primary concern was with its implications for intergroup processes such as conflict, prejudice, and discrimination. The primary way in which this was achieved was through work that he did with Turner to develop social identity theory in the late 1970s. In line with points made earlier, this theory centres on the insight that when people define themselves in terms of a given group membership they (1) strive to determine the meaning and standing of the group through social comparisons with relevant outgroups and (2) seek to define their ingroup favourably by differentiating it positively from those outgroups. As an example, if Matthew defines himself as Australian, then he is likely to try to work out what being Australian means by comparing Australia with other countries and he will generally be motivated to make comparisons that lead him to see Australia as better than other countries.

What is assumed to drive these processes is the motivation to enhance positive identity (Tajfel & Turner, 1979). Positive identity manifests itself as high collective self-esteem associated with membership in a particular group (i.e., the self-esteem derived from group belonging), but is also more generally reflected in higher life satisfaction and less psychological distress – in short, enhanced well-being. This means, for example, that when (and to the extent that) Matthew's sense of self is defined by a given social identity, his well-being will be boosted or dampened to the extent that the group with which that identity is associated does well or badly (either in his own eyes or in the eyes of others). Accordingly, his well-being may be lifted if Australia wins the Cricket World Cup (as it did in 2015), but it may take a hit if Australia is rebuked by the Human Rights Commission for its treatment of asylum seekers (something else that happened in 2015). This can be formalised in terms of the following hypothesis:

H3 (the group circumstance hypothesis): When, and to the extent that, a person defines themselves in terms of a given social identity, their well-being will be affected by the state and circumstances of the group with which that identity is associated.

More specific corollaries of this are:

H3a. When the group that defines a person's social identity is enhanced in some way (e.g., by success, high status, or advancement), social identity becomes a beneficial psychological resource and tends to have positive consequences for their well-being.

H3b. When the group that defines a person's social identity is compromised in some way (e.g., by stigma, low status, or failure), the capacity for social identity to function as a beneficial psychological resource is reduced, and this will tend to have negative consequences for their well-being.

A large body of work supports these hypotheses. For example, early work by Nyla Branscombe and Daniel Wann showed that the well-being (measured as self-esteem) of Americans who identified highly with their country or with a particular sports team was reduced when those groups did poorly or were threatened by outgroups (Branscombe & Wann, 1994; Wann & Branscombe, 1990). Likewise, longitudinal research by Kathleen Ethier and Kay Deaux (1994) showed that the well-being of Hispanic students fell once they entered tertiary educational institutions in which their identity was devalued.

It is not the case, however, that the consequences of events for people's group-based well-being are determined simply by what fate holds in store for the groups they identify with. This is because as much as group-relevant events determine well-being, so, too, the motivation for positive identity is often an important driver of behaviour. So when Branscombe and Wann's American participants were threatened by a Russian outgroup, they felt bad, but this also motivated them to engage in group behaviour to restore their positive identity – in this case through retaliatory derogation of that outgroup. Likewise, the highly identified Hispanic students in Ethier and Deaux's sample restored their positive identity by engaging more enthusiastically in cultural activities that celebrated their Hispanic heritage.

Along similar lines, Jason Crabtree and colleagues observed that because mental health support groups are stigmatised, this tends to have negative implications for those who identify with them. At the same time, however, identification with such groups also motivates their members to work together to challenge negative stereotypes of the ingroup and to resist the stigma to which they are subjected (a point we will return to in Chapter 13; Crabtree, Haslam, Postmes, & Haslam, 2010). This point can be formalised as follows:

H4 (the identity restoration hypothesis): People will be motivated to restore positive identity when this is compromised by events that threaten or undermine their social identities (e.g., group failure, stigma, low status, or loss of group membership).

According to social identity theory, the form that this attempt at positive identity restoration takes will vary as a function of the specific circumstances that the individual and the group confront. In particular, the theory points to the importance of two sets of factors (Tajfel & Turner, 1979; see also Ellemers, 1993; Ellemers & Haslam, 2012). The first of these is the perceived *permeability* of group boundaries – that is, whether or not group members feel that it is possible to leave the group and hence believe that *personal mobility* is possible. If it is (i.e., if group boundaries are permeable), then an obvious way for a person to deal with the threat that the group's fate poses to their positive identity is simply to leave. They can do this either physically (e.g., by walking out of the door) or psychologically (e.g., by disengaging from the group). This, for example, is what happens when fair-weather fans stop identifying with their team (and going to games) once it stops being successful. As work in Spain by Fernández, Branscombe, and colleagues has shown, it also happens when people who suffer from skeletal dysplasias that lead them to have disproportionately short stature (in the form of dwarfism) feel that they can escape the stigma and discrimination they face through limb-lengthening surgery (Branscombe, Fernández, Gómez, & Cronin, 2012; Fernández, Branscombe, Gómez, & Morales, 2012). And, as we will see in Chapter 9, it can also happen when a person who is in a substance-abusing group decides to try to exit the group because they see that the group is ruining their life (Best et al., 2016; Dingle, Stark et al., 2015; Dingle, Cruwys, & Frings, 2015). Stated formally, then, it can be hypothesised:

H5 (the mobility hypothesis): When circumstances threaten, undermine, or preclude positive social identity, if people perceive group boundaries to be permeable, they are likely to respond to the threat to positive identity through strategies of personal mobility.

One of the factors that determines these perceptions of permeability is social identification itself. This is because people are less likely to think that it is possible to leave a group if the group means a lot to them. If you are the fan of a particular football club, for example, it is, of course, always possible not to buy a season ticket, but this becomes harder if you are a die-hard fan whose identity is bound up with the club. More poignantly, these same dynamics can be observed in cycles of violence where the desire to leave an abusive relationship is tempered by identification with the group in which that relationship is embedded (e.g., a family, a cult, a gang; Campbell, 1987). In this regard, a key factor that feeds into identification (and hence the desire to exit across a permeable group boundary) is the *status* of the group in question. This means that even if a boundary is perceived to be permeable, people are less likely to want to leave a group that has high status. Amongst other things, then, this helps explain why it proves harder for people to leave abusive marital relationships in communities where marriage is associated with high status (Zink, Regan, Jacobson, & Pabst, 2003).

Where group boundaries are perceived to be *impermeable*, a second set of factors comes into play. Here the group's unfortunate circumstances are seen to be impossible to escape, and social identity theory argues that how people respond to or cope with this situation depends on whether or not the position of the ingroup is seen to be *secure* – in the sense of being both *stable* and *legitimate*. If it is, then group members are predicted to try to restore a sense of positive social identity through a process of *social creativity*.

This is seen, for example, when groups choose to measure their performance by selectively using metrics (e.g., particular types of 'league tables') on which they do well (Elsbach & Kramer, 1996; Platow, Hunter, Branscombe, & Grace, 2014). In the health domain this is also what Fernández, Branscombe, and colleagues observed among people suffering from skeletal dysplasias in the United States, where limb-lengthening surgery is less commonly available than in Spain. Here those who had this condition were much more likely to try to cope with stigma and group-based discrimination by denying their inferiority – in particular, by working creatively to replace negative stereotypes and labels (e.g., "dwarf") with more positive ones ("Little People"; Branscombe et al., 2012, p. 124). This, then, is the basis for the following hypotheses:

H6 (the creativity hypothesis): When circumstances threaten, undermine, or preclude positive social identity, if people perceive group boundaries to be impermeable but group relations to be secure, they are likely to respond to the threat to positive identity through strategies of social creativity.

However, when the quest for positive social identity is thwarted and the position of an ingroup is seen to be impermeable and *insecure* (i.e., unstable and/or illegitimate), then its members are more likely to embrace strategies of *social competition* that involve trying to produce *social change*. Amongst other things, this may involve participation in political action designed to win improved rights or better treatment for one's ingroup. This has been seen, for example, in the trajectory of actions taken by groups campaigning for disabled people's rights in developed countries over the past three or four decades (e.g., Hernandez, Balcazar, Keys, Hidalgo, & Rosen, 2006; Schlaff, 1993). With a growing sense that the disadvantage their members experience is not only unfair but can also be overcome, these groups' actions have become increasingly confrontational. This leads to the following hypothesis:

H7 (the competition hypothesis): When circumstances threaten, undermine, or preclude positive social identity, if people perceive group boundaries to be impermeable and group relations to be insecure, they are likely to respond to the threat to positive identity through strategies of social competition.

The over-arching point that emerges from the analysis provided by social identity theory (and from H3 to H7) is that individuals' internalisation of particular social identities is critical for understanding how they respond to the circumstances faced by the groups to which those identities relate. For example, how a woman responds to evidence of gender discrimination and the impact that this has on her well-being will depend, in the first instance, on whether or not she sees herself as a woman who shares social identity with other women (Ellemers, 2001). But at the same time, we also see that the tendency to define oneself, and act, in terms of social identity, as well as the meaning of this identity, depends on perceptions of the prevailing social structure. As was seen at the start of the 20th century, women are much more likely to band together to confront the adverse effects of sexism once they see their position in society to be illegitimate and possible to change.

In this way, social identity theory starts to give us an insight into when and how social (rather than personal) identities have important implications for health and well-being. We say "starts", though, because although social identity theory offers insight into the causes and consequences of social identity (especially for intergroup relations), these elements were subsequently specified more precisely, and with much broader applicability, by self-categorization theory.

Self-categorization theory: the psychology of group behaviour

If one looks back over H3 to H7, it is apparent that social identity theory is primarily concerned with the way in which people's behaviour is shaped by the situation that their ingroup finds itself in vis-a-vis other groups. Primarily, then, it is a theory of *intergroup* relations. It is clear, however, that there is a broader set of questions that relate to the functioning of social and personal identity and social groups more generally. When do we define ourselves in terms of social identity? What determines which particular social identity defines our sense of self in any given context? What are the consequences of defining the self in terms of a particular social identity?

The depersonalisation process

It was to answer such questions that Turner and his colleagues developed self-categorization theory in the 1980s and 1990s. At the outset a core goal of the theory was to explain what it was, psychologically, that allowed people to engage in group behaviour. Traditional answers to this question had pointed to the importance of interdependence and mutual attraction, but Turner found these unsatisfactory. For a start, this was because these elements were absent in the minimal group paradigm, and yet this produced clear evidence of group behaviour (in the form of ingroup favouritism). Other work, dating back to a series of famous studies conducted in boys camps in the United States by Muzafer Sherif and his colleagues (see Sherif, 1956; Platow & Hunter, 2017), also showed that when it comes to predicting people's behaviour in intergroup contexts, personal liking and friendship are often trumped by a sense of shared (or non-shared) group membership.

As we have seen, Turner thus argued that it was social identity that provided the psychological platform for group behaviour. Beyond this, he also argued that group behaviour arose from the *process* of defining oneself in terms of social identity – a process he termed *depersonalisation*. This refers to the fact that as one's social identity becomes more important, or more *salient*, how one sees the world, and how one acts, is determined less by the sense of oneself as a unique individual ('I') and more by the sense of oneself as a group member ('us'). More particularly, depersonalisation is a process of *self-stereotyping* through which the self comes to be understood in terms of a social category membership that is shared with other ingroup members.

For example, once a doctor – let's call her Karlie – enters a hospital, she will tend to stop seeing herself simply as a unique individual and start to define herself as someone who shares category membership with some people (e.g., other doctors) but not with others (patients, administrators). Moreover, this will have a profound impact on her behaviour. For example, on the street, Karlie would probably never dream of asking a complete stranger to remove their clothes or to tell her their medical history; however, *as a doctor* it might be a problem if she failed to do this. Formally, then, it is hypothesised:

H8 (the norm enactment hypothesis): When, and to the extent that, a person defines themselves in terms of a given social identity, they will enact – or at least strive to enact – the norms and values associated with that identity.

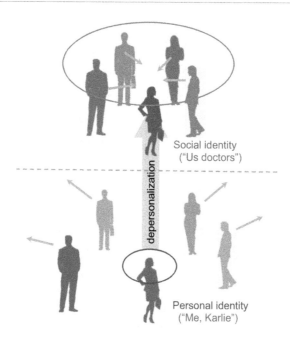

Social identity
("Us doctors")

depersonalization

Personal identity
("Me, Karlie")

Figure 2.3 The process of depersonalisation

Note: Depersonalisation involves transitioning from thinking about the self in terms of personal identity (as 'I') to thinking about the self in terms of social identity (as 'we'). Here, through a process of *self-stereotyping*, the self and other ingroup members (in this case, other doctors) come to be seen as members of the same social category (as "us doctors").

The process of depersonalisation is represented schematically in Figure 2.3. Note, too, that whereas in everyday language the terms 'depersonalisation' and '(self-)stereotyping' tend to have negative connotations, within self-categorization theory they are understood to be much more neutral – referring simply to the process through which the self comes to be seen as categorically *interchangeable* with other ingroup members. In the case of Karlie, this might mean that although outside the hospital her actions diverge sharply from those of her colleagues, within its walls they are likely to become much more aligned (being shaped by their shared identity as doctors and by the business of *doing* what doctors do). Moreover, there is no sense in which this process is inherently problematic – indeed, it is a *necessary* part of *being* a group member (in this case, a doctor). In particular, it is important to note that depersonalisation does not involve a *loss* of self; rather, it involves a *redefinition* of self. Karlie does not stop being Karlie when her identity as a doctor becomes salient, but the nature of her personhood changes. She does not stop knowing what she likes and dislikes or having thoughts and feelings; it is just that *what* she likes, thinks, and feels changes.

Determinants of social identity salience

The process of depersonalisation describes *how* people come to see themselves in terms of social identity, but it does not explain *when* or *why* this occurs. What is it that makes social identity salient? And what is it that makes a *particular* social identity salient? For example, what leads a woman to see herself in some contexts as a doctor and in others as a mother? And what determines what exactly it means for her to be a doctor or a mother?

Building on insights both from social identity theory (e.g., as specified in H3 to H7) and from cognitive psychology, self-categorization theory answers these questions by understanding the functioning of the self as reflecting a process of *social categorization*. Following influential work by Jerome Bruner (1957), the salience of a given identity (whether personal or social) is seen to be determined by the interaction of two factors: the *fit* of a particular self-categorization and a person's *readiness* to use it (Oakes, 1987; Oakes, Haslam, & Turner, 1994).

The first of these factors means that a person is more likely to define themselves as a member of a given group if this self-categorization allows them to make sense of themselves in the context at hand. This in turn depends upon two factors: (1) differences among ingroup members being perceived to be smaller than differences between ingroup members and outgroup members (the principle of *metacontrast*, also known as *comparative fit*; see Figure 2.4) and (2) patterns of category difference corresponding to prior expectations about what it means to belong to those categories (known as *normative fit*; see Figure 2.5). This means, for example, that a person is more likely to define themselves as depressed and as sharing group membership with other depressed people if (1) the differences between depressed people appear to be smaller than the differences between depressed and non-depressed people and (2) the nature of these differences maps on to their expectations about depressed and non-depressed people (e.g., if the former seem to be less happy than the latter).

The second factor, perceiver readiness, refers to the fact that a person is more likely to define themselves as a member of a given group if they are predisposed to use a particular social identity as a basis for self-definition. A person is more likely to understand themselves to be depressed if they have a history of being diagnosed with depression and of accepting this diagnosis or if they live in a culture

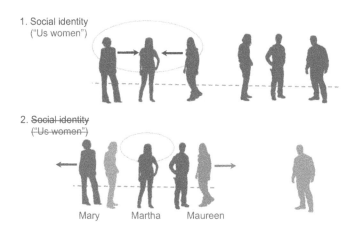

Figure 2.4 The principle of comparative fit

Note: Martha is more likely to define herself in terms of a social identity that she shares with Mary and Maureen – as "us women" – in Context 1 (top) than in Context 2 (bottom). This is because in Context 1 the differences between the three women are small in comparison to the differences between them and the other people (men) who are psychologically present in this context. By the same token, she is also more likely to define the men in terms of a social identity that she does not share – as "them men" – in Context 1 than in Context 2 (Haslam & Turner, 1992; Haslam, Oakes, Turner, & McGarty, 1995).

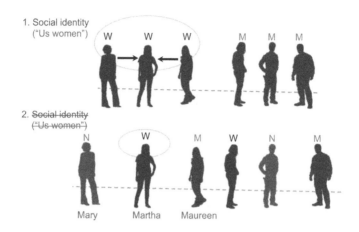

1. Social identity ("Us women")

2. Social identity ("Us women")

Mary　　Martha　　Maureen

Figure 2.5 The principle of normative fit

Note: W signifies behaviour consistent with Martha's expectations about women's behaviour.
M signifies behaviour consistent with Martha's expectations about men's behaviour.
N signifies behaviour consistent with Martha's expectations about neither women's nor men's behaviour.
Martha is more likely to define herself in terms of a gender-based social identity that she shares with Mary and Maureen – as "us women" – in Context 1 (top) than in Context 2 (bottom). This is because in Context 1 the behaviour of women and men is more consistent with her content-related expectations about gender categories.

where it is more common, and more acceptable, to see oneself as depressed (Chang, Jetten, Cruwys, & Haslam, 2017).

This process of social identity salience is represented schematically in Figure 2.6. The key points to note here are that, in the present, a given social identity becomes salient to the extent (1) that it is both comparatively and normatively fitting and (2) the perceiver has used that identity as a basis for self-definition in the past. Going forward, the enactment of the identity then creates a state of *social identification* that makes the identity available as a resource for the future.

Social influence

As alluded to in H8, when (and to the extent that) people define themselves in terms of a given social identity, they generally strive to live up to the norms and values associated with that identity. But this raises the question of how exactly they work out what these norms and values are. If Karlie defines (or wants to define) herself as a doctor, to whom should she turn to discover what this involves? The obvious answer is to other people who share this identity – in this case, to other doctors. Indeed, she is likely to turn to those people who best exemplify that identity, or who, in the language of categorization theory, are most *prototypical* of it (Rosch, 1978).

Like fit (see Figures 2.4 and 2.5), prototypicality has both comparative and normative elements – being determined by the extent to which a person is perceived to be more different from outgroup members than from ingroup members and in ways that are consistent with perceivers' normative expectations (Turner, 1985). Karlie is therefore more likely to see a particular doctor, Jean, as prototypical of the category 'doctors' if Jean appears similar to other doctors but different from patients and administrators, and in ways that are in line with Karlie's expectations about these different categories.

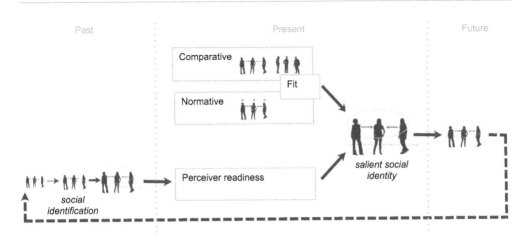

Figure 2.6 The process through which social identity becomes salient

Note. At a given point in time, a particular social identity (e.g., as "us women") becomes salient, and hence is a basis for perception and action, to the extent that it is comparatively and normatively fitting *and* has been enacted in the past and so is ready to be invoked. The process of enacting the identity also feeds into a state of *social identification* that contributes to perceiver readiness and increases the likelihood of the social identity becoming salient again in the future (for evidence of the role these processes play in the salience of gender identities, see Blanz, 1999; Haslam, 2004; Palomares, 2004).

So in Figure 2.5 this would mean that Martha is more prototypical of 'us women' than Mary or Maureen (because she is the woman who is the least different from other women and most representative of women's norms), but that Mary is more prototypical than Maureen (because she is more different from men and more representative of women's norms).

The reason why people who are more prototypical of a given social identity exert more influence over their fellow group members is that they best represent – and can be assumed to know the most about – the identity in question (Turner, 1985). Moreover, in this, such people are in a position to play *leadership* roles in helping group members to understand what a given group membership both means and entails (Haslam, Reicher, & Platow, 2011; Reicher, Haslam, & Hopkins, 2005).

Support for these ideas comes from a large body of work in the social identity tradition. Amongst other things, this shows that health communication is more effective when communicators and recipients share social identity than when they do not. For example, Daphna Oyserman and her colleagues have shown that when members of ethnic minority groups in the United States are encouraged to focus on their ethnic identity, they are more likely to reject messages to eat healthily that are presented by white middle-class sources because here the outgroup status of those sources is highly salient, and hence their ability to define 'what we should do' is limited (Oyserman, Fryberg, & Yoder, 2007; see also Tarrant, Hagger, & Farrow, 2012). More generally, this same logic helps us understand the *therapeutic alliance* between practitioners and clients as something that is social identity based. It also explains why health treatment that occurs across social category boundaries (e.g., of ethnicity, culture, and class) tends to be less satisfactory and less successful than treatment that occurs within those boundaries (Cooper et al., 2003; Martin, Garske, & Davis, 2000; Tucker & Kelley, 2000).

Such patterns can be formalised in terms of the following two hypotheses:

H9 (the influence hypothesis): When, and to the extent that, people define themselves in terms of shared
social identity, they will be more likely to influence each other.
H10 (the prototypicality hypothesis): People will have more influence in defining the meaning of a
given social identity to the extent that they are seen to be representative of that identity.

Applying the social identity approach to health

Even though their relevance is not yet fully fleshed out, the hypotheses presented above relate to principles of social identity and self-categorization theories that have obvious relevance to issues of health and health psychology. In this context, it is worth noting, however, that it was not until the turn of the millennium (30 years after the first work on social identity theory and 20 years after the first work on self-categorization theory) that the theories started to be applied in earnest to the domain of health (e.g., Haslam, Jetten, Postmes, & Haslam, 2009; Jetten, Haslam, & Haslam, 2012). Moreover, as we will see in the chapters that follow, although the process of exploring the applicability of these hypotheses to different health-related topics has served to test these theories' core principles, it has also extended them in important ways. As a result, this work has served to consolidate *distinctive* principles of the social identity approach to health (e.g., Gallagher, Muldoon, & Pettigrew, 2015; Haslam, 2014; Haslam, Jetten, & Haslam, 2012). In the remainder of this chapter it is therefore useful to spell out these principles because, as with the previous hypotheses, they will inform much of what is to follow.

Social identities are an important health-related resource

As we will see, two areas of health in which social identities have proved particularly important to health are those of *recovery* (e.g., Haslam, Holme, Haslam, Iyer, & Jetten, 2008; Jones & Jetten, 2011) and *resilience* (e.g., Drury, 2012; Williams & Drury, 2009). This work reinforces one key point which was not envisaged in original formulations of social identity and self-categorization theories – namely that social identities are an important psychological *resource* (Greenaway, Cruwys, Haslam, & Jetten, 2016; Jetten, Haslam, Haslam, Dingle, & Jones, 2014). One consequence of this is that, beyond the point that social identity is generally beneficial for health, it is also the case that the *more* social identities a person has, the more benefit they should experience because these give them access to more health-related resources – at least to the extent that those identities are important for them and compatible with each other (Iyer, Jetten, Tsivrikos, Postmes, & Haslam, 2009).

This prediction has been supported in studies with a range of different samples. These include patients recovering both from stroke (Haslam, Holme et al., 2008) and from depression (Cruwys et al., 2013b), students moving to university (Iyer et al., 2009), adults adjusting to becoming older (Haslam, Cruwys, & Haslam, 2014a), and sportspeople recovering from physical exertion (Jones & Jetten, 2011). Studies of various populations by Jetten and her colleagues (2015) also show that people experience elevated self-esteem to the extent that they acquire more social identities. Such work speaks to the following hypothesis:

H11 (the multiple identities hypothesis): Providing they are compatible with each other, important
to them, and positive, the more social identities a person has access to, the more psychological
resources they can draw upon and the more beneficial this will be for their health.

It also follows from this analysis that, as resources, social identities can be *actively managed* – in particular, by service providers – with a view to improving the health of particular groups. This point is brought home by a growing number of intervention studies which point to the tangible benefits that flow from activities which help to develop, maintain, or bolster the social identities of service users.

For example, a range of studies that have been carried out in care homes (which will be discussed in more detail in Chapter 7) have shown that residents experience better cognitive, mental, and physical health if their lives are organised in ways that help them build social identity with other residents (Haslam, Haslam et al., 2010; Haslam, Haslam, Knight et al., 2014b; Haslam, Haslam, Ysseldyk et al, 2014c; Knight, Haslam, & Haslam, 2010). Likewise, as we will see in Chapters 4, 8, 9, and 15, for vulnerable populations in the community (e.g., those who are homeless or recovering from substance abuse), the process of bringing people together in groups is found to improve their mental health and to provide a platform for recovery (Best et al., 2016; Cruwys, Haslam, Dingle, Jetten et al., 2014c; Haslam, Cruwys, Haslam, Dingle, & Chang, 2016c) – providing that the content of the social identities that people derive from group membership is positive (Dingle et al., 2015).

Importantly, this same point also applies to service providers themselves, as they, too, should benefit from activities and processes that serve to increase their sense of shared social identity. In line with this point, studies have found that the motivation and well-being of hospital workers is enhanced where managers take steps to foster, rather than undermine, their shared identity. Indeed, this is something that is true for workers in general (O'Brien et al., 2004; Steffens Haslam, Kerschreiter, Schuh, & van Dick, 2014). Relatedly, work by Kirstien Bjerregaard and colleagues also indicates that the training experiences and outcomes of carers are enhanced to the extent that the training process engages with and serves to consolidate, rather than compromise, team-based social identification (Bjerregaard, Haslam, & Morton, 2016). Indeed, an approach that takes these ideas to heart has been shown to have beneficial consequences for the leadership capacity of health professionals in general (Haslam, Steffens et al., 2017).

Psychological resources that result from shared social identity

The idea that social identities are psychological resources is central to most of the issues that we will explore in the chapters that follow. But what exactly does this mean? And what precise form do these resources take? To prepare the ground for what is to follow, we can answer these questions by exploring four of the most important psychological resources that flow from internalised group memberships.

Connectedness and positive orientation to others

The first psychological resource that is derived from social identity pertains to perceptions of *social connection* – the sense that one is psychologically close to, and yoked with, other people. As a copious amount of health research has shown, this has profound implications for health (e.g., Berkman & Syme, 1979; Cacioppo & Patrick, 2008; Cruwys, Haslam, Dingle, Haslam, & Jetten, 2014b; Haslam, Cruwys et al., 2016c; Putnam, 2000; Saeri, Cruwys, Barlow, Stronge, & Sibley, 2017; Sani, 2012). For example, if one looks back to Figure 2.3, one can see that, as individuals, the five people have no necessary bond to each other. However, as group members who recognise that they share social identity, their similarity and interconnectedness become much more apparent and much more significant. A key reason for this is that a sense of shared social identity transforms others who are *different from the self* into fellow ingroup members who are *part of the self* (Turner, 1985).

This observation is nicely illustrated in work by Hani Alnabulsi and John Drury (2014) that explored feelings of connectedness amongst pilgrims at the Hajj in Mecca – a massive religious festival attended each year by over 2 million Muslims (see Figure 2.7). Here the more people identified with the large crowd of people participating in the pilgrimage, the more at one they felt with their fellow pilgrims, the more supported they felt by them, and the safer they felt as a result. Thus, whereas the density of the throng was experienced as a problem for those who did not identify strongly with the crowd, this was not the case for those with high levels of identification.

However, the process of coming to see others in terms of shared social identity does not only change abstract perceptions of similarity and connectedness, it also changes our openness and receptivity to others. In particular, this is seen in perceptions of liking and trust and in the desire for mutual

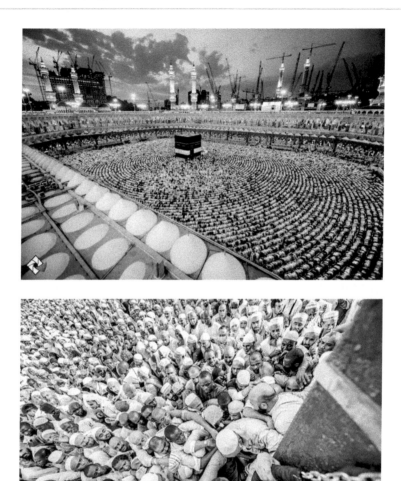

Figure 2.7 Pilgrims attending the annual Hajj at Mecca

Note: Research by Alnabulsi and Drury (2014) shows that the more people feel that they share social identity with other pilgrims, the more positive their experience of the event.

Source: Wessam Hassamin

communication and contact. Indeed, even in minimal group contexts, once people start to relate to others as members of their ingroup (e.g., as fellow over-estimators), they tend (1) to view them more positively and to see them as more trustworthy (Doise et al., 1972; Foddy, Platow, & Yamagishi, 2009; Güth, Levati, & Ploner, 2008; Platow, Haslam, Foddy, & Grace, 2003) and (2) to respond more positively to their communication (Greenaway, Wright, Reynolds, Willingham, & Haslam, 2015; see also Hewett, Watson, Gallois, Ward, & Leggett, 2009).

This is even more true in non-minimal contexts. For example, in a simulated prison experiment (that we will discuss in more detail in Chapter 5), Reicher and Haslam (2006a) observed that as the sense of social identity increased among the members of one group (the Prisoners), so their levels of mutual liking and trust increased; yet as social identity declined in the other group (the Guards), its members became more suspicious of each other and more paranoid (Haslam, Reicher et al, 2016; see Chapter 13). For the Prisoners, the prison thus became a site for engagement and enjoyment, whereas for the Guards it became increasingly alienating and frightening. Similar patterns have been observed in a range of group contexts, including schools (e.g., Bizumic, Reynolds, Turner, Bromhead, & Subasic, 2009), workplaces (e.g., Wegge, Van Dick, Fisher, Wecking, & Moltzen, 2006), and residential care homes (e.g., Gleibs et al., 2011b; Haslam, Haslam, Knight et al., 2014b). This, then, is the basis for the following hypothesis:

H12 (the connection hypothesis): When, and to the extent that, people define themselves in terms of shared social identity, they will be more likely to perceive themselves as similar and connected and to be positively oriented towards (e.g., trusting of) each other.

Meaning, purpose, and worth

The significance of perceptions of connectedness and trust, of course, is not simply cognitive but also behavioural. That is, as well as shaping how we think and feel, they feed into what we do. More particularly, social identity is a major determinant of *social interactions* – how people get together and do things. Indeed, as we have argued, to the extent that they share a sense of social identity, what people do is largely determined by the content of their identity. Thus, those who share an identity as members of a work team work together, those who share an identity as members of a choir sing together, and those who share an identity as members of a family participate in family events together. Moreover, social identification means that people don't just 'do' these things, but that they do them willingly and with passion – so that their actions have a quality that Émile Durkheim (1912/1915) referred to as 'effervescence' (Hopkins et al., 2016).

Note, too, that, in reality, groups also spend much (in many cases most) of their time *working towards* particular collective outcomes – organising a conference, rehearsing for a choral performance, planning a wedding, and so on. This is likely to impact positively on their members' well-being (even if they are not in the presence of other group members) because it not only channels their attention and energy, but also gives them a sense of common direction and purpose. This was something Durkheim (1897/1951) famously noted when he observed that the incidence of suicide declines sharply during wartime. Through his forensic research he came to attribute this to the fact that "great popular wars rouse collective sentiments, stimulate partisan spirit and patriotism, political and national faith alike, and, concentrating activity toward a single end, at least temporarily cause a stronger integration of society"[2.1] (p. 208). At the same time, the process of contributing to common goals is likely to be valued and valorised by other ingroup members and hence is likely to make one's efforts seem worthy and worthwhile. On this basis, then, we can hypothesise:

H13 (the meaning hypothesis): When, and to the extent, that people define themselves in terms of shared social identity, that identity will focus their energies and imbue them with a sense of meaning, purpose, and worth.

Social support

Reference to the collective activities that groups engage in alerts us to the fact that social identity does not simply affect individuals' behaviour in isolation, but also structures the way that they engage and interact with each other. More particularly, as people come to define themselves in terms of shared group membership, they are motivated to engage with others in ways that serve to advance interests associated with the identity they share. One of the most obvious ways they can do this is by trying to help each other out – a motivation that becomes more pronounced the more that other group members are perceived to be in difficulty. Again, this flows from the fact that here the other person is not seen as 'other' but as 'self'. This point is made lyrically by the Hollies in their ballad, "He Ain't Heavy, He's My Brother". Challenging the idea that those in need of help should be seen and treated as 'other', the song recognises shared identity as a basis for seeing their welfare as a vital concern rather than as a burden.

Empirical evidence that speaks to the underlying processes here comes from another sizeable corpus of social identity literature (see Haslam, Reicher, & Levine, 2012). For example, carefully staged field experiments by Mark Levine and colleagues showed that when a Manchester United fan saw another Manchester United fan trip and fall, they typically rushed over quickly to offer assistance, whereas when a Liverpool supporter (or someone wearing a plain shirt who therefore didn't appear to support any team) tripped over, they were more likely to look away or pretend not to notice (Levine, Prosser, Evans, & Reicher, 2005). Likewise, in the context of international aid, Levine and Thomson (2004) showed that how much financial support people provide to victims of a disaster (as well as how sympathetic they are to the victims' plight) depends very much on their sense that they share identity with those victims. For example, someone living in the UK was likely to donate more money to support disaster relief in Italy when they were encouraged to define themselves as European rather than as British. This was because, as Europeans, Italian and British people share social identity in a way that they do not as citizens of different nations. Likewise, as we will discuss further in Chapter 5, an important feature of Levine and colleagues' (2005) research was that it showed Manchester United fans would offer as much support to a Liverpool supporter as to a Manchester United supporter if they had been encouraged to define themselves as football fans rather than as supporters of a particular team.

Importantly, too, these same self-categorization processes structure people's responses to any social support that they receive – so that help is construed more positively when it is provided by ingroup rather than outgroup members (Haslam, Reicher, & Levine, 2012). This point has been confirmed in studies of workplace supervision by Ellemers and her colleagues in which advice that is given by an ingroup supervisor is experienced as supportive and useful, but exactly the same advice from an outgroup supervisor is experienced as interfering and unwanted (Ellemers, Van Rijswijk, Bruins, & De Gilder, 1998). In sum, then, one can hypothesise:

H14 (the support hypothesis): When, and to the extent, that people define themselves in terms of shared social identity, they will (1) expect to give each other support, (2) actually give each other support, and (3) construe the support they receive more positively.

Control, efficacy, and power

Finally, it is also the case that involvement in collective projects will tend to furnish people with a sense of *control*. At a group level, this should imbue people with a sense of being in charge of their destiny and of having power in the world (Turner, 2005). As we saw when discussing H6 and H7, this is something countenanced by social identity theory where, when positive social identity is threatened, group members attempt to recover this through either social creativity or social competition. More generally, we see that social identity creates in a group a sense that it is not just watching the world from the sidelines but actively making – and in a position to make – its own history (Drury & Reicher, 2005). As we will see in the chapters that follow, this can be especially important for individuals suffering from clinical conditions (e.g., dementia, autism, anxiety) who might otherwise succumb to a sense of helplessness and powerlessness (Clare, Rowlands, & Quin, 2008; Crabtree et al., 2010), but who can be motivated by an emergent sense of shared social identity to 'fight back'. Importantly, too, as studies by Chris Cocking and John Drury (e.g., 2004) have shown, when they do, benefits can be derived from an empowering sense of shared social identity, regardless of how successful the group's fight actually is.

What is true at the level of the group also has implications at the level of the individual (Postmes & Jetten, 2006). Accordingly, a sense of shared social identity also has the capacity to imbue group members with a sense of *personal control* over their lives. This is a point that has been corroborated in a large programme of research by Katharine Greenaway and colleagues (2015). For example, their analysis of data from the World Values Survey (encompassing 62,000 people in 47 countries) shows that people report a greater sense of personal control to the extent that they identify highly with their community, with their nation, or with humanity as a whole. Another study also showed this to be true for members of both political parties in the United States immediately after the 2012 presidential election – even for the Republicans who had the distressing experience of losing.

This observation is particularly significant for issues of health because a large body of research attests to the fact that a sense of personal control is a cornerstone of well-being. Indeed, within the *World Happiness Report* control is identified as one of the "six pillars" of life satisfaction (Helliwell, Layard, & Sachs, 2013). Typically, this pillar is thought to have largely personal origins, but Greenaway's work suggests that it can have its basis in social identities and social identifications – suggesting that a strong sense of "me" flows from a strong sense of "us" (see also Jetten, Haslam, Pugliese, Tonks, & Haslam, 2010b). Putting these observations together then, we can hypothesise:

H15 (the agency hypothesis): When, and to the extent that, people define themselves in terms of shared social identity, they will develop a sense of efficacy, agency, and power.

Conclusion

This chapter has covered a lot of ground and at some pace. As a result, we recognise that the process of engaging with the various ideas we have laid out is likely to have proved quite demanding – especially for those who are new to the social identity approach. We recognise too that much of the challenge here arises from the fact that these ideas are at odds with the prevailing orthodoxies that we outlined in Chapter 1. In particular, this is because they challenge the dominant model of the self that prevails in psychology (and in Western society as a whole) which sees the true nature of the person as residing in their immutable individuality, and hence which sees pathways to health as largely requiring engagement with, and mobilisation of, this individuality and an associated sense of personal identity.

The alternative view that we have set out does not question the importance of individuality or personal identity for our sense of personhood or for our behaviour. However, it suggests that this is most likely to have an impact on health and well-being where it emerges *out of*, rather than independently of, meaningful group memberships (Greenaway et al., 2015; Jetten et al., 2015). Indeed, more generally, we suggest that people's internalised group memberships – that is, their social identities – can be an essential source of psychological robustness and resilience. In large part this is because, as we have seen, social identities constitute key psychological resources of the form summarised in Figure 2.8. Moreover, as well as being psychological, these resources have important *material* consequences for the groups they are members of and for the social world that those groups are part of.

This can be seen clearly in each of the three examples with which we started this chapter. In Sardinia, the residents of the mountain villages are observed to have a fierce and proud sense of their shared and distinctive identity (Pinker, 2015); at the Magh Mela pilgrims revel in the opportunity to live out their shared religious faith (Tewari et al., 2012); in outback Australia resilient farmers report feeling a strong sense of belonging with others in their community that helps them to cope with the adversity of drought and hardship (McLaren & Challis, 2009; McPhedran & De Leo, 2013b; Schirmer, Mylek, Peel, & Yabsley, 2015). In all these cases it is not simply personal resilience or hardiness that protects health; rather this seems to flow from depersonalised connections between people that are a source of support, solidarity, and strength.

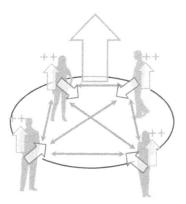

1. Connection and positive orientation to others

2. Meaning, purpose, and worth

3. Effective social support

4. Control, efficacy, and power

Figure 2.8 Key resources that flow from shared social identity

Note: To the extent that individuals define themselves in terms of shared social identity, they should (1) feel connected and positively oriented towards each other; (2) have a sense of meaning, purpose, and worth; (3) provide each other with effective social support; and (4) develop a sense of control, efficacy, and power. These psychological resources in turn have material consequences for the groups of which they are a part.

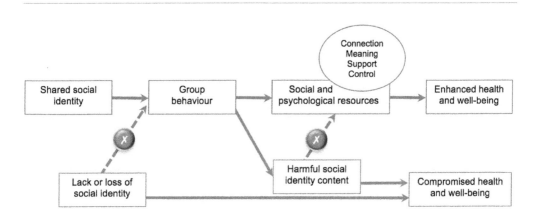

Figure 2.9 The social identity approach to health

Note: This figure represents key relationships between social identification, group behaviour, and health. Social identification that increases access to psychological resources generally serves to enhance health. However, when such identity is lacking or lost or promotes harmful behaviour, then this will tend to compromise health.

Source: Based on Haslam, Haslam et al. (in press)

In making these points, though, it is important also to acknowledge that the relationship between groups, social identity, and health is not straightforward. In particular, it would be dangerous and misleading to conclude that the message of this chapter (or this book as a whole) is that groups are an unalloyed good such that "groups = social identity = health". Not least, this is because, as the schematic representation in Figure 2.9 suggests, when groups fail, or are stigmatised, or develop destructive norms, pathways to health become complicated. The same is true for individual group members who find social identification hard to achieve – for example, because they are at the margins of a group or because they identify with multiple groups that have conflicting norms. Accordingly, one does not have to scour history books or newspapers too hard to find examples of groups whose social identities have been a major impediment both to the health of their own members and to the health of people in other groups. In this regard, then, much of the power of the social identity approach to health is that it allows us to understand these negative dynamics as well as those that are more positive.

At this point in our journey, though, the case that we have assembled to support such claims is formulated primarily in the form of hypotheses and propositions. The task before us is therefore to show how, in the process of exploring specific health topics, these hypotheses and propositions can be tested and how they can be leveraged to improve both theory and practice. Fortunately, this has been the primary goal of researchers who have advanced the social identity approach to health over the course of the last decade. Accordingly, the path ahead is well lit and it is increasingly well trodden. Like pilgrims on the road to Allahabad, we need not be afraid that we are travelling alone.

Points for practice

On the basis of the arguments presented in this chapter, it is possible to identify a range of points that are relevant to the work of health practitioners. Of these, the following four are perhaps the most important:

1. *Group life is a major determinant of health and well-being.* The key reason for this is that in lots of different ways, groups make life worth living and they are what we live for. So when a person's group life is fulfilling, this typically has a range of positive consequences for their mental and physical health. However, when it is compromised in some way, they become more vulnerable.
2. *The social identities that underpin group behaviour determine the impact of group life on health and well-being.* The precise impact that a particular group has on a person's health and well-being will depend on the nature of the social identity that underpins that group membership. For this reason, it is important to look closely at the norms, values, and practices that are associated with relevant social identities, as well as strength of social identification, in order to understand the specific implications of a given group membership.
3. *A range of processes that are central to health and well-being – including trust, control, and support – are not properties of a person but rather products of group dynamics.* Where there are deficiencies in these things that need to be understood and addressed, it is therefore necessary to look beyond the individual and to take stock of the broader social context in which they are embedded.
4. *The therapeutic alliance between practitioners and their clients has its basis in shared social identity.* Research points to the importance of the relationship between therapists and clients for the success of therapy, but tends to analyse and explain this in terms of 'qualities' of the two parties and their relationship. The social identity approach suggests instead that this alliance arises from a process in which those parties come to see themselves as sharing an interest in 'us'. Promulgating a sense of 'us' is therefore often very important to the success of any given therapy or treatment.

Resources

Further reading

To find out more about the social identity approach to health and well-being, the following publications are probably the obvious place to start.

① Turner, J. C., Oakes, P. J., Haslam, S. A., & McGarty, C. (1994). Self and collective: Cognition and social context. *Personality and Social Psychology Bulletin, 20*, 454–463.

There are lots of good summaries of social identity and self-categorization theories, but this is one of the best (and easiest to obtain) short introductions, and it is a classic paper in its own right. It explains the origins and consequences of a collective sense of self (i.e., social identity) and the importance of this for psychology as a whole.

② Haslam, S. A., Jetten, J., Postmes, T., & Haslam, C. (2009). Social identity, health and well-being: An emerging agenda for applied psychology. *Applied Psychology, 58*, 1–23.

This paper was one of the first to spell out the implications of social identity and self-categorization theories for issues of health and well-being and to define a research agenda which would go on to explore these implications. It was also the introduction to a special issue on the topic that contained a number of other important papers on this theme.

③ Jetten, J., Haslam, C., & Haslam, S. A. (Eds.) (2012). *The social cure: Identity, health and well-being*. New York, NY US: Psychology Press.

This edited volume was the first to assemble the work of various research groups around the world who were investigating the relationship between social identity and health. A number of the chapters are classics in their own right, and the book also provides the platform and rationale for the present volume.

④ Jetten, J., Haslam, S. A., Cruwys, T., Greenaway, K., Haslam, S. A., & Steffens, N. R. (2017). Advancing the social identity approach to health and well-being: Progressing the social cure research agenda. *European Journal of Social Psychology, 47*, 789–802.

This paper discusses recent developments in social cure research framed around the 15 hypotheses that we presented above. The special issue that it introduces also contains a range of other papers which showcase the many different ways in which the social identity approach to health can be applied and extended.

Video

① Search for "Introduction to social identity theory" to see a short video by Kevin Durrheim in which he discusses some of the foundational assumptions of social identity theory. www.youtube.com/watch?v=Tf5_gWa3h2g   (11 minutes)
② Search for "You are the groups you belong to" to watch a short video made by the Canadian Institute for Advanced Research in which Alex Haslam talks about the importance of groups for our sense of identity. www.youtube.com/watch?v=BmGfLemCBY4   (12 minutes)
③ Search for "Haslam BPS Glasgow" to see a the video of a keynote talk given by Alex Haslam at the British Psychology Society's Division of Clinical Psychology Conference in 2013 in which he introduces the social identity approach to health. www.youtube.com/watch?v=TWWZd8lrraw   (50 minutes)

Websites

ⓘ www.icsih.com/icsih-3-talks/ This site contains information about the 3rd International Conference on Social Identity and Health (ICSIH-3) that was held in Brisbane in June 2016. Amongst other things, it contains slides from 45 talks that were given by delegates from around the world on topics relevant to the material covered in this chapter and those that follow.

Note

1 Note, however, that this issue is complex because although what Durkheim referred to as 'egotistical suicide' declines in war, those in the military are also more likely to commit 'altruistic suicide' by sacrificing their lives for the good of their group, as per the connection hypothesis (H12; Davies & Neal, 2000).

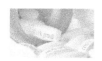

Chapter 3
Social status and disadvantage

Wherever people live together, hierarchies quickly develop. Because of their income, wealth, education, living conditions, skills, gender, ethnicity, geographical location, or social standing more generally, some individuals and some groups find themselves at the top of the hierarchy while others occupy lower-status positions. The rank that people have in society or in particular groups also affects important outcomes in life: access to resources, education, housing, quality of employment, and the extent to which they can exert power and social influence over others.

Even though social status, social rank, social class, and socio-economic status (SES) are not identical concepts and all refer to different divisions in society, in this chapter, we will refer to them as 'social status' for short. Importantly for our current purposes, this general social status concept is also a major determinant of health and well-being. Typically, we find that people at the bottom of a particular status hierarchy have the poorest health and those at the top have the best health. This so-called "*health gradient*" (Marmot, 2004, 2015) is not only found when examining various health risk factors (such as smoking, obesity, high blood pressure, or lack of exercise), but also is strongly associated with the prevalence of illnesses (such as depression, heart disease, diabetes, and cancer). Notably too, SES is a powerful predictor of mortality (for reviews see Braveman, Cubbin, Egerter, Williams, & Pamuk, 2010; Marmot, 2004, 2015; Putnam, 2000; Syme & Berkman, 1976; Wilkinson & Pickett, 2009). As Figure 3.1 shows, the statistics are stark. In Australia, for example, the richest 20% of the population live on average six years longer than the poorest 20% (Friel, 2014).

In this chapter we will focus on the reasons why social status (and in particular the lack of social status that is associated with social disadvantage) has such a profound effect on health and well-being. Even though the root causes of social disadvantage are many (including low levels of education, adverse early-life experiences, disability, stigma, and discrimination), in this chapter we will home in on the health-related effects of disadvantage (e.g., those relating to living in a deprived community, poor housing, or housing instability). In that sense, social disadvantage is more than a lack of access to financial and economic resources and involves multiple forms of social exclusion (see Cruwys et al., 2013a; Saunders, 2008). The negative health effects of stigma and discrimination will then be the focus of the next chapter.

An astute reader may ask why we would be interested in attempting to develop psychosocial explanations of the health gradient (see Figure 3.2). Is it not the case that there are straightforward non-psychosocial explanations for this relationship? For example, might it not be explained simply by the fact that poor people have less access to the health system and so do not get appropriate help for their mental and physical health conditions? Likewise, might it not simply be the case that those with lower education have poorer health than their more educated counterparts because they lack knowledge about how to live a healthy life and/or are more likely to engage in risky health behaviour (e.g., excessive alcohol consumption, drug taking)?

Although there is some logic to this reasoning (see Compton & Shim, 2015), findings from a range of studies suggest that these economic factors do not fully account for the health gradient (see Marmot, 2015; Sapolsky, 2004; Wilkinson & Pickett, 2009). This is for a number of reasons. First, the gradient can be found in all countries, and it is unaffected by the extent to which health care is affordable and accessible to all citizens. Second, the gradient exists even for diseases where preventative health or quality of health care is less relevant (e.g., juvenile diabetes; see Sapolsky, 2004). A health gradient is also present in mental illnesses (e.g., depression, schizophrenia, anxiety) – conditions where it is

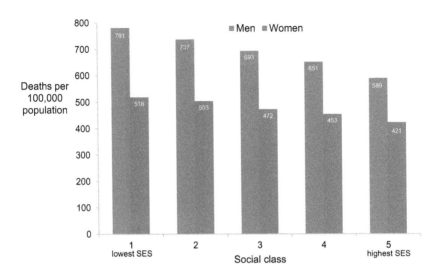

Figure 3.1 The health gradient

Note: This graph plots death rates among 15- to 64 year-old Australians between 2009 and 2011 as a function of socio-economic status (SES). This shows two clear main effects: men and members of low SES groups are much more likely to die than women and members of high SES groups.

Source: Australian Institute of Health and Welfare (2014)

clear that there is not a straightforward biological or genetic cause (Syme & Berkman, 1976; e.g., see Chapters 8 and 13). Third, and perhaps more intriguingly, data suggest that worse health is not only observed for those below a particular poverty line or education level. Instead, the health gradient is linear: with every increment of wealth and education, health improves. As we will explain further, this means that the health of people in the top 5% income bracket is better than that of those in the 5% income bracket just below them. And their health in turn is better than that of those in the 5% income bracket just below them, and so on. Put differently, even for those groups for whom all basic economic and financial needs are well met and where it is unlikely that there are substantial differences in education or key health services, we find that differences in wealth and income matter for health and well-being. This suggests that social disadvantage is about a lot more than just "having enough money".

In an attempt to better understand the psychosocial determinants of the health gradient, we start this chapter with a review of the biological and social determinants of health. Building on work by social scientists who have highlighted the important role that social capital and control play in determining our health, we explain how this is linked to a social identity analysis of health. In particular, we will outline how our social group memberships are integral to the development of social capital and a sense of control. Indeed, we argue that how we manage our social group memberships (and the social identities associated with them) holds the key to a better understanding of these processes.

One of the key insights of this chapter is that the way social status affects health may be quite different depending on whether people find themselves in a stable versus more unstable situation. Instability in particular threatens health, but it does so differently for people of high and low status. For

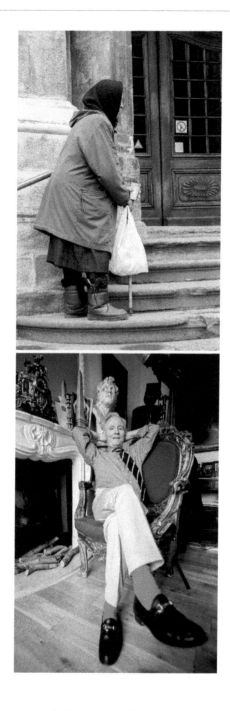

Figure 3.2 Wealth inequality: a cause of ill health for both the poor and the rich

Note: A large body of evidence shows that wealth inequality has a significant negative impact on the health of all members
of a given society (e.g., see Wilkinson & Pickett, 2009). It is easy to understand why this is the case for those who
are poor, but it is less obvious why this is also true for those who are wealthy.

Source: Pixabay

high-status groups, health declines when their social status is threatened; whereas for low-status groups health declines when there are insufficient resources or opportunities to improve their status. We will start to unpack this issue by first exploring different forms of status threats (in particular, related to situations where status is unstable, illegitimate, or when group boundaries are not permeable). After this, we will explore how status affects our health when we are going through major life changes such as moving countries or entering university. More specifically, we present research which shows that health disparities come to the fore when people undergo important life transitions that involve identity change. To integrate and elaborate these points, we then introduce the *social identity model of identity change* (SIMIC) – a model that has broad relevance to the themes of this book.

Current approaches to the health effects of social status

Physiological models

In an attempt to gain insight into the biological aspects of the relationship between social status and health, we first need to look at animal studies. According to this research, there is a very basic reason why status affects health: low status in a particular hierarchy evokes a strong biological stress response. Across numerous animal species, research has shown that subordinate animals both secrete more stress hormones and can show a lack of, or a blunted, stress response (e.g., in rats; Blanchard et al., 1995, guinea pigs; Sachser & Prove, 1986, and in squirrel monkeys; Manogue, Leshner, & Candland, 1975). Moreover, if the stressor is not dealt with effectively and the stress response remains chronically high, health is negatively affected, resulting in – amongst other things – immune suppression, gastric ulcers, loss of muscle mass, and reproductive suppression (Creel, 2001).

Interestingly, however, this work suggests that the heightened stress response for subordinate animals compared to dominant animals is not straightforward. It depends on which type of physiological stress response is examined, the type of stressor that the animal is exposed to, and importantly, the situation in which the animal finds themselves when stress responses are recorded (see Creel, 2001). For example, at baseline levels (in situations that do not evoke stress), dominant squirrel monkeys have lower levels of cortisol (a stress hormone) than subordinate animals. However, a study of squirrel monkeys by Kirk Manogue and colleagues showed that after exposure to different types of stressors (e.g., a live snake, physical restraint), dominant male squirrel monkeys showed greater reactivity to stress than subordinate male monkeys – with the latter showing a more sluggish physical response after exposure to a stressor (Manogue, Leshner, & Candland, 1975). This physical reactivity is likely to be adaptive when confronted with a stressor: the stressor triggers a rapid response among dominant animals, and this is arguably functional because it is aimed at resolving the stressful situation.

Findings are more straightforward when examining cardiovascular responses to stress among subordinate and dominant animals. Although stress has been found to negatively affect cardiovascular function among many different types of animals, subordinate status amplifies these effects. Among a range of different animals, subordinate status is associated with elevated resting blood pressure, higher levels of cholesterol, and more vascular damage than found in dominant animals (for a review see Sapolsky, 2004).

Even though the negative relationship between subordinate status and health among animals is well established, the challenge lies in explaining this relationship. There is some indirect evidence of the mechanisms that might be at work here. In particular, classic work suggests that poor health among subordinate animals appears to result from low predictability and lack of control, lack of other outlets for frustration and aggression, and lack of social support (Weiss, 1970). Indeed, each of these factors has been found to be related to a biological stress response (see Creel, 2001; Sapolsky, 2004).

Importantly, however, social context matters here. For depending on the nature of the animal group and the circumstances the group finds itself in, both lower- and higher-ranked animals may experience low predictability, control, and lack of social support. This in turn has a negative impact

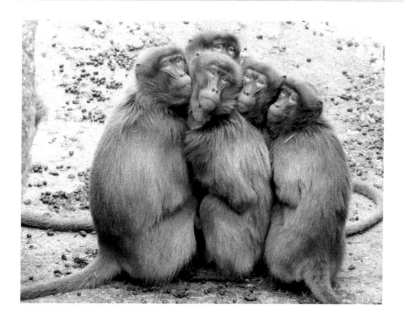

Figure 3.3 Social support can attenuate the heath-threatening effects of low status

Note: Studies of monkeys show that although subordinate animals tend to have higher cortisol levels than dominant ones, this difference is attenuated when members of the subordinate group provide each other with social support (Abbott et al., 2003).

Source: Pixabay

on their health (Goymann & Wingfield, 2004). For example, when dominant status is insecure (e.g., because ranks within a group change on a regular basis), dominant animals in the group experience the least control and predictability and they constantly need to compete to defend their position. It has been repeatedly observed that in such contexts, dominant status is no longer associated with health benefits. For example, Deborah Gust and her colleagues studied the formation of a new group among nine rhesus monkeys that were housed together after being relocated from elsewhere (Gust et al., 1991). They found that although all animals showed a stress response in the initial stages, once the dominance structure was established, the stress response remained high for the dominant group and continued to be higher for this group than for the subordinate animals nine weeks later.

There is also evidence that the higher stress response (leading to poorer health) among subordinate or more vulnerable animals is not found when there are high levels of social support among the subordinate group (Boccia et al., 1997). This was demonstrated by David Abbott and his colleagues in a comparative analysis of various primates living in captivity (rhesus, cynomolgus, talapoins, squirrel monkeys, and olive baboons; Abbott et al., 2003). Here subordinates only showed higher concentrations of the stress hormone cortisol than dominant animals when they had lower opportunities for social support (see Figure 3.3).

Although there are always issues when seeking to generalise from animal models (Shapiro, 1998), there are two important lessons for our understanding of status and disadvantage that we can take from this biological research. First, it suggests that the health-related problems that flow from low status are not inevitable. Second, it suggests that improving one's status is not the only way to address those problems. In particular, this is because it appears that the harmful health effects of stress can be remediated through social solidarity. This is a point that resonates with evidence relating to the role of group processes in ameliorating stress more generally that we discuss in greater depth in Chapter 5.

Human biological models

Although the animal research is instructive, it cannot fully capture the health effects of social status in humans. Recently, researchers have started to do this. Some of the trailblazing work in this regard was conducted by Jim Blascovich (2008) in work on the *bio-psychosocial model of challenge and threat* (BPM-CT). Focusing on the measurement of threat, Blascovich proposed that people are more likely to experience threat when the demands of the situation they face outweigh the resources that they bring to the situation to deal with these demands. For example, giving a speech is more threatening when facing a tough audience (i.e., a highly demanding situation) and one does not have much time to prepare (i.e., having limited resources). In contrast, when resources match or exceed demands (e.g., if a person has had days to prepare for a speech and the audience is friendly and encouraging), then the person is more likely merely to feel challenged rather than threatened. Importantly, threat and challenge are associated with different types of physiological response – with "unhealthier" responses (associated with higher blood pressure, slower heart rate recovery) more likely when a situation evokes threat rather than challenge.

Important for our current purposes, Daan Scheepers and Naomi Ellemers (2005) provided the first evidence of differences – albeit complex ones – in the physiological responses of members of high- and low-status groups. This study used a minimal group paradigm in which participants were randomly allocated to one of two groups, ostensibly on the basis of their perceptual style, and told that one group (detailed perceivers) had higher status than the other (holistic perceivers; see Chapter 2 for a discussion of this paradigm). Blood pressure (which tends to be elevated in response to threat; Blascovich & Mendes, 2000) was measured multiple times. The first time was when participants were initially told that their group had high or low status and, here, those in the low-status group had higher blood pressure than those in the high-status group. Blood pressure was measured a second time when participants were told that they were going to engage in a range of tasks that would define their status for the rest of the experiment. Now blood pressure was higher for those in the high-status group. Consistent with findings from animal studies, then, it appears that when high-status group members become aware that they may lose their social standing, they have a stronger stress response than their low-status counterparts. In contrast, as we will discuss in more detail later, for low-status group members, the possibility that status relations might improve was appraised more positively, and here their status was associated with a challenge rather than a threat response (i.e., lower blood pressure; see also Scheepers, Ellemers, & Sintemaartensdijk, 2009).

These findings make it clear that there is more to health disparities between groups of different status than merely physiological differences between subordinates and dominants. In other words, there is no genetic or biological difference between subordinate and dominant groups (in either animals or humans) that makes either group healthier or fitter for survival at birth. Moreover, it appears that biological stress responses that are associated with poor health are not simply a function of differences in social status. Instead, studies that have examined changing status hierarchies indicate that the relationship between social status and health is shaped in important ways by social context and, in particular, reflects the dynamics of *experienced and anticipated intergroup relations*.

This in turn suggests that to explain physiological responses to social status, we need to move beyond biology and focus on the environment and social inequality. Interestingly, when we do, we find corroborating evidence that many of the factors that were identified above (notably, the predictability of the environment, control, and social support) play an important role in producing the health gradient. It is this literature that we review next.

Sociological and epidemiological models

A vast body of work by sociologists and epidemiologists has documented the capacity for status inequalities to produce the health gradient in a range of different societies and populations. The following statistics are illustrative of the findings from this work and are presented by Michael Marmot (2015) in his best-selling book *The Health Gap*:

- In the poorest parts of Baltimore (where there have been many riots in recent years), life expectancy for men is currently 63 years. In the richest part of Baltimore it is 83 years.
- In the poorest parts of Tottenham in North London (one of the places where the 2011 London riots started) the life expectancy for men is 17 years lower than it is for men living in affluent suburbs such as Kensington and Chelsea. In Glasgow between 1998 and 2002 life-expectancy gaps for men were even more pronounced; whereas men's life expectancy was 82 in upmarket Lenzie, it was only 54 in the poor parts of Calton. This difference has reduced from 28 years to around 20 years in 2015, yet remains stark for residents in a single city.
- In Australia today, middle-aged people with fewer than 12 years of education have a 70% higher mortality risk than the most educated Australians. Meanwhile, the difference in the life expectancy of Indigenous and non-Indigenous people in Australia is 11 years. A 2012 report by Australia's National Centre for Social and Economic Modelling concluded that "Australia suffers the effects of a major differential in the prevalence of long-term health conditions. Those who are most socio-economically disadvantaged are twice as likely to have a long-term health condition as those who are the least disadvantaged" (Brown, Thurecht, & Nepal, 2012, p. vii).

Although the magnitude of these effects is stark, as we noted earlier, one might still explain them away by arguing that they all involve extreme comparisons: between the poorest and the wealthiest in a particular location or the least educated and the highest educated. Moreover, because there are many differences between these groups, aside from those that involve social status, other explanations for these differences cannot easily be ruled out. For example, they could reflect the influence of different lifestyles, cultures, or family structures.

One very influential research programme that sought to address some of these concerns was conducted by Marmot with British civil servants in Whitehall (2004; 2015; see Figure 3.4). The first study was a large prospective examination of 18,000 male civil servants between the ages of 20 and 64, assessed over a period of ten years starting in 1967. Starting two decades later, a second study focused on the health of 10,308 civil servants aged 35 to 55 of whom around two-thirds were men. Clearly the public servants who were participants in these studies had much in common (e.g., they were all employed, not poor, and had comparable social backgrounds). Nevertheless, in the first study, Marmot found clear evidence of a health gradient such that the higher their employment grade, the longer employees lived. Indeed, men at the bottom of the hierarchy were more than four times more likely to die in the course of the study than the men at the top.

Importantly too, for all men, data were collected on a range of health behaviours, and this allowed the researchers to control for risk factors such as obesity, smoking, reduced leisure time, physical activity, prevalence of underlying illness, and blood pressure. These risk factors are important to control for because men with lower status generally score worse on these factors, and each is associated with poorer health in its own right. Inclusion of these risk factors in the analysis accounted for 40% of the variance in health outcomes, so they were clearly important. However, even after controlling for these factors, there was still a substantial health gradient. For example, the risk of cardiovascular disease was still 2.1 times higher for those in the lowest employment grade than for those in the highest.

There is one further important point that these data drive home. This is that when we talk about the implications of social status for health, we should not simply be concerned about *absolute* level of disadvantage. Instead, we should be looking at the degree of inequality between those who are

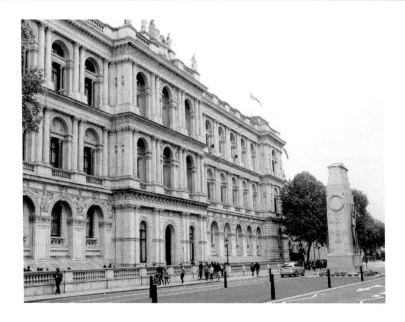

Figure 3.4 Civil service buildings in Whitehall, London

Note: Michael Marmot's (2004, 2015) studies of British civil servants showed that even in this relatively advantaged and homogeneous group there was a substantial health gradient such that higher-ranking employees had far better health outcomes than lower-ranking ones.

Source: Pixabay

most disadvantaged and those who are the most advantaged within a particular community or society (also known as *relative* disadvantage). This observation accords with a classic social identity principle that we discussed in Chapter 2: social disadvantage cannot be objectively established, but depends largely on comparisons with others in the immediate context (Tajfel & Turner, 1979). In other words, *regardless of how large objective differences in status or wealth actually are, to the extent that they are perceived to be large, they will have an adverse impact on the perceiver's health.*

So how, then, are we to explain the Whitehall findings? Interestingly, Marmot's explanation for the results is quite similar to the one provided to explain findings from the animal studies that we reviewed earlier (see Sapolsky, 2004). Specifically, he suggests that workers in lower employment grades had lower predictability and control in their work and in their lives more generally than their higher employment grade counterparts and that it was this lack of control and predictability that was the source of their poor health (Marmot, 2004; 2015; Vaananen et al., 2008; see also Martin, 2016).

Other researchers interested in the social determinants of health have argued that the health gradient can be explained by the amount of *social capital* in a particular group or society. Based on work by the Organization for Economic Co-operation and Development (OECD), Robert Putnam (2000, p. 41) defines social capital as "networks together with shared norms, values and under-standings that facilitate co-operation within or among groups". The key idea here is that member-ship in groups affects individuals because it confers benefits (Hawe & Shiel, 2000). Social capital is often measured in terms of trust and the number of ties within a particular group or society. It is higher when individuals are more likely to trust each other and when ties between members in a community are tighter and when there are more frequent interactions between them (i.e., when there are high levels of social cohesion; Helliwell, 2006; Helliwell & Barrington-Leigh, 2012; Oh, Chung, & Labianca, 2004).

Consistent with our hypothesis that group memberships are important psychological resources (the multiple identities hypothesis, H11), researchers in the social capital tradition have highlighted a number of ways in which social capital promotes health and well-being. Of particular importance here is the distinction that is often made between *bonding* and *bridging* capital. Bonding capital relates to relationships between people. It reflects trust and social cohesion, and also resembles shared social identity (as defined in Chapter 2). High bonding capital is often also seen as a pre-requisite for the development of bridging capital – which is defined as the ability of an individual to take on new group memberships and/or their ability to maintain their memberships in important groups (Johnstone, Jetten, Dingle, Parsell, & Walter, 2016, see also Kim, Subramanian, & Kawachi, 2006).

Importantly, the distinction between bonding and bridging capital is useful in helping us understand the health gradient. This is because people with higher status in groups typically have more bonding capital in being better able to sustain an active social life and more opportunities to develop a network of group memberships (Ball, Reay, & David, 2003; Bourdieu, 1979/1984). Moreover, the more social capital one has, the easier it is to extend social capital (because strong group memberships are a good platform for developing further strong group memberships; Hawe & Shiel, 2000), and this means that individuals with high bonding capital also tend to develop more bridging capital. Speaking to this point, a large body of evidence suggests that the more social groups a person belongs, to the happier and healthier they tend to be (Cohen & Janicki-Deverts, 2009; see also Haslam, Holme, et al., 2008; Iyer, Jetten, Tsivrikos, Postmes, & Haslam, 2009; see Jetten, Haslam, Iyer, & Haslam, 2010a, for an overview).

Yet even though this account sheds light on the processes underlying the health gradient, it has also been argued that because the concept of social capital has tended to be used both broadly and loosely, its explanatory power has been weakened (Hawe & Shiel, 2000). A key part of the problem here is that it is quite difficult to specify precisely what social capital is, and hence to measure it (Whiteley, 1999). This is a challenge that we will return to in the second part of this chapter.

Despite these conceptual and measurement concerns, research into the social determinants of health has been important for several reasons. Not only has it shown that social status, poverty, and disadvantage are profound predictors of health, but it has also helped to drive a growing recognition among policy makers that these social factors matter and need to be addressed. It has also led to changes in the type of recommendations that are provided to the general public about how to stay healthy and well. So whereas standard formulations – in particular, those informed by the biomedical model that we discussed in Chapter 1 – have focused on behaviours that individuals should engage in to improve their health (e.g., of the form identified in the "ten traditional tips for better health" presented in Table 3.1), research on social determinants has led us to focus more on the ways in which individuals' social environment needs to be improved (see the somewhat tongue-in-cheek "ten alternative tips for better health" in Table 3.1).

Such insights present a radical departure from traditional health models and fit well with the social identity approach to health that we present in this book. The social determinants approach also aligns well with the policy implications that emerge from the social cure approach (e.g., see Haslam, Jetten, & Haslam, 2012; Jetten, Haslam, Haslam, Dingle, & Jones, 2014). For when health is understood as being determined in large part by the social environment in which a person finds themselves, then responsibility for that person's health lies not with them alone but also with the groups, communities, and societies to which they belong. Although very simple, this is a point that has enormous policy implications (e.g., see Agich, 1982; World Health Organization & United Nations Children's Fund, 1978).

Table 3.1 Two different lists of top ten tips for health

Ten traditional tips for better health

1. Don't smoke. If you can, stop. If you can't, cut down.
2. Follow a balanced diet with plenty of fruit and vegetables.
3. Keep physically active.
4. Manage stress by, for example, talking things through and making time to relax.
5. If you drink alcohol, do so in moderation.
6. Cover up in the sun, and protect children from sunburn.
7. Practice safer sex.
8. Take up cancer-screening opportunities.
9. Be safe on the roads: follow the Highway Code.
10. Learn the first aid ABCs: airways, breathing, circulation.

Ten alternative tips for better health

1. Don't be poor. If you can, stop. If you can't, try not to be poor for long.
2. Don't live in a deprived area. If you do, move.
3. Don't be disabled or have a disabled child.
4. Don't work in a stressful, low-paid manual job.
5. Don't live in damp, low-quality housing or be homeless.
6. Be able to afford to pay for social activities and annual holidays.
7. Don't be a lone parent.
8. Claim all the benefits to which you are entitled.
9. Be able to afford your own car.
10. Use education to improve your socio-economic position.

Note: The first of these lists was developed by England's chief medical officer, the second was developed by researchers interested in social determinants of health at the Townsend Centre for International Poverty Research (cited in Raphael, 2000, p. 403).

The social identity approach to social status and health

As suggested in the previous section, social identity theorising (e.g., as outlined in Chapter 2) is well placed to build upon work into the social determinants of health. Not only can it help us to better understand some of the findings in this literature, it can also help us more precisely target efforts to flatten the health gradient that this work identifies. For instance, having recognised that lack of control is at the core of the health gradient, a social identity analysis can help us understand what makes disadvantage so disempowering and how control can be increased through strategies that build social identification (e.g., after Greenaway et al., 2015). It can also shed light on when those who are socially disadvantaged are most likely to feel disempowered (e.g., after Drury & Reicher, 2009).

These are ideas that the remainder of this chapter will now explore in greater detail. As we noted in the previous chapter, our approach starts from the assumption that groups can differ in many ways, but that the differences that are probably most consequential are those that relate to social status (Mullen, Brown, & Smith, 1992; Otten, Mummendey, & Blanz, 1996; Sachdev & Bourhis, 1987). This was certainly an understanding that informed the development of social identity theory, as it sought to explain the general behavioural consequences of psychological group membership (Tajfel & Turner, 1979) and it has proved no less important in understanding the implications of social identities for health and well-being (e.g., as suggested by Haslam et al., 2009).

Social identities are important determinants of social status

Within social identity theory, status is defined as the position of a group in the social hierarchy of a given society or culture *relative* to other groups (i.e., relevant outgroups). Status is thus not fixed, but always determined in comparison to other groups. This is an important point because it helps us appreciate the complexities of the health gradient. For example, a person in a poor suburb of Baltimore may be objectively wealthier and more educated than a relatively advantaged person in Bangladesh, but *compared to others in their city or in their country*, they are likely to be disadvantaged on these dimensions, and it is this *relative standing* that will determine their health outcomes. This, then, helps to explain why, on some indicators, their health is actually worse than that of the average person in Bangladesh (see Marmot, 2015).

Status can be achieved on different dimensions. For example, high status can reflect a group's superior skill, knowledge, physical strength, or power. But of particular relevance here, high status often reflects a group's superior wealth, education, and social standing more generally. And because our personal identity is defined in important ways by the groups to which we belong, the status of those groups not only affects the self-esteem and well-being we derive as a *group member* (e.g., collective self-esteem; Crocker & Luhtanen, 1990; Luhtanen & Crocker, 1991) but also our *personal* self-esteem and well-being (Jetten et al., 2015). In line with the identification hypothesis (H2), this is especially true if individuals identify highly with their social group such that it is internalised as an important aspect of self (i.e., so that this *self-categorization* furnishes them with a sense of *social identity*; Turner, Hogg, Oakes, Reicher, & Wetherell, 1987).

A key premise of the social identity approach is that group members strive to compare themselves positively with other groups on relevant dimensions of comparison (Turner, 1975). If the comparison with other groups is favourable, they achieve or maintain a positive identity, and this has positive implications for their well-being and self-esteem (in line with the group circumstance hypothesis, H3a). However, when the comparison is negative and emphasises their ingroup's lower standing, it is more difficult to achieve a positive identity, and this will tend to compromise well-being and self-esteem (H3b). Consistent with these hypotheses, there is now an abundance of evidence that higher (perceived) group status is beneficial for individuals' well-being and health. In particular, it is associated with higher self-esteem, life satisfaction, and general well-being and lower levels of anxiety and depressive symptoms (Anderson, Kraus, Galinsky, & Keltner, 2012; Begeny & Huo, 2016; Sani, Magrin, Scrignaro, & McCollum, 2010; Singh-Manoux, Marmot, & Adler, 2005; Smith, Tyler, & Huo, 2003).

Evidence for the processes underlying this effect is provided by the research of Fabio Sani and his colleagues. They studied two populations: prison guards in Italy and families in Scotland (Sani, Magrin, Scrignaro, & McCollum, 2010). Drawing on social identity theorising, the researchers reasoned first that people should identify more strongly with high- (rather than low-) status groups because these are more likely to provide them with a sense of positive identity. Second, they argued that because identification generally promotes health and well-being (due to it being a psychological resource that people can fall back on when facing challenges in their life, as outlined in the previous chapter), then health and well-being should be higher among members of high-status groups. In line with this reasoning, in both populations higher subjective ingroup status was associated with greater psychological health (in the form of lower perceived stress, lower depression, and greater satisfaction with life). And in both cases this effect was explained by higher identification with ingroups that were perceived to be of high status.

Important as social status is, a key insight from social identity theory is that low social status or disadvantage will not *always* be associated with lower self-esteem. Indeed, even though self-categorization as a member of a socially disadvantaged group will tend to compromise self-esteem – and hence have negative consequences for well-being – this does not mean that people who have low status will simply resign themselves to their dismal fate and give up on the search for a positive identity. On the contrary, and consistent with the identity restoration hypothesis (H4), in such situations social identity theory predicts that people will continue to be motivated to engage in identity management strategies that help them achieve the best possible outcomes for themselves and/or for their group. Indeed, it is precisely because members of low-status groups will search (and often therefore find) avenues to improve their fate that there are no straightforward relationships between social status and well-being (measured as self-esteem, see Martiny & Rubin, 2016; Rubin & Hewstone, 1998). To see why this is the case, we can explore a few of these avenues and see how they lead to different outcomes.

Resisting identification with disadvantaged groups

One way for members of socially disadvantaged groups to protect their well-being is to deny that they belong to the group in question. To illustrate how this might work, consider the case of someone who is homeless. In light of their perilous position in society, it is not surprising that people experiencing homelessness have mental and physical health problems that are considerably more pronounced than those of the rest of the general population (Chamberlain & McKenzie, 2006; Johnson & Chamberlain, 2011). Indeed, poor health is sometimes the reason why people become homeless and it is certainly exacerbated by the experience of becoming and being homeless (Busch-Geertsma, Edgar, O'Sullivan, & Pleace, 2010; Johnson & Chamberlain, 2008).

When Zoe Walter and colleagues (Walter, Jetten, Parsell, & Dingle, 2015b) interviewed a large number of people who met the definitional criteria for homelessness, many (55%) described themselves as homeless. More surprising was the fact that nearly a third of respondents (31%) refused to describe themselves in this way. Some of the reasons they gave for this refusal are presented in Table 3.2.

Importantly for our argument, those who rejected the 'homeless' self-categorization reported higher personal well-being and better mood than those who accepted the label, independent of the duration of their homelessness (Walter et al., 2015b). These findings point to the importance of how one self-defines, or self-categorizes, for well-being and also show that people do not passively accept labels that might seem to describe their situation objectively. Instead, for some of these participants at least, self-categorization was an active process of identity negotiation in which they *resisted* externally imposed labels, presumably in an attempt to protect their self-worth and well-being (see also Parsell, 2011).

There are also other ways in which members of low-status groups can escape the negative well-being consequences of their group membership, at least psychologically, without actually leaving the group. In three studies with naturally occurring and laboratory-created groups, Sonja Roccas (2003) showed that group members tend to identify more with a group if a different group (to which they also belonged) is both salient and lower in status. One can interpret these findings as showing that because most of us belong to multiple groups, we can strategically emphasise our membership of those particular groups that are higher in status. Belonging to this higher-status group not only gives us a *relatively* positive identity (and remember that relativities matter here), but at the same time it reduces

Table 3.2 Examples of alternative self-categorizations in the face of homelessness

Defining homelessness as different from, and worse than, one's current situation
> *"To me homeless is on the street. This is a hostel, it's a refuge, it's a roof over your head, a shower, food, so I wouldn't say I was homeless. I've got somewhere to go everyday to sleep, so I wouldn't say I'm homeless"* (male, age 44).
> *"I did a little bit of time on the streets. Compared to that no. Struggling yeah, but not homeless"* (male, age 24).

Rejecting a homeless self-categorization because one has alternative housing options
> *"I could have some options if I really want them but no, I'm not really homeless . . . but I choose to live here because it's the safest place to be"* (female, age 43).

Rejecting a homeless self-categorization because one has found a "home" in the homeless shelter
> *"It might be a homeless shelter, but it doesn't feel like one. . . . So, basically I'm not homeless, I feel like this is my home"* (female, age 19).

Note: The table identifies the different ways in which respondents who met criteria for homelessness negotiated their self-categorization.

Source: Based on Walter et al. (2015b)

---

the negative effects that belonging to lower-status groups has on health and well-being. Indeed, even though well-being was not measured in these studies, Roccas speculated that because people had other social groups to which they could turn to achieve a positive identity, this might be one reason why there is not an overwhelmingly negative relationship between group status and self-esteem (see also Diener & Diener, 1996). At the same time, we can also see that the capacity for alternative group memberships to afford opportunities for strategic self-enhancement is one further reason why there is a reliable relationship between multiple group memberships and psychological health (as noted earlier; e.g., see Jetten et al., 2010a, for an overview).

Leaving disadvantaged groups

Of course, a more direct way of dealing with the esteem- (and, thus, health-) related threats associated with belonging to a low-status group is simply to leave it (Ellemers, 1993; Tajfel & Turner, 1979). However, an obvious reason why people do not always take this route is that it is not always open. In particular, this is because the likely success of this strategy depends very much on the extent to which boundaries between groups are *permeable*, and thereby allow for *individual mobility* (as suggested by the mobility hypothesis, H5; Ellemers & van Rijswijk, 1997; Ellemers, van Knippenberg, & Wilke, 1990; Lalonde & Silverman, 1994; Wright, Taylor, & Moghaddam, 1990).

But even if individual mobility *is* an option, it often turns out to be a double-edged sword. For even though the health of those who are able to cross boundaries and join a higher-status group may increase, costs are associated with going down this path. For instance, those who engage in individual mobility and decide to leave the disadvantaged group may be penalised by the group for being disloyal (Branscombe, Wann, Noel, & Coleman, 1993), for being a traitor to the cause, or even for being an impostor because they claim to be something they are not (Warner, Hornsey, & Jetten, 2007). Moreover, the high-status group they join may not treat them especially well (e.g., looking upon them as an upstart, a 'Johnny-come-lately', or a 'blow in'; De Nooy, 2016) and they may only be allowed to occupy a 'token' position in the group (Branscombe & Ellemers, 1998). In both these scenarios, a person's personal standing will be diminished, and this is likely to have negative implications for their health and well-being.

A study by Tom Postmes and Nyla Branscombe (2002) of African Americans in the United States who were living and working in predominantly White communities provides powerful insights into these dynamics. On the basis of social identity theory, these researchers hypothesised that minority group members who attempt individual mobility in this way may suffer from the dual handicap of being rejected both (1) by their new ingroup (Whites) on grounds that they are 'different' and (2) by their former ingroup (Blacks) on grounds that they are 'deserters' or 'traitors'. Moreover, they reasoned that this latter response might be accentuated by the fact that, in seeking acceptance from their new ingroup, members of minorities feel obliged to denounce their former group membership. In short, as suggested by the mobility hypothesis (H5) when members of minority groups attempt to become part of the majority by engaging in an individual mobility strategy, they may gain social status by moving up the social hierarchy, but also in the process be cut off from their former group and, importantly, the health benefits that this group can provide (e.g., in the form of social support).

When boundaries between groups are more impermeable (e.g., if group membership is based on ethnicity), the strategies that members of low-status groups engage in to achieve a more positive identity (and thus higher well-being) are likely to be quite different – again in ways predicted by social identity theory (Tajfel & Turner, 1979). In this situation it is not easy (and it may in fact be impossible) to improve one's status by leaving the low-status group behind, but this does not always lead to disempowerment (and hence a reduction in well-being). If they share a strong sense of social identity with one another, members of low-status groups are likely to provide each other with social support and solidarity, and this will help to buffer them from the negative consequences of their social status for well-being.

This is a finding that emerges from the animal studies that we reviewed earlier (e.g., Abbott et al., 2003, see Figure 3.3), but there is now considerable evidence of the same process in other branches of psychological research. For instance, Jetten and colleagues (2015; see also Walter, Jetten, Dingle, Parsell, & Johnstone, 2015a) found that former residents of a homeless shelter who went on to belong to multiple important groups showed increased personal self-esteem and well-being as they were tracked over time. In this study, all the participants were asked to list their friends and close others by name (i.e., to list their interpersonal ties) and to list the important groups they belonged to (i.e., the ones they identified with) when they first moved into a homeless shelter (Time 1). They were also asked to do the same three months later (Time 2) and then again nine months after that (Time 3). Interestingly, participants' self-esteem was not predicted by the number of interpersonal ties that they had at Time 1 nor by any increase in number of interpersonal ties over time. Rather, the best predictor of self-esteem 12 months after leaving the shelter was the number of important *groups* that people belonged to at Time 1. Clearly then, important groups matter as they have unique powers to protect us from the health-disrupting ravages of low status.

The aforementioned research by Postmes and Branscombe (2002) also provides evidence of the specific role that group-based social support plays in countering the negative health effects of social disadvantage. For whereas African Americans who had engaged in individual mobility had poorer health outcomes because they had lost social support by leaving their minority group behind, those who continued to live and work in Black communities reported receiving more social support, being more accepted by their ingroup, and having enhanced levels of psychological well-being. From this we can see that the positive effects of group membership are most apparent when members of minorities are not forced to discard their group membership and assimilate to the majority, but are able to simultaneously maintain their social identity as members of that minority in systems that are pluralist (Berry, 1997; Hornsey & Hogg, 2000). This is because under such conditions – where individuals are not required to relinquish valued social identities –they are best placed to benefit from the social support that groups provide (as proposed by H14, see also Chapter 5).

In this regard, one of the most comprehensive explorations of responses to low social status was provided by the BBC Prison Study (Reicher & Haslam, 2006a; see Figure 3.5). In this, 15 men were randomly assigned to either a high- or a low-status group – Guards or Prisoners – within a simulated

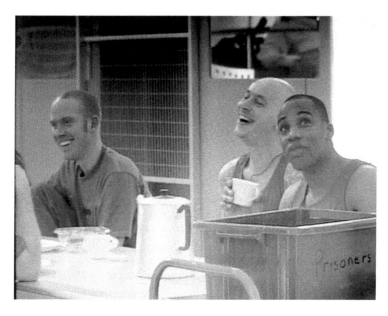

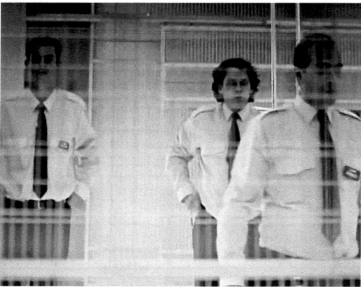

Figure 3.5 Prisoners and Guards in the BBC Prison Study

Note: At the start of the study the high-status Guards had better mental health than the low-status Prisoners. However, as the Prisoners' sense of shared social identity increased (after promotion was no longer possible and group boundaries were impermeable), they started working together to improve their situation, and their psychological health and well-being improved markedly. At the same time, the Prisoners' actions contributed to a reduced sense of shared social identity among the Guards and, as a result, their health and well-being declined.

Source: Reicher and Haslam (2006a); see also www.bbcprisonstudy.org

prison environment and their behaviour was then studied closely over a period of 8 days. Informed by the principles of social identity theory, the design of the study involved manipulating factors that were expected to have an impact on the Prisoners' degree of social identification and examining the impact of this on both groups' behaviour as well as on the functioning of the prison system as a whole. At the study's outset, participants were led to believe that the boundaries between the two groups were permeable and hence that it was possible to be promoted from Prisoner to Guard. At this stage it was expected that Prisoners would adopt an individual mobility strategy and pursue a self-enhancement strategy of working individually to gain favour with the Guards (in line with the mobility hypothesis, H5). However, after one seemingly fortunate prisoner had been promoted in this way, group boundaries were made impermeable by ruling out further opportunities for promotion. It was expected that this would increase Prisoners' social identification and encourage collective responses to their situation (in line with the competition hypothesis, H7).

As predicted, social identification among the low-status group (Prisoners) increased once group boundaries were impermeable. Importantly too, once it was no longer possible for individuals to transition between groups, the Prisoners started to explore ways to improve their status collectively. In particular, they worked together to undermine the Guards' authority and to formulate plans to overthrow their regime. Indeed, ultimately this resistance contributed to a breakout that made the Guards' regime unworkable and brought the study to a premature end (for a broader discussion of the psychology of resistance, see Haslam & Reicher, 2012). In the process of arriving at this outcome, the Guards also became increasingly apprehensive about their authority, and this, combined with the Prisoners' insurgency, contributed to a steady decline in their sense of shared social identity.

As we will explore later in Chapters 5 and 13, these processes also had a significant bearing on the participants' health and well-being. Most particularly, as the Prisoners' sense of shared identity increased, they became less stressed, less depressed, and less paranoid. On the other hand, as the Guards' sense of shared identity declined, they became more stressed, more depressed, and more paranoid. So, whereas at the start of the study the Prisoners' low status had negative implications for their health and well-being, as they came together to improve their status collectively, things improved markedly, and it was now the high-status Guards whose health and well-being were threatened.

Social identification is beneficial for well-being even in disadvantaged groups

Whereas the BBC study showed that group identification provides important resources to respond to devaluation and thereby improve psychological health, one could argue that it is also the case that these benefits for well-being came to the fore at a time in the study when the Prisoners were resisting the Guards' power and authority. Were the Prisoners still seeing themselves as a low-status group at this point? Perhaps not, and by the time they were breaking out of their cells, status relations may, in their own mind, have effectively reversed so that it was the Guards who were now in the low-status position.

If this is true, then it leaves unanswered the question of whether it is generally the case that when low-status members turn to their group for social support this will prove to be good for their psychological health. The significance of this question arises from the fact that there is something quite ironic about turning to a low-status group for support when membership of that group was itself the cause of the original threat to health and well-being. As Niamh McNamara, Clifford Stevenson, and Orla Muldoon (2013) observe:

> The paradox of community deprivation is therefore that although the community identity can provide resources to cope with the daily challenges and stresses faced by disadvantaged communities, the stigmatisation of disadvantage itself can undermine this resource by reducing collective support and cooperation as well as inhibiting engagement with external services and other communities.
>
> (p. 393)

Indeed, bearing this in mind, one might well ask why members of disadvantaged groups do not simply disengage from them and turn to *other* groups to help them cope with the threats to well-being that they face?

Even though this might be an intuitively appealing strategy (and one that people certainly pursue sometimes; see Roccas, 2003), there is now a growing body of evidence that group identification delivers health benefits *even in disadvantaged communities which offer limited social resources*. For example, in a study of immigrants in Switzerland, Mouna Bakouri and Christian Staerklé (2015) found that higher perceived disadvantage was associated with feeling there were more barriers to taking control of one's life and that this predicted lower self-esteem. However, it was also clear that bonding identities (consisting of existing social relationships in the form of interpersonal connections and group memberships) buffered this relationship. That is, the negative effect of perceived barriers to control was less pronounced for people who reported having more bonding identities. Looking to explain this relationship, the researchers found that this was because bonding identities increased the immigrants' sense of self-efficacy (rather than their sense of being supported). This is again consistent with our argument that one of the reasons why social identities are important psychological resources is that they serve to empower otherwise disadvantaged groups (in line with the agency hypothesis, H15).

In a similar vein, in a household survey conducted in disadvantaged areas of Limerick in Ireland, Niamh McNamara and her colleagues (2013) found positive effects of identifying with the community on well-being. Further analyses showed that this relationship was accounted for by the greater perceived collective efficacy of those who identified more strongly with the community. Respondents' better well-being was thus explained by a sense that they were coping collectively with challenges that their community as a whole were facing.

Other work has also reinforced this point that identifying with others who are similarly devalued can enhance efficacy and empowerment in disadvantaged groups. In a study of African Americans, it was found that higher identification with one's racial ingroup was associated with a greater sense that its members would provide social support (Outten, Schmitt, Garcia, & Branscombe, 2009). Higher group identification also predicted a stronger belief that the group could cope effectively with disadvantage, and again it was these perceptions of collective efficacy (rather than perceptions of social support) that predicted self-esteem and life satisfaction.

In sum, despite the fact that devaluation is an obvious stress factor in and of itself, those who turn to the devalued group generally appear to experience (1) higher levels of collective efficacy (believing that their groups can counter some of the challenges it faces) and (2) higher social support. Both of these factors have been found to boost health and well-being – although which is the most potent resource appears to vary from group to group.

As a final thought, it is also important to bear in mind that although membership in higher-status groups usually confers more health benefits than membership in lower-status groups, this is not true in all circumstances. Consistent with some of the animal research that we reviewed earlier in this chapter, it appears that those who are privileged, powerful, and wealthy are likely to become less healthy if their status position is threatened and becomes unstable. This was seen among the Guards in the BBC Prison Study, and it was also seen in the research of Scheepers and colleagues (2009) that we discussed earlier in which only high-status groups who feared losing their status displayed a physiological stress response (see also Scheepers & Ellemers, 2005). As the Prisoner who was promoted to be a Guard in the BBC Prison Study found out, even if one were to try to join a more advantaged group with a view to improving one's health and well-being, this would not always have the desired results.

Social identity resources facilitate adjustment to life transitions

Ironically, despite the fact that those who are socially disadvantaged are often most motivated to acquire a more positive identity, it is also this group that tends to struggle most whenever they face life transitions and changes. Indeed, members of low-status groups experience their disadvantage most profoundly when they are undergoing life transitions (Bakouri & Staerklé, 2015). Before we outline why this is the case, we first review a large body of research in the social identity tradition that has examined how social identity is implicated in life transitions and changes more generally.

The social identity model of identity change (SIMIC)

Life transitions can have both positive and negative outcomes. Transitions can be positive when they provide individuals with new opportunities and experiences. For example, a promotion at work may mean an increase in salary, job responsibilities, and overall prestige. Similarly, entering university provides students with an opportunity to extend their knowledge and develop critical thinking skills. On the other hand, life transitions can be a negative experience when they involve such things as becoming unemployed, being forced into early retirement, or being diagnosed with a life-threatening illness.

When an important social identity is threatened or changed, this has a range of negative consequences for well-being, and these are well-documented in the literature (e.g., see Breakwell, 1986; Haunschild, Moreland, & Murrell, 1994). Amongst other things, when we can no longer retain membership in a valued group – either because we change or the group does – this tends to be disorienting and stressful (e.g., Jetten, O'Brien, & Trindall, 2002). Indeed, as we will see in later chapters (e.g., Chapters 7 and 8) the social identity loss that this entails can precipitate significant cognitive decline and depression.

Yet despite the recognition that identity change and/or loss tends to have negative consequences for health and well-being, it turns out that group identification also plays a key role in protecting people against these negative consequences. In particular, this is because the negative consequences of identity change will generally be limited when individuals are able to join a new group and thereby take on a *new* social identity. Here the new sense of identification that this affords – and the various positive consequences that flow from this (as discussed in Chapter 2) – will tend to counteract the sense of identification that has been lost. For instance, threats to well-being will be minimised if employees quickly take on the identity of a new work team when their old work team is disbanded, or if university students quickly identify as a university student after losing their secondary-school identity. More generally, an important way in which people protect long-term well-being in the face of identity loss is by joining groups to help them adjust to and 'get over' the loss. Speaking to this point, and as we will discuss in later chapters, *support groups* are widely recognised as helping people cope effectively with such things as bereavement, injury, illness, and trauma (Wuthnow, 1994).

Over the course of the last decade, these processes of adjustment to social identity change have been theorised and integrated within the *social identity model of identity change* (SIMIC; Haslam, Holme et al., 2008; Jetten, Haslam, Haslam, & Branscombe, 2009). As we outlined in the previous chapter, because the self is defined in important ways by our membership in social groups, losing an identity or experiencing a permanent change in the meaning of the identity is likely to affect our sense of self in important ways (Hopkins & Reicher, 1996). Moreover, regardless of whether it leads to desired or undesired outcomes, change itself may adversely affect well-being because it requires adjustment on the part of those who undergo it (Ethier & Deaux, 1994; Hopkins & Reicher, 1996; Jetten et al., 2002). Change, then, is associated with uncertainty and often requires the individual to reorient themselves to the world.

Another reason why identity change is challenging is that those who undergo it need to start defining themselves as members of the new group that they have joined. Indeed, changes to social identities often require a redefinition of the meaning of identity for the self as well as a reformulation of the relationship between oneself and others in the group. As represented schematically in Figure 3.6, SIMIC identifies a number of processes that hinder or facilitate this process of adjustment in the face of major life events and transitions (Haslam, Holme et al., 2008; Jetten et al., 2009).

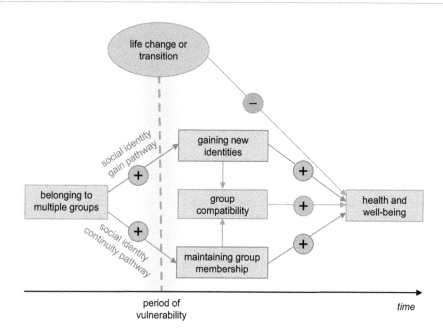

Figure 3.6 The social identity model of identity change (SIMIC)

Note: SIMIC identifies two key pathways that help people cope with identity change in the face of major life transitions and events. The first is a *social identity gain* pathway associated with the acquisition of new group memberships; the second is a *social identity continuity* pathway associated with the maintenance of pre-existing group memberships. Both pathways are more likely to be accessible the more group memberships a person had prior to the life transition. The impact of the two pathways on health and well-being also depends on the compatibility of the social identities they involve.

Source: Based on Jetten et al. (2009)

First, the adverse impact of change will be minimised when individuals are able to *maintain* valued social identities (the *social identity continuity pathway*). However, this is not always possible, and change may require individuals to give up or move away from old group memberships ('unfreezing'; Lewin, 1948). This is often a difficult process because, even if those old identities are negative and problematic (e.g., being an addict or unemployed), people are often unwilling to give up identities that have been important in defining themselves in the past. Indeed, losing one's grounding is stressful in part because it is associated with a break from that which we know best. Indeed, when the connection between the past and the present becomes interrupted, this loss of *self-continuity* in itself presents a threat to individuals' well-being (Sani, 2008; Sani, Bowe, & Herrera, 2008).

Second, adjustment will also depend on a person's ability and willingness to take on a *new* social identity in the new situation that they find themselves (the *social identity gain pathway*). Taking on a new identity not only provides a new sense of grounding and belonging, but it also forms the basis for receiving and benefiting from new sources of social support (Haslam, O'Brien, Jetten, Vormedal, & Penna, 2005; Iyer et al., 2009). More generally, joining new groups after important life transitions can protect and sometimes even reverse the negative effects of change because, to the extent that those groups provide a basis for self-definition, the resources they provide access to are likely to make the experience of entering a new phase in life a positive opportunity for personal growth, rather than a stressful experience of loss (see Haslam, Jetten, Haslam, & Postmes, 2009).

Third, successful adaptation to identity change depends very much on the features of a person's pre-change social identity network. Previous research has shown that two aspects of this identity network are particularly important in determining the way that identities promote successful adjustment to important life transitions (Iyer et al., 2009; Jetten, Haslam, Pugliese, Tonks, & Haslam, 2010b). First, the extent of a person's social connections before the life transition are likely to be an important predictor of their ability to cope successfully with identity change (see Iyer, Jetten, & Tsivrikos, 2008; Jetten & Pachana, 2012; Jetten et al., 2015). In particular, we have argued that *multiple group memberships* provide people with more *social identity capital* and that this protects well-being in times of change because when people belong to multiple groups, this increases the likelihood of them being able (1) to maintain some group memberships post-transition (and thereby benefit from the social identity continuity pathway) and (2) to use their old identity network as a platform for building new identities (and thereby benefit from the social identity gain pathway). Second, when predicting adjustment to change, it is not just the number of identities that matters, but also the relationships among them. In particular, this is because identity change can strain relationships – and therefore compromise well-being – when new identities are not *compatible*.

A large body of research now provides strong support for various components of SIMIC. In particular, there is abundant evidence that maintaining strong social identities helps to protect health and well-being in the context of significant life changes (Haslam, Holme et al., 2008; Iyer & Jetten, 2011; Sani et al., 2008). For example, a study of people who had recently had a stroke found that life satisfaction *after* the stroke was appreciably higher for those who had belonged to more social groups *before* their stroke (Haslam, Holme et al., 2008). Other studies have reported similar effects on well-being among students transitioning to university (Iyer et al., 2009), women becoming mothers (Seymour-Smith, Cruwys, Haslam, & Brodribb, 2017), and older adults retiring from work (Steffens et al., 2016). We will discuss many of these studies in more detail in later chapters (e.g., Chapter 7 on ageing and Chapter 8 on depression), but in all these cases, belonging to multiple groups is observed to predict increased resilience and better mental health (see also Linville, 1985, 1987; Thoits, 1983). Importantly too, effects are not limited to measures of psychological well-being, but are also found on indices of physical health and mortality.

There is now also considerable evidence that health and well-being are enhanced by the *acquisition* of new social identities in times of change. For example, longitudinal studies that we will discuss next and in later chapters show that joining new groups is beneficial in helping people to overcome depression (Cruwys et al., 2013b; Cruwys, Haslam, Dingle, Haslam, & Jetten, 2014b, see also Chapter 8) or to recover from acquired brain injury (Jones, Williams et al., 2012; see Chapter 11).

The ability to gain new group memberships is particularly important when individuals embark on life changes where they aim to lose problematic social identities. This is the case, for example, if they belong to groups defined by drug or alcohol addiction (Dingle, Stark, Cruwys, & Best, 2015) or by violence (Williams et al., 2010). Here developing new social networks and joining new groups that promote recovery and avoid violence is found to be crucial for recovery from substance dependence and avoiding serious injury. As we will discuss further in Chapter 9, when it comes to substance abuse, it is also apparent that when individuals form new social networks with non-users, the chances of them staying clean are far higher.

But it is not only those who struggle with serious negative life changes who benefit from acquiring new group memberships in the context of life transitions. In longitudinal research studying students entering a British university, Aarti Iyer and her colleagues found that the more groups that students belonged to before they moved, the more likely it was that they would quickly adopt and start to identify with their new student identity (Iyer et al., 2009). This in turn was associated with higher well-being and lower depression. Likewise, Katharine Greenaway and colleagues found that university students who gained group memberships in their final (and most challenging) year of study were more likely to report having their global needs for control, belonging, self-esteem, and meaning in life satisfied (Greenaway, Cruwys, Haslam, & Jetten, 2016). And as with all the other studies we have discussed in this section, in both these cases, these patterns remained statistically reliable when controlling for other potentially relevant factors (e.g., a person's financial circumstances).

In sum, then, it appears that the two key pathways identified within SIMIC – the social identity gain pathway and the social identity continuity pathway – delineate two very effective ways in which people can tackle the challenges of major life transitions. At the same time, though, in a final twist to our story, it is also the case that these two pathways are not equally accessible to everyone. On the contrary, it turns out that one of the main factors that stops people accessing them is social disadvantage. We will draw this chapter to a close by considering the reasons for this – and thereby also bring our analysis full circle.

Disadvantage can be a barrier to successful social identity change

Why then is identity change particularly hard for members of lower-status groups? There are a number of reasons for this. First, classic developmental research shows that well-being is determined in important ways by a person's feelings of control over the goals and events in their life, including the sense that they are in a position to shape their own environment (Bandura, 1982). As discussed earlier in this chapter, this is where those in higher-status positions have an advantage over their lower-status counterparts: for their access to various social and material resources means that they have more control over their lives and are in a better position to determine their own fate than those at the bottom of the social ladder. Members of lower-status groups are also more likely to face barriers and constraints in the course of pursuing their goals for a better future, and they are less likely to find themselves in the optimal environment for realising those goals.

Moreover, as a number of researchers have observed, these fundamental differences in control are most likely to come to the fore and to have the effect of reproducing inequalities in the context of important life transitions (Bakouri & Staerklé, 2015; Heinz, 2009). For example, in a classic study of people with cancer in Boston, 1- and 3-year survival rates were found to be much lower for low-income than for higher-income groups even after controlling for type of tumour, stage of cancer at diagnosis, age, or type of treatment received (Lipworth, Abelin, & Conelly, 1970). In what follows, we will explore the dynamics that contribute to these steeper health gradients for members of disadvantaged groups in three different transitional contexts: (1) in education as people move between institutions, (2) in housing as people endeavour to break out of homelessness, and (3) in whole communities that undergo major upheaval.

Education contexts

Education is one domain in which the health gradient is particularly pronounced. In particular, this is seen when students enter university. As George Akerlof and Rachel Kranton (2000) observe, even though "individuals may – more or less consciously – choose who they want to be . . . the limits on this choice may also be the most important determinant of an individual's economic well-being" (p. 3).

This point is well illustrated by the work of Iyer and colleagues (2009) that we referred to in the previous section. This study surveyed British undergraduate students entering university and found that, before they came to university, students from lower SES backgrounds reported belonging to significantly fewer social groups than their higher SES counterparts. This finding accords with other research which has found that people from higher-class backgrounds are more likely to develop rich social networks composed of multiple groups (Ball et al., 2003; Bourdieu, 1979/1984).

In line with SIMIC, this difference proved important once the students had entered university. For as we noted earlier, those students with fewer group memberships were less adept at managing this transition successfully. In particular, because they had belonged to fewer groups previously, low SES students were less well placed to take on the new identity as a university student, and this was associated with substantially lower well-being (see also Jetten, Haslam, & Barlow, 2013).

Entering university is more difficult for students from disadvantaged backgrounds for other reasons too. In particular, and consistent with SIMIC, even though gaining an education represents a good investment in one's future (as suggested by research into the social determinants of health; e.g., see Table 3.1), it is more likely to be incompatible with the previous identities of low SES students than is the case for their more affluent counterparts. Unsurprisingly, then, students from disadvantaged backgrounds tend to feel less comfortable in educational institutions and they are more likely to drop out (Friel, 2014; Rubin, 2012). Moreover, as we noted earlier, those who strive to enhance their personal status through individual mobility may encounter double discrimination when new and old groups are incompatible – for they may be rejected both by the group they try to leave behind and by the group they try to join (Postmes & Branscombe, 2002). Furthermore, in this case the self-*dis*continuity between the past (as a member of groups for whom universities are foreign places) and the present (as a university student) is more marked, and this also stands in the way of taking on the new identity as a university student.

Consistent with this reasoning, in a study of young people aspiring to go to university, Jetten and colleagues found that the more entering university was perceived by respondents to be incompatible with their SES background, the less prepared for university they reported being and the lower their expected level of identification was (Jetten, Iyer, Tsivrikos, & Young, 2008; Jetten, Iyer, & Zhang, 2017). A second study showed that this story was not any different for those who had recently entered university. Individuals identified more highly with the university when their social background was compatible with the new context that they were entering. There was also evidence that the less willing students were to take on the new identity in the long run, the less likely they were to endorse the belief that a university degree is an effective individual mobility strategy. These findings are somewhat depressing, in that they suggest that individual mobility strategies appear most costly to those who stand to gain the most from them.

Related findings emerge from a longitudinal study of the transition of Hispanic students into two Ivy League American universities conducted by Kathleen Ethier and Kay Deaux (1994). This examined the way that university entry affected these minority group students' ethnic identity over their first year at university. From this, the researchers identified two paths of identity negotiation, each with quite different implications for well-being.

The first pathway was more typical for those students who started with lower initial ethnic identification but also did not come to identify with the university (i.e., who did not go down SIMIC's identity gain pathway). As with the students in Jetten and colleagues' (2008) study, these students perceived entry into university as more of a threat to their ethnic identity (presumably because their Hispanic identity was incompatible with a university student identity), and they were more stressed during the transition. This resulted in even lower ethnic identification and lower self-esteem.

The second pathway had more positive outcomes. Consistent with the social identity continuity pathway of SIMIC, some of the students chose to engage in ethnic activities at university, thereby establishing continuity between their past and present identities. This type of behaviour was associated with stronger ethnic identification at the end of their first year at university. Notably though, this pathway was more likely to be chosen by students who had high ethnic identification initially. Interestingly too, Ethier and Deaux (1994) point out that the ethnic identity of these students *did* change over the course of this year. For example, although before entering university many students' ethnic identity was shaped by interactions with their family and the communities in which they lived, once they were at university they sought out people and took part in activities that were consistent with a Hispanic identity on campus. Nevertheless, because these students were able to 'remoor' (i.e., re-attach) their old identity, add new meaning to it, and connect it to supportive elements in the new environment, positive effects of identity continuity ensued. In other words, because they experienced identity continuity during the change, the students felt less threatened by the transition and adjusted better to it.

Whatever path they take, though, it is clear that the barriers for lower SES or minority group students entering mainstream educational institutions are substantial. The irony here is that getting a good education (e.g., by going to university) is widely recognised as a way to improve one's life conditions and, by extension, one's health and well-being (Marmot, 2004; Putnam, 2000; Siegrist & Marmot, 2006). Accordingly, it would appear that this *upward mobility* function is least accessible to the people who need it most. In this way too, we see that barriers to education have a disproportionately negative impact (e.g., in terms of health and well-being) on those who are disadvantaged (see also Jetten et al., 2017).

Again, though, while students from lower SES backgrounds typically need to negotiate multiple obstacles on their path to a good education, there are also reasons to believe that this does not have to be the case. In particular, this is because these obstacles can be addressed through various forms of structural change (e.g., to student funding; see Rubin & Wright, 2017). An example of how this can work is provided by research with the children of rural workers in China. Historically, these children were an extremely disadvantaged group within the Chinese educational system – having little or no access to resources that would make higher education possible. In particular, this was because they were forced to attend schools that were under-resourced and provided only basic schooling relative to the facilities enjoyed by children of city workers (Huang & Xu, 2006). However, in 2011 the government introduced legislation that outlawed segregation in education and required urban authorities to provide rural workers' children with access to mainstream public schools.

For a while during this transition, segregated schools and integrated schools continued to exist alongside each other. Airong Zhang and colleagues (Zhang, Jetten, Iyer, & Cui, 2013) saw this as an opportunity to compare the self-esteem of children in different school systems. As one would expect, in both the old (segregated) and the new (integrated) schools, rural workers' children reported lower self-esteem than city children (i.e., the advantaged group). However, the self-esteem of rural workers' children in integrated schools was significantly higher than that of rural workers' children in segregated schools. Knowing that one's group might be able to engage in collective mobility was thus heartening for the lower-status children in the integrated schools, and their well-being clearly benefitted from the availability of *"cognitive alternatives"* to the status quo (Tajfel, 1978, p. 93). These same ideas were tested more formally in two further studies in which these perceptions of cognitive alternatives were measured (Study 1) and manipulated (Study 2). Both studies showed that students had higher self-esteem to the extent that they perceived there to be cognitive alternatives to the educational status quo.

Together, then, these lines of research show that although it may be more difficult for students from lower SES backgrounds to take advantage of life transitions than it is for their higher SES peers, the gap in their educational experience – and hence in their health and well-being outcomes – can be narrowed by appropriately targeted socio-structural change. If one is interested in narrowing this gap, the big questions for any given society are thus how willing its leaders are to devise, defend, and deliver such changes (Marmot, 2015). More generally too, we see that the primary obstacles to improvement in the health and well-being of those who are disadvantaged are not psychological but political.

Housing contexts

The barriers that the most disadvantaged people in society encounter when they undergo change are also apparent when it comes to housing. Whereas having a roof over one's head is a given for most of us, it again turns out that those who are most in need of this basic necessity are also least equipped to acquire it. Again, though, looking at this life challenge through the lens of identity change is useful because it helps explain who is most likely to escape homelessness and who is not. In particular, work by Walter and her colleagues has documented the profound benefits of social connectedness not just to the physical and mental well-being of homeless people, but also to their ability to break the cycle of homelessness (Walter et al., 2015a).

Although no-one disputes that this is a complex and difficult process, it is generally the case that individuals who are homeless are not in the best position to join groups. This is because they tend to have fewer social connections than those who are not homeless and relatively few opportunities to develop new group memberships by building on existing social networks (i.e., to develop bonding capital). Nevertheless, in a study of 119 clients of homelessness services in Australia, Walter and colleagues found that group-based social support still played a critical role in people's ability to transition out of homeless shelters and into secure housing (Walter et al., 2015a). In particular, the more that people came to identify with the service that provided the homeless shelter (i.e., the more bridging identity capital that they built), the more they were able to benefit from the support that that service provided and ultimately to remain in stable housing.

This finding is all the more remarkable given that research suggests that shelters can be hotbeds for the development of negative social relationships as well as relationships that undermine people's efforts to escape homelessness (e.g., because some residents engage in drug use or criminal activities; Auerswald & Eyre, 2002; Snow & Anderson, 1993). This means that staying in shelters can sometimes be more dangerous than sleeping in public places (Fitzpatrick & Jones, 2005).

In this context, it is thus important to distinguish between positive and negative sources of social support and to recognise that whereas some forms of social identification will have positive implications for health and well-being, others will not (see also Chapter 9). This conclusion is consistent with a recent study that examined resilience among women living in trailer parks in the United States (Notter, MacTavish, & Shamah, 2008). Here the researchers found that positive turning points were related to residents' ability to build effectively on support from positive groups while also distancing themselves from negative group influences. Consistent with this, Walter and colleagues' research found that these interactional patterns were associated with residents perceiving there to be, and using, more opportunities at the service. This in turn fed into better well-being when they came to leave (Walter et al., 2015b).

Here again, then, we see that social identity capital proves critical to the process of successfully negotiating change in ways predicted by SIMIC. And while again we see that members of disadvantaged groups (in this case homeless people) start with a profound disadvantage – because they have poorer initial networks and hence a limited social support base – social identity processes nevertheless play a key role either in cementing these disadvantages or in helping their most pernicious effects to be ameliorated. Critically though, we also need to acknowledge the role that *other groups* – and the support they provide (or do not provide) – play in this process. This reinforces the point that the fate of disadvantaged groups is never entirely in their own hands. In particular, it is determined in no small part by the treatment they receive from those who are more advantaged.

Community contexts

Disadvantage does not just hamper the attempts of particular subgroups in society to come to grips with change. It also affects whole communities. Speaking to this point, influential research by Michael Chandler and Christopher Lalonde (1998) examined youth suicide rates in Indigenous communities in Canada and showed that rather than being a simple reflection of poverty and disadvantage, these were powerfully determined by the group culture of the communities and, in particular, by the way that this had been shaped by governmental authorities.

Of course, given the fact that these Indigenous communities are the poorest group in North America, poverty is an important contributor to the high rates of youth suicide rates that are seen in these communities relative to those in the general population. However, Chandler and Lalonde's (1998) research also makes it clear that this is not the full explanation of the problem. In particular, this is because while all the communities that they examined were poor, there was very substantial variation in their rates of reported youth suicide. Indeed, 90% of suicides occurred in just 12% of the communities, whereas in about half of the 111 communities that were studied there had been no suicides for

5 years. Many Indigenous communities were therefore doing just as well as the most affluent non-Indigenous communities in terms of this particular health statistic. What, though, was going on in the communities where youth suicide was a particular problem?

According to Chandler and Lalonde (1998, 2008), the answer to this question is found by looking at the extent to which these communities had been able to maintain a sense of *collective continuity* (see also Chandler, Lalonde, Sokol, & Hallett, 2003). As they argue, this sense of collective continuity is particularly important for young people transitioning from childhood to adulthood. To support their claims, the researchers examined the prevalence of six markers of collective continuity in each of these communities (e.g., participation in land claims, self-governance, establishment of cultural facilities, community control over education). They found that suicide rates within Indigenous communities were dramatically increased when these communities had been managed in a way that disrupted the connection with the past and when they had not been able to hold on to their cultural history. In fact, the observed 5-year suicide rate fell to zero when all six of these protective factors were in place in any particular community.

This is an important point with which to draw this chapter to a close, speaking as it does to the importance of the social identity continuity pathway that is central to SIMIC. Indeed, consistent with our analysis, the authors themselves conclude by observing that:

> Where all of this leaves us is with a deep conviction that a better understanding of the problem of suicide in First Nations communities can only be had by focusing attention on the interface between personal and cultural change.
>
> (Chandler & Lalonde, 1998, p. 19)

Conclusion

There is a growing recognition that when it comes to the negative effects of social status on health and well-being "it does not have to be like this" (see Friel, 2014; Marmot, 2015). Precisely because there are no biological or genetic reasons for systematic differences in health and well-being on the basis of social status, these differences also are increasingly seen as unfair and unacceptable. In the words of Sharon Friel (2014, p. 161):

> Pursuit of health equity recognises the need to redress the inequitable distribution of these resources. Creating a fairer distribution of the resources relates to freedoms and empowerment at the individual, community, and whole country level. Empowerment is affected by three core things: basic material requisites for a decent life, control over our lives, and voice and participation in the policy decisions that affect the conditions in which people are born, grow, live, work, age and die.

She goes on to note that "these dimensions of empowerment are influenced by public policy and the way in which society, at the international, national and local level, chooses to run its affairs" (p. 161, see also Marmot, 2015).

Moreover, as Leonard Syme and Lisa Berkman first noted in 1976, the health gradient cannot be tackled by individuals on their own. Instead, these researchers argue that it requires large-scale action that targets whole communities. We agree, and our analysis is consistent with this conclusion. Moreover, the consensus that is emerging on this point is important because recognising that social status and disadvantage *do not need* to affect our health and well-being should encourage us all to participate in efforts to flatten the health gradient.

Importantly, though, we think that understanding the important role that group memberships and social identities play in creating this gradient is also critical to these efforts. The reason for this is that just as multiple group memberships and social identity capital are the key psychological resources that are conferred by wealth and privilege, so, too, they are key resources that are compromised by poverty and disadvantage. Accordingly, investment that focuses on (re)building these resources is likely to be particularly well targeted and peculiarly beneficial.

Points for practice

The key insight of this chapter is that for members of disadvantaged communities, their group membership is both the problem and a resource that they can draw from to counter negative effects on health and well-being. Given this, the following three points can assist those working with members of these groups.

1. *Avoid the need for the individual to self-categorize as belonging to a disadvantaged group.* When members of disadvantaged communities do not feel forced to categorize as members of a disadvantaged group they do not want to belong to (e.g., as homeless), the very fact that they can negotiate their identity the way they want contributes not only to health and well-being, but also empowers them when interacting with services.
2. *Do not assume a person's health and well-being status on the basis of their 'objective' social status.* Because *relative* disadvantage, the permeability of boundaries between status groups, and inequality within a particular society are such important predictors of health and well-being, an individual's objective social status (as determined by income, occupation, and education) should always be judged in context. What is more, because social status is relative, it is not fixed and determined by birth, but open to change (e.g., via interventions from health care workers).
3. *It is essential to recognise the identity-related barriers that members of disadvantaged groups encounter when they undergo important life transitions.* For example, recognising that a person belonged to very few groups before they faced an important life change (e.g., illness, retirement) or that they belong to a disadvantaged group and have limited group resources to fall back on to help manage such a change is likely to be very important in working out how best to support them.

Resources

Further reading

The following provide a good introduction to work that explores the links between social status and health.

① Marmot, M. (2015). *The health gap: The challenge of an unequal world*. London, UK: Bloomsbury.

   This book represents a comprehensive, accessible, and well-written overview of research on the health gradient.

② Iyer, A., Jetten, J., & Tsivrikos, D. (2008). Torn between identities: Predictors of adjustment to identity change. In Sani, F. (Ed.). *Self-continuity: Individual and collective perspectives* (pp. 187–197). New York: Psychology Press.

This chapter provides an overview of predictions derived from the social identity model of identity change (SIMIC). It shows that social identity processes have an essential role to play in adjustment to life changes.

③ Sani, F. (2008). *Self-continuity: Individual and collective perspectives*. New York: Psychology Press.

This edited book brings together work by researchers in a wide range of fields – all of which speak to the important contribution of personal and collective-level continuity to health and well-being.

Audio and video

① Search for "Marmot Boyer Lectures" to listen to the 2016 lecture by Prof. Michael Marmot on "Health inequality and the causes of the causes". www.abc.net.au/radionational/programs/boyer-lectures/boyer-lecture-health-inequality-and-the-causes-of-the-causes/7763106.   (57 minutes)

② Search for "Wilkinson Spirit Level Ted talk" to watch a 2011 TED talk by Richard Wilkinson on "How economic inequality harms societies". This provides an overview of ideas presented in more detail in the influential book *The Spirit Level* that he wrote with Kate Pickett in 2009. www.ted.com/talks/richard_wilkinson   (17 minutes)

Websites

① www.who.int/social_determinants/thecommission/finalreport/key_concepts/en/. This World Health Organization site provides a rich resource for anyone interested in the social determinants of health. It contains publications, evidence for the social gradient of health, and training tools on how to implement insights to practice.

② www.bbcprisonstudy.org This is the official website for the BBC Prison Study. It contains a range of materials and resources that are relevant to the issues explored in this chapter.

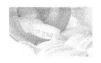

Chapter 4

Stigma

Sticks and stones will break my bones, but words will never hurt me

Old English children's rhyme.

When we were at school many of us would have learned this rhyme and perhaps recited it to deter those who taunted or made fun of us. The saying is based on the premise that other people's taunts are incapable of hurting us. Unfortunately, this is not true, and there is now considerable evidence that discrimination and exclusion hurt us psychologically. Importantly too, such treatment can have broader detrimental effects on our long-term physical and mental health.

Consider, for example, the case of the Indigenous Australian Rules football player, Adam Goodes, who was unable to continue playing after he had faced months of booing from fans of the opposing team while on the field – booing which, according to some, was racially motivated. The strain that the continued booing caused initially led Goodes to take a period of indefinite leave from the game – as part of an attempt to escape the negative attention he was receiving. Goodes did briefly return to the field after an outpouring of support from fans. However, it appears that the negative treatment that was meted out to him on the field was a major reason for him taking early retirement in 2015 (see Figure 4.1).

In the previous chapter, we focused on the ways in which disadvantage feeds into negative health outcomes. Here we turn our attention to groups that face stressors other than disadvantage – those who (often in addition to disadvantage) face discrimination and exclusion because they belong to a stigmatised group. Facing negative treatment and discrimination because of one's membership in such a group is extremely challenging in and of itself. However, as we have intimated, there is now a large body of evidence showing that it has a powerful negative effect on health. So what are these effects? And what is the best way to deal with them?

Stigma and its effects on health

In his classic book *Stigma* the sociologist Erving Goffman (1963) describes the origin of the term stigma in ancient culture. In both Greek and Roman cultures, those who were considered different, morally delinquent, or blemished were often subjected to skin burning or cutting that left them with a permanent mark, referred to as a *stigma*. This made their inferior status clear to everyone. In later centuries, Christians continued this tradition and started also using it for people who were physically different and disabled, and also to identify slaves.

Goffman was one of the first researchers to formally explore the consequences of stigma and stigma-related exclusion. He distinguished three broad categories of stigma: those relating to (1) physical deformities; (2) "blemishes of individual character" arising from "mental disorder, imprisonment, addiction, alcoholism, homosexuality, unemployment, suicidal attempts, and radical political behaviour"; and (3) stigma on the basis of category or group memberships such as nationality, religion, or race (1963, p. 14). Irrespective of the category, all who are stigmatised are typically perceived and responded to in terms of their stigma and not in terms of other attributes and behaviours they may possess. Because of this, stigma is associated with discrimination and negative evaluations on the

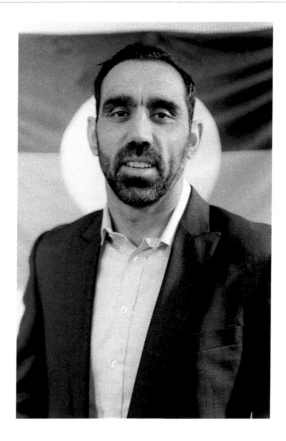

Figure 4.1 The Australian Rules football player Adam Goodes in front of the Aboriginal flag

Note: A distinguished Australian Rules football player and former Australian of the Year, Goodes' playing career ended in controversy following his decision to retire from the game after being targeted by sustained booing from fans – booing which he perceived to be racially motivated.

Source: Wikipedia

basis of group or category membership in which there is no recognition of an individual's or group's skills, abilities, or qualities – these are overlooked, ignored, or otherwise pushed to the background. Consistent with this, Goffman (1963, p. 3) defines stigma as an attribute of an individual or group that extensively discredits the individual, reducing him or her "from a whole and usual person to a tainted and discounted one" (see also Major & O'Brien, 2005).

Stigma-related discrimination can take many different forms. It can range from subtle forms of exclusion, ostensibly aimed at protecting the individual (e.g., excluding older adults from fitness clubs when they are physically frail) to more blatant manifestations (e.g., when an individual is less likely to be hired for a job because of their ethnicity). Stigma-related discrimination and exclusion can also differ in their pervasiveness (e.g., the extent to which exclusion on the basis of group membership is widespread, frequent, and impacts on many areas of life). Pervasive discrimination affects every aspect of an individual's life (e.g., systemic exclusion of particular groups from society in areas of employment, housing, and health care – as suffered by Jews, homosexuals, and gypsies in Nazi Germany) whereas the impact of some forms of discrimination are more limited (e.g., the practice of women paying more for dry cleaning and haircuts than men).

Regardless of these differences, there is growing awareness, and increased condemnation, of discrimination on the basis of group membership. However, it is also clear that such discrimination is not a problem that can be relegated to the past. For example, women continue to be disadvantaged in many areas of life. In the labour force, for example, they still face significant inequality when it comes to receiving equal pay for equal work, and they face barriers to advancement that take the shape of both "glass ceilings" (an inability to access leadership positions) and "glass cliffs" (an inability to access high-quality leadership positions; see Barreto, Ryan, & Schmitt, 2009; Ryan & Haslam, 2007).

What is more, in the case of gender discrimination, even though many countries now outlaw exclusion on the basis of gender (e.g., the 1984 Australian Sex Discrimination Act or affirmative action programmes in the United States that require federal contractors to ensure that there is no gender bias in their hiring and promotion decisions), not all countries have legislation in place requiring equal treatment of men and women. For example, a recent report by the World Bank and International Finance Corporation (2012) observed that out of 141 studied countries, the majority (103) still imposed differential gender-based legal treatment in at least some areas of life. Moreover, even if a country has legislation in place to protect those who encounter discrimination, this does not mean that the legislation eliminates all forms of discrimination that women experience (Gunderson, 1989).

Although there is now considerable awareness of problems associated with racism and sexism, there are also forms of exclusion that have only recently attracted attention. For example, ageism is not only widespread (Angus & Reeve, 2006) but it is also endorsed in many spheres of society (Hummert, Garstka, Shaner, & Strahm, 1994). In a similar vein, prejudice and bias against those who are overweight are still very prevalent (Crandall, Eshleman, & O'Brien, 2002; Tarrant, Hager, & Farrow, 2012; Spahlholz, Bear, Köning, Riedel-Heller, & Luck-Sikorski, 2016; see also Chapter 10). Likewise, discrimination on the basis of marital status (i.e., 'singlism' against those who are unmarried, single, separated, or divorced) has only recently been recognised but is widespread and pervasive (see Figure 4.2; Morris, Sinclair, & DePaulo, 2007).

Nevertheless, what all of these forms of stigma have in common is that they are increasingly challenged in society on the grounds that everybody *should* be treated equally regardless of their ethnicity, religion, gender, or sexual preference. Importantly too, for our present purposes, aside from fairness and justice concerns that propel people to challenge discrimination on the basis of group membership, the case for combatting stigma is also increasingly made with reference to health. Indeed, the fact that stigma is harmful to health and well-being means that there are compelling medical, not just moral, reasons why one would want to tackle racism, sexism, and other forms of stigma-related discrimination.

Consistent with this point, there is now growing evidence that although many factors contribute to the health deficits associated with belonging to stigmatised groups, exposure to stigma and

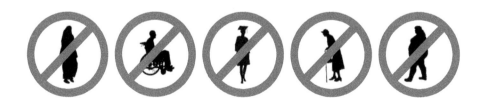

Figure 4.2 Signs of stigma-related exclusion

Note: More traditional forms of discrimination (in terms of ethnicity, disability, and gender) on the left alongside more recently identified forms (in terms of age and weight) on the right.

discrimination is one of the most important (e.g., Paradies et al., 2015; Matheson, McQuaid, & Anisman, 2016; Schmitt, Branscombe, Postmes, & Garcia, 2014). For instance, the pervasive discrimination experienced by people who are homeless – particularly discrimination that restricts access to accommodation and goods and services – has been found to contribute significantly to the high rates of poor health found among members of this group (Lynch & Stagoll, 2002; Phelan, Link, Moore, & Stueve, 1997).

As we will outline further, because stigma typically involves discrimination and exclusion on the basis of group membership, an understanding of group membership and social identity is critical to understanding when and how stigma affects health. Indeed, group membership is not only the reason why people face exclusion, but it can influence how well people cope with such exclusion. This is rather ironic because it implies that for those who are members of a stigmatised group, their group membership is both a cause of negative health effects *and* the key to helping them counter those negative effects. In other words, group membership can be both a curse *and* a cure to that same curse. This accords with one of the key hypotheses that we put forward in Chapter 2 – that *because it is the basis for meaningful group life, social identity is central to both good and ill health* (the social identity hypothesis, H1).

Quantifying the relationship between stigma and health

Before discussing the different theoretical approaches to understanding the relationship between stigma and health, one can ask the question *just how harmful is* stigma and discrimination for health and well-being? In other words, what is the magnitude of this relationship? A number of meta-analyses have answered this question by quantifying the impact that discrimination has on health.

In one such meta-analysis, Elizabeth Pascoe and Laura Smart Richman (2009) focused on both physical and mental health outcomes among those facing discrimination. They drew on data from 36 studies investigating the relationship between discrimination and physical health – including risk factors related to cardiovascular disease; physical conditions such as hypertension, pelvic inflammatory disease, diabetes, yeast infections, and respiratory conditions; and general indicators of illness (such as nausea, pain, and headaches) – and reports of symptoms on general health questionnaires. They found negative associations between discrimination and these health indicators in 83% of the analyses. However, these negative effects only reached an acceptable level of significance in 42% of cases. Their examination of mental health included 110 studies and revealed an overall correlation (r) of $-.20$ between discrimination and mental health (Pascoe & Smart Richman, 2009). Further analyses of the relationship between discrimination and specific mental health outcomes showed a significant negative relationship with depressive symptoms, psychiatric distress, and general well-being.

A more recent and more comprehensive meta-analysis by Michael Schmitt and colleagues (2014) reached similar conclusions. This analysed 328 studies that examined the relationship between discrimination and mental health outcomes indexed by measures of self-esteem, depression, anxiety, psychological distress, and life satisfaction. Overall, there was a negative and significant correlation between perceived discrimination and mental health ($r = .23$). Interestingly, though, effect sizes were larger for disadvantaged groups ($r = .24$) than for advantaged groups ($r = .10$). This finding is important because it suggests that the experience of being the target of discrimination is different for members of advantaged groups (e.g., White people) and disadvantaged groups (e.g., Black people). Importantly too, Schmitt and colleagues found that the negative well-being effects of discrimination were more pronounced for particular types of minorities. For example, there were stronger relationships between perceived discrimination and well-being for sexual minorities, people with mental illness, people with a physical disability, and people stigmatised as overweight than for those who face discrimination based on gender or race.

These findings correspond with results of a subsequent meta-analysis by Yin Paradies and colleagues (2015) which examined the relationship between stigma and health for one specific form of group-based exclusion – racism (i.e., exclusion and negative treatment on the basis of ethnicity and/

or race). This found that racism was significantly related to poorer health, but that the relationship was stronger for mental health outcomes (as evident in measures of depression, anxiety, psychological stress; $r = -.23$, $k = 227$; where k is the number of studies) than for physical health ($r = -.09$, $k = 50$) and general health outcomes ($r = -.13$, $k = 30$). Interestingly, and consistent with observations in Schmitt and colleagues' meta-analysis, the relationship between racism and poor health was not the same for all ethnic groups. Instead the mental health impact was greater for Asian Americans and Latino Americans than for African Americans. Furthermore, the relationship between racism and physical health was stronger for Latino Americans than for African Americans.

It thus appears that if one wants to understand the relationship between stigma and health, it is important to consider not only whether groups are advantaged or disadvantaged within society (as in the Schmitt et al., 2014, meta-analysis), but also the specific intragroup and intergroup relations that determine the position of the stigmatised group in society (as in the Schmitt et al., 2014 and Paradies et al., 2015 meta-analyses). We will elaborate on this point in the second part of this chapter.

Current approaches to stigmatised group membership

Interestingly, although a great deal of research in social psychology and sociology has traditionally examined perceptions of those who are stigmatised, it is only recently that the focus has shifted to examining how people who face discrimination or exclusion on the basis of group membership respond to, and cope with, stigma (Crocker, Major, & Steele, 1998; Major et al., 2002a; Major, Quinton, & McCoy, 2002b). Stigma and discrimination are considered to have a negative impact on health for a number of reasons. First and foremost, they reduce access to, and the benefits of, employment, housing, and education. These in turn directly limit opportunities, affect the access and affordability of health care, and are associated with reduced health literacy (Sentell & Halpin, 2006). People can also experience unfair treatment in health care directly (e.g., Paradies, Truong, & Priest, 2014), and discrimination can erode the quality of close relationships (e.g., Doyle & Molix, 2014) and broader social networks (Brondolo, Libretti, Rivera, & Walsemann, 2012).

There are also other ways in which stigma impacts negatively on health – and many of these are psychological and physiological in origin. Along these lines, researchers have used a stress and coping approach to explain when and why stigma is associated with poor health (Major et al., 2002b). According to this view, stigma represents a significant stressor that challenges individuals' well-being in at least three ways (Pascoe & Smart Richman, 2009; see Figure 4.3). *First*, being the target of

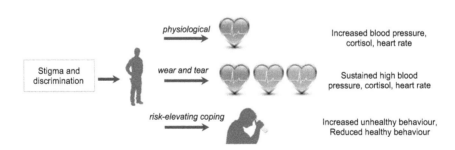

Figure 4.3 Three pathways from stigma and discrimination to ill-health

Note: The first pathway involves a direct stress response that is adaptive in the short term but carries some risk. The second pathway involves a sustained response to ongoing stress that makes chronic stress much more likely. The third pathway involves forms of coping which increase willingness to engage in behaviours that negatively affect health.

stigma and discrimination triggers a direct stress response in the body. This includes elevated blood pressure, increased cortisol levels, and increased heart rate – physiological responses which are adaptive in reaction to short-term physical challenges (e.g., they help you to run away from an attacker) but can nevertheless increase the risk of health consequences such as anxiety disorders and cardiac arrest (Matheson & Anisman, 2012). *Second*, stigma affects health if this physiological stress response is sustained, as this causes wear and tear on the body. Here the nature of discrimination as a stressor – being pervasive, uncontrollable, and lasting over prolonged periods – makes it particularly likely that a chronic stress response will occur. Over time this is associated with an increase in vulnerability to physical and mental illness (Gee, Spencer, Chen, Yip, & Takeuchi, 2007). In particular, this is because sustained physiological responses lead to higher systolic and diastolic blood pressure (Steffen, McNeilly, Anderson, & Sherwood, 2003) and can increase the risk of cardiovascular disease (Brondolo et al., 2008). In line with this analysis, exposure to discrimination has also been found to predict a greater risk of obesity, breast cancer, and high blood pressure (Williams & Mohammed, 2009). *Third*, stigma impacts negatively on health because many individuals cope with the stress associated with discrimination and stigma by engaging in behaviours that negatively affect health. For example, they may turn to drugs and alcohol or may reduce their participation in healthy behaviours such as exercise (Pacoe & Smart Richman, 2009).

The meta-analyses that we reviewed earlier not only found meaningful differences between groups in how much stigma affects health (a finding we return to later in this chapter), but also noted considerable variation within groups. This suggests that those who confront stigma and discrimination may respond to it in quite different ways. On the one hand, there are examples of individuals who appear unaffected and untouched by the negative treatment they receive. Indeed, in line with Friedrich Nietzsche's (1888) observation that "that which does not kill me makes me stronger", they may become hardier by enduring the suffering associated with their stigma. Others, however, respond to stigma and discrimination with shame, self-hate, withdrawal, low self-esteem, and anxiety (Corrigan, Watson, & Barr, 2006). There are also those who become angry and upset about their treatment and challenge any type of behaviour or response that they suspect may be stigma related. Accordingly, this raises the critical question of what it is that leads some people to be strong (possibly stronger) and able to cope well in the face of stigma, but others to experience despair and suffering. To answer this question, researchers have traditionally turned to individual-difference explanations and to situational factors that shape these various reactions. We will discuss these in turn.

The dispositional model: the role of personality and individual differences

Unsurprisingly perhaps, when seeking to understand who stands firm in the face of stigma and who succumbs to it, many researchers have pointed to the importance of individual differences or personality factors. In this regard, several personal characteristics have been identified as candidate variables, including an individual's stigma sensitivity, individual differences in justice-related beliefs, and an individual's domain identification and specific goals and motives (Major & O'Brien, 2005).

Starting with *stigma sensitivity*, it has been argued that some individuals are simply more sensitive to being stigmatised than others. Rejection sensitivity is typically measured by presenting participants with scenarios of the following form:

> Imagine that you are in class one day, and the professor asks a particularly difficult question. A few people, including yourself, raise their hand to answer the question.

or

> Imagine that you are in a restaurant, trying to get the attention of your waitress. A lot of other people are trying to get her attention as well.

Next, participants are asked to indicate to what extent they would be concerned or anxious that they would receive a negative outcome because of, for example, their race (on a scale with response options ranging from *very unconcerned* to *very concerned*). A second question would then ask them to estimate the likelihood that in each scenario the other person would engage in rejecting behaviour towards them on the basis of their race (on a scale with response options ranging from *very unlikely* to *very likely*).

Research has found that individuals who endorse such items (i.e., who score high on 'stigma sensitivity') are also more likely to make an attribution that this is due to stigma, compared to individuals who score lower in stigma sensitivity (Mendoza-Denton, Purdie, Downey, Davis, & Pietrzak, 2002). Such individuals are also more likely to expect negative treatment from outgroup members at both a personal and a group level (Pinel, 1999). There is also some evidence that rejection sensitivity predicts health outcomes. For example, Steve Cole, Margaret Kemeny, and Shelley Taylor (1997) observed that for gay men with HIV, there was a positive correlation between being sensitive to rejection by the broader community and the acceleration of HIV symptoms and mortality. However, this relationship was only found for men who had disclosed their sexuality. This pattern of accelerated HIV progression was not observed among rejection-sensitive men who had chosen to hide their sexuality.

There is also evidence that people are more negatively affected by discrimination when they experience it in a domain that they identify strongly with. Here, because of individual differences in the extent to which the person cares about their standing in a particular domain (e.g., one that is sporting or academic), they are more likely to care about how they are treated and to see themselves as targets of discrimination (Sellers & Shelton, 2003), and this in turn is likely to have negative health effects.

Researchers have also suggested that health outcomes are affected by individual differences in the extent to which we seek to *justify* exclusion. More specifically, it is argued that some individuals are more likely than others to believe that the world is fair and just (Lerner & Miller, 1978) and that we live in a fair and meritocratic society (Sidanius & Pratto, 1999). The reasoning goes that the more an individual endorses these so-called 'legitimising ideologies' (believing that the world is fair and meritocratic), the more likely they are to believe that those who face stigma (including themselves) must have done something to deserve the exclusion they encounter. As a result, these ideologies lead people to downplay the seriousness of exclusion and, if they are on the receiving end, to justify their own negative treatment. In effect, they make sense of their bad experiences by thinking "I must be a bad person to have deserved all this".

What is not clear, however, is whether greater endorsement of such legitimising ideologies is beneficial or damaging for health. Studies that have investigated this issue report mixed findings. In particular, this is because the relationship between support for legitimising ideologies and well-being varies depending on the specific group under investigation. For example, individual differences in the belief that the world is a just and fair place have been found to be negatively related to self-esteem among African Americans, but this relationship is reversed for European Americans (Jost & Thompson, 2000; see also Rankin, Jost, & Wakslak, 2009; Schaafsma, 2013).

Individuals also differ in the extent to which they perceive they have *control* over their own outcomes, including bad outcomes such as exclusion (Weiner, 1985). Typically, people are held responsible for outcomes that are seen to be under their control. As a result, stigma is often perceived as controllable – and hence more justified – when it is seen to be linked to specific behaviours, as might be the case for people who are obese, addicted to drugs or alcohol, single mothers, or fall victim to AIDS. In all these cases, because stigma is seen to be under the individual's control, it is seen as avoidable. As a result, individuals are more likely to be blamed for negative health outcomes in ways that prove deleterious to their health and well-being (Gneezy, List, & Price, 2012).

Importantly, these individual differences not only affect the responses of onlookers who witness discrimination (e.g., determining whether they challenge a perceived wrong or see people's treatment as deserved), but also affect the responses of those who are excluded. For example, it has been found that the more that women endorse a belief that the world is fair and just, the less likely they are to perceive themselves to be personally discriminated against, and the less likely they are to interpret ambiguous negative outcomes and situations as being due to sexism (Major et al., 2002a, b).

Yet although these factors may at times account for people's responses to stigma, the individual-difference approach also has some very significant weaknesses.

First, it cannot account for a number of the meta-analytical findings that we discussed earlier. For example, Schmitt and colleagues (2014) observed that the relationship between discrimination and well-being is weaker for advantaged groups than for disadvantaged groups. But why would these two types of groups differ systematically on individual difference indicators? Are health outcomes worse for disadvantaged group members because they are more likely to believe in a just world and more likely to believe that people are in control of their own outcomes than people in advantaged groups? If anything, the opposite appears to be true. For generally it is clear that members of advantaged groups are more likely to endorse legitimising ideologies than their disadvantaged counterparts (see Sidanius & Pratto, 1999). And, as the work we reviewed earlier shows, if groups hold these beliefs when they are advantaged in society (e.g., Whites in the United States; Jost, & Thompson, 2000; Rankin et al., 2009), then belief that the world is fair and just is associated with better health and well-being. Yet the opposite pattern is found among disadvantaged groups such as African Americans – where endorsement of legitimising ideology tends to lead to poorer health. It thus appears that the relationship between endorsement of ideological beliefs and health is far from straightforward and certainly cannot be explained by individual differences alone.

Second, individual-difference approaches are limited because they focus on appraisals of negative *personal* outcomes. However, the evidence suggests that it is often not a person's personal experience of discrimination that affects their health, but rather their perception that their group is the target of discrimination. For example, in a sample of homeless individuals, Melissa Johnstone and her colleagues found that lower well-being was predicted by perceptions of *group-based* discrimination, whereas perceived personal discrimination was unrelated to well-being (Johnstone, Jetten, Dingle, Parsell, & Walter, 2015). Other studies show diverging or even opposing relationships between personal perceptions and group-based perceptions. For example, a recent study of unemployed people in Belgium showed that participants had higher self-esteem to the extent that they perceived unemployed people to be discriminated against as a group. However, in contrast to this, the same individuals had lower self-esteem the more they felt personally discriminated against because of their unemployment (Bourguignon, Yzerbyt, Teixeira, & Herman, 2015). This again suggests that even though individual-difference variables may contribute to some well-being and health outcomes, on their own they tell an incomplete story.

There is a third puzzle that remains unresolved by individual-difference accounts. Recall the finding by Schmitt and colleagues (2014) that the negative well-being effects of discrimination differed across a number of minority groups (e.g., so that there are stronger relationships between perceived discrimination and well-being for sexual minorities than for those who face discrimination based on gender or race). How can we explain this? It seems unlikely that this reflects the fact that members of particular minority groups differ substantially from members of other groups in terms of their individual differences. It seems equally implausible that differences in individuals' beliefs in a just world and legitimising myths could account for the variability in the negative effects of racism that Paradies and colleagues (2015) observed in their meta-analysis. Instead, then, we suggest that these differing patterns of relationship may be better explained by attending to group dynamics associated with particular intragroup and intergroup relations. In recognition of this, researchers have increasingly turned their attention to the following questions: Under what circumstances do victims of discrimination attribute their treatment to their stigmatised group membership? And how do *situational factors* determine people's attempts to cope with discrimination?

The situational model: concealing stigma

In an attempt to do justice to the broader context in which stigma is experienced, researchers have homed in on particular features of the stigmatised group membership. In particular, they have focused on whether stigma is *concealable*. The reason for this is that it is argued that when group members can conceal their stigmatised group membership, they are more likely to avoid prejudice (Frable, Blackstone, & Scherbaum, 1990), and there is evidence that this in turn may protect their health and well-being. This suggests that, in some cases, hiding stigmatised identities may protect health – presumably because it reduces exposure to discrimination. However, it turns out that hiding stigmatised group membership is not always protective of health and that significant health costs can be associated with long-term concealment. For example, among HIV-infected gay men, long-term hiding of sexual identity has been found to be related to increased vulnerability to infectious diseases such as pneumonia, bronchitis, sinusitis, and tuberculosis (Cole, Kemeny, Taylor, & Visscher, 1996).

It thus appears that there are no straightforward answers to the question of whether concealing a stigmatised identity is protective of health or not. Even though individuals who hide stigma are less likely to be targets of discrimination, as we will outline in greater detail later, it is also clear that those who hide stigma are less likely to receive and benefit from the social support of other group members. As a result, the long-term health consequences of hiding one's membership of a stigmatised group may be rather negative (see also Beals, Peplau, & Gable, 2009).

The social identity approach to stigma and health

Although the literature that examines situational factors such as concealability has acknowledged that important group-related factors affect the relationship between discrimination and health, to date, this research has tended to focus largely on single processes and factors. This means that when it comes to explaining the health-related consequences of stigma, little consideration has been given to the broader social context in which it occurs. However, we would argue that to fully understand the complex relationship between stigma and health, we need to go beyond an analysis of group characteristics and situational factors in isolation. In particular, we would contend that much is to be gained by developing a coherent theoretical framework that clarifies the role of social identity and self-categorization processes in the relationship between group membership and health.

This is also important from an applied perspective. For it is only when we start to recognise that group dynamics can affect the relationship between stigma and health that we can understand why some groups are more successful in countering the negative effects of stigma on health than others and why there are also important variations within a group's response to stigma (e.g., Williams & Mohammed, 2009). As well as advancing theory, we contend that the social identity approach to health provides a practical framework for engaging with these applied issues.

Social identity affects coping with stigma and discrimination

Building on the recognition that social identities play a part in the maintenance of well-being, an important question that remains to be answered is how people who face discrimination on the basis of group membership (e.g., because of their ethnicity, gender, or class) use identities as a resource to protect well-being. Interestingly, recent research suggests that when people are confronted with group-based discrimination, they do not necessarily downplay the importance of the group identity that the discrimination targets. On the contrary, it appears that group-based rejection can sometimes lead them to nurture and embrace the excluded identity even more (e.g., Branscombe, Schmitt, & Harvey, 1999; Jetten, Branscombe, Schmitt, & Spears, 2001). Indeed, this insight provides the basis for the *rejection-identification model* (Branscombe et al., 1999; Schmitt & Branscombe, 2002, see Figure 4.4).

The starting point for this model is the observation of a significant negative correlation between the experience of discrimination and respondents' well-being. In other words, as the group circumstance hypothesis (H3b) suggests, being a victim of discrimination is harmful to health. Importantly, though, as the identity restoration hypothesis (H4) argues, *people will also be motivated to restore positive identity when this is compromised by events that threaten or undermine their social identities.* In line with this reasoning, Nyla Branscombe and her colleagues (1999) noted that when people

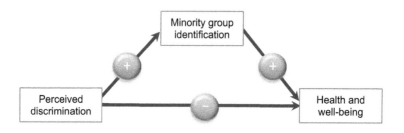

Figure 4.4 The rejection-identification model

Note: Perceived discrimination has a direct negative effect on health and well-being. However, this direct negative effect is counteracted by a positive indirect path whereby (1) perceived discrimination is positively associated with minority group identification and (2) enhanced minority group identification positively affects health and well-being.

Source: Based on Branscombe et al. (1999)

recognise they are victims of group-based discrimination, this is also found to predict increased levels of ingroup identification. Moreover, they found that this heightened ingroup identification can buffer minority group members from the negative effects of discrimination – in particular, because it is a basis for increased *social support* (as suggested by H14; see also Chapter 5). In that sense, 'suffering out loud' is found to increase respondents' sense of shared group membership, and this provides a platform for them to work together, both to cope with their situation and to start doing something to improve it.

Significantly, then, Schmitt and Branscombe's (2002) isolation of the rejection-identification mechanism again demonstrates that social identity is central to the dynamic that turns negative social experiences into positive opportunities and that transforms negative personal emotions into positive social energy. In this way, identification with a minority group may serve not only as a buffer against environmental threats (e.g., discrimination, exclusion, poverty), but also as a key *resource* that can be mobilised in managing and combating exclusion and discrimination. Such increased identification in response to perceived discrimination has clear psychological benefits that at least partially counteract the negative effects of perceived discrimination on well-being (Jetten et al., 2001).

The importance of group-based support for well-being is most clearly observed when individuals lose that support. As social identity theory predicts, and as argued in H5 (see Chapters 2 and 3), when members of minority groups attempt to become part of the majority, they typically pursue a personal identity-based strategy of individual mobility. However, a downside of this strategy is that it cuts them off from social identity and its benefits. This is a point that emerges from research by Postmes and Branscombe (2002) which found that African Americans who attempt to assimilate with White people (e.g., by leaving predominantly Black neighbourhoods and moving into those that are predominantly White) are more likely to feel psychologically abandoned by their former ingroup (other African Americans) on grounds that they are 'deserters' or 'traitors'. Moreover, this feeling can be accentuated by the fact that in seeking acceptance from their new ingroup, members of minorities may strategically align themselves with members of the new group (Jetten, Branscombe, Spears, & McKimmie, 2003; Jetten, Hornsey, Spears, Haslam, & Cowell, 2010) or they may feel obliged to denounce their former group membership in order to 'prove' that they are not imposters. In contrast, Postmes and Branscombe (2002) found that Black Americans who live and work in separated rather than integrated communities report receiving more social support, being more accepted by their ingroup, and having enhanced levels of psychological well-being.

There is now considerable evidence that group identification facilitates coping with discrimination among stigmatised minorities as varied as southern Italians facing discrimination from their northern compatriots (Latrofa, Vaes, Pastore, & Cadinu, 2009; McNamara, Stevenson, & Muldoon, 2013), immigrant groups (Jasinskaja-Lahti, Liebkind, Jaakkola, & Reuter, 2006), multiracial groups (Giamo, Schmitt, & Outten, 2012), people with body piercings (Jetten et al., 2001), women (Redersdorff, Martinot, & Branscombe, 2004), and older adults (Garstka, Schmitt, Branscombe, & Hummert, 2004). It thus appears that individuals are more likely to be able to cope successfully with stigma when they can band together with other members of their minority group and collectively address their difficulties rather than being left to deal with them on their own. This is because it is only when they act in terms of shared social identity that individuals can draw upon the psychological resources that group membership provides.

This insight can also help us explain some of the mixed findings that we reported earlier in relation to the question of whether hiding stigma is beneficial for health or not. We can best illustrate this with reference to research by Fernando Molero and colleagues which studied people living with HIV in Spain (Molero, Fuster, Jetten, & Moriano, 2011). These researchers found evidence of two pathways via which people can respond to stigma associated with being HIV positive – both of which are represented schematically in Figure 4.5. First, they found that the more that participants believed that people with HIV face group-based discrimination, the more inclined they were to hide their stigmatised group membership. This in turn reduced perceptions of personal discrimination and protected well-being. However, the second pathway points to a downside of this concealment strategy. For perceived group-based discrimination was also positively related to social identification with others who had HIV and this, in turn,

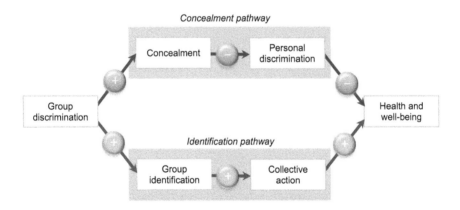

Figure 4.5 Dual pathways from group-based discrimination to well-being

Note: The concealment pathway (at the top of the figure) suggests that group discrimination may increase people's tendency to hide their stigmatised group membership. This reduces the likelihood that the individual will face personal discrimination. In turn, lower personal discrimination is associated with higher well-being. The identification pathway (at the bottom) suggests that the perception of group-based discrimination leads individuals to turn towards the stigmatised group, enhancing their identification with this group. This then increases the individual's willingness to tackle group-based discrimination together with others (i.e., through collective action) and is associated with enhanced well-being.

Source: Based on Molero et al. (2011)

was positively related to collective action intentions and well-being (in line with the agency hypothesis, H15). The latter pathway is also consistent with research which shows that negative effects of conceal-ment for health arise from (1) the cost of inhibiting emotional expression and (2) the loneliness and isolation that it leads to (see also Barreto, Ellemers, & Banai, 2006; Newheiser & Barreto, 2014).

It thus appears that people are in a better position to draw from the resources that membership in stigmatised groups provides (i.e., in terms of social support) when they respond collectively to stig-ma-related threats. However, for such a collective response to occur, group members need to recognise that the discrimination they face is (1) group-based and (2) illegitimate (Jetten, Iyer, Branscombe, & Zhang, 2013). We will explore these two conditions next in the process of outlining how social identity affects the appraisal – and thus the experience – of discrimination.

Social identity affects the appraisal of stigma

We noted earlier that before group members can work out how they are going to respond to discrimination, they first need to know that they are being discriminated against on the basis of their group membership. In other words, they need to respond 'yes' to Question 1 in Figure 4.6. This may sound straightforward, but it is not always easy to establish whether or not one has been a victim of

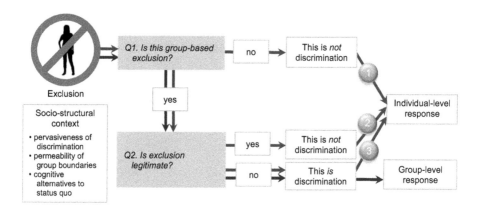

Figure 4.6 Responses to exclusion

Note: There are three situations in which individual-level responses to group-based discrimination prevail: *first*, when members of disadvantaged groups do not perceive their exclusion as group-based ("No" to Q1), which thus elim-inates opportunities for challenging the group's negative identity as a collective (Path 1); *second*, when members of disadvantaged groups perceive that there is a valid reason for excluding them on the basis of group membership ("Yes" to Q2, Path 2); and, *third*, when collective responses are undermined because discrimination is rare, bound-aries between groups are permeable (i.e., allowing for individual mobility), and when there are no clear alternatives to the status quo ("No" to Q2, Path 3).

In contrast, collective responses are most likely when exclusion is perceived as group based ("Yes" to Q1) when there is no apparent valid reason for the group-based exclusion ("No" to Q2), discrimination is pervasive, group boundaries are impermeable, and/or there are clear cognitive alternatives to the status quo. Importantly, it is only when there is a group-based response to discrimination (e.g., heightened identification with the minority group) that the socially curative effects of group membership can be unlocked, buffering minority group members from the negative effects of discrimination on health and well-being (through increased *social support* as suggested by H14).

Source: Based on Jetten et al. (2013)

discrimination (DePaulo & Morris, 2006; Gurin, 1985; Major et al., 2002b; Simon & Klandermans, 2001). A key reason for this is that in many contexts we can experience ambiguous and negative outcomes for a range of reasons other than group-based discrimination. Did I fail to get the job because I am a woman – or because the other candidates were better? Was that person unpleasant to me because I am a Muslim – or because they were having a bad day?

It is also clear that identification with the stigmatised group itself plays an important role in determining whether exclusion is seen to be group based. In particular, evidence suggests that victims are more reluctant to understand their negative outcomes as evidence of "discrimination" when (1) their identification with the devalued group is relatively low, (2) when there are no clear boundaries between groups (e.g., as can be the case with age), (3) when exclusion is based on attributes that people tend to think of as individual features rather than group features (e.g., one's weight or marital status; DePaulo & Morris, 2006), or (4) when the devalued group membership is not salient.

Consistent with the last of these points, research has found that women are more likely to recognise group-based discrimination when their gender group membership has first been made salient (Foster & Matheson, 1999; Hafer & Olson, 1993). Presumably, this is because the salience of the group for victims makes it more likely that they make intergroup comparisons that highlight the distinction between 'us' and 'them' (see Major & Testa, 1989; Postmes, Branscombe, Spears, & Young, 1999). It is also the case that there are a range of situations in which group salience will tend to be low for victims of discrimination and hence where they are less likely to detect it than might otherwise be the case. These include (1) when negative treatment is received from a fellow ingroup member (e.g., another woman) rather than from an outgroup member (Inman & Baron, 1996), (2) when the perpetrator does not fit the stereotype of a typical outgroup 'villain' (Baron, Burgess, & Kao, 1991), or (3) when the exclusion is not seen as a typical instance of discrimination (e.g., Swim, Mallett, Russo-Devosa, & Stangor, 2005). In this case, then, stigma only 'sticks' and only affects individuals as group members (either positively or negatively) to the extent that they make sense of their treatment through the lens of their membership in the relevant stigmatised group. This speaks to the identification hypothesis (H2) – that *a person will experience the health-related benefits or costs of a given group membership only to the extent that they identify with that group*.

As Figure 4.6 suggests, the second question that structures people's experience of discrimination relates to their sense that their treatment is legitimate or illegitimate (Jetten et al., 2013; Major & Schmader, 2001). At first blush, this might seem like an odd question. When, one might ask, would group-based exclusion ever be seen as legitimate? In fact, though, one does not have to look too far to find examples. Indeed, many forms of group-based exclusion are not at all contentious. The fact that we routinely prohibit young people from buying alcohol, driving a car, or voting are clear examples of our willingness to use group membership as a basis for exclusion and to see this as quite reasonable. However, there are also situations where it is far less clear that group membership provides an appropriate basis for exclusion. In today's society, for example, many people still consider it legitimate for women to be excluded from the priesthood, for gay couples to be denied the right to marry or adopt children, and for prisoners to be denied the right to vote. But equally, for other people, these same practices are seen to be profoundly wrong.

When negative differential treatment is not appraised in group-based terms (i.e., where the answer to Question 1 in Figure 4.6 is "no") or when exclusion is perceived as being to some extent legitimate (where the answer to Question 2 is "yes"), disadvantaged group members are less likely to see their treatment as a reflection of group-based discrimination. Importantly, this also means that they will tend to prefer individual-level responses to their low-status group membership and associated discrimination (i.e., pursuing a strategy of individual mobility) over group-level responses (e.g., collective protests against differential treatment). This is consequential for health outcomes because, as we argued earlier, it is only when members of stigmatised groups *band together* with other members of their own or another group (i.e., when they identify with them and strive to deal collectively with their disadvantage; see Dixon et al., 2015) that the beneficial health effects of group membership are unlocked. Indeed, in line with the group circumstance hypothesis (H3b), when discrimination is appraised (by both the advantaged and the disadvantaged group) as legitimate, we predict that *the capacity for social identity to function as a beneficial psychological resource is reduced and that this will tend to have negative consequences for health and well-being.* In contrast, when members of both the advantaged and the disadvantaged group appraise discrimination as illegitimate, individuals are more likely to act in terms of shared social identity and to feel collectively empowered to address the disadvantages that their group is facing. As a result (and consistent with H3a), under these circumstances, *social identity becomes a beneficial psychological resource and tends to have positive consequences for their health and well-being.*

Features of the broader socio-structural context affect responses to stigma

As indicated in Figure 4.6, it is nevertheless the case that the decisions victims of discrimination make about how to respond to their treatment do not occur in a vacuum. That is, even when devalued group members judge that their differential treatment is group based and that there is no valid reason underlying such treatment, it does not necessarily mean that they will collectively challenge the exclusion. This is because a number of features of the broader socio-structural context also affect whether or not an instance of discrimination is appraised as arising from one's stigmatised group membership, and this will determine whether a group-level response is judged to be appropriate.

Pervasiveness of discrimination

First, when discrimination is perceived to be pervasive and widespread (rather than rare), it is more likely that group members will see the boundaries between groups as sharply drawn (Schmitt & Branscombe, 2002; Schmitt, Branscombe, & Postmes, 2003). If that is the case, it becomes clear that "people like me" are treated differently from "them". These enhanced perceptions of intragroup similarity and intergroup difference will in turn generally strengthen intergroup categorization and group salience (Drury & Reicher, 2000; Turner, Hogg, Oakes, Reicher, & Wetherell, 1987). In such cases, it is therefore more likely that differential treatment will be appraised as group based, and therefore seen to require a group-based response.

Support for this reasoning is provided by a study by Donna Garcia and her colleagues which investigated responses to gender discrimination (Garcia, Schmitt, Branscombe, & Ellemers, 2009). This started by asking female participants to indicate to what extent they believed that gender discrimination was pervasive. After this, the women were presented with an unfair hiring decision in which a highly qualified female lawyer was denied partnership in her firm in favour of a less qualified male. Participants were then randomly allocated to a condition in which they were presented with one of three responses on the part of the woman in question: (1) she chose not to protest the decision, (2) she protested the decision by pointing to collective disadvantage (the hiring decision was unfair to women), or (3) she protested by arguing that the decision was unfair to her individually. Participants were then asked to indicate their liking for the female lawyer and to rate the appropriateness of her response. Results showed that those participants who perceived gender discrimination to be more pervasive were more in favour of collective responses to group-based exclusion and were also more inclined to like the female protester and to judge her protest as appropriate (regardless of whether she employed an individualistic or a collective protest strategy). Moreover, it was precisely under these conditions that the non-protester was evaluated most negatively. In short, then, it appears that seeing discrimination as pervasive is a pre-cursor to being drawn towards other ingroup members who want to help you fight it, and to distance yourself from those who do not.

A second factor that is important when determining whether discrimination is perceived as group based concerns the extent to which boundaries between groups are seen to be permeable or impermeable. This question of permeability often focuses on the extent to which individuals can control whether or not they belong to the stigmatised group. That is, can they leave the group and join another one that does not face stigma and exclusion? For example, smokers might see group boundaries between smoking and non-smoking groups to be permeable because people can decide to quit smoking (see Jetten, Schmitt, Branscombe, Garza, & Mewse, 2011). In such cases stigma is therefore perceived as more controllable because it is possible to leave the stigmatised group behind.

How then do members of groups whose stigma is controllable respond to discrimination? Evidence suggests that answers to this question are not straightforward (see Jetten & Branscombe, 2009). On the one hand, it has been argued that where society views stigma as controllable, this enhances the perception that it is the person's own fault that they are stigmatised. In this context it is harder for a person to cope with their negative treatment. For example, overweight people or smokers who believe that being overweight or smoking is under their own control may perceive that any exclusion and discrimination they experience is more legitimate because they think that their circumstances are a reflection of their own personal weakness (e.g., reflecting a lack of willpower to diet or quit smoking). Social identity theory would suggest for these people the boundaries between groups (of those who are 'overweight' vs. 'thin', of smokers vs. non-smokers) are permeable. It follows that when there are thought to be plenty of opportunities for individual mobility, group members who fail to escape their stigmatised group are themselves to blame for being targets of discrimination (Ellemers, van Knippenberg, & Wilke, 1990; Garstka et al., 2004). This leads to the prediction that perceived controllability of stigmatised group membership would be associated with self-hate and low self-esteem.

However, and in contrast to this prediction, there is also evidence that opportunities to leave a devalued group behind are often unrelated to people's use of individual mobility strategies and do not necessarily lead to self-loathing. Just because you can leave a stigmatised group does not mean you will always feel bad if you do not leave (Tajfel, 1978). Consistent with this view, it has been found that group identification tends to be higher among members of groups where membership is controllable and self-selected than when membership is not under the individual's control (Ellemers, Kortekaas, & Ouwerkerk, 1999; Perreault & Bourhis, 1999). An example of this process emerges from research by Jetten and colleagues (2001) with people who had chosen to have body-piercings. Even though these individuals could take out their piercings to avoid discrimination, the researchers found that if respondents felt they were subjected to discrimination as a result of their body piercings, they were *more* likely to justify having body piercings on identity grounds (e.g., "I do this because it's an important part of who I am") and more likely to identify with others who had body piercings.

Cultural differences can also affect whether people perceive group boundaries to be permeable or not and thus whether stigma is perceived as controllable. This point emerges from research by Branscombe and colleagues (Branscombe, Fernández, Gómez, & Cronin, 2012) in Spain and the United States with people suffering from skeletal dysplasias that cause dwarfism that we touched upon in Chapter 2. This showed that boundaries were perceived to be more permeable in Spain (where health care covers limb-lengthening surgery) than among people suffering from this illness in the United States (where health care does not cover limb-lengthening surgery). This in turn affected the way the illness was perceived and the coping strategies that people used to respond to discrimination. More specifically, Saulo Fernández and colleagues (2012) showed not only that there was greater use of individual mobility strategies in Spain than in the United States, but also that in Spain there was a negative correlation between the success of the surgery (i.e., the longer people's limbs had become) and people's perceptions of discrimination. In other words, in Spain successful attempts at individual mobility reduced the negative impact of the discrimination that these dysplasia sufferers faced. In contrast, in the United States (where boundaries were perceived to be more impermeable), there was no such correlation between height and discrimination. Here, though (and only here), greater contact with other people with skeletal dysplasias buffered the negative effects of discrimination on respondents' perceived quality of life. It thus appears that in the United States (unlike Spain) because individuals with dysplasia perceived the boundaries between their group and taller people to be impermeable, they were more likely to resort to collective-level coping mechanisms in order to protect their health and well-being.

More generally, then, what we see is that the perceived permeability of group boundaries has important consequences for the strategies that people use to deal with stigma. However, the precise nature of this impact is also conditioned by features of the groups in question, particularly as these relate to the broader society in which the groups are embedded. What this means is that in order to understand the health-related consequences of efforts to deal with stigma, one needs to engage closely with what permeability *means* for group membership. Sometimes permeability will signal opportunities to escape stigma that will be good for health if they are successful but bad if they are not. But sometimes too, permeability can be a cue to dig one's heels in and join with others to resist pressure to become part of the non-stigmatised majority – a strategy that is nevertheless more common when boundaries are impermeable. Here stigma (e.g., associated with smoking or unhealthy eating) can be worn as a badge of pride, and group members gain a sense of identity and purpose precisely through their defiance.

Cognitive alternatives to the status quo

A final socio-structural factor that determines whether exclusion is appraised as being group based relates to perceptions that there is a possibility for discrimination to be eradicated in the future. Henri Tajfel (1978) used the term *"cognitive alternatives* to the status-quo" to describe such perceptions and defined these as arising in situations where minority group members become aware that "the existing social reality is not the only possible one and that alternatives to it are conceivable and perhaps attainable" (Tajfel, 1978, p. 93). The general point here, then, is that people are more likely to define themselves as a group and to work together to challenge stigma if they have a sense that their efforts are likely to bring fruit in the form of *social change*. In part, this reflects the fact that, in line with one of social identity theory's core hypotheses (the identity restoration hypothesis, H4; Tajfel & Turner, 1979), people are motivated to have positive rather than negative social identities (e.g., as possible winners rather than certain losers).

This was an issue that Airong Zhang and colleagues explored in research that looked at how students from low socio-economic backgrounds in rural China responded to disadvantage that severely limited their opportunities for education and hence for self-development (Zhang, Jetten, Iyer, & Cui, 2013; see also Jetten, Iyer, & Zhang, 2017). As we discussed in the previous chapter, historically, this has been a major issue in China with children from rural backgrounds routinely being denied access to high-quality education (Afridi, Li, & Ren, 2015). Across a range of school contexts, the researchers found that students were more likely to seek out educational opportunities, and to report higher self-esteem as a result, when new political policies served to communicate a sense that social change was now possible.

Consistent with the competition hypothesis (H7), such patterns suggest that perceptions of cognitive alternatives to the status quo tend to enhance people's willingness to engage in collective strategies to overcome stigma and that these can have both direct and indirect benefits for health and well-being. The direct effects flow from the change that such efforts can produce (e.g., better education); the indirect effects flow from the positive consequences of the process through which this is achieved (e.g., a sense of hopefulness, optimism, and self-efficacy; Reicher & Haslam, 2012). As leaders of the U.S. Civil Rights movement recognised, the rallying cry "we shall overcome" is as valuable for the sense of possibility it creates as it is for the change it ultimately produces (see Figure 4.7; Finlayson, 2003).

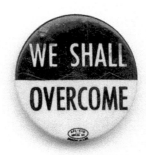

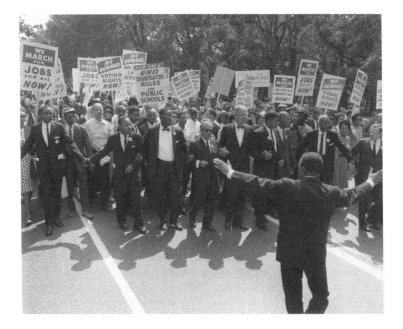

Figure 4.7 Cognitive alternatives have important direct and indirect benefits for health and well-being

Note: When people sense that there are possibilities for stigma and discrimination to be challenged and removed, they are more likely to come together to try to make this happen. This will have direct benefits by helping to address the problem, but also indirect benefits in giving them a sense of hope, optimism, and collective self-efficacy.

Source: The authors; Wikipedia

Social identity affects engagement with health services

In addition to group-based and identity factors that determine how minority members appraise and experience stigma and discrimination, there is evidence that membership in a stigmatised group affects people's engagement and utilisation of health care services. In particular, there is evidence that members of stigmatised groups either avoid or delay engaging with mental and physical health care services (Hommel, Madsen, & Kamper, 2012; see also Pendleton & Bochner, 1980). This can reflect fear of rejection, concerns about confirming negative stereotypes (the phenomenon of *social identity threat*; Branscombe et al., 1999; see Chapter 7), or simply a sense that 'these services are not for the likes of us" (Haslam, Reicher, & Levine, 2012).

Illustrative evidence emerges from research that found that Black women who identified strongly with their race were more likely to feel anxious in a health care setting than their White counterparts (Abdou & Fingerhut, 2014). This effect was particularly pronounced when there were cues in the context that made negative racial stereotypes salient (e.g., when there was an advertisement on the wall of a virtual doctor's waiting room that depicted Black women who had an unplanned pregnancy or AIDS). Clearly this heightened anxiety and an associated sense that one is 'not in the right place' may be a barrier to members of stigmatised minorities seeking out medical and other health professional care when they need it.

What is more, there is evidence of considerable mistrust in interactions between members of stigmatised groups and medical health professionals (Cuevas, O'Brien, & Saha, 2016; López-Cevallos, Harvey, & Warren, 2014) that is inimical to the development of shared identification. More generally, 'us' versus 'them' dynamics between health professionals and their clients can lead to suboptimal interactions in health care settings for at least two reasons. First, health professionals may treat clients from stigmatised groups differently than members of non-stigmatised groups (e.g., people of higher socio-economic status) with whom they would be more likely to share identity. As evidence of this point, Michelle Ryn and Jane Burke (2000) surveyed physicians after they had interacted with Black and White patients and asked them to estimate their levels of drug abuse, compliance with medical advice, intelligence, educational level, and rationality. Results showed that Caucasian doctors rated African American patients as less intelligent, less reliable, less likely to take medical advice, and more likely to engage in risky behaviour than fellow Caucasian patients. Furthermore, doctors (who are typically from higher SES backgrounds) rated patients from lower SES backgrounds more negatively than their higher SES counterparts in terms of their estimated levels of self-control, irrationality, and intelligence. In addition, lower SES patients were rated as less likely to be compliant with treatment plans, less likely to want to have a physically active lifestyle, and more likely to be at risk of having inadequate social support than higher SES patients. Importantly too, these effects for race and SES remained even after controlling for social demographic factors such as patient age, gender, socio-economic status, and degree of illness. Along related lines, other research shows that doctors tend to interact less with patients who are members of outgroups (e.g., as defined by ethnicity and class) than with those who are members of ingroups (Pendleton & Bochner, 1980). When they interact with members of stigmatised minorities, doctors have also been found to dominate the conversation and to provide less information than they do when they are dealing with ingroup patients (Dovidio et al., 2008; St. Claire & Clucas, 2012).

Second, and partly as a result of these same suboptimal interactions, members of stigmatised minority groups are less likely to listen to, and trust, doctors who are not members of their group (Dovidio et al., 2008). Evidence thus suggests that African American patients tend to be less satisfied with consultations, to be less likely to book an appointment, and to have lower rates of medical compliance when they have consultations with Caucasian rather than African American physicians (Williams, 2005). And although it is difficult to examine the long-term consequences of poor doctor–patient relationships (in part because where these are bad, the relationship is non-existent), it seems likely that low levels of mutual trust have ongoing impact on the health of those who are members of stigmatised minority groups. In this way, rather than being curative, their exposure to medical health services can sometimes prove toxic.

Conclusion

We started this chapter with the observation that for those who belong to stigmatised groups, their group membership is often both a curse and the cure to that curse. Indeed, it is precisely because these individuals belong to groups that are tainted that it is much harder to derive a positive identity from their social group memberships than it is for an individual who belongs to a group that is more main-stream, or that benefits from a privileged status in society.

However, it is also clear that members of stigmatised groups hardly ever accept their fate at face value. Moreover, it is clear that it is often the stigmatised group itself that proves crucial in determining whether stigma drags a person (and their health) down or else is the means by which they (and their health) are lifted up. In particular, there is now abundant evidence that when individuals turn towards a stigmatised group, identify with it, and draw social support from its members, their health will be protected against some of the more negative consequences of discrimination. Importantly though, groups are not equally suited or well placed to provide the psychological resources that individual members need to counter the negative effects of stigma on health and well-being. Accordingly, in order to understand the implications of stigma for health and well-being, theorists and practitioners need to attend to both group-specific factors (e.g., related to identity content) and the broader socio-structural context (e.g., to observe the pervasiveness of discrimination, the permeability of group boundaries, and the presence of cognitive alternatives to the status quo). For it is these elements which ultimately deter-mine whether stigma serves to erode or to enhance social identity – and hence whether it is implicated in a recipe for ruin or a road to recovery.

Points for practice

Working with clients who are members of stigmatised groups is often a major challenge for health practitioners. One reason for this is that practitioners themselves often come from priv-ileged (or at least non-stigmatised) groups and so professional services are delivered across an intergroup divide. In this context, the following three points are important to bear in mind.

1. *Social identification can provide an important basis for members of stigmatised groups to come together and challenge their stigma in ways that are beneficial for their health.* It fol-lows that health professionals can help to redress some of the problems that stigma causes by providing opportunities for stigmatised clients to develop social identification.
2. *If members of stigmatised groups are aware of, and embrace, cognitive alternatives to the status quo, this is likely to have positive consequences for their health and well-being.* One of the reasons for this is that having a sense of cognitive alternatives encourages people to work with others to overcome their challenges rather than to resign themselves to discrim-ination and disadvantage.
3. *It is essential to recognise and try to address the identity-related barriers that members of stigmatised groups experience when interacting with health care services.* These barriers come in a range of forms, but relate to the fact that the social identities of health care users and providers are often very different. Sweeping these differences under the carpet or imag-ining that they do not exist is unlikely to contribute to therapeutic progress.

Resources

Further reading

The following papers provide a good introduction to work that explores the links between stigma, discrimination, and health.

① Branscombe, N. R., Schmitt, M. T., & Harvey, R. D. (1999). Perceiving pervasive discrimination among African Americans: Implications for group identification and well-being. *Journal of Personality and Social Psychology, 77*, 135–149.

This paper introduces the rejection–identification model in the context of an examination of African Americans' experiences of discrimination.

② Jetten, J., Iyer, A., Branscombe, N. R., & Zhang, A. (2013). How the disadvantaged appraise group-based exclusion: The path from legitimacy to illegitimacy. *European Review of Social Psychology, 24*, 194–224.

This review examines the conditions that lead to discrimination being seen as illegitimate rather than legitimate. It shows that social identity theory provides a good way of understanding this process as well as its consequences for health and well-being.

③ Paradies, Y., Ben, J., Denson, N., Elias, A., Priest, N., Pieterse A., . . . Gee, G. (2015). Racism as a determinant of health: A systematic review and meta-analysis. *PLoS ONE, 10*(9), e0138511.

This meta-analysis systematically examines a wealth of evidence concerning the relationship between racism and health. It examines data from nearly 300 studies and shows that the experience of race-based discrimination has a range of negative consequences for both mental and physical health, but also that the strength of this relationship varies across different ethnic groups.

Video

① Search for "stigma and mental illness" to watch a video by the IWK Health Centre and the Mental Health Commission of Canada (MHCC) on the impact of stigma related to mental illness on diagnosis and health. The video also addresses the importance of social support: www.youtube.com/watch?v=LTIZ_aizzyk   (11 minutes)
② Search for "stigma social and self" to see a short video that talks about the importance of social support for countering the negative effects that social stigma has on mental health on well-being. www.youtube.com/watch?v=_jz7yo7L3Z0   (11 minutes)
③ Search for "stigma of brain injury and rehabilitation" to watch a one-hour video which explores of the consequences of stigma for people with brain injury (an issue that we also explore in Chapter 11): www.youtube.com/watch?v=WBU5K4lgCw0   (65 minutes)

Websites

The following articles on the way that stigma causes isolation and suffering and the way that social support can be essential to overcoming the negative health effects of stigma are worth reading:

① https://theconversation.com/how-australias-discrimination-laws-and-public-health-campaigns-perpetuate-fat-stigma-80471. In this piece, the author, Dr Cat Pausé, outlines the consequences of fat stigma and describes how discrimination against overweight individuals is legitimate in the Western world.
② www.vice.com/en_us/article/ywgqgg/for-older-hiv-positive-people-social-support-can-save-lives. Older people who are HIV positive often face isolation. This article stresses

the importance of social support provided by buddy programmes whereby volunteers are paired with someone who is HIV positive.

③ http://newsinfo.inquirer.net/870725/standing-up-for-little-people. This article on people with achondroplasia that causes dwarfism sheds light on the problem of stigma for individuals who have this condition. The article also covers how people with the condition find support at the annual summits organised by the organisation "Little People of America".

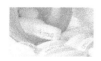

Chapter 5

Stress

Life is full of potential sources of stress. These range from everyday hassles such as preparing for an exam, managing multiple demands on one's time, or dealing with a difficult boss, through to far more substantial challenges such as being exposed to constant abuse, undergoing major surgery, or having a job that routinely puts you in life-threatening situations. Reflecting on such experiences, it is clear too that there is a large amount of variability in the way that people deal with them. This is seen, for example, in some of our own early research on stress in which we were interested in the stress-related experiences of people going through some of the more substantial challenges mentioned above – specifically, patients undergoing heart surgery and bomb disposal officers whose work involved constant exposure to danger (see Figure 5.1; Haslam, O'Brien, Jetten, Penna, & Vormedal, 2005). Surprisingly perhaps, many of the people we studied reported finding the experience of these most demanding of circumstances far less stressful than one might expect. Typically, though, those who responded most positively reported receiving a lot of support from their family or from colleagues.

Such observations raise a range of intriguing questions. What leads different people (or the same person at different times) to vary in the degree to which they find exactly the same situation stressful? How do people succeed in coping with the stress that certain life events entail? And speaking specifically to the issues of social identity that we are concerned with in this book as a whole, what role do groups play in this process?

As we will see, and as the earlier examples attest, groups and associated social identities turn out to be critical to this story. In particular, this is because they shape not only the way that we understand potentially stressful events, but also the way we respond to them. And as our research with surgical patients and bomb disposal officers suggested, a key reason for this is that the support they provide turns out to be a major determinant of whether we succumb to stress or else overcome it.

Current approaches to understanding stress

The biomedical model: the importance of physiology and adaptation

Stress can be defined as the *strain* that is imposed on a person by *stressors* in the environment that are perceived to be in some way threatening to the self. These stressors can take many different forms, including poor living or working conditions, adverse life events, fraught relationships, or unreasonable demands. Moreover, such threats can prove difficult – and in extreme cases impossible – to bear. From the inception of work on stress in the 1930s, a major goal of researchers has thus been to understand exactly how people respond to the slings and arrows that life throws at them.

Early work that had this goal was informed by a *biomedical model* which took the view that, as they are exposed to increasing strain, people (and organisms more generally) go through a defined series of stages. The work of the physiologist Hans Selye (1946, 1956) was particularly influential in this regard. This argued that stress responses entail three distinct phases which form part of what he termed the *general adaptation syndrome* (GAS).

The first of these phases is one of *alarm* (or shock) in which the person registers a threat and experiences a state of physiological arousal. This in turn triggers a second stage of *countershock* in which they become more aroused in the context of attempting to counteract the stressor. Depending on the success of such attempts, this can then develop into *resistance*. A key point, however, is that this second stage places heavy demands on the person because it requires them to expend mental

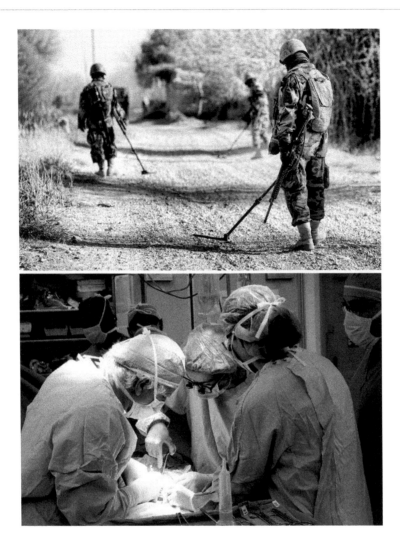

Figure 5.1 Stressful experiences? Doing bomb disposal work and undergoing heart surgery

Note: Unsurprisingly, both these experiences have the potential to be a major source of stress. However, research by Haslam et al. (2005) shows that this tends to be lower among people who identify with relevant groups and who, as a result, perceive themselves to receive greater social support.

Source: Crown copyright; Pixabay

and physical resources – what Selye termed *adaptation energy* – to try to restore equilibrium to their physiological system. If they succeed, the overall experience of stress can actually be positive and the person achieves a state that is referred to either as *salutogenesis* or *eustress* (the opposite of distress). However, if they fail, or the resistance process continues for too long, then the person enters a third *exhaustion* phase in which their adaptation energy is depleted, equilibrium cannot be restored, and they are no longer able to function effectively.

Bleak as this picture is, the developmental pattern outlined by Selye (1956) is certainly one that many people do go through – not least as they struggle with the demands of the modern life. In particular, since the 1970s, a massive literature has built up which identifies exhaustion as one component of a chronic form of stress referred to as *burnout*. The other two components of the burnout syndrome are *lack of accomplishment* and *callousness* (or depersonalisation), and when combined with exhaustion these are seen to represent a potent threat both to individual health and group functioning (e.g., Jackson, Schwab, & Schuler, 1986; Maslach & Jackson, 1981). Moreover, because exhaustion is so corrosive for the physiological system – compromising neurochemical, hormonal, and immunological functioning – it can also lead to a range of adverse long-term health outcomes. These include heart disease, stroke, kidney damage, failure of the digestive and immune systems, and even cancer and early death (Eyer & Sterling, 1977; Sklar & Anisman, 1981).

Although the picture that the medical model paints is pretty bleak, it is worth noting that there is nothing inevitable about the three-stage GAS process outlined by Selye. Most obviously, this is because if the resistance process proves successful, then people's overall experience of stress can actually be positive. This, indeed, is a pattern that Peter Suedfeld has observed in studies of groups who willingly expose themselves to extreme stressors (e.g., mountain climbers, polar explorers, astronauts; Palinkas & Suedfeld, 2008; Suedfeld, 1997). More generally too, one might question whether a life that was entirely stress free would actually be worth living.

Nevertheless, the question of what determines whether people are able to successfully resist particular stressors is largely unresolved by the biomedical model. When do people crack up under strain and when do they triumph over it? And, more particularly, why?

The dispositional model: the role of personality and individual differences

Apart from anything else, asking the above questions invites us to acknowledge that stress is not simply a physiological process but also a psychological one. And in asking why some people succumb to stress and others do not, one obvious answer is that some people are simply made of sterner stuff.

In this vein, there is a long tradition of research in psychology that has sought to investigate the role of individual differences as predictors of stress. One particularly significant contribution was made in the 1950s by two cardiologists, Meyer Friedman and Ray Rosenman. As legend has it, in their work they were struck by the fact that the people who reported to their clinic with various heart-related problems were defined not so much by their medical history (e.g., whether or not they exercised or smoked) but whether or not they were of a particular *type* (Friedman & Rosenman, 1974). More specifically, they observed that people with coronary heart disease (CHD) tended to be more hostile, aggressive, demanding, irritable, and ambitious than their other patients. Friedman and Rosenman dubbed this constellation of attributes the *Type A* behaviour pattern (TABP) and contrasted it with the more laid-back and relaxed behaviour pattern that they referred to as *Type B* (TBBP).

More recently, this analysis has been refined somewhat, with researchers arguing that rather than being distinct types, TABP and TBBP are two ends of a continuum. It is also suggested that the reason people at one end of this are more prone to illness is that they have more intense and hostile reactions to various life stressors (Motowidlo, Packard, & Manning, 1986). Nevertheless, the underlying argument remains that some people have a more intense (and hence potentially stress-inducing) approach to life than others and that this therefore puts them at greater risk of serious illness. Indeed, on the basis of their ground-breaking 8-year study Friedman and Rosenman (1959) concluded that having TABP approximately doubled a person's likelihood of being diagnosed with CHD.

Yet despite the fact that it has been a major focus for research on stress and health for nearly 50 years, evidence linking TABP to poor health outcomes is mixed at best. To some extent this stems from a lack of clarity about how best to measure the construct and from evidence that different methods of assessment produce different results – partly because various components of the construct (e.g., hostility and ambitiousness) do not correlate highly. It also reflects the fact that, however it is measured, the relationship between TABP and relevant outcomes (e.g., stress and health) is both quite variable and generally low. Adding to this, the research proved to be very controversial once it emerged that Friedman and Rosenman's work had been heavily funded by the tobacco industry. The funding was provided because this line of research could be used to support the argument that the link between smoking and heart disease is unclear because studies generally fail to control for TABP (Landman, Cortese, & Glantz, 2008).

Seeking to resolve some of this controversy, Myrtek (2001) conducted a meta-analysis of all prospective studies that had attempted to link TABP to hostility and heart disease. Tellingly, this showed that TABP accounted for almost none (0.03%) of the variance in CHD. Moreover, although there was a significant relationship between TABP and hostility, TABP accounted for only 2.2% of the variance in hostility – a figure "so low that it has . . . no practical meaning for prediction and prevention" (Myrtek, 2001, p. 245).

Findings such as these have meant that in recent years research seeking to understand the relationship between personality, stress, and health has diversified considerably. This has involved consideration of a broad array of candidate personality factors that might be implicated in people's experience of stress. Principal amongst these are (1) hardiness (Funk, 1992), (2) self-efficacy (Bandura, 1982), (3) self-esteem (Dumont & Provost, 1999), and (4) neuroticism (Gunthert, Cohen, & Armeli, 1999). Again, though, relationships between measures of these constructs and stress are "typically not very strong" (Semmer & Meier, 2003, p. 83). Moreover, there is some circularity in the argument that stress is explained by a person's possession of such characteristics, since in many ways the characteristics themselves simply describe what it is that needs to be understood. So, for example, a person's agreement with the item "I have a hard time making it through stressful events" (from Smith et al.'s, 2008, brief resilience scale; see Appendix for further details) does not *explain* their stress, it merely describes and measures it. Relatedly, where personality factors are involved in the stress process, it also seems likely that this will often be as an *outcome* rather than as input. So, for example, it may not be neuroticism that makes a person stressed, but the experience of stress that makes them neurotic. Thus although research in this tradition provides us with a useful set of terms for talking about a person's stress (e.g., "he's very hardy", "she's very Type A"), it leaves unanswered the all-important question as to what it is that makes a person have particular stress-related characteristics in the first place.

The situational model: the role of life events

If stress is not the result of dispositional factors, one obvious alternative is that it results from the situations in which people find themselves. Along these lines, we might not be surprised to discover that a young woman was more stressed when she was preparing for an important exam than when she was lying on the beach, or that a police officer was generally more stressed than a librarian. Speaking to such observations, a number of researchers have sought to develop methods for quantifying the amount of stress that is associated both with particular life events and with particular professions. This quasi-actuarial activity has led to the construction of various tables in which a range of events and occupations are ranked in terms of their inherent stressfulness.

Of the former, one of the most well known and still very widely used is Thomas Holmes and Richard Rahe's (1967) *Social Readjustment Rating Scale* (SRRS). This was constructed by asking a convenience sample of nearly 400 participants (most of whom were White Protestants) to rate a list of 43 events in terms of the amount of readjustment they required relative to the anchor of "marriage", which was given an arbitrary value of 50. On the basis of the data they collected, the authors were therefore able to construct a table which ranked events in terms of the degree to which they demanded more or less readjustment relative to this anchor – with those at the top demanding more readjustment and hence being more likely to be a source of illness-inducing stress.

Holmes and Rahe's (1967) table makes for quite interesting reading, and is partially reproduced in Table 5.1. From this, one can see that marriage itself came seventh in a table that was topped by

Table 5.1 Selected events in the Social Readjustment Rating Scale

Ranking	Life event	Mean value
1.	Death of spouse	100
2.	Divorce	73
3.	Marital separation	65
4.	Jail term	63
5.	Death of close family member	63
6.	Personal injury or illness	53
7.	Marriage (anchor)	50
8.	Fired at work	47
9.	Marital reconciliation	45
10.	Retirement	45
11.	Change in health of family member	44
12.	Pregnancy	40
19.	Change in number of arguments with spouse	35
24.	Trouble with in-laws	29
26.	Wife begins or stops work	26
27.	Begin or end school	26
32.	Change in residence	20
35.	Change in church activities	19
41.	Vacation	13
42.	Christmas	12
43.	Minor violations of the law	11

Source: Holmes and Rahe (1967)

the death of a spouse and divorce. Interestingly, marital reconciliation also figured prominently, as did change in (rather than simply frequency of) the number of arguments that a person has with their spouse. Vacations and Christmas are towards the bottom of the list, but it is apparent that these were not seen as entirely stress free.

The SRRS has been, and continues to be, enormously influential, and like other instruments of this form, it has proved to have general utility for practitioners in helping them to assess general levels of risk. For example, knowing that a person's partner has died allows one to know that they are likely to be experiencing considerable distress and that they are at increased risk of depression (e.g., Clayton & Darvish, 1979). Moreover, a large number of prospective studies have shown that the more events on the SRRS that a person experiences within a given time frame (e.g., a year), the more likely they are to report psychological and psychosomatic symptoms of stress (e.g., Myers, Lindenthal, & Pepper, 1971; for a recent review see Thoits, 2013).

Nevertheless, such an approach has a number of problems (Dohrenwend, 2006). Some are procedural (e.g., How recent or severe does an event need to be to be reported? How representative is a given instance of a particular class of event?), some are psychometric (e.g., What does a given value actually mean? To what extent are events independent?), and some arise from the fact that scales of this form are always the product of a particular culture at a particular point in time (e.g., for Holmes and Rahe, one in which particular attitudes towards marriage and women's employment prevailed). At a deeper level too, it is apparent that the general patterns that such tables reveal are hard to interpret without a specific understanding of the lives of the people to whom they apply. For example, the amount of stress involved in getting married must surely depend on the nature of the relationship between the people involved. And this, too, must change as a function of other contextual factors (e.g., the nature of people's relationships with their families, the cost, the weight of cultural expectations).

Together, these various problems have meant that despite the inherent plausibility of the link between adverse life events and stress, as Peggy Thoits (2013) observes, "correlations between life change and psychological (and physical) disorder have been disappointingly low" (p. 42). One way in which researchers have attempted to overcome this problem is to break down the various events and experiences that contribute to stress in a particular domain (e.g., the school, the home, the office) into their constituent parts. In the workplace, for example, beyond crude indices which suggest that being a miner or a police officer is generally more stressful than being a vicar or a librarian (Cooper, 1995), researchers have identified distinct categories of experience that contribute to stress. Illustrative of this approach, Susan Cartwright and Carey Cooper (1997) identify six distinct sets of factors that contribute to work-related stress: (1) intrinsic job features (e.g., working conditions), (2) organisational roles (e.g., those entailing responsibility and ambiguity), (3) work relationships (e.g., with one's boss or one's peers), (4) career development (e.g., being promoted, moved, or made redundant), (5) organisational factors (e.g., the culture and leadership), and (6) the work–home interface (e.g., as a source of balance, or conflict).

Despite the appeal of such an approach, the problems identified earlier reappear at whatever level of abstraction one chooses to focus on. In a workplace context, this can be illustrated by reflecting on classic research on the link between working conditions and well-being conducted by the pioneering organisational psychologist Hugo Münsterberg at the start of the 20th century. Part of Münsterberg's research was conducted in factories where one might imagine that various features of the work – such as having to perform the monotonous task of packing light bulbs into cartons inside a dreary warehouse – would be a recipe for high levels of job dissatisfaction and stress. Yet when Münsterberg (1913) interviewed the factory workers, he found enormous variability in their responses to this work, with one woman finding it "really interesting" and "full of constant variation" (even though she packed 13,000 bulbs a day; p. 196). At the same time, Münsterberg noted that many people who supposedly had very exciting jobs (e.g., as teachers, doctors, and lawyers) reported finding their work extremely dull. The important point that he took from all this was that what matters for stress is not so much the *objective* features of a given situation, but rather a person's *subjective* experience of it. He also noted that the groups that people are part of have an important role to play in this experience as a result of their capacity to "enhance the consciousness of solidarity amongst the labourers and their feelings of security" (1913, p. 234). Again, then, such insights reinforce the point that it is impossible to understand stress without engaging fully with its social psychological underpinnings.

The transactional model: the role of appraisals of threat and support

Although Münsterberg's observations are not widely heralded, they anticipated major developments in theorising about stress that only took place in the latter part of the same century. Moving away from the idea that certain events are inherently stressful, these focused on the fact that people's *perceptions and cognitions* are central to the experience of stress and that they are both fluid and negotiable.

The trailblazing work in this area was conducted by Richard Lazarus in the 1960s, later in collaboration with Susan Folkman (e.g., Lazarus, 1966, 2006; Lazarus & Folkman, 1984). The starting point for this was research which involved monitoring the blood pressure and self-reported stress levels of participants who had been asked to watch films of people in traumatic situations (e.g., having an accident in an industrial workshop). These were pretty gruesome and therefore potentially quite distressing to watch. Certainly, this was the experience of participants in control conditions who watched the films without being told anything more about them. However, in various experimental conditions, Lazarus and colleagues gave participants information which encouraged them to see the films as less threatening. For example, in the 'denial' condition of one study (Lazarus, 1966) participants were told that the people in the film were simply actors, whereas in an 'intellectual' condition they were told that the people were actors and that the film had been made to teach people about workplace safety. As expected, participants in these two conditions – and particularly those in the intellectual condition – showed fewer signs of stress than those in a control condition.

For Lazarus, the key point that these studies made was that the stress-related implications of a particular stimulus situation are not a direct product of its objective features. Instead, he argued that the experience of stress is always heavily structured by a person's *cognitive appraisal* of a given stressor (see also Tomak, Blascovich, Kelsey, & Leitten, 1993). This insight ultimately led to the formulation of the *transactional model of stress* (Lazarus & Folkman, 1984). This argues that stress depends on two particular forms of appraisal that occur in response to a potentially self-threatening stimulus situation. *Primary appraisal* involves a person working out whether a given stimulus is threatening to their well-being. *Secondary appraisal* involves them working out whether or not they are able to cope with such a threat. Accordingly, upon exposure to a potentially stressful stimulus, a person will only experience stress when primary appraisal leads them to think that the stimulus is harmful or threatening and when secondary appraisal leads them to think that they do not have the necessary coping resources to deal with the harm or the threat (see Figure 5.2).

Both primary and secondary appraisal are complex evaluative processes. Both reflect a person's understanding of themselves and their environment, but secondary appraisal also involves their assessment of coping resources and options (e.g., opportunities for denial or avoidance) and of likely outcomes (Lazarus & Folkman, 1984). It is worth noting too that coping strategies are not always effective. Indeed, some – in particular, denial and avoidance which involve failing to deal directly with the stressor – can ultimately increase stress in the long run (Carver, 1995). Nevertheless, a negative stress

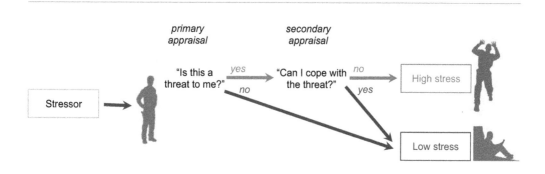

Figure 5.2 A schematic representation of the transactional model of stress

Note: Rather than being sequential, primary and secondary appraisal are dynamically interrelated. This means that just as primary appraisal has a bearing on secondary appraisal, so too secondary appraisal can affect primary appraisal (because feeling that you are not able to cope with a threat tends to make it more threatening). However, in the interests of simplicity, this link is not shown in this figure.

response is most likely when a person perceives their coping resources to be inadequate. Amongst other things, this is because primary and secondary appraisal are not independent but feed into each other. This means that just as stress-enhancing primary appraisal ('This is threatening') can promote stress-enhancing secondary appraisal ('I can't cope'), so too stress-enhancing secondary appraisal ('I can't cope') can promote stress-enhancing primary appraisal ('This is threatening').

One of the most important foci for work on secondary appraisal is research that explores the role of *social support* as a key process that helps people to cope with stress (Aspinwall & Taylor, 1997; Cohen & Wills, 1985; Underwood, 2000). More specifically, it is argued that there are four key forms of support that people (e.g., friends, family, or health professionals) can provide that help to ameliorate a person's stress (House, 1981). First, they can provide *instrumental* support by giving material resources or financial assistance; second they can provide *emotional* support, for example, by affirming a person's sense of self-worth; third, they can provide *companionship* through affiliative social contact; fourth, they can provide *informational* support such as practical information about the nature of their problems and ways to address them.

When they are effective, these various forms of support can result in people feeling that they are cared for and valued by others and that they are "part of a network of mutual assistance and obligations" (Taylor, 2007, p. 145). Nevertheless, despite the potential for coping to be facilitated in this way, evidence suggests that the actual impact of social support is decidedly mixed. For example, a meta-analysis by Ralf Schwarzer and Anja Leppin (1991) examined the relationship between social support and health and coping in 88 studies that included over 60,000 participants. Although a majority of these studies found that a person's receipt of social support was associated with positive health outcomes, around one-fifth of them revealed the opposite pattern. Moreover, most relationships were very small. Indeed, in around 80% of studies social support explained no more than 1% of the variance in coping and health.

One key reason why the receipt of support is not a good predictor of successful coping is that it is not particularly highly correlated with *perceptions* of support. Indeed, a meta-analysis of 23 studies by Mason Haber and colleagues (2007) found that the size of the average correlation between received and perceived social support was only moderate ($r = .35$; Haber, Cohen, Lucas, & Baltes, 2007). In other words, variation in how much social support a person receives only explains about 12% of the variation in how much social support they actually experience receiving. As the authors conclude, this makes it "unlikely . . . that received support is the primary constituent factor in perceived support" (Haber et al, 2007, p. 139). Amongst other things, this can be because "behaviours that are designated a priori as supportive may not be subjectively desirable to the recipient, perhaps because they are performed begrudgingly, or by persons not otherwise perceived as supportive" (Procidano, 1992, p. 2).

However, when the actions of other people *are* seen as supportive, they turn out to be quite a good predictor of effective coping. This point emerges from influential research into people's responses to natural disasters conducted by Fran Norris and Krzysztof Kaniasty (1996). Their research investigated people's stress in the wake of two devastating hurricanes – Hurricane Hugo and Hurricane Andrew – that hit the United States in early 1989 and 1992. What they found was that the relationship between the amount of support people received and their level of distress was fully mediated by perceptions of received support. In other words, it was only when support was actually perceived to be supportive that it played a role in ameliorating stress. Likewise, a systematic review by Sheldon Cohen and Thomas Wills (1985) confirmed that it is not the *actual* availability of support that promotes coping, but its *perceived* availability.

Evidence of the importance of perceived support is again consistent with the basic tenets of the transactional approach which speak to the capacity for the very same set of circumstances to induce very different stress reactions – not just in different people but in the same person at different times. In this, it highlights some of the core problems with simple dispositional or situational models and affirms Hamlet's observation – after Rosencrantz and Guildenstern objected to his suggestion that Denmark seemed like a prison – that "there is nothing either good or bad, but thinking makes it so".

This point is nicely illustrated by Suedfeld (1997) in an examination of changes in attitudes towards flotation tanks over time. In the 1950s these were thought to be the ultimate tool for subjecting another person to stress because they were thought to deprive them of sensory experience and thereby strip away their identity. For example, Donald Wexler and his colleagues saw them as ideally suited for investigation of the origins of psychosis and had to equip the tanks with panic buttons and pay anxious participants handsomely to encourage them to enter them (Wexler, Mendelson, Leiderman, & Solomon, 1958). Yet in the 1990s the tanks were rediscovered as relaxation tools, ideal for transporting people away from their everyday woes. As a result, today people are happy to lay out large sums of money for the privilege of using them as an integral part of upmarket stress-management programmes. Indeed, whereas Wexler and colleagues' research saw flotation tanks as ideal places to induce stress, more recent research suggests they are ideal places to escape it (Kjellgren, Lyden, & Norlander, 2008; Suedfeld & Bow, 1999).

Speaking to the idea that there are important *cultural* influences on perceptions of particular stimuli as stressful, it is worth noting too that there are a range of syndromes whereby – at a given place and time – groups of people come to *share* specific stress-related complaints. This is seen in the spread of so-called 'mass psychogenic illnesses' such as sick building syndrome (SBS; Redlich, Sparer, & Cullen, 1997) and repetitive strain injury (RSI; van Tulder, Malmivaara, & Koes, 2007). In the case of sick building syndrome people in the same work environment typically report headaches, respiratory difficulties, and nausea; in the case of repetitive strain injury, they experience aches and pain in the upper limbs. Although these conditions undoubtedly have physical substrates, it is also apparent that their spread and amplification follow the contours of shared identity (e.g., within a particular workplace or community; Kirmayer, 1999).

At one level, of course, epidemics of this form can simply be attributed to people's common experiences (e.g., of poor working conditions). In other words, such conditions undoubtedly have a grounding in objective features of the environment. At the same time, though, it appears that context-specific *group processes* – in particular, those of social interaction and social influence – lead to particular experiences being given a common label and acquiring specific meanings within a given community at a particular point in time (Bartholomew & Wessely, 2002). This in turn points to the fact that there is a significant *social* dimension to stress but one that tends to be somewhat under-theorised in the transactional model (Folkman & Moskowitz, 2004; Haslam, 2004). Accordingly, although the transactional approach makes an essential contribution to the field, there is scope for its insights to inform broader theoretical analysis that integrates and explains both personal and social aspects of the stress process.

The social identity approach to stress

Social identity is a determinant of primary stress appraisal

As we noted earlier, the key strength of the transactional model is that it offers a clear and compelling conceptualisation of stress as a psychological process in which people's subjective experience is central. Nevertheless, as Folkman and Moskovitz (2004, p. 758) acknowledge, a shortcoming of the approach is that the analysis of the person that lies at the heart of the model is relatively individualistic. That is, in common with most stress research, it focuses primarily on appraisal as a process that relates to personal identity. This means that questions of primary and secondary appraisal are phrased largely in the first-person singular ("Is this a threat to *me*?", "Can *I* cope with the threat?; see Figure 5.2).

In this regard, as we discussed in Chapter 2, one of the first points that the social identity approach alerts us to is that appraisal can also relate to a person's social identity, and hence these same questions can also be phrased in the first-person plural (i.e., "Is this a threat to *us in the bomb squad* – or to me *as a member of the bomb squad*?", "Can *we* cope with the threat?"). Moreover, it seems reasonable to suppose that in a range of contexts it is answers to these sorts of questions that will be of primary importance in determining a person's stress-related response. For example, the reason that Australian soldiers travelled to Europe to take part in the First World War was not because the Kaiser and his armies were a personal threat to them, but rather because they threatened an important social identity that they perceived themselves as sharing with other members of the British Empire. Likewise, for an infantryman on the front line, appraisal of his ability to cope with any threat is likely to be informed more by assessment of the resources and strategies of his military unit than by an assessment of those that he alone has at his disposal.

More formally, this leads us to hypothesise that stress appraisal will vary as a function of self-categorization. More specifically, to the extent that features of the prevailing social context lead a person to self-categorize in terms of a given social (rather than personal) identity (i.e., as specified in Chapter 2, see Figures 2.3 and 2.4), their primary and secondary appraisals should be shaped more by the circumstances of a relevant ingroup than by their personal circumstances.

One of the first studies to explore this possibility was conducted by Mark Levine and Steve Reicher (1996) and involved them asking sports science students to report how distressing a range of different physical injuries would be and how much each would adversely affect their lives. Some of these injuries were particularly threatening to the participants' sport identities (e.g., a damaged knee), whereas others were particularly threatening to the identity of the women participants (e.g., a facial scar). Before providing these ratings, though, the experimenters introduced a manipulation of social identity salience that involved some of the students being told that the study was intended to compare the responses of men and women (thereby making their gender identity salient), whereas others were told that it involved comparing sports people with other professionals (thereby making their sports identity salient).

Levine and Reicher hypothesised that participants' primary appraisal of the different injuries would vary as a function of the experimental manipulation so that a given injury would be perceived as more distressing when it threatened a salient social identity. Their findings provided clear support for this prediction (see also Levine, 1999, Experiment 1). In particular, when their identity as sports science students was salient, both women and men saw injuries that were threatening to women to be quite trivial, but when gender identity was salient, women perceived these same injuries to be much more distressing, whereas men saw them as more trivial.

Findings from a series of subsequent studies supported similar conclusions (Levine, 1999). Amongst other things, these served to demonstrate that responses to identity-related threats depend on the specific meaning that an identity assumes in a given setting. Thus, in an experiment where men in a rugby club were asked to evaluate the seriousness of a range of injuries, the men were again keen to downplay the seriousness of injuries that would be threatening to women, but this was especially apparent when they thought their responses were being compared to those of 'new age' men. Levine argued that this was because here the rugby players perceived their distinctive male identity to be under threat and hence were especially keen to emphasise their own masculinity by downplaying the seriousness of these threats.

A related point emerges from some of our own research to which we have alluded already. This examined how members of different occupational groups appraise the stresses of their work (Haslam et al., 2005) – specifically, how bomb disposal officers and bar staff feel about the challenges of diffusing bombs or working in noisy bars for long periods. As we noted at the start of this chapter, one of the most striking findings of the study was that bomb disposal officers reported finding the business of diffusing bombs to be particularly *un*stressful (compared to doing bar work and compared to the way bar staff felt about this activity). One reason for this was that it was an activity that they had habituated to and *normalised* as a group (as a form of *acceptance coping*; see Britt, Crane, Hodson, & Adler, 2016). A second reason was that dealing with bombs was something that affirmed these participants' social identity – as members of a distinctive and elite professional group – and hence made them feel good about themselves.

Such findings point to the limitations of situational approaches that attempt to quantify the stress of a given life event or a given profession independently of people's actual experiences. At the same time, a more subtle point that emerges from this work is that beyond simply being subjective, stress appraisal can be (and often is) *inter-subjective* in the sense that it is structured by social identities that are *shared* (to varying degrees) with other people. One further consequence of this is that appraisal should also be affected by the appraisals of other people, as well as by who those people are. In other words, appraisal should be subject to *social influence* along the lines of hypotheses that we set out in Chapter 2 (i.e., H9 and H10).

This proposition was initially tested in a study that two of us conducted with Anne O'Brien and Elissa Jacobs which involved students completing a range of potentially stress-inducing mathematical exercises in a limited time (Haslam, Jetten, O'Brien, & Jacobs, 2004). Along the lines of Lazarus and Folkman's (1984) classic studies, we were interested in how participants' experiences of stress varied as a function of the ways in which they were encouraged to appraise the task. This was manipulated by asking them to watch a video before they did the exercises in which a woman who had supposedly performed them previously described her experience. In one 'threat' version of the video she said that she had found the tasks very stressful, but in another 'intellectual' version she indicated that she had found them to be quite enjoyable – seeing them as character building rather than threatening in any way. Critically, though, some participants were told that the woman in the video was a fellow student like them (i.e., an ingroup member), whereas others were told that she was someone with a stress disorder (an outgroup member).

Along the lines of the transactional model, participants were predicted to find the exercises more stressful when the content of the video had primed the students to appraise them as threatening. But it was also predicted that this would only be true when participants saw the woman in the video to be representative of a salient ingroup. This is what was found. Thus participants generally reported greater anxiety and physiological arousal when the video presented a threat message rather than an intellectual one – but this effect was only statistically significant when the person presenting the message was an ingroup member.

A similar pattern was also subsequently observed by Jetten and colleagues in a study where ingroup–outgroup membership was defined in terms of gender (Jetten, Haslam, Iyer, & Haslam, 2010a) and in a study of physiological responses to pain in which reassurance was (or was not) provided by students who were studying the same or a different subject than participants (Platow et al., 2007; see Chapter 12). Further physiological evidence to support a social identity analysis was also provided in a more recent study by Johanna Häusser and colleagues (Häusser, Kattenstroth, van Dick, & Mojzisch, 2012). This found that when they had to perform a stressful public-speaking exercise (as part of the widely used Trier Social Stress Test for groups; Von Dawans, Kirschbaum, & Heinrichs, 2011), students' cortisol levels were significantly lower – indicative of a lower level of stress – if their social (rather than personal) identity had previously been made salient through a task that reinforced their connection to fellow students.

Challenging the view that stress appraisal is determined by information in the abstract, such findings suggest that it is a more nuanced process in which the cognitive processing of information is structured by the meaning that information has in relation to a perceiver's currently salient identity. This means that the success of attempts to encourage a person to construe a potential stressor in a particular way does not depend simply on the quality of the information they have access to. Instead, it also depends both on that information being seen to be relevant to a salient identity and on the source of that information being perceived to be representative of that identity (and hence to be qualified to inform perceivers about relevant features of their social world; Turner, 1991).

The fact that these conditions are not always met helps to explain why campaigns and treatments that are designed to reduce stress by promoting positive appraisal do not always meet with success. Indeed, they can sometimes backfire. An example of this happening occurred in the 1980s when the British government led by Margaret Thatcher published *Protect and Survive*, a pamphlet designed to explain to citizens how they might deal with the threat of nuclear attack. Rather than quell fear, the pamphlet fuelled it, partly because it alerted the public to the possibility that the actions of the government were increasing rather than reducing this threat (Cordle, 2012; see also Kearon, Mythen, & Walklate, 2007).

We noted earlier that a key determinant of secondary appraisal – the ability to cope with a given stressor – is a person's perception that they are in a position to benefit from social support (e.g., Cohen & Wills, 1985; Underwood, 2000). The relevance of the social identity approach to this issue should be apparent from our discussion in Chapter 2 where we noted that social support is one of the key resources that can be seen to flow from shared social identity. Formally, then, H14 stated that when and to the extent that people define themselves in terms of shared social identity, they will both give each other more support and construe the support they receive more positively. The reason for this is that where they categorize themselves as members of the same group, people are motivated to help each other out – and to respond positively to that help – because this serves to advance the collective identity they share.

In Chapter 2 we discussed examples of research that support this hypothesis. In particular, we alluded to work which shows that people tend to give more assistance to those who are in difficulty (e.g., a person who has an accident; a group that has experienced a natural disaster) to the extent that they see them as members of an ingroup rather than an outgroup (Levine, Prosser, Evans, & Reicher, 2005; Levine & Thompson, 2004). Recall, for example, Levine and colleagues' (2005) research, where an initial study showed that Manchester United fans were much more likely to lend assistance to a person (a male confederate) when he tripped and fell in front of them if that person was wearing a Manchester United top rather than a Liverpool top or a plain shirt. Along related lines, Tamara Butler (2016) has also shown in an online game-playing paradigm that when identification with others is manipulated experimentally, this feeds into participants' *requests* for social support and, through this, has an impact on their stress and well-being.

Again, though, it is worth noting that the self-categorization process that underpins such acts is potentially fluid, and hence the inclination to support others will change as the nature of one's social identity is redefined. This point is nicely illustrated in a second study undertaken by Levine and his collaborators. This employed the same paradigm as the first experiment, but here, prior to seeing the accident unfold in front of them, the experimenters asked participants questions that served to make salient their identity as football fans rather than as fans of one *particular* team. Responses to the confederate in the Manchester United shirt and in the plain shirt were essentially the same as those observed in the first experiment. Now, though, participants proved as willing to help the confederate in the Liverpool shirt as they were to help the Manchester United fan. Here, then, because the social identity that was important to participants was that of football fan, what determined the level of support they gave to the confederate was his being a football fan (or not), not his status as a supporter of a specific team.

Our research with bomb disposal officers and bar staff also provides evidence that when a person defines themselves as a member of a particular group, they are more likely to receive – and, importantly, to *feel* that they receive – support from other people who share the same social identity. Here, then, employees' social identification with their work colleagues emerged as a strong positive predictor of the amount of social support they reported receiving at work ($r = .67$). Moreover, this appeared to have a positive bearing on respondents' well-being in so far as it was a strong negative predictor of their overall stress levels ($r = -.63$; as was social support, $r = -.69$). At the same time, statistical analysis suggested that the relationship between social identification and stress was partially mediated by social support. In other words, in line with H14, and as shown schematically in Figure 5.3, it appears that social identification protects people from stress in part because it provides them a basis for being – and perceiving themselves to be – in a position to receive social support.

This same conclusion was also supported by another study to which we have already alluded in which we worked with Norwegian colleagues to explore stress among patients recovering from heart

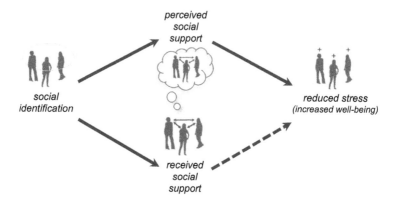

Figure 5.3 Perceived and received social support are mediators of the relationship between social identification and stress

Note: A point that this figure underlines is that receiving support and perceiving support are not the same thing. That is, when a person is given support, they will not always see it as supportive. Indeed, in the absence of shared social identity between support providers and recipients, these two things will often be uncorrelated. It is also the case that a person's *perceptions* of social support tend to be a better predictor of stress than the actual receipt of it.

surgery in an Oslo clinic (Haslam et al., 2005, Experiment 2). In this instance patients' sense that they shared social identity with their family and friends was a strong predictor of the amount of support they perceived themselves as receiving while in hospital ($r = .58$) and of both the amount of stress they experienced as a result of their hospitalisation ($r = -.34$) and their satisfaction with life in general ($r = .42$). In this case statistical analysis suggested that the relationship between social identification and both stress and life satisfaction was fully accounted for by the (perceived) receipt of social support. Moreover, beyond this, the study also provided evidence that patients' social identification with hospital staff contributed to these same positive outcomes. Thus, as well as confirming the role that a sense of shared social identity plays in ameliorating stress, such patterns speak to the important role that this identity-based *therapeutic alliance* between health practitioners and their clients plays in positive health outcomes (as noted in Chapter 2).

The model presented in Figure 5.3 has been also supported by research in a number of other contexts. In particular, within the organisational domain, a meta-analysis conducted by Nik Steffens and colleagues showed the relationship between work-based social identifications and stress to be highly reliable (Steffens, Haslam, Schuh, Jetten, & van Dick, 2016; for a review see van Dick & Haslam, 2012). This analysis looked separately at social identification with workteams and with an organisation as a whole and found both to be predictive of reduced stress (across 58 studies and 102 effects, including nearly 20,000 people; both $rs = .21$). Speaking again to the importance of inter-subjective aspects of stress, the former relationship was also significantly stronger to the extent that all members of a given workteam *shared* the same degree of social identification.

Yet despite this broad level of support for a social identity approach to stress, two important nuances to this analysis should be kept in mind when considering the model presented in Figure 5.3.

First, just as social identification is a basis for social support, it is also the case that the experience of receiving social support should have the capacity to strengthen the social identification of those who benefit from it (meaning that in Figure 5.3 the arrows between social identification and social support are bi-directional). This possibility was confirmed in research by Ilka Gleibs and colleagues which examined care home residents who were going through the process of joining new groups (Gleibs et al., 2011a; discussed in more detail in Chapter 7). More generally, then, it would appear there is the potential for an 'upward spiral' whereby social identification promotes social support and this in turn promotes social identification (Reicher & Haslam, 2006b).

A second important nuance relates to the fact that, as noted in Figure 5.3, there is often a disconnection between the subjective and objective features of support, such that, as we discussed earlier, (1) the relationship between the receipt of support and recipients' well-being tends to be highly variable and generally quite weak (Schwarzer & Leppin, 1991) and (2) stress is predicted more by a person's subjective experience of support than by its objective availability (Cohen & Wills, 1985; Norris & Kaniasty, 1996). In part, these patterns can be seen to arise from the fact that the providers and recipients of support do not always act in terms of the same social identities. For example, as Europeans, Germans may attempt to provide material support to Greeks, but if those Greeks are acting in terms of their national identity rather than as Europeans (perhaps because they feel their national identity is under threat or because they see the support as an attempt to manoeuvre their country into a position of weakness), they may regard this behaviour with distrust and be suspicious of the motives behind it. Here, then, the mismatch of social identifications will mean that the support does not have its intended impact, and indeed it may trigger a reaction among the support provider that leads them to revert to a more narrowly defined social identity (e.g., as German rather than European).

More generally, then, as large programmes of work by Arie Nadler (e.g., 2010) and Butler (2016) have shown, there are good reasons why social support will not always be well received and why people are often inclined to be wary of those who offer them help. Again, the key point here is that social support is likely to have its most positive impact when providers and recipients share the same social identity and hence have the same framework for interpreting it (Haslam, 2004; Haslam, Reicher, & Levine, 2012; Postmes, 2003). Accordingly, often the most important (and difficult) part of any support attempt is convincing the recipient that the source of support has their interests at heart. This is a point that resonates with evidence that therapists who are seen to be honest, respectful, warm, interested, and open tend to achieve better therapeutic outcomes than those who are not because they are better able to build a therapeutic alliance with their clients (Ackerman & Hilsenroth, 2003). As we noted in Chapter 2, from a social identity perspective, we can see this alliance as revolving around a sense of shared identity in which these positive therapist characteristics are those that people typically attribute to ingroup members (Doise et al., 1972). Indeed, in these terms, whether or not a person perceives themselves to share identity with a therapist may be no less important for the success of the therapy they deliver than the therapy's actual content.

Social identity can transform the experience of stress

Evidence that shared social identity provides a basis for effective social support starts to get to the heart of the qualitative difference between stress that is experienced by people as individuals and stress that is experienced by them as group members. As we have seen, a key reason for this is that identity-based social support has the capacity to underpin effective coping and thereby counteract the negative effects of stress. Beyond this, though, it is also the case that social support has the capacity to *fundamentally transform* the nature of people's stress-related experience – in particular, by turning personal distress into collective eustress, in ways suggested by Figure 5.4. As John Cacioppo and colleagues observe: "a focus on 'we' rather than 'me' has risks but . . . it can also buffer the effects of traumatic stressors [people] may confront and help them learn and grow from those stressors" (Cacioppo, Reis, & Zautra, 2011, p. 44).

Some powerful examples of this process are provided by Suedfeld (1997) in accounts of the ways in which groups of Arctic explorers and prisoners of war (POWs) have succeeded in overcoming the most abject and unforgiving conditions and used their common experiences as a basis for shared

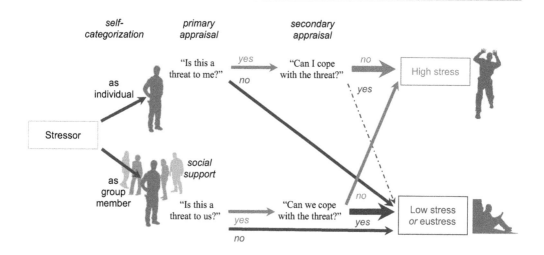

Figure 5.4 A schematic representation of the ways in which stress appraisal is moderated by self-categorization

Note: As in Figure 5.2, rather than being sequential, primary and secondary appraisal are dynamically interrelated. A key difference that self-categorization as a group member makes to the appraisal process is that because this is the basis for receipt of effective support, it tends to increase people's ability to cope with stress and hence makes positive secondary appraisal more likely.

inspiration and enrichment. For example, when discussing the experiences of POWs in Vietnam he draws on observations by William Sledge and colleagues that:

> Many . . . underwent years of torture, deprivation, solitary confinement and brainwashing attempts. In all these situations, prisoners survived by drawing upon support from each other, upon their religious, patriotic, and moral values, and upon self-discipline in setting hygienic standards, daily routines, and the like. In one study 61 percent of ex-Vietnam PoWs reported having higher optimism, self-insight and better social relationships than they had had previously.
>
> (Sledge, Boydstun, & Rahe, 1980; cited in Suedfeld, 1997, p. 334)

This is not to say that social identity-based social support will always produce such positive effects. Indeed, in line with basic principles of social identity theory that we discussed in Chapter 2, these should only materialise if a group is motivated and able to positively reinterpret or reframe the nature of the stress experience (e.g., by having access to specific cognitive alternatives).

More specifically, how exactly groups understand their experiences of stress should vary as a function of structural, contextual, and ideological factors that shape their preferred strategy for self-enhancement in ways outlined by social identity theory. For example, a high-status group that is working hard to maintain or enhance its position may interpret the stressors to which it is subjected as uplifting and character building, whereas a low-status group that wants to challenge the legitimacy of a high-status group may interpret the stressors to which it is subjected as illegitimate and unreasonable (Terry & O'Brien, 2001). On top of real differences in the forms and intensity of stressors that different groups are subject to, these differences in motivation may also help to explain why perceptions of stress typically follow the contours of psychological group membership (in ways suggested by research on mass sociogenic illnesses such as sick building syndrome) and often vary systematically as a function of a group's status within society as a whole.

This possibility is spelled out more formally in the *integrated social identity model of stress* (ISIS; Haslam & Reicher, 2006). This specifies the way in which the strategic responses to status inequality explored within social identity theory can be translated into a framework for understanding the basis of different coping responses to stress. Indeed, Haslam and Reicher (2006) argue that this translation makes perfect sense in light of the fact that social identity theory was formulated to account for variation in responses to social structural conditions that are aversive to self (i.e., stressful; e.g., see Branscombe et al., 1999; Haslam, 2004; Schmitt & Branscombe, 2002).

A schematic representation of the ISIS model is presented in Figure 5.5. In line with social identity theory (Tajfel & Turner, 1979), this presents an analysis that is grounded in structural and social psychological dynamics and which sees individual or collective coping styles as *outcomes* of those dynamics. More specifically, the model suggests that where individuals feel that a given social structure provides opportunities for them to escape stressors associated with their low status (through a strategy of personal mobility), they are unlikely to define themselves and act in terms of shared social identity and should seek to achieve positive outcomes for the self through a strategy of individual *avoidance*. Where there are no such opportunities but status relations are perceived to be secure (i.e., legitimate and stable), those who are subjected to status-related stressors should be more likely to display social creativity in the form of individual or collective *denial*. However, when there is no way to escape stress and status relations are *in*secure, shared social identification is more likely to dispose individuals to embrace cognitive alternatives that involve active and collective *resistance* to the stressors they face (Haslam & Reicher, 2012).

The ISIS framework is consistent with a large body of research that has explored the ways in which minority group members cope with the stress of stigma, discrimination, and prejudice (as reviewed in the previous two chapters). In particular, it is consistent with work that has supported Nyla Branscombe and Michael Schmitt's rejection–identification model in which minority group members' recognition of prejudice is a basis for social identification that then provides them with a platform for mutual support that can be mobilised in attempts to tackle stress and overcome injustice (Branscombe et al., 1999; Schmitt & Branscombe, 2002; Schmitt, Spears, & Branscombe, 2003).

However, the most comprehensive test of ISIS was provided by the BBC Prison Study that we discussed in some detail in Chapter 3 (Reicher & Haslam, 2006a). Here, as social identification increased among the Prisoners over the course of the study, this led them to support each other more and, as a result, to tackle more effectively the range of stressors that life in the simulated prison exposed them to (e.g., in the form of restricted living space, poor food, limited privacy, and boredom). At the same time, as the Prisoners came together as a group, their strategy of social competition made them increasingly willing to impose strain on the Guards (notably by undermining their authority and subjecting them to humiliation and bullying). This contributed to a decline in social identification among the Guards that led to them becoming increasingly distressed. Consistent with the analysis we presented in the previous section, a key reason for this was that they withdrew from each other's company and failed to provide each other with the support necessary to maintain their authority and resist the various threats presented by the Prisoners. Ultimately too, their failure to run the prison effectively led to full-blown burnout (of the form described by Maslach & Jackson, 1981). Thus not only were they exhausted, but they had also lost any sense of accomplishment and had become increasingly callous.

These patterns can be seen in the quantitative psychometric and physiological data presented in Table 5.2, but they are also apparent in the wealth of qualitative data that the study generated. For example, the state of the Guards is exemplified by the following exchange in which they were trying to decide how to deal with various breaches of prison rules that had occurred after the boundaries between groups had been made impermeable and the Prisoners had started to rebel against the system:

TAg: OK, . . . they've got their privilege hour coming up.
FCg: Fuck their privilege hour, all of them.

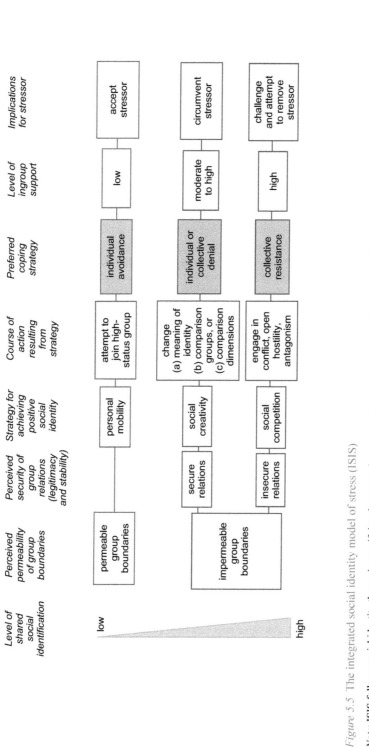

Figure 5.5 The integrated social identity model of stress (ISIS)

Note: ISIS follows social identity theory in specifying that strategic responses to stressors vary as a function of social-structural conditions (specifically, the perceived permeability of group boundaries and the security of status-based group relations). First, where individuals feel that it is possible to escape stressors associated with their low status, they are likely to pursue a strategy of individual *avoidance*. Second, where there are no such opportunities but status relations are seen to be secure, individuals are likely to respond to those stressors through socially creative *denial*. However, third, when stressors are seen to be inescapable and status relations are insecure, individuals are more likely to engage in collective *resistance* in which they work with others to try to remove the stressors they confront.

Source: Haslam and Reicher (2012). Reproduced with permission from SAGE publications

TAg: That's fine, that's fine.
FCg: End of story.
TAg: Well, we have to give them a bit of er. . .
TQg: Tell everybody. . .
TAg: 'Cause they've been locked up. . .
TMg: We haven't even tried punishing the person who's made the mistake first. Before we go down the road of punishing. . .
BGg: Don't jump the gun, chaps.
TMg: . . . people who haven't made the mistake. . .
TAg: Nah, we'll give them the privilege hour
TMg: I think we should just try . . .

(Haslam, Reicher, Koppel, & Mirsky, 2006, p. 50)

What is striking here is the fact that, because they lack a sense of shared identity, the Guards' contributions to the discussion are disconnected and disjointed and, as a result, they are unable to develop a coherent strategy for dealing with the stressors presented by the Prisoners' insurrection. Indeed, the exchange captures almost perfectly the state of burnout described by Christina Maslach and Michael Leiter (1997, p. 49) in which:

The loss of community is evident in greater conflict among people, less mutual support and respect, and a growing sense of isolation. A sense of belonging disappears [and] people work separately rather than together.

This contrasts markedly with discussions among the Prisoners that were taking place at approximately the same time:

JEp: I'm enjoying meself.
PPp: I'm having a great time, I'm really having a great time. I'm happy as a pig in shit. Tomorrow is going to be even funnier.

(Haslam, Reicher, Koppel, & Mirsky, 2006, pp. 43–44)

Table 5.2 Social identification and stress in the BBC Prison Study

Group:	Guards		Prisoners	
Study phase:	**Day 2**	**Day 6**	**Day 2**	**Day 6**
Measure				
Social identification	1.00	0.17[a]	0.63	1.29[a]
Burnout	2.23[a]	3.17[ab]	2.38	2.29[b]
Exposure to bullying from outgroup	1.36[a]	3.50[ab]	1.21	1.71[b]
Cortisol ($\sqrt{mg}$/10 ml)	1.28[a]	1.80[a]	1.33[b]	1.59[b]

Note: Cells in the same row with the same superscript ([a] or [b]) are significantly different.

Source: Haslam and Reicher (2006)

Conclusion

As well as its capacity to integrate multiple forms of qualitative and quantitative data, as a study of stress, what is distinctive about the BBC Prison Study is that it allowed for an integrated examination of the complex roles that social identification and unfolding intragroup and intergroup dynamics play in the stress process. On the one hand, the experiences of the Prisoners exemplify the ways in which an emergent sense of shared social identity can allow individuals to resist strain and to turn adversity into advantage. On the other hand, the experiences of the Guards show how the erosion of social identity exposes individuals to stress and how, when this contributes to collective failure, it can ultimately pave the way to chronic burnout.

More significantly still, by providing a longitudinal analysis of the multiple processes that contribute to both resistance and exhaustion, the study also supports a theoretical framework that allows us to understand the social psychological dynamics that underpin the physiological and personal aspects of stress (e.g., as described by Selye, 1946). Importantly, within standard studies of stress, these underpinnings are typically concealed because researchers' preferred methodologies privilege static, individualised understandings of these processes often in relation to relatively trivial stressors (Cooper, Dewe, & O'Driscoll, 2001). Once released from these constraints, we see that stress-related physiological trajectories are not set in stone and that there is no sense in which stress responses are a fundamental expression either of personality or biology (e.g., as suggested by Rosenman et al., 1964).

It is therefore a mistake to think of stress primarily as a problem of biology, physiology, or personality; just as it is a mistake to think of it simply as a problem of culture, context, or environment. Instead – and consistent with the social identity approach to health in general – we would argue that stress should be seen as one aspect of an array of interwoven social and psychological processes that shape the conditions of group life and the sense of identity and community that this provides. These conditions have two important consequences. First, they determine whether stressors change us (for the worse) or whether we attempt to change them (for the better). Second, they determine whether the stress process as a whole is experienced as positive and enabling (i.e., as *eu*stress) or as negative and disabling (as *dis*tress). It also follows that to the extent that stress constitutes a problem (as it often does), it is therefore these conditions that we need to interrogate and endeavour to improve. The distinctive value of the social identity approach is that it provides powerful tools for such interrogation.

Points for practice

From the arguments outlined in this chapter, it is possible to abstract four key points that are especially relevant to practitioners working in the area of stress:

1. *Group life and the social identities that underpin it are major determinants of primary stress appraisal.* That is, whether or not a stressor is perceived as threatening will often depend on the meaning of that stressor for a perceiver's currently salient social identity.
2. *Groups and the social identities that underpin them are a major source of effective social support.* This is not only because social identity is a basis for people to give and receive support, but also because, when it is shared, social identity is a basis for support to be interpreted positively – thereby bringing its objective and subjective features into alignment.
3. *Groups have the capacity to transform otherwise negative stress experiences into positive ones.* When people tackle stressors alone, it can be hard for them to see how those stressors can be overcome. However, groups that are composed of people who share social identity allow people to develop a social change belief system that, together with social support, provides a basis for them to engage in collective stress resistance. This resistance will not always succeed, but where it does, it can change distress into eustress.

4.   *Groups are both a major source of stress and a key means by which stress is overcome.* In many ways this is a summary of the preceding points and also the key message to emerge from this chapter.

Resources

Further reading

If you want to find out more about the social identity approach to stress, the following papers are a good place to start.

①   Levine, R. M., Prosser, A., Evans, D., & Reicher, S. D. (2005). Identity and emergency intervention: How social group membership and inclusiveness of group boundaries shapes helping behaviour. *Personality and Social Psychology Bulletin, 31*, 443–453.

This paper looks at the way in which helping behaviour is structured by shared identity and how this behaviour changes as the nature of that shared identity is redefined.

②   Haslam, S. A., & Reicher, S. D. (2006). Stressing the group: Social identity and the unfolding dynamics of responses to stress. *Journal of Applied Psychology, 91*, 1037–1052.

This paper presents an analysis of the stress-related dynamics that arose from relations between Prisoners and Guards in the BBC Prison Study. It also sets out the key principles of the integrated social identity model of stress (ISIS).

③   Haslam, S. A., Reicher, S. D., & Levine, M. (2012). When other people are heaven, when other people are hell: How social identity determines the nature and impact of social support. In Jetten, J., Haslam, C., & Haslam, S. A. (Eds.), *The social cure: Identity, health, and well-being* (pp. 157–174). Hove, UK: Psychology Press.

This book chapter reviews a large body of work that speaks to the nuanced relationship between social identity and social support. It explores in some detail why support does not always lead to positive health outcomes.

Video

①   Search for "Ryan Work-life balance" to watch a TEDx talk by Michelle Ryan in which she discusses the relationship between social identity and the stress of work–life imbalance. www.youtube.com/watch?v=79tRTivyMSM   (32 minutes)

A longer version of this was also presented as a keynote lecture at the 2014 conference of the British Psychology Society's Division of Clinical Psychology. www.youtube.com/watch?v=8I7U9b_PV5A

②   Search for "McGonigal stress" to watch a TED talk in which Kelly McGonigal talks about the complex relationship between stress and health. Amongst other things, she notes (1) that when people come to see stress as something positive, this can have positive consequences for their health and (2) that social connection is a basis for stress resilience www.ted.com/talks/kelly_mcgonigal_how_to_make_stress_your_friend   (14 minutes)

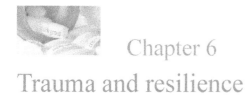

Chapter 6

Trauma and resilience

Case study 6.1 Siegfried Sassoon

Unlike the other case studies in this book, we can identify Siegfried Sassoon by name (see Figure 6.1) because his life story is a matter of public record – primarily as a result of his celebrated poetry (see Egremont, 2014; Sassoon, 1983). Born into a wealthy British family at the end of the 19th century, he studied history at Cambridge (but left in 1907 before getting a degree) and later enlisted to fight in World War I. At the start of the war he was passionate about the Allied cause, having been caught up in the patriotic fervour whipped up to counter threats to the British Empire. Yet as the war wore on, he was confronted first-hand with human carnage on a colossal scale through his engagement on the Western Front, and he became increasingly disillusioned. Having lost many friends in the fighting as well as his younger brother, and even though he had been awarded the Military Cross for bravery, he became a pacifist and lobbied widely for an end to the war. These actions were interpreted by his seniors as treasonous. Yet rather than put him on trial in 1917 they sent him to a hospital outside Edinburgh to be treated for *neurasthenia* or *shell shock* (later termed *combat stress reaction*, but known today as *posttraumatic stress disorder* [PTSD]). This diagnosis was applied to around 10% of all British officers and encompassed a broad range of symptomatology. In Sassoon's case, the diagnosis was based on symptoms of depression and evidence of the range of self-destructive actions he had undertaken (including those for which he had been decorated and which had earned him the nickname 'Mad Jack'). It was also a convenient way of dealing with the political challenges that his insurrection presented to military authorities.

In the previous chapter we examined people's responses to stressors and strains that they experience as part of their daily life. Many of these were associated with challenging situations – for example, working in a demanding job or having a serious medical condition – but by and large they were related to experiences that were part of people's normal everyday lives. Sometimes, though, stressors come in an altogether more extreme and frightening form. Consider, for example, the London commuters who were victims of the 7/7 terrorist bombings in 2005, or the communities in Chile that were rocked by violent earthquakes in 2010, or the residents of Northern Ireland caught up in 'the Troubles' in which over 3,000 people were killed and nearly 50,000 injured in acts of violence between 1969 and 2002, or the hundreds of thousands of soldiers caught up in trench warfare in northern France during World War I (see Figure 6.2). In each of these contexts individuals were directly exposed to horrific scenes of carnage and destruction that were very much out of the ordinary. Moreover, many more people ended up being traumatised by these events because they resulted in someone they loved being killed or seriously injured.

Traumatic events such as these are profoundly disturbing and, unsurprisingly, they have the capacity to seriously compromise the mental health of those who experience them or who they directly

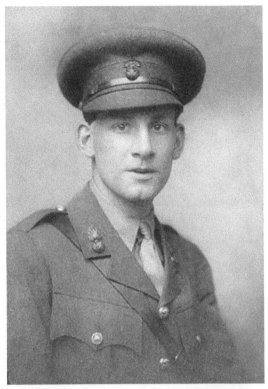

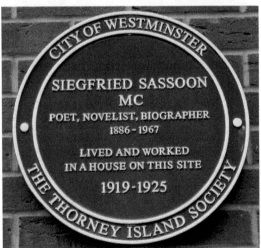

CITY OF WESTMINSTER

SIEGFRIED SASSOON
MC
POET, NOVELIST, BIOGRAPHER
1886-1967

LIVED AND WORKED
IN A HOUSE ON THIS SITE
1919-1925

THE THORNEY ISLAND SOCIETY

Figure 6.1 Siegfried Sassoon and the commemorative plaque outside his London home

Note: Sassoon was a celebrated war poet who, in common with many of his fellow combatants, received treatment for *neurasthenia* or *shell shock*. This was later termed *combat stress reaction*, but is known today as *posttraumatic stress disorder* (PTSD). This diagnosis was based on symptoms of depression and evidence of acts of self-destruction.

Source: Wikipedia

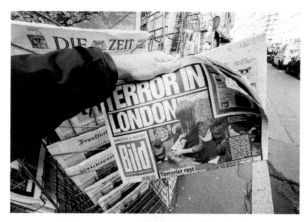

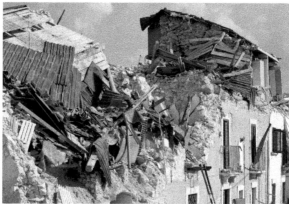

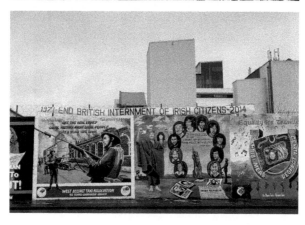

Figure 6.2 Examples of traumatic events: terrorism, natural disaster, and intergroup conflict

Note: Such events are profoundly disturbing and, unsurprisingly, have the capacity to seriously compromise the mental health of those who are affected by them. Nevertheless, people respond to trauma in a range of different ways. Moreover, because they often involve and affect social groups, social identity processes play a major role in shaping these responses.

Source: Shutterstock; Angelo Giordano, Pixabay; Shutterstock

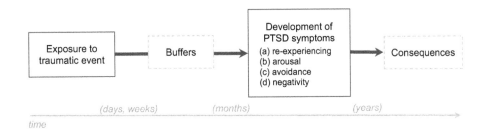

Figure 6.3 The development of posttraumatic stress disorder (PTSD)

Note: DSM-IV defined two criteria as essential for the diagnosis of PTSD: (1) exposure to a traumatic event and (2) the intense response to that event (in the form of fear, helplessness, and horror; American, Psychiatric Association, 1994). Recognising that the development of PTSD is more nuanced than this (and that an intense response can occur in the context of the exposure itself), in DSM5, diagnosis focuses on four clusters of symptoms: (1) re-experiencing, (2) arousal, (3) avoidance, and (4) negativity. It is widely recognised that a range of factors can buffer people from developing PTSD and that its development can also have a wide array of consequences. It is important to note too that a strong stress response is normal in the days and weeks following a traumatic event. Accordingly, it is only if this response becomes prolonged (so that it is apparent more than one month after the event) that a diagnosis of PTSD would be considered.

affect. Indeed, it is common for people who endure extreme trauma to report the experience as 'life changing'. In line with this point, posttraumatic stress disorder (PTSD) was one of the more significant conditions to be added to the third edition of the *Diagnostic and Statistical Manual of Mental Disorders* (DSM-III; American Psychiatric Association, 1980). As suggested in Figure 6.3, this defined a condition in which, after experiencing, witnessing, or otherwise being confronted by a traumatic event that involved or threatened death, serious injury or harm, a person goes on to have an extreme stress response that centres on feelings of "intense fear, helplessness or horror" (American Psychiatric Association, 1994, pp. 427–428; see also Resick, Monson, & Rizvi, 2014).

An important point to make here is that it is entirely normal for people to have a strong response to traumatic events. Accordingly, they will only be diagnosed with PTSD if that response is *prolonged*. Over time, too, the diagnosis of PTSD has become more nuanced, so that the most recent diagnostic manual, DSM5, focuses on four clusters of symptoms: (1) re-experiencing the event (e.g., as flashbacks and intrusive thoughts), (2) heightened arousal (e.g., hyper-vigilance; sleep disturbances; or aggressive, reckless, or self-destructive behaviour), (3) avoidance, especially of situations that trigger reminders of the event, and (4) negative thoughts and mood (e.g., a distorted sense of blame of self or others).

PTSD came to prominence in the context of the mental health problems experienced by veterans of the 1955–1975 Vietnam War and its subsequent inclusion in DSM-III (1980). Nevertheless, researchers (e.g., Birmes, Hatton, Brunet, & Schmitt, 2003) have pointed to discussion of PTSD-like symptomatology in the writings of the ancients (e.g., Homer's *Iliad*, where Achilles "went on grieving for his friend [Patroclus] whom he could not banish from his mind, and the all-conquering sleep refused to visit him"; Morris, 2015, p. 72) and of Shakespeare (e.g., in the hallucinations and nightmares of the protagonists in *Macbeth*). However, the first systematic accounts of PTSD emerged in the context of soldiers' experiences of shell shock in World War I (Jones & Wessley, 2005). (e.g., see Loughran, 2012; Motion, 2009; Shepherd, 2002):

Powerful as these soldiers' testimony is, it is worth observing that the sequence of events associated with the emergence of PTSD (as set out in Figure 6.3) is a focus for intense debate and controversy (McNally, 2003; Muldoon & Lowe, 2012). This has two particular foci: conceptual and empirical. Speaking to the first of these, it is important to note that the diagnosis of PTSD is not intended to be used liberally as a way of describing people's reactions to expected and predictable events, upsetting as these may be (e.g., the death of a pet, watching distressing news stories, failing an exam). Nevertheless, as a range of commentators have observed, over time, the terms 'trauma' and 'PTSD' have been associated with "conceptual bracket creep", such that they are applied to an ever-increasing realm of human experiences (McNally, 2003, p. 231; see also Drury & Williams, 2012; N. Haslam, 2016). McNally, for example, questions the appropriateness of believing that PTSD might be triggered by overhearing sexist jokes in the workplace (a case discussed by Avina & O'Donohue, 2002) and argues that this was certainly not what was intended by the architects of DSM-III whose primary focus was on the psychological legacy of intense trauma (e.g., as caused by war or rape; Yehuda & McFarlane, 1995).

A second controversy is empirical and relates to the fact that, as we observed when discussing stress in the previous chapter, the path from traumatic experience to negative stress response is not certain. To be sure, there are many people whose lives (and minds) are destroyed by horrific life events. Moreover, it is clear that repeated or sustained exposure to trauma is likely to be very damaging to mental health (in part because it erodes victims' coping resources; e.g., Matheson, Jorden, & Anisman, 2008; Turner & Lloyd, 1995). Events in Haiti – where residents had to endure a devastating cyclone in 2010, then a major outbreak of cholera (introduced by UN aid workers), and then another cyclone in 2016 – bear tragic testimony to this fact (Dai et al., 2016).

But there is nothing that makes PTSD an inevitable response to horrendous experiences. This can be seen from Figure 6.4 which plots no fewer than seven different posttraumatic mental health trajectories that were identified in a review of the literature by Jonathan Bisson and colleagues (Bisson, Cosgrove, Lewis, & Roberts, 2015; for related evidence of variability in PTSD trajectory, see Bryant et al., 2015). These include three patterns that were ultimately associated with high PTSD symptomatology (emerging immediately, gradually, or after delay) but also three that ultimately led to few or no adverse symptoms (either because these declined soon after the event, or because they were minor or never arose at all). Importantly too, epidemiological studies suggest that of people who experience traumatic events, only a minority (around 10% to 30%) go on to have a full clinical presentation of PTSD, although it is also notable that prevalence rates differ markedly both (1) across cultures (being higher in the United States than most other countries) and (2) as a function of the nature of the trauma (being higher for events that affect individuals and/or are perpetrated by other humans, for example, sexual abuse and assault, than for events that affect large groups and/or are due to non-human causes, for example, natural disasters; Resick et al., 2014).

Speaking further to the massive amount of variability in people's responses to trauma, in a systematic review of 39 studies, Alex Linley and Stephen Joseph (2004) observe that a sizeable proportion of people who have traumatic experiences report that these ultimately contributed to their psychological development – in the form of *posttraumatic growth* (Colville & Cream, 2009; Tedeschi & Calhoun, 2004). Indeed, the modal proportion of different populations who reported some degree of growth was 69% (although this varied between 3% and 98% across studies).

These various observations raise a range of intriguing issues that we will attempt to grapple with in this chapter. Most obviously, we will try to understand the psychological processes that shape responses to traumatic experiences and that determine whether things that nearly kill us ultimately make us weaker or stronger. As we will see, social identity processes are a large part of the story here. This is for the simple reason that groups and group life are routinely bound up with collective

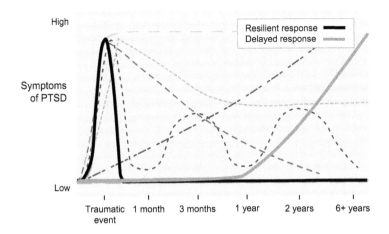

High

Resilient response ▬▬
Delayed response ▬▬▬

Symptoms
of PTSD

Low

Traumatic   1 month   3 months   1 year   2 years   6+ years
event

Figure 6.4 Examples of different trajectories of PTSD symptoms after exposure to trauma

Note: These trajectories are associated with responses to a single traumatising event. They become even more complex and varied in cases of repeated exposure to trauma (e.g., as experienced by victims of childhood sexual abuse).

Source: Bisson, Cosgrove, Lewis, & Roberts (2015)

experiences and understandings of trauma. Importantly too, these experiences and understandings have a central role to play in the historical and political development of groups and societies. This means that such things as war, mass catastrophe, and widespread abuse are not generally things that groups experience and then simply forget about. Instead they tell stories (or in the case of Siegfried Sassoon write poems) to help them and other members of their group make sense of those experiences. Where such stories cannot be told, or only told with shame, they can be devastating. But if group members are able tell them with pride, they can turn out to be a significant source of personal and collective enrichment.

Current approaches to trauma and resilience

Biological models

In seeking to explain why only some people fall victim to the psychological toll of trauma, many researchers have pointed to individual differences in biological susceptibility. In particular, because it is clear that PTSD is a response that reflects the functioning of the *sympathetic nervous system* – that is, that part of the autonomic nervous system that processes adaptive fight or flight responses – the emergence of the condition can be seen to reflect weaknesses in this system (Kolb, 1987). In this regard, one influential biological model posits that people who succumb to PTSD are distinguished from those who do not by their *allostatic dysregulation* – that is, by the difficulty they experience in responding adaptively to a range of social stimuli. Amongst other things, this is evidenced by increased activation of the sympathoadrenal system (the system which is responsible for connecting the sympathetic nervous system to the adrenal medulla) in response to memory-evoking cues of traumatic events. Consistent with this model, research by Miles McFall and his colleagues found that Vietnam veterans who were suffering from PTSD had increased levels of adrenaline in their blood plasma as well as elevated heart rate and blood pressure after being exposed to violent war-related images, whereas control participants showed no such effects (McFall, Murburg, Ko, & Veith, 1990). In a similar vein, a study of childhood trauma victims showed that levels of urinary cortisol, adrenaline, and noradrenaline (both produced by the adrenal glands in response to distressing events) were highly predictive of PTSD symptomatology (although, for reasons that were not clear, this was true for boys – with r's between .41 and .52 – but not for girls; Delahanty, Nugent, Christopher, & Walsh, 2005).

Related to this, a second biological model argues that PTSD is associated with a *dysfunctional memory system* in which both short- and long-term memory are disrupted in complex ways. Both the amygdala (which is responsible for processing emotions and memory) and the prefrontal cortex (which is involved in working memory and attention) are involved in this system (Elzinga & Bremner, 2002), and people suffering from PTSD have been found to have both heightened amygdala responsivity and a hyporesponsive prefrontal cortex (Shin, Rauch, & Pitman, 2006). There is also consistent evidence that the hippocampus (which is involved in memory recall; Patai et al., 2015) is implicated in PTSD. In particular, this brain structure tends to be smaller than normal and to have damaged cortisol receptors in those who suffer from this condition (Cruwys & O'Kearney, 2008; Hutterer & Liss, 2006; Stam, 2007; Weiss, 2007). Indeed, evidence of hippocampal atrophy has been found in a wide range of groups, including studies of women suffering from PTSD as a result of childhood sexual abuse (Bremner et al., 2003) and Vietnam veterans suffering from PTSD as a result of their wartime experiences (Hedges et al., 1993; for meta-analytic confirmation of this pattern, see Smith, 2005).

Studies of nervous and memory systems such as these provide compelling evidence that adverse responses to trauma (particularly in the form of PTSD) have meaningful biological correlates. In particular, these appear to be related to a tendency for sufferers (1) to be in a state of hyperarousal and hypervigilance in which stimuli are interpreted as threatening to the self, and therefore as requiring a fight or flight response, and/or (2) to have reduced sympathetic nervous system reactivity, and/or (3) to have memory systems which make benign experiences hard to register and remember but traumatic experiences hard to forget. Unsurprisingly too, these disturbances also interfere with other biological systems – including those that regulate relaxation and sleep (Sheikh, Woodward, & Leskin, 2003).

Nevertheless, most of the neurobiological research on trauma has documented the processes underpinning symptoms, rather than identifying the determinants of PTSD (e.g., McFall et al., 1990). In particular, rather than differences in the operation of biological processes being the *cause* of adverse responses to trauma, it seems highly likely that these are, to some extent, primarily their *consequence*. In other words, it may be in part *because* (for whatever reason) a person is haunted by past trauma that relevant biological systems have difficulty 'switching off' and 'letting go' rather than just the other way round. Indeed, it seems likely that there is a complex interplay between physiology and traumatic experience in which each of these things has the capacity to shape the other.

Speaking to this complexity, although it is clear that traumatic events have the capacity to exert profound changes on the biological systems that regulate stress and memory, it is also apparent that there is huge variation in the way these systems respond to these events that cannot be fully explained in biological terms. Moreover, there is good evidence for the "top down" regulation of these stress and memory systems by higher-order brain systems (particularly the medial prefrontal cortex) which accords with evidence that people's interpretations of events, emotions, and memories play a huge role in their neurobiological response (e.g., Rauch, Shin, & Phelps, 2006; Shin et al., 2006; Tomita, Ohbayashi, Nakahara, Hasegawa, & Miyashita, 1999).

This complexity in turn means that pharmaceutical approaches to PTSD treatment are unlikely to provide a full solution to the problems it causes. In line with this conclusion, although reviews suggest that drugs which attempt to regulate the functioning of the sympathetic nervous system (e.g., antidepressants) can be helpful in the initial stages of treatment to help counteract some of the most disruptive symptoms (e.g., Friedman, Donnelly, & Mellman, 2003), their capacity to deliver long-term benefits appears to be limited. Thus, as Friedman (1997, p. 361) observed two decades ago, "dramatic responses to medication have been the exception rather than the rule" and – despite pursuing at least nine different lines of pharmacological attack (see Ravindran & Stein, 2009) – there is little to suggest that things have changed much in the intervening period (Wilson, Friedman, & Lindy, 2012).

At the same time, the fact that some non-pharmaceutical interventions to tackle the adverse consequences of trauma *do* prove to be successful (as we will discuss later) suggests that a full account of the role that biological factors play in the development of PTSD needs to be informed by an appreciation of the way in which they interact with psychosocial factors. This indeed is the conclusion endorsed by most researchers working in this area (e.g., Wilson, Friedman, & Lindy, 2012). Nevertheless, as with other mental health conditions (e.g., depression, see Chapter 8) and as we argued in Chapter 1, it is clear that a lot more could be done to ensure that physiological research is integrated within a full-blown bio-psycho-*social* model.

Psychoanalytic models

One limitation of the biological models discussed in the previous section is that they focus more on the physiological consequences of adverse responses to trauma than on the psychological dimensions. However, for the scholars and practitioners who were first interested in understanding these adverse responses, it was their psychological dimensions that struck them as most important and most distinctive. In particular, this was true for the French neurologist Jean-Martin Charcot, who argued that trauma lies at the heart of all mental illness – or what he and his students referred to as *hysteria*.

As these ideas developed, they laid the foundations for *psychoanalytic* models of trauma which argued that trauma has the capacity to fundamentally undermine an individual's sense of self in ways that have profound consequences for their psychological and social functioning (e.g., Ulman & Brothers, 2013). Indeed, although we do not consider psychoanalytic approaches elsewhere in this volume, they are worth considering here precisely because they were the first to explore questions of self and identity in the context of mental illness. It is also the case that it is in the realm of trauma that psychoanalytic approaches to health have probably received the most attention – both in academic debate and in popular imagination (Brett, 1993; Seltzer, 1997).

The most influential contribution to psychoanalytic thinking around trauma was made by one of Charcot's students – Sigmund Freud. In his book *Beyond the Pleasure Principle*, Freud (1920) famously proposed that trauma arises when the intensity of a particular stimulus is so overwhelming that a person cannot defend themselves against the psychological impact of that stimulus. As a result, the person is flooded with impulses that they are unable to manage and their psychological functioning is compromised. He also argued that a lack of preparedness leads sufferers to repeatedly go back to their traumatic experiences (e.g., through intrusive thoughts and hyperarousal) in an effort to prepare themselves for the trauma they subsequently experienced. As he put it:

> In the case of quite a number of traumas, the difference between systems that are unprepared and systems that are well prepared . . . may be a decisive factor in determining the outcome; though where the strength of a trauma exceeds a certain limit this factor will no doubt cease to carry weight. The fulfilment of wishes is, as we know, brought about in a hallucinatory manner by dreams, and under the dominance of the pleasure principle this has become their function. But it is not in the service of that principle that the dreams of patients suffering from traumatic neuroses lead them back with such regularity to the situation in which the trauma occurred. We may assume, rather, that dreams are here helping to carry out another task, which must be accomplished before the dominance of the pleasure principle can even begin. These dreams are endeavouring to master the stimulus retrospectively, by developing the anxiety whose omission was the cause of the traumatic neurosis.
>
> (Freud, 1920/1953, p. 155)

In this formulation, then, the ongoing torment that trauma sufferers experience in the course of reliving their experiences is understood to be a manifestation of the challenges they face in trying to retrospectively prepare themselves for a horrific event for which they had actually been unprepared.

As his thinking on these matters developed, Freud became especially interested in World War I veterans who continued to be haunted by their exposure to wartime trauma in the form of neurasthenia (shell shock). He recognised, though, that his earlier writing did not fully account for the symptoms of this condition. Not least, this was because these analyses had tended to see trauma as having primarily sexual origins and as being related primarily to early childhood experience (Lifton, 1988). Accordingly, he elaborated his theorising to include the idea of *repetition compulsion* in which, among adults, traumatic experiences are continually relived as part of an – often futile – effort to master them and to resolve internal conflict within the self. Indeed, Freud argued that war created such intense trauma because it presented soldiers with profound identity challenges that were hard to make sense of and resolve. As he put it:

> The conflict . . . between the soldier's old peaceful ego and his new warlike one . . . becomes acute as soon as the peace-ego realises what danger it runs of losing its life owing to the rashness of its newly formed, parasitic double. It would be equally true to say that the old ego is protecting it from a mortal danger by taking flight into a traumatic neurosis or to say that it is defending itself against a new ego which is threatening its life. Thus the pre-condition of the war neuroses, the soil that nourishes them, would seem to be a national [conscript] army; there would be no possibility of their arising in an army of professional soldiers or mercenaries.
>
> (Freud, 1939/1953, p. 209)

There is still a great deal of debate both around what Freud actually thought about trauma and around the status of the evidence on which his thinking was based (e.g., Cohen, 1980). Many contemporary researchers are also dismissive of his contribution, not least because the focus on the role of dreams, fantasies, and primitive impulses fails to engage with – and can be seen to make light of – the 'hard reality' of traumatic experiences (Migone, 1994). Although, as we will see, the nature of combatants' military identity proves important for the trajectory of their mental health (e.g., Harvey et al., 2011; Hoge, Auchterloniek, & Milliken, 2006; Magerøy, 2009; Sundin et al., 2010); the very specific prediction that it is not possible for professional soldiers to experience trauma-related 'neurosis' is also plainly false (Jones & Wessley, 2005).

Nevertheless, for all this, Freud's writings on trauma serve as a key reference point for psychoanalytic and popular thinking on the subject to the present day (Brett, 1993). An obvious reason for this is that he was the first person to closely interrogate the psychology of trauma and to delineate some of its distinctive features. Beyond this, though, it is also the case that many of Freud's observations have stood the test of time and anticipated insights provided by later cognitive and neuroscientific research (Bromberg, 2003). In particular, this is true of his core observation that the adverse effects of trauma centre on the acute difficulties that people have in reconciling their experiences with a meaningful worldview and associated sense of self (Lifton, 1988; Resick & Schnicke, 1992). It is also the case that these insights have paved the way for treatments such as *narrative therapy* in which victims of trauma-related disturbance work with therapists to try to engage constructively with the past (rather than simply repress it) and re-create a positive and coherent sense of themselves and of their place in the world (Kaminer, 2006; McPherson, 2012; Tuval-Mashiach et al., 2004).

Cognitive and behavioural models

The fact that the validity and utility of psychoanalytic approaches to trauma is contested means that the approach is often overlooked by mainstream texts and courses on trauma. Yet it is nevertheless the case that some of the issues flagged by the approach are widely recognised as important within mainstream psychological theorising. In particular, the idea that experiences of trauma can compromise the functioning of the self has been a focus in efforts to advance *cognitive models* of trauma over the course of the last two decades.

Early attempts to address the role of cognition in trauma-related conditions were informed by a *learning model*. In line with Hobart Mowrer's (1960) two-factor theory of learning, this argued that negative symptomatology following trauma was a form of conditioned response in which, first, classical conditioning leads a previously neutral stimulus to become associated with an unconditioned stimulus (the traumatising event) that evokes discomfort or fear. As an example, Edna Foa and her colleagues discuss the case of Vietnam War veterans whose traumatic experiences became associated with various sounds (e.g., bangs), smells (e.g., burning), and objects (e.g., trucks; Foa, Steketee, & Rothbaum, 1989). Following this, operant conditioning can reinforce learned responses such as avoidance by reducing the discomfort arising from the presence of the conditioned stimulus. War veterans, for example, might learn to avoid going out in public because this protects them from exposure to triggers (the conditioned stimuli) that reawaken memories of their traumatic experiences.

Researchers generally agree that a learning model can help to explain the development of some of the extreme emotional and behavioural responses that are observed in trauma-related disorders (Foa et al., 1989; Resick et al., 2014). However, they note that it does not explain the full suite of symptoms – in particular, failing to account for those that relate to memory disturbance. As a result, they have tended to favour cognitive models which argue that the negative consequences of trauma (especially in the form of PTSD) derive from dysfunctional information processing precipitated by the extreme nature of a person's traumatising experiences.

Particularly influential in this regard is Anke Ehlers and David Clark's (2000) model which sees PTSD as arising from disturbance to two inter-related cognitive systems, as represented in Figure 6.5. The first of these reflects problems of *appraisal* that limit a person's ability to construe the precipitating event as time limited and context specific. These are similar to, but more extreme than, the problems of stress-related appraisal that we discussed in the previous chapter (e.g., see Figure 5.2). This means that rather than a person being able to consign their traumatic experience to the past ("that was then, this is now"), they experience it as an ongoing and global threat to self. These "maladaptive" appraisals

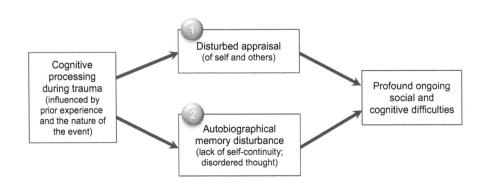

Figure 6.5 The two cognitive systems implicated in PTSD

Note: The model suggests that the difficulties associated with PTSD arise via two pathways: one which involves faulty appraisal (e.g., a person having an unrealistic sense of their own responsibility for outcomes), the other which involves faulty memory (e.g., a person being unable to recall occasions when they acted positively).

Source: Based on Ehlers and Clark (2000)

are observed to have multiple foci and to take a range of different forms – from a sense on the part of the sufferer that they are irreparably damaged ("I'm dead inside", "I'll never be able to relate to people again") to a sense that the world they inhabit is irreparably toxic ("Nowhere is safe", "You can't rely on other people"; Ehlers & Clark, 2000, p. 322).

The second form of cognitive disturbance that Ehlers and Clark's model identifies relates to evidence that PTSD sufferers have difficulty integrating the traumatic event into their *autobiographical memory*. So whereas in the normal course of our daily lives we are able to make sense of our experiences – including those that are negative – with reference to a range of expectations (e.g., "if you play a lot of contact sport you are likely to get injured"), in the case of severe trauma, this is no longer possible. Here, then, the event is so extreme that it shakes a person's sense of themselves and the world to the core. In particular, in ways anticipated by psychoanalytic theory, this is because it compromises their sense of *self-continuity* (Lifton, 1988). This difficulty in reconciling one's experience with one's identity is also associated with a range of other disturbances to memory, including flashbacks, poor memory organisation, excessive rumination, and heightened sensitivity to stimuli that prime the original trauma (Resick et al., 2014).

Multiple lines of research support these cognitive models by providing evidence of differences in the cognitive functioning – especially the appraisal and autobiographical memory – of trauma sufferers and control participants (e.g., Gil, Calev, Greenberg, Kugelmass, & Lerer, 1990; McNally, Lasko, Macklin, & Pitman, 1995; Vasterling, Brailey, Constans, & Sutker, 1998). Research has also shown that cognitive disturbances (especially those that affect social judgement and memory) are good predictors of long-term symptomatology. For example, to the extent that trauma leads a person to develop a view that the world is inherently unsafe or to ruminate excessively about why the trauma they suffered happened to them, they tend to experience ongoing difficulty leading a normal life (Ehring et al., 2008). In particular, and unsurprisingly, they are likely to find social interaction incredibly challenging, sometimes to the point where they avoid it altogether (Orsillo, Heimberg, Juster, & Garrett, 1996).

Models of this form have tended to lead psychologists to see trauma-related conditions (notably PTSD) primarily as cognitive problems. As a result, they have also developed and embraced treatments that have a similarly cognitive focus. In particular, many of the most widely recommended treatments centre on attempts to restore the appraisal and memory systems that are observed to be compromised following trauma. In particular, this is the goal of *cognitive behavioural therapy* (CBT) for PTSD which, as originally formulated, focuses on (1) educating people about the ways in which trauma can impair cognition, (2) encouraging them to gradually and safely relive their traumatic experiences through imaginal exposure, (3) facilitating more adaptive appraisals of those experiences through cognitive restructuring, and (4) attempting to manage anxiety through relaxation and the development of relevant coping skills (Harvey, Bryant, & Tarrier, 2003).

Although early studies were compromised by a lack of appropriate controls and a tendency not to study those populations most at risk of profound disturbance (e.g., war veterans), recent reviews provide good evidence that CBT can be an effective treatment for PTSD (e.g., see Cusack et al., 2016; Resick et al., 2014). At the same time, though, as Patricia Resick and colleagues point out, the resource-demanding nature of CBT limits its capacity to serve as an intervention to help manage large-scale trauma. Moreover, in the case of the trauma arising from natural disaster (e.g., floods, earthquakes), John Thoburn and Chasity O'Connell (2016) suggest that – especially when they are administered by outside experts – cognitive and behavioural interventions in general can create more problems than they resolve due (1) to the precious resources they consume (e.g., as a result of the need to transport and accommodate therapists) and (2) to the problems that arise from treatment being administered by experts who lack, or are seen to lack, local cultural knowledge.

The latter point also resonates with Resick and colleagues' (2014, p. 84) observation that many of the positive effects that result from treating PTSD with CBT (and other cognitive and behavioural therapies) arise from its "non-specific" features. As with other forms of psychotherapy, these include the nature of the relationship between therapist and client. In particular, it is clear that where trauma arises from a person's treatment at the hands of another group (e.g., as in war or rape), the identity of the therapist (e.g., as civilian or male) will have a bearing not only on the outcome of therapy, but also on people's willingness to participate in it (e.g., Keller, Zoellner, & Feeny, 2010).

It is also the case that as this work has advanced, researchers have had cause to question the value of some of the cognitive components that underpin particular interventions. In particular, there is now evidence that the process of imaginal exposure in which victims are encouraged to relive their trauma can sometimes backfire, especially if this occurs early in the therapeutic process and the circumstances of the trauma were complex (Dorahy et al., 2016). Relatedly, research has challenged the belief that it is always a good idea to debrief people after trauma (Rothbaum & Davis, 2003), with influential reviews by Bisson and his colleagues indicating that *critical incident stress debriefing* (which involves discussing a traumatic incident in the immediate aftermath) is as likely to do harm as to do good (and most likely to have negligible impact on adjustment; Bisson, 2003; Rose, Bisson, Churchill, & Wessely, 2002). As a result, contemporary guidelines recommend that therapists encourage trauma victims to revisit their experiences only after their condition has stabilised and they have developed the internal and external resources (in particular, relevant support networks) to help them negotiate threatening aspects of the process (e.g., Australian Centre for Posttraumatic Mental Health, 2007; Cloitre et al., 2011; Litz, Gray, Bryant, & Adler, 2002).

Beyond this, it is also the case that forms of treatment that aim to take people away from their trauma (rather than zero in on it) can also be effective. This is true, for example, of the Seeking Safety programme (Najavits, 2002) in which the primary emphasis is on removing people (e.g., women who have been abused or people with substance use problems) from the site of their trauma and placing them in a positive group context where they receive support and exposure to a new way of life (e.g., without abuse or drugs; Lenz, Henesy, & Callender, 2016).

Together, these various points suggest that although cognitive behavioural models provide a very useful framework for understanding the nuanced ways in which a person's thoughts and emotions can be disrupted by trauma, they are not especially good at accounting for the important role that social factors play in shaping the course that trauma recovery takes – either within a therapeutic context or outside it. In particular, it would appear that there is considerable scope for these models to be enriched by a theoretical framework which recognises the social dimensions of trauma and resilience as also lying *at the heart of the process* and sees them as integral not only to treatment outcomes, but also to the processes by which these are achieved.

The social identity approach to trauma and resilience

The literature on psychological reactions to trauma speaks to the fact that this is a complex and multi-faceted topic. Indeed, for this reason it is hard to summarise and do justice to it in a short review. Nevertheless, for all this complexity, three points emerge quite clearly from the material we have covered in the previous sections. The first, and most important, is that *when trauma has an adverse psychological impact, this is because it fundamentally compromises a person's social sense of self and their relationship to the world at large*. Indeed, in ways that are not immediately obvious in the case of more general stressors (as reviewed in the previous chapter), we would argue that problems created by trauma can therefore often be understood as problems of social identity. Traumatic events often have the capacity to undermine a person's sense of self-continuity and their sense of meaningful and positive connection to others (Pennebaker & Keough, 1999). Accordingly, trauma can also compromise all that a strong sense of self achieves. In particular, as proposed in Chapter 2 (e.g., in the meaning and agency hypotheses, H13 and H15), it can undermine feelings of control, confidence, efficacy, self-esteem, meaning, and purpose.

Second, by the same token, it is also the case that resilience in the face of trauma is typically associated with processes that help to restore, maintain, or enhance a person's sense of self and their sense of meaningful connection to others. In this way, effective intervention – whether psychological or behavioural, and whatever its specific theoretical underpinnings – can often be seen to achieve its effects through a process of *identity revitalisation*. In particular, this occurs where the trauma itself is the basis for the development of *new social identities* – in particular, those that are shared with other survivors (as also seen with recovery from addiction; Dingle, Cruwys, & Frings, 2015; see Chapter 9, and brain injury, see Chapter 11).

In teasing out these points, however, a third important point becomes apparent. This is that, to date, theorising around the identity-related aspects of responses to trauma has focused almost exclusively on sufferers' personal identities. This focus can be traced back to Freud's (1939/1953) assertion that trauma is an issue of ego conflict, but it is seen today in work on narrative therapy and autobiographical memory which attends primarily to the difficulties that sufferers experience *as individuals* and that typically looks at the problems these create 'from the inside out' (e.g., such that problematic cognitions are seen to interfere with productive social experiences). However, in line with the central theme of this book, we can see that there is scope for also seeing the problematic effects of trauma as reflecting the difficulties this creates for a person's sense of *social identity* 'from the outside in' (e.g., such that problematic social experiences are seen to interfere with productive cognitions). Here, then, we can hypothesise that social identity threat is an important determinant of trauma-related psychological difficulties. It would follow, too, that *social identity development* might also be part of the effective resolution of trauma and more generally play a key role in structuring people's resilience (and potentially their growth) in the face of trauma. These, then, are the key propositions that have informed social identity research in this area and that we will explore in the sections that follow.

Social identity is central to the experience and appraisal of traumatic events

Although these will not always relate to a group membership that is chosen, it is often the case that, to some extent, people experience trauma *because* of their group membership. For example, soldiers in World War I and Vietnam were exposed to trauma because they were in particular armies and regiments; likewise, victims of earthquakes and floods are exposed to trauma because of the countries and communities in which they live. Indeed, more generally, one fundamental reason why social identity often plays a major role in the psychology of trauma is that this is something that people often experience *in groups*. Certainly it is possible to be an isolated victim of trauma, but it is apparent that many of the examples that we have discussed up to this point affect large numbers of people not just one or two in isolation. Indeed, even when trauma is experienced by a person in isolation (as in the case of rape or other forms of interpersonal violence), it often has a group-based dimension – which means that members of particular groups (e.g., women, members of minority groups) are much more likely to be victims.

In many cases the level of a person's social identification with a particular group will also be important to the specific nature of these experiences. For example, a soldier may choose to put themselves in harm's way, or a town resident may decide not to move out of a flood zone, or a person may not leave an abusive relationship, because the strength of their identification with the group in question (their country, town, or family) is very strong or because they have no other viable groups to join. Indeed, this point emerges from research by Amy Bombay and her colleagues with Aboriginal communities in Canada (Bombay, Matheson, & Anisman, 2011, 2014). This found that intergenerational transition of trauma – in which the effects of the historical discrimination and abuse that their cultural group experienced were transmitted from one generation to the next – was higher to the extent that Aboriginal heritage was central to the identity of community members. As these researchers note, this association can be seen to arise from multiple processes, but it seems likely to reflect the fact that those for whom Aboriginal identity is important are more likely (1) to be exposed to discrimination and abuse (and hence experience trauma) and (2) to feel the effects of discrimination and abuse more keenly (i.e., as a threat to their identity and hence be more traumatised by it). Importantly then, when a person does suffer trauma, identification with the group can also intensify the problems – and, in particular, the sense of personal conflict – that this creates. This is because the identification reflects and has created affinity for the group, and yet it appears that this affinity has ultimately been the cause of personal harm. A large task of any treatment therefore has to be to try to repair the sense of group-based safety and trust that the traumatic event has typically compromised (e.g., see Resick & Schnicke, 1992).

In ways suggested in Figure 6.6, we can thus see that social identities are often implicated in *exposure* to trauma and, equally, that they often also have a bearing on the trajectory of trauma *impact*. More particularly, the theoretical principles that we set out in Chapter 2 suggest that group dynamics and norms – particularly those that relate to *social support* – will play a key role in determining (1) whether and how individuals are buffered and protected from a particular source of trauma, (2) how exactly they respond to the trauma, and (3) what the consequences and outcomes of the trauma are. As we will see in the sections that follow, there is now quite a large empirical literature which bears these points out in a range of different ways.

Some of the work that speaks most clearly to the capacity for social identity to shape people's experience and appraisal of traumatic (or potentially traumatic) events has been conducted by John Drury and his colleagues in the context of a wide range of disasters and emergencies (e.g., Drury, Cocking, & Reicher, 2009b; Drury, Novelli, & Stott, 2015). In one of these researchers' early studies they examined how people's experience of mass emergencies was shaped by the extent to which the situations in which they arose were associated with high or low levels of shared identification among victims (Drury et al, 2009b). The participants in this study were British residents who had been involved in a range of different events – including the bombing of Harrods in 1983, the fire at Bradford City's football stadium in 1985, the sinking of the cruise ship *Jupiter* in 1988, the deaths of 96 Liverpool supporters at Hillsborough in 1989 (see Figure 6.7), and the crush that occurred at a Fatboy Slim beach party in 2002.

On the basis of their interviews, the researchers established whether the specific context of each event, as experienced by participants, was associated with a high or low level of shared identification among those who were there. Importantly, then, although the groups of people who were attending

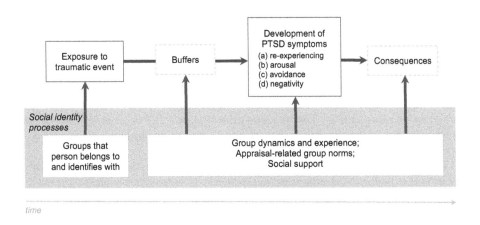

Figure 6.6 Ways in which social identity processes can shape the development of posttraumatic stress disorder (PTSD)

Note: Social identities are often implicated in exposure to trauma as well as its impact. In particular, group dynamics, group norms, and social support play a role in determining (1) whether individuals are buffered from trauma, (2) how they respond to the trauma, and (3) what the consequences of the trauma are.

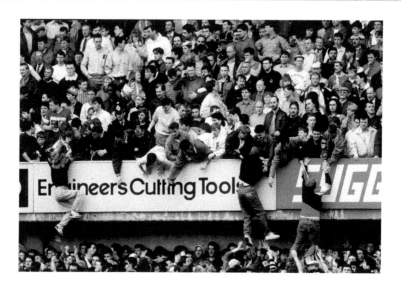

Figure 6.7 The 1989 Hillsborough disaster

Note: The worst sport-related disaster in British history unfolded when police opened a gate at the side of the stadium to relieve overcrowding outside the stadium. This led to an influx of Liverpool supporters into an enclosed space in which 96 people were crushed to death and over 700 injured. The trauma of survivors – especially among families of the victims – was intensified by press coverage which claimed that the disaster was the fault of callous and unruly fans. An initial coroner's inquest concluded in 1991 that the deaths were 'accidental', but in 2016 a second inquest, for which the families had campaigned for more than a decade, returned a verdict of 'unlawful killing' arising from gross negligence on the part of senior police officers.

Source: www.birminghammail.co.uk/news/midlands-news/19-people-refuse-help-hillsborough-11421704

these events tended to be unknown to each other, the researchers observed that there was variation in the degree to which it was psychologically meaningful for their participants to self-categorize in terms of shared group membership (e.g., in ways suggested by Figure 2.5). For example, some of the party-goers attending the Fatboy Slim beach party were judged as having had high shared identification with the rest of the crowd, whereas others had low shared identification.

The key question in which Drury and colleagues were interested was how these differences in participants' level of shared social identification (as assessed by an independent judge) played out in their experiences of the unfolding disaster. Here one of the most striking findings was that low identifiers were much less likely than high identifiers to report having felt a sense of solidarity with the people around them (see also Alnabulsi & Drury, 2014, as discussed in Chapter 2; Novelli, Drury, Reicher, & Stott, 2013). Associated with this, as things started to go wrong, low identifiers were much more likely to report experiencing a sense of panic and to perceive others as experiencing panic. In contrast, high identifiers were more likely to report themselves and others as behaving in a calm and orderly fashion, as in the following recollections from a passenger on *Jupiter*:

> [Passengers] just followed the queue because maybe that was the way out . . . It was very orderly very noisy but very orderly and people calling out and this teacher very calmly saying 'come on, just keep going get going get going.'

> (Drury et al., 2009b, p. 497)

Importantly too, a sense of shared identity with others was also associated with increased perceptions of mutual support and helping (as suggested by the support hypothesis, H14). So whereas respondents who were in situations in which there was a low level of shared social identity tended to feel that this was a situation of 'everyone for themselves', those in situations where there was a high degree of shared social identity reported feeling a strong sense of togetherness and solidarity – to the point where they were prepared to put others (including strangers) *before* themselves. This is illustrated by the following statements – the first from another *Jupiter* passenger, the second from a supporter at Hillsborough:

> As soon as I could get my arms out I was helping people and pushing them up, yeah, absolutely it was . . . yeah it was only you felt that 'cos I mean it's only when you look back you just feel 'oh I could have done that', I mean you look back, I mean everyone did help each other and I don't think there was anyone that . . . could really look back and say I didn't do anything to help anybody.
>
> The behaviour of many people in that crowd simply trying to help their fellow supporters was heroic in some cases. So I don't think in my view there was any question that there was an organic sense of unity of crowd behaviour . . . It was clearly the case that people were trying to get people who were seriously injured out of that crowd, it was seriously a case of trying to get people to hospital, get them to safety . . . I just wish I'd been able to . . . to prevail on a few more people not to . . . put themselves in danger.
>
> (Drury et al., 2009a, p. 497)

More recently, similar patterns were confirmed by Drury and colleagues in a more forensic study of the 2002 Fatboy Slim beach party (Drury, Novelli, & Stott, 2015; Study 1). This was an event held on Brighton Beach that had originally been expected to attract around 65,000 revellers but which, for a range of reasons (including unexpectedly good weather) ended up attracting around 250,000 (see Figure 6.8). Unsurprisingly, this led to a dangerously high concentration of people on the beach – a situation that became even more dangerous once the tide started to come in.

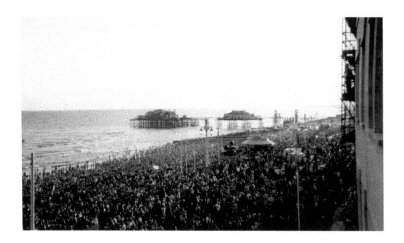

Figure 6.8 The 2002 Fatboy Slim beach party in Brighton

Note: Attended by around 250,000 people (four times more than expected), the crush that this created represented a serious threat to party-goers' health. Drury and colleagues (2015) argue that disaster and ensuing trauma were only averted because shared social identity allowed participants to self-organise and self-regulate in response to impending threats (e.g., the incoming tide).

Source: Wikipedia

Although the unfolding situation threatened the lives of many thousands of people, it transpired that only 150 people reported minor injuries. In this way, disaster – and hence people's exposure to potential trauma – was averted (which may explain why the event is not more widely known about outside the live events industry). The key question, of course, is 'How?' On the basis of survey responses from 48 people who were caught up in the unfolding drama, Drury and colleagues' key conclusion was that this was the result of the same dynamics as outlined in their previous work, in which a high level of shared identification among the crowd on the beach led to high levels of order and calm, even in the face of impending calamity. In particular, statistical analysis showed that high social identification was associated with a high level of *collective self-regulation* and that this was mediated by an expectation of support from others, as well as trust in the crowd. This accords with the reflections of the party-goers themselves, as illustrated by the following comment:

> I'm absolutely of the opinion that it was the crowd that stopped the disaster . . . none of the barriers, none of the coppers, none of the stew- stewards, none of the alleged things that were put into place . . . to protect the crowd I don't think any of that mattered, I think it was the crowd that kept everything together.
>
> (Drury et al., 2015, p. 540)

In this and much of their other research, a secondary concern of Drury and colleagues was to explore whether participants' understandings and representations of behaviour at the event differed from those of onlookers, including members of the emergency services charged with ensuring public order and safety. This was indeed the case. More specifically, what the researchers found was that whereas the accounts of participants tended to tell a story of identification-based order, those of the emergency personnel tended to refer to the *dis*orderliness of the crowd and to its *lack* of control. In this way, the latter aligned with a widespread belief that crowds are inherently dangerous and unruly – a belief that can be traced back to the influential writings of Gustave Le Bon at the end of the 19th century (Le Bon, 1895; see Reicher, 1987; also Drury, Novelli, & Stott, 2013). Moreover, the crowd's unruliness was seen by the officials as something that had been extremely threatening to their well-being at the same time that they asserted that public safety had only been achieved through their own acts of bravery. As one police chief inspector put it:

> Many officers have been traumatised. Some of them have been verbally and physically abused by members of the public while they are trying to help people in distress.
>
> (Drury et al., 2015, p. 540)

As Drury and colleagues note, the primary goal of their research was not to establish which of these different sets of accounts was correct. Rather, it was to show that different groups of people tend to have very different understandings of (potentially) traumatic events and that a standard LeBonian account of crowd (and group) behaviour – which sees this as inherently threatening to health and which tends to be embraced by members of the emergency services – is very much at odds with the social psychological reality of participants (for a related discussion see Bottrell, 2007, 2016). Nevertheless, in line with social identity theorising, the researchers show that of these two accounts it is only the former which explains the capacity for groups to respond adaptively to impending disaster. Indeed, far from being inherently problematic, their findings suggest that shared identity can allow group members to self-regulate and self-organise in ways that ward off trauma rather than deepen it.

Social identity is central to the experience of posttraumatic stress

As we noted earlier in this chapter, it is probably in military contexts that the psychology of trauma – and in particular of PTSD – has been of greatest interest to researchers. Indeed, the main body of work that has investigated PTSD from a social identity perspective has been carried out in Northern Ireland in the context of 'the Troubles' associated with sectarian conflict between Protestants and Catholics and between the British army and various paramilitary groups. This conflict lasted over 30 years and affected a broad swathe of the country's residents – to the extent that a representative survey of Northern Ireland residents by Orla Muldoon and Ciara Downes (2007) indicated that around 10% had symptoms suggestive of PTSD.

Interestingly, as well as showing that residents who had PTSD symptoms were likely to have had more direct experience of sectarian violence than those without PTSD symptoms, Muldoon and Downes' survey showed that the former group were likely to have lower levels of national identification. This suggested to the researchers that a person's national identification (as either Irish or Northern Irish) might be protecting them from the worst effects of trauma. Accordingly, they embarked on a more extensive programme of work in which they sought to explore more thoroughly the role of social identity processes in the development of posttraumatic stress.

The first of these studies involved surveying 3,000 residents who lived in Northern Ireland and the border regions of the Irish Republic (the key region on which intergroup conflict was focused; Muldoon, Schmid, & Downes, 2009). The survey replicated the results of the earlier study, in showing that exposure to conflict was a significant predictor of compromised well-being. Beyond this, though, it also showed that national identification (as either British or Irish) was heavily implicated in this relationship. More specifically, experiencing violence tended to *increase* national identification and, perhaps counterintuitively, this in turn tended to increase well-being. Interestingly though, respondents who saw themselves as Northern Irish – a national identity that can be seen as more inclusive of the traditionally oppositional political positions associated with the conflict (Lowe & Muldoon, 2014) – did not demonstrate this same identity protection. The key point that the researchers took from this was that identities associated with the conflict appeared to provide an *interpretative lens* through which conflict was given meaning and therefore became less traumatising. Put differently, their findings suggest that *people are more likely to be traumatised by the violence that flows from intergroup conflict if they do not define themselves in terms of a social identity that allows them to make sense of that conflict.* So whereas a sense of the importance of 'us' and 'our cause' makes conflict worth enduring, without this, the conflict and its consequences are much harder to live with.

These were issues that the same research team elaborated upon further in another study in Northern Ireland, this time exploring the relationship between *perceived intergroup threat* and well-being (Schmid & Muldoon, 2015). Using a random sample of 2,000 residents, this found that among those residents who were most exposed to conflict, there was both a direct and an indirect relationship between perceived threat and well-being. On the one hand, the direct relationship showed that respondents' health was worse the more threatened they felt by the conflict. On the other hand, though, the indirect effect suggested that the more threatened respondents felt, the more they identified with their ethno-religious ingroup (Protestant or Catholic), and the *better* this was for their health.

On the basis of these findings the researchers argued that social identification is an important *coping mechanism* for subpopulations who are exposed to high levels of conflict and violence in the context of intergroup threat. This was an analysis that Katharina Schmid and colleagues tested further in another study of Northern Ireland residents (N = 221; Schmid, Muldoon, & Lowe, 2017). This differed from earlier studies in having a longitudinal design which allowed the researchers to be more confident making causal inferences. Again, though, the findings ultimately supported the same theoretical conclusions: that threat drives social identification which in turn serves to protect well-being in populations that are exposed to political violence.

Very similar conclusions have also been drawn by researchers who have studied the relationship between social identity, trauma, and health in other theatres of conflict. In particular, this is true of work by Blerina Kellezi and Steve Reicher that has examined the health and well-being of Albanian communities affected by the 1999 war in Kosovo – a war in which 10,000 people died and nearly half a million people were forced to flee their homes. In the first of their studies, the researchers studied a group of refugees who had directly experienced at least one extreme event in the war and examined the relationship between (1) their appraisal of conflict-related trauma as more or less identity affirming and (2) their health and well-being (Kellezi, Reicher, & Cassidy, 2009). As one might expect, levels of anxiety and depression in the sample were generally quite high. Importantly, though, the results showed that participants' mental health varied significantly as a function of the degree to which they saw the conflict as identity-affirming. More specifically, those refugees who agreed more with the statements "Only through fighting could we build a Kosovo Albanian Nation" and "The war had to be fought for the good of the nation" were less likely to have been psychologically scarred by the conflict. Moreover, these patterns were mediated by social support such that where identity had been affirmed by the conflict, respondents reported having received more support from their community and having better mental health as a result.

One of the wretched features of war, however, is that the protagonists' interest in promoting health and well-being is usually highly circumscribed. In particular, this means that combatants are generally more interested in destroying the hearts and minds of their enemies than in lifting them up. In this regard, one implication of the foregoing analysis is that if a group's goal is to accentuate rather than ameliorate trauma-related stress (and sadly this is often the case), then a powerful way to do this is by breaking down the identity-based bonds among group members. This is a point that Kellezi and Reicher (2012) make in the context of a discussion of the ways in which perpetrators of war crimes often target their malevolence in ways that do precisely this. For example, Nazi perpetrators routinely sought to humiliate Jews in ways that *dis*affirmed their social identity (e.g., by making them eat pork), knowing that this would break them down both individually and collectively (e.g., Sofsky, 1993). Likewise, commentators have observed that rape is a particularly potent weapon in war because it creates a sense of shame among victims that erodes family bonds and these family bonds are a key source of community strength and resilience (e.g., Ramanathapillai, 2006). Indeed, as Ruth Seifert (1996, p. 35) observes, in war, rape can be seen to constitute a "second front" because:

> War crimes against women . . . have cultural functions. They destroy the physical and psychological existence of the women concerned and, moreover, inflict harm on the culture and collective identity of the whole group, ethnicity, or nation under attack.

These darker identity dynamics are also brought to light by Kellezi and Reicher's work with Kosovan refugees. In particular, extended interviews with men and women who had endured a range of traumatic experiences pointed to ways in which the impact of these depended upon the degree to which they lent themselves to stories that could be told with pride or else could not be told at all. On the one hand, then, when a traumatic experience could be retold as part of a virtuous story of one's contribution to the group, it tended to be construed positively and to have positive implications for well-being – not least because victims were supported by other ingroup members who were happy to hear the story. This was the case, for example, when a woman told of how "I hid my son inside my breast, and I thought 'let the bullets take me, only my son should survive". Here, then, the victim's story was made bearable by the capacity to share it with ingroup members. Indeed, as Ali Aslan Yildiz and Maykel Verkuyten (2011) have pointed out, by cultivating a sense of *inclusive victimhood*, the collective retelling of traumatic events can help to build social identity and thereby promote both solidarity and well-being.

On the other hand, though, Kellezi and Reicher (2012) observed that there was no such positive pathway if traumatic experiences could not be recounted in this way (for related evidence, see Pennebaker, 1993). This was the case for all the victims of rape that they interviewed, but, to a lesser extent, it was also true if members of an interviewee's family had died as civilians (rather than soldiers) and hence were seen by other members of their community as cowards rather than heroes. In both cases, then, strong group norms made the victim's story 'unspeakable'. And because there was no capacity for them to recruit the support of others through retelling their stories, this made their trauma unbearable.

Evidence from drug rehabilitation contexts also points to the fact that PTSD symptomatology can itself be a barrier to the development of social identities that might facilitate recovery. Indeed, this is the key point that emerges from a longitudinal study by Ken Herington and his colleagues of 152 adults entering residential drug and alcohol treatment in a therapeutic community (Herington, Dingle, & Perryman, 2017). This found that experiences of interpersonal maltreatment were widespread among participants: 66% reported emotional abuse in their lifetime, 48% reported physical abuse, and 23% had experienced sexual abuse. As a result, on admission there was a high level of PTSD symptomatology in the sample (with the mean level above the cut-off for PTSD diagnosis), and the level of this symptomatology was negatively associated with retention in treatment ($r = -.28$). Looking to identify factors that might explain this relationship, the researchers found that among those participants who were available for follow-up seven months after discharge, PTSD symptom severity at admission was negatively correlated with their adoption of a substance misuse "recovery" identity ($r = -.35$), their perception of support from their recovery groups ($r = -.34$), their adoption of a "non-user" identity ($r = -.40$), and their perceptions of support from non-using social groups ($r = -.31$). It thus appears that PTSD symptoms acted as a barrier to the formation of recovery and non-user identities, and thereby obstructed the path to long-term positive outcomes (a point we return to when discussing addiction in Chapter 9).

Together, then, the various programmes of research discussed in this section all point to the fact that social identity (or lack of it) has a powerful role to play in determining how trauma is appraised, spoken about, and dealt with, and hence what its implications are for victims' mental health. The latter links in this chain are entirely consistent both (1) with physiological models which suggest that the functioning of stress and memory systems is structured "top-down" by brain systems implicated in the interpretation of events, emotions, and memories (e.g., Rauch et al., 2006; Shin et al., 2006) and (2) with cognitive models which suggest that the stress-related effects of trauma are mediated by appraisal (as in Figure 6.5; e.g., Ehlers & Clark, 2000; Lazarus & Folkman, 1984). Importantly, though, social identity scholarship supports the claim that these appraisals are themselves structured by internalised group memberships. In particular, in the case of trauma that results from intergroup conflict, positive appraisal of that trauma is more likely to the extent that perceivers identify with a group that is implicated in the conflict and *through interaction with other ingroup members* come to see the costs of that conflict as a price they are prepared – even proud – to pay. The corollary of this, though, is that for those who do not identify in this way and who cannot draw on group support (for whatever reason), the depredations brought about by conflict will generally prove to be altogether more distressing. Not least, this is because they are more likely to be suffered in silence and in solitude.

Social identity is a basis for resilience and posttraumatic growth

Although the study of the impact of trauma tends (for obvious reasons) to focus on its capacity to be a source of psychological damage, in recent years a large number of commentators have appealed for a more balanced approach to the issue (e.g., Linley & Joseph, 2004). Their appeals are based on the fact that, on the whole, human beings prove remarkably resilient in the face of trauma – even when it is of the most extreme form. This is an observation that Rebecca Solnit (2009) explores compellingly in her powerful book *A Paradise Built in Hell* which details the ways in which communities that experience catastrophic disasters manage not simply to recover but to *thrive*.

Such resilience is seen, for example, in the case of the 2005 London bombings that we mentioned at the start of this chapter. In these, 52 people were killed and around 700 people were injured after bombs were detonated on three underground railway carriages and a bus. In the former case, one might expect that after a bomb had gone off below ground – in darkness, surrounded by carnage, and with emergency services unable to reach the victims for hours – the scene would be one of utter chaos and extreme psychological distress. Yet when Drury and colleagues interviewed survivors, they observed that this was far from the case (Drury, Cocking, & Reicher, 2009a; see also Williams & Drury, 2009, 2011). Generally speaking, this meant that there was more calm than panic, more quiet leadership than mayhem, more resilience than trauma.

These interviews also revealed a number of other interesting findings. The first was that, in line with patterns observed in other disasters that we discussed earlier (e.g., Drury et al., 2009a, 2009b), those who were in the bombed carriages reported a strong sense of connection with and among their fellow travellers.

This is remarkable in itself, because anyone who has ever travelled on the Tube knows that the experience is usually associated with a marked *lack* of connection between passengers. Indeed, as London tourist guides make clear, the general norm is to keep to oneself, to pretend not to notice others, and to studiously avoid eye contact (e.g., Ensall, 2014; see Figure 6.9). Drury and his colleagues argue, however, that although such behaviour is the norm, after the bombs had gone off victims were rapidly brought together by their emergent sense of *common fate*. As Drury (2012, p. 202) notes, this sense of shared group membership emerged because, in ways suggested by the principle of meta-contrast (e.g., see Figure 2.3), "the social 'figure and ground' shift[ed] from 'me in contrast to others' to 'us in contrast to the emergency.'"

Drury and colleagues' interviews also suggested that, where it occurred, this emergent sense of shared identity had cognitive and relational implications for victims. Cognitively, people described how it gave them a sense of shared purpose and goals (in line with the meaning hypothesis, H13); relationally, it was a basis for a sense of both solidarity (e.g., associated with an expectation to give and receive help, as per the support hypothesis, H14) and validation (e.g., associated with feelings of consensus and trust, as per the connection hypothesis, H12). Moreover, the researchers argue that, for those who experienced them, these cognitive and relational elements combined to *empower* survivors as a group (as per H15) in ways that allowed them to be collectively resilient. Some sense of this combination of elements is provided by the following statement from one of the survivors:

> I felt that we're all in the same boat together [ ] and then for the feelings that I was feeling could well have been felt by them as well 'cos I don't think any normal human being could just calmly sat there going oh yeah this is great [ ] it was a stressful situation and we were all in it together and the best way to get out of it was to help each other . . . yeah so I felt exactly I felt quite close to the people near me.
>
> (Drury et al., 2009a, p. 82)

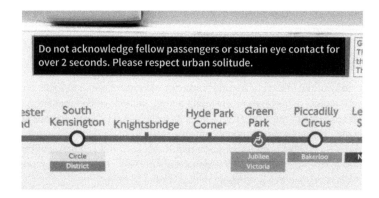

Figure 6.9 A sign of everyday social disconnection on the London Underground

Note: Spoof notices such as this appeared mysteriously on the London Underground in 2012. They speak to the fact that it is normal for travellers to be psychologically disconnected from each other. However, research by Drury and colleagues (2009) found that commuters who were on the carriages that were bombed by terrorists in 2005 very quickly developed a strong sense of shared social identity. This was a basis for them to provide each other with support and for collective resilience.

Source: The authors

Drury (2012) integrates these various elements within the *social identity model of collective resilience* that is reproduced in Figure 6.9. The critical point to note here is that, in contrast to models which see resilience as an aspect of personal identity (i.e., the psychology of the person *as an individual*), resilience is here seen as a *collective* process that is only made possible by an internalised sense of shared social identity (see also Cacioppo et al., 2011, p. 44). Stated more baldly, as a participant in a recent field study of resilience among primary care givers recognised, "You can't be resilient on your own, can you?" (Matheson, Robertson, Elliott, Iversen, & Murchie, 2016).

Following on from these early studies, more recent work by Drury and colleagues has provided further support for their model of resilience. In particular, a survey of 1,240 survivors of the 2010 earthquake in Chile provided broad support for the claim that an emergent sense of common fate among survivors led them to develop a strong sense of shared identity and that this fed into the provision and receipt of support as well as a sense of collective efficacy (Drury, Brown, González, & Miranda, 2016). This study also elaborated upon previous work in several interesting ways. In particular, it showed (1) that the expectations of support that derived from shared social identity were pivotal to emergent group dynamics that allowed for coordinated efforts to help survivors and (2) that the experience of seeing other ingroup members 'pitching in' to help survivors provided onlookers with a strong motivation to pitch in themselves. Indeed, this meant that even if those onlookers had not been able to do physical work themselves, they had worked hard to sustain those who were.

Aspects of the social identity model are also supported by recent research that Loris Vezzali and colleagues have conducted with children who have lived through earthquakes in Italy (Vezzali, Drury, Cadamuro, & Versari, 2015; see also Vezzali, Cadamuro, Versari, Giovannini, & Trifiletti, 2015). Here though, as well as supporting claims that shared social identity is a basis for engaging with and helping

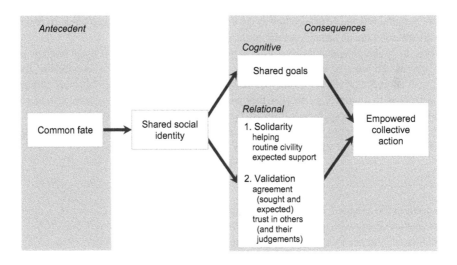

Figure 6.10 The social identity model of collective resilience

Note: The key feature of this model is that it sees resilience as arising from a sense of shared social identity that flows from an emergent sense of common fate. This is because shared social identity has cognitive and relational consequences that allow for empowered collective action.

Source: Based on Drury (2012)

other ingroup members, the researchers observed that the experience of PTSD symptoms (as reported by the children) was actually a precursor to this sense of shared identity. So rather than PTSD creating a desire to dissociate from one's ingroup (which might be expected, based on the pattern of symptoms often described), it actually appeared to do the opposite – by creating a sense of common hurt and a strong sense of connection to other ingroup members. This indeed aligns with other studies of the experience of sharing pain (e.g., Bastian, Jetten, & Ferris, 2014a) that we will explore in greater depth in Chapter 12.

Yet as well as allowing people to *cope* with the challenges of trauma, it is also the case that the emergent sense of social identity that collective trauma can create has the capacity to help individuals and communities *move forward* (Cacioppo, Reis, & Zautra, 2011). This point is confirmed by a study of nearly 400 survivors of the 2015 Nepal earthquake undertaken by Muldoon and colleagues 6 months after this had devastated large areas of the country – killing 9,000 people, injuring over 20,000, and leaving more than 3 million people homeless (Muldoon et al., 2017). As in Drury and colleagues' work, the researchers found that, although levels of PTSD were very high, a sense of shared social identity was an important determinant of responses to the earthquake. In particular, this was because survivors with a stronger sense of shared social identity also reported having a stronger sense of collective efficacy.

At the same time, though, Muldoon and colleagues' study showed that the sense of shared identity was higher in some communities than in others and that this was an important predictor of the earthquakes' psychological impact (i.e., on victims' PTSD symptomatology) as well as communities' material response. This indeed is a point that accords with sociological and epidemiological research which shows that pre-trauma levels of social capital are an important predictor of responses to natural disasters (e.g., Nakagawa & Shaw, 2004) in ways suggested by the social identity model of identity change (SIMIC, Haslam, Holme et al., 2008; Jetten, et al., 2009; see Chapter 3). In this case, shared social identity tended to be higher in communities whose members were from higher rather than lower Hindu castes (Chhetri and Brahim vs. Janajatis and Dalits). It was in these communities, then, that people were not only less likely to succumb to the effects of PTSD but also more likely to report post-traumatic growth after the devastation of the earthquake.

However, as Muldoon and colleagues (2017) observe, at the same time as these findings point to the psychological and material benefits of being in a high-status group, they also underline the costs of belonging to an under-privileged group. Not only, then, were members of lower-caste groups more likely to be exposed to trauma (e.g., because they had inferior housing), but they were also more likely to have difficulties dealing psychologically with its consequences due to their low levels of shared identity. So where for the more privileged group the trauma could provide opportunities for growth, for the disadvantaged group it was more likely only to compound their misery.

Conclusion

With death in the terrible flickering gloom of the fight
I was cruel and fierce with despair; I was naked and bound;
I was stricken: and beauty returned through the shambles of night;
In the faces of men she returned; and their triumph I found.
(Siegfried Sassoon, *The Triumph*, 1918[6.1])

If you want to gain insight into the psychological impact of trauma, you could do worse than start by reading the war poems of Siegfried Sassoon. This, indeed, was very much his purpose in writing them – to try to communicate, and work through, the agonies of martial conflict on a terrifying scale and the struggle to find any semblance of light in the "terrible flickering gloom". Within them, there are many observations that align with the analysis we have presented in this chapter. Most notably, his poems tell (1) of the collective enthusiasm that led him to enlist (e.g., "We are the happy legion for we know/ Times but a golden wind that shakes the grass"; *Absolution, 1915*, Sassoon, 1983, p. 15), (2) of the sense of disillusionment he experienced as the recruiting slogans proved hollow (e.g., "They hoped the show'd be finished before long/ And cursed it for a senseless, bloody stunt"; *The Optimist*, 1917, Sassoon, 1983, p. 74), (3) of the symptoms of stress he experienced in the face of relentless slaughter (e.g., "Those whispering guns – O Christ, I want to go out/ And screech at them to stop – I'm going crazy;/ I'm going stark, staring mad because of the guns"; *Repression of War Experience*, 1917, Sassoon, 1983, p. 74), and, finally, (4) of the efforts to work though his mixed emotions with fellow veterans after the armistice ("I can't talk easily about the War/ I ask you guarded questions, naming men/ Who've come through safe and sound; and when we hit/ On someone who's been killed or badly maimed/ We're silent for a while and prod the ground"; *A Last Word*, 1917, Sassoon, 1983, p. 138).

The particularities of Sassoon's experiences also speak to the role of social identity processes in trauma. Most especially, just as it was social identity that led him to put himself in harm's way, so, too, it led to his acute stress and depression, and so, too, it fed into the politics surrounding his treatment for shell shock (where his hospitalisation was partly an attempt to manage the problems that his emergent pacifism created for military authorities). So although his were a singular set of traumas, they resonate so forcefully because they are shot through with the terrors – and ultimately the salvation – of the collective.

This, then, has been the primary objective of this chapter: to show that while we tend to scrutinise (and pathologise) the psychological effects of trauma through a concentrated focus on the individual victim, these effects can sometimes be better understood (as well as easier to make sense of and to seek to resolve) once we appreciate them as having powerful group-based determinants. Amongst other things, this appreciation also allows us to understand why treatment for traumatic stress is typically more effective when it is administered by insiders rather than outsiders, why trauma is typically easier to bear (and treat) when it is experienced in a group and in the service of a collective cause, and why (providing it is sensitive to such social identity dynamics) treatment can be particularly effective when it is delivered in groups and recognises them as a source of psychological strength (Başoğlu et al., 1996, 1997; Drury & Winter, 2004; Katona & Brady, in press; Resick et al., 2014).

At the same time, though, it is important to note that the efficacy of group-based interventions for PTSD is chronically under-studied (Sloan, Bovin, & Schnurr, 2012). Nevertheless, there is growing empirical evidence that insights from social identity theorising can improve trauma-related intervention (see Carter, Drury, Rubin, Williams, & Amlôt, 2015; Williams & Drury, 2009), and this promises to be a very fertile agenda for future research.

As with other conditions that are discussed in this book, it would therefore appear that although internalised groups memberships are often the cause of psychological problems, they can also be a very important resource to draw upon as people attempt to work their way through those problems. Most significantly, this is because they are central to the process through which individuals regain control of the personal identity narrative that they often lose hold of as a result of trauma. It is this process that then allows the trauma of the past to be reconciled with the present (rather than repressed) and thereby open up opportunities for personal development.

And so it was that, after he had worked through the horrors of his experiences on the Western Front (not least through correspondence with his fellow war poets), Siegfried Sassoon was ultimately able to lay his own demons to rest and announce:

War's a mystery.
Beyond my retrospection. And I'm going
Onward, away from that Batallion history
With all its expurgated dumps of dead:
And what remains to say I leave unsaid.
(Sassoon, *A Footnote on the War*, 1918[6.1])

The point here, then, is that no amount of cognitive reflection could ever allow Sassoon to understand the experiences that had caused his trauma. What he could do, though, was develop a new life "away from that Batallion history". As he reflected at the time:

> The fact is that five years ago I was, as near as possible, a different person to what I am tonight. I, as I am now, didn't exist at all. Will the same thing happen in the next five years? I hope so.

More particularly, Sassoon came to see his post-war recovery from trauma as a process of putting his former identities behind him (letting "the whispering wraiths of my dead selves repass"; Egremont, 2014, p. 275) and developing new ones. This is something he did with some success through his subsequent work as a celebrated editor, author, and political activist. And while there is always a danger in generalising from any individual case, it would appear that this forging of positive new social identities is a common – perhaps general – feature of recovery from trauma. Since it is such an important issue, the question of how this might best be achieved is therefore one that we will explore further in the chapters that follow.

Points for practice

1. *Social identities that precede, or emerge in the context of, traumatic events can protect people from some of their adverse psychological effects because groups that people identify with provide them with cognitive and emotional resources that help them to make sense of those events and to give them meaning.* This is seen most clearly in the context of war-related trauma, where disidentification will often mean both (1) that traumatic events appear meaningless and (2) that victims are not able to draw upon support from ingroup members to help them deal with the intellectual, emotional, and practical challenges that they face. Although more research is needed to confirm this point, it would thus appear that working with such identities should be a focus for therapeutic intervention.

2. *When responding to traumatic events, it is important not to undermine social identities that are a basis for effective response and resilience.* This is a corollary to the previous point, but it is one that is especially relevant for representatives of agencies that provide institutional responses to emergencies (e.g., health professionals, emergency service workers, insurance agents), as these can all too easily undermine survivors' own group-level responses (which are likely to be critical for long-term outcomes).

3. *Efforts to 'talk through' trauma will be more productive if they help to create or rebuild a sense of shared social identity.* Indeed, unless they do this, their benefits may be limited (as is often found following critical incident stress debriefing) – especially if the conversation is with someone who is perceived by the victim to be an outgroup member.

4. *Shared identity can be the basis for mobilising support and facilitating posttraumatic growth following a traumatic event.* Several lines of research point, in particular, to the role that new group memberships – including those that emerge in the context of the traumatic experience (e.g., as a Vietnam veteran, or a survivor of institutional abuse) – can play in providing trauma victims with psychological and material resources (e.g., social support, a sense of purpose, opportunities for collective self-actualisation) that underpin positive forms of self-development. Again, then, this means that cultivating these should be a particular focus for posttraumatic intervention.

Resources

Further reading

In their review of the social determinants of resilience among trauma victims (particularly in the military), Cacioppo and colleagues conclude that "[i]dentifying the features of individuals, relationships, and group structures and norms that promote social resilience – and determining effective interventions to build social resilience – represent some of the most important challenges facing . . . contemporary behavioral science" (Cacioppo et al., 2011, p. 43). Happily, since this was written, social identity researchers have made considerable headway in rising to this challenge. The following publications exemplify the efforts of research groups that have made the most significant contributions to this effort.

① Drury, J. (2012). Collective resilience in mass emergencies and disasters. In J. Jetten, C. Haslam, & S. A. Haslam (Eds.), *The social cure: Identity, health and well-being* (pp. 195–215). Hove, UK: Psychology Press.

This book chapter provides an overview of John Drury's programmatic work on resilience in the context of emergencies and disasters – with a particular focus on the London bombings. Although these ideas have been elaborated in more recent work, this is a good introduction to this line of work.

② Kellezi, B., & Reicher, S. (2012). Social cure or social curse? The psychological impact of extreme events during the Kosovo conflict. In J. Jetten, C. Haslam, & S. A. Haslam (Eds.), *The social cure: Identity, health and well-being* (pp. 217–234). Hove, UK: Psychology Press.

This chapter (which follows on from Drury's in *The Social Cure*) presents an integrated overview of the authors' work with war survivors in Kosovo. This clarifies the nuanced ways in which social identity can both attenuate and exacerbate the psychological effects of trauma.

③ Muldoon, O. T., & Lowe, R. D. (2012). Social identity, groups, and posttraumatic stress disorder. *Political Psychology, 33*, 259–273.

This article provides a rich discussion of the way in which social identity processes feed into the complex political dynamics of PTSD as a clinical and social phenomenon, drawing heavily on the first author's programmatic research with colleagues in Northern Ireland.

Video

① Search for "John Drury power of crowd" to watch a TEDx talk by John Drury which challenges negative conceptions of crowd psychology (after LeBon, 1895) and points to the ways in which crowds can actually be a positive force in society – not least because the sense of shared identity within them is a basis for mutual support, collective empowerment, and social change. www.youtube.com/watch?v=9fVPQ6X4Fw8   (14 minutes)

② Search for "Why soldiers miss war" and watch Sebastian Junger give an excellent TED talk in which he discusses why soldiers can have difficulty adjusting to life after combat. The answer, he suggests, is that they miss the intensity of conflict and the "intense experience of connection" to their fellow soldiers – things that are hard to re-create in civilian life. He also talks about the experience of PTSD and explains why it can be those who are most traumatised by war who miss it most. www.ted.com/talks/sebastian_junger_why_veterans_miss_warwww.youtube.   (13 minutes)

Websites

ⓘ   www.mind.org.uk/information-support/types-of-mental-health-problems/post-traumatic-stress-disorder-ptsd/#.WYKO9__5iNU. MIND is a leading mental health charity in the UK, and this website provides a good introduction to the topic of PTSD.

Note

1 These and other quotations below are the copyright of Siegfried Sassoon. They are reproduced with permission from the estate of George Sassoon.

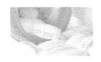

Chapter 7

Ageing

What makes for a long and healthy life? This is a question that has been of particular interest to generations of researchers involved in the longest-running studies on the factors that predict successful ageing – the Grant and Glueck studies at Harvard University. These studies tracked the lives of two groups of men, Harvard graduates and disadvantaged inner-city youth from Boston, over a period of 75 years from 1938 to the present day (Landes, Ardelt, Vaillant, & Waldinger, 2014; Vaillant, 2002, 2012). Clearly there were vast differences between the two groups of participants: one included many people who went on to have illustrious careers (including President Kennedy), whereas the fortunes of the other tended to be less celebrated. Nevertheless, the studies' definitive finding was that, regardless of differences in such things as wealth and intellect, the key to healthy ageing lies in building and maintaining strong and close relationships with other people. As George Vaillant writes in his book about the study, *Triumphs of Experience*: "the most important contributor to joy and success in adult life is [social] attachment" (Vaillant, 2012, p. 370). Robert Waldinger, the program's most recent director, stresses that good relationships are also protective of brain health, with data showing that memories stayed sharper for longer among those who were more socially connected. Moreover, he argues that it is the quality, not simply the quantity, of social relationships that matter for health. Importantly too, these researchers are not alone in making these claims. Many others investigating this same question in more representative populations of older people have reached the same general conclusion (e.g., Bassuk, Glass, & Berkman, 1999; Ertel, Glymour, & Berkman, 2008; Giles, Anstey, Walker, & Luszcz, 2012; Seeman et al., 2011).

This question of what makes for healthy ageing becomes all the more important when we consider the unprecedented rate at which societies today are ageing. Global projections in the United Nations *World Population Ageing Report* estimate that the number of people aged over 60 years will increase from 841 million in 2013 to over 2 billion in 2050 (United Nations, 2013). Indeed, the changing shape of population distributions – which is illustrated clearly in Figure 7.1 – means that by 2047, people over 60 years of age are projected to outnumber those who are under 15. This trend is even more pronounced in poorer countries – with the expectation that by 2050 about 80% of the people in the world who are aged over 60 will be living in less developed regions (compared to 50% in 1965 and 65% today; United Nations, 2013, p. 15).

These changing demographics present major health challenges. For longer life expectancy brings an increased risk of illness and disease – primarily of chronic and degenerative forms. Indeed, as we note in Chapter 14, these are now the leading causes of disability and death around the world, and each comes with a range of costs. Take, for example, those associated with managing dementia. The estimated worldwide costs of managing dementia was in the region of US$604 billion worldwide in 2010 and these are estimated to rise by 85% in 2030 (Wimo & Prince, 2010). Moreover, beyond medical costs, for those who provide unpaid care there is an emerging social cost that is now being recognised. This is because although unpaid care is a source of economic savings (amounting to $5 billion annually; Access Economics, 2009), it comes at the cost of the carer's own health and well-being. With current figures suggesting that one in five older people will develop dementia, there is thus an urgent need to find effective and efficient ways of addressing the needs both of those who need care and those who do the caring (Bjerregaard, Haslam, Mewse, & Morton, 2015).

In line with these trends, recent years have seen a shift in priorities when it comes to managing healthy ageing – from a focus on people's survival to a focus on building resilience and quality of

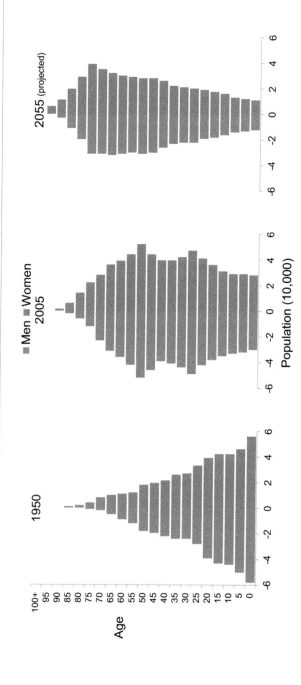

Figure 7.1 Representations of the ageing population in Japan

Note: These figures chart the changing shape of population distributions over time. It can be seen that over time the shape is changing from a pyramid (on the left, where most people are young and few are old) to a kite (in which more people are old than young). Although Japan's population is ageing faster than that of many other countries (and hence is a particular cause for concern), similar patterns are seen in most developed countries (e.g., see United Nations, 2013, p. 10).

Source: Created from data collated by the Japanese National Institute of Population and Social Security Research www.ipss.go.jp/index-e.asp

life. This has been accompanied by a burgeoning of resources – interest groups and their various organs – that offer an array of tips for successful ageing. Many of these highlight the importance of such things as managing blood pressure, reducing cholesterol, losing weight, quitting smoking, and cutting down alcohol consumption. These reflect theoretical approaches to healthy ageing which emphasise the biological and medical dimensions of illness. These approaches are certainly vital in managing health, but it is also notable that they routinely overlook the importance of social factors of the form revealed to be so critical by researchers such as Vaillant and Waldinger. And even when they are addressed, these social factors tend to be treated more as an 'optional extra' than as something that is in any way fundamental to sustained health and well-being. As a consequence, the health-promoting potential of these social processes is far from fully realised when it comes to optimising health in ageing populations. This is a shortcoming that the present chapter attempts to correct. It does this primarily by elaborating on the ways in which a social identity approach can inform improved understanding and management of older people's health. However, before we can make the case for this approach, we need to start by reviewing the modes of thinking and practice that currently dominate the field.

Current approaches to ageing

Medical and biological approaches

Given the prevalence of chronic disease in older adults, the traditional emphasis on medical management is not surprising. As we will discuss further in Chapter 14, chronic diseases are long-term health conditions that are persistent and tend to have a progressive and deteriorating course. Prominent among these are cardiovascular conditions (e.g., heart disease, stroke), dementia, cancers, respiratory disease (asthma, chronic obstructive pulmonary disease), diabetes, arthritis, chronic pain, and depression. Many chronic diseases are partially determined by health behaviours such as smoking, poor diet and nutrition, low levels of physical activity, and harmful alcohol use – all of which contribute to obesity, high blood pressure, and high cholesterol.

Generally speaking, chronic conditions can be controlled, but not cured, and it is common to use prescribed medication to ease symptoms. One problem, though, is that such medication is expensive. As a result, the cost of pharmaceuticals for older adults is placing an increasing burden on both individuals and health care systems. By way of illustration, figures from the United States on their ageing baby boomer generation show that spending on drugs for chronic conditions increased by 17.5% in the 12 months between 2004 and 2005 and accounted for about 20%, or $40 billion, of all prescription medication spending in 2005 (Institute for Safe Medication Practice, 2007). It is no surprise, therefore, that these costs prove to be prohibitive for many – especially those who are poor or who have limited access to public health care (e.g., Piette, Heisler, & Wagner, 2004).

These challenges are compounded by the fact that many older adults have multiple chronic conditions, each of which might require a different medication regimen. Consistent with this, Australian statistics indicate that among people aged between 65 and 74 years of age, about half had five or more chronic conditions that required treatment (Australian Institute of Health and Welfare, 2012). However, each additional medication brings with it an exponential increase in the risk of adverse reaction (Gujjarlamundi, 2016), in part due to age-related physiological changes. For instance, slower drug absorption and action increase the risk that drugs will interact in ways that compromise their potential for beneficial effect. Medication can also have psychological side effects, affecting mood, cognitive orientation, and alertness, or more seriously, triggering a psychotic episode. As just one example of this, there is a risk that beta-blockers prescribed for cardiovascular disease might produce confusion, depression, and disorientation (Siegler, Elias, & Bosworth, 2012). Furthermore, the interactive effects of multiple drug regimens – referred to as *polypharmacy* – are so complex that they are not only unknown but also essentially unknowable (Hajjar, Cafiero, & Hanlon, 2007).

Although exceedingly common among older adults, polypharmacy is therefore far from ideal. Accordingly, *preventative* approaches offer a better solution to challenges of chronic disease. Primary among these are programmes that encourage positive lifestyle changes – for example, helping people to quit smoking, to follow a diet low in saturated fats, to maintain a healthy weight, and to keep physically active (see also Chapters 10 and 14 on eating and physical health conditions). All of these strategies are pursued to promote older adults' health, but the factor that has arguably received the most attention recently is physical activity. This is because the beneficial effects of exercise extend to multiple health domains – from improving physical fitness and stamina, to enhancing mental health, preventing cognitive decline, and slowing neurodegenerative disease (Berchicci, Lucci, & Di Russo, 2013; Kramer, Erickson, & Colcombe, 2006).

What has been harder to pinpoint, however, is the critical ingredient that produces all these benefits. To date, research has focused largely on the biological changes associated with regular physical activity. Testament to this, there is a vast literature that explores its positive effects on things such as cardiorespiratory fitness (e.g., Kramer et al., 1999), neural growth (e.g., van Praag, Schubert, Zhao, & Gage, 2005), neural connectivity (Voss, Prakash, Erikson et al., 2010), cognitive function (Bixby et al., 2007; Colcombe & Kramer, 2003; Etnier & Chang, 2009), muscle mass (e.g., Greiwe, Cheng, Rubin, Yarasheski, Semenkovich, 2001), and immune function (Pedersen & Hoffman-Goetz, 2000).

But are the benefits of exercise for older adults entirely reducible to biology and physiology? One reason for thinking that they might not be is that reviews of the ageing, cognitive health, and exercise literatures show that most interventions that seek to promote physical activity are conducted in *groups*. This makes it difficult to differentiate the physiological from the social ingredients of intervention. In the case of a yoga class, for example, is it only the yoga that delivers the benefits? Might not the class, or group itself, also have a role to play?

Hitherto, such questions have not been a major focus for research. Nevertheless, a handful of studies have compared the benefits of programmes that promote exercise to those that involve some form of group activity, entailing social interaction (e.g., Boström et al., 2015; Emery & Gatz, 1990) or cognitive stimulation (e.g., Fabre, Chamari, Mucci, Massé-Birron, & Préfaut, 2002). These have involved healthy older adults but also people who are more vulnerable to physical and cognitive decline.

One of these studies was conducted by Gustav Boström and his colleagues and involved comparing the effects of high-intensity physical activity with a non-exercise control on mental health outcomes in a vulnerable population of older people with dementia in residential care (Boström et al., 2015). The physical activity involved a range of exercises that aimed to improve balance, lower limb strength, and mobility for 45 minutes every other week day over a period of 4 months. The control activity was a seated social group activity that engaged residents in conversation, singing, and listening to readings and music. There was about 70% adherence in both conditions, with those in the exercise group gradually increasing the intensity of their physical activity during the program. Notably, though, while there was improvement in depression symptoms in both conditions 4 and 7 months later, there was no difference between the conditions. Nor was there a difference when looking at subgroups of dementia type and depression severity. This study suggests that a social group activity may be as effective as individual exercise in improving mental health. It may well also be the case that among group-based exercise programmes social participation is a key element, as findings from another study suggest that "much of the positive effect of exercise on depression in past research is due not only to improved aerobic fitness but also to the social aspect of the exercise conditions" (McNeil, LeBlanc, & Joyner, 1991, p. 488).

This is an important point because exercise may not be an option for everyone. Indeed, with increasing age people's risk of physical disability also increases, and this may prevent them from engaging in as active a lifestyle as they would like. This raises the obvious question of what intervention we might offer people who are less physically active to help them manage chronic illness effectively. This is a question that we will return to later in this chapter.

Psychological approaches

Psychological approaches to healthy ageing tend to focus on those factors that help older people understand and cope with the challenges that ageing can pose to their health. The more influential of these have examined the role of personality and social isolation on health and longevity and have explored ways to modify behaviour with a view to improving health outcomes.

The role of individual differences

Prominent among work that has sought to identify psychological determinants of healthy ageing is evidence that individual differences have the capacity to predict how long we will live. Here work has tended to focus on the 'big five' personality traits – dimensions that capture people's *openness* to experience, their *conscientiousness* and dependability, their *extraverted* approach to stimulation seeking, their *agreeableness* towards others, and their *neurotic* emotional tendencies. Conscientiousness, in particular, and broader traits of hostility, perfectionism, and optimism (Fry & Debats, 2009; Kern & Friedman, 2008; Smith & Spiro, 2002; Weiss & Costa, 2005) are all associated with health risk and survival. Along these lines, it has been argued that those of us who are more hostile, for example, are more prone to stress than other personality types and that cynical and distrusting types are at increased risk of developing dementia (Neuvonen et al., 2014). As discussed in Chapter 5, other research suggests that the constellation of traits that form the Type A personality (characterised by competitive, outgoing, ambitious, impatient, and aggressive behaviours) negatively affect physical health outcomes (Friedman & Rosenman, 1974; Miller, Smith, Turner, Guijarro, & Hallet, 1996).

Yet there are some inconsistent findings in this area, and studies of the relationship between these traits and mortality often report small effects. Higher scores on the trait of neuroticism, for example, seem to be protective of health in some studies (Weiss & Costa, 2005), but are associated with an increased risk of premature death (Fry & Debats, 2009; Shipley, Weiss, Der, Taylor, & Deary, 2007) and of mental and physical health decline in others (Laney, 2009). Likewise, conscientiousness has been associated with both adaptive (thoroughness, reliability, self-discipline) and maladaptive (e.g., over-concern with mistakes, self-criticism, and self-doubt) thoughts and behaviours. As we noted in Chapter 5, meta-analyses of the impact of Type A behaviours on health also reveal mixed results. Whereas some studies indicate that Type A personality is a risk factor for coronary heart disease (Booth-Kewley & Friedman, 1987), other research shows no clear relationship between the two (Matthews, 1988). On the basis of these data, it is difficult to ascertain which traits are good or bad for our health, leading some to question whether there is a meaningful relationship here at all (Haslam, Jetten, Reynolds, & Reicher, 2013).

Nevertheless, there have been a number of attempts to use knowledge of personality type to target those skills required to manage health-related risk, in ways that have been an important focus for intervention in substance misuse (e.g., Conrod, Castellanos-Ryan, & Strang, 2010; Loxton, Bunker, Dingle, & Wong, 2015). Such approaches have yet to be applied to manage the health of older adults, and there are questions about when one might intervene. As chronic health conditions tend to be more common later in life when traits are well established, at what point would we deem that a particular trait (e.g., conscientiousness) becomes sufficiently maladaptive (i.e., resulting in over-concern with mistakes, self-criticism, and self-doubt) to warrant therapeutic attention? There is, however, some evidence that personality change is possible in this population, at least when it comes to increasing openness to new experiences. For example, research by Joshua Jackson and colleagues showed that a 16-week programme of cognitive stimulation with inductive reasoning training and crossword and Sudoku puzzles was associated with an increase in the trait of openness in older adults (Jackson, Hill, Payne, Roberts, & Stein-Morrow, 2012). Presumably though, similar increases might be observed with other forms of intervention, which do not involve direct moulding or re-framing particular traits. Overall then, despite considerable enthusiasm for this approach in some quarters (e.g., Ferguson, 2013), at this point it is not clear how useful a personality approach can be in managing the health-related concerns that are common to older adults.

The role of behaviour change

As already suggested, a more practical approach to the management of health in ageing has focused on efforts to modify behaviour. The focus here is largely on improving healthy lifestyle habits – such as promoting physical activity, healthy eating, and reduced alcohol use. Behaviour change clearly has relevance across the lifespan, although several approaches are increasingly advocated for use with older adults specifically. In particular, *motivational interviewing* (MI) is one approach that is rapidly gaining popularity. This aims to explore and enhance a person's motivation to change unhealthy behaviour (Miller & Rollnick, 2002) and has been shown to improve behaviours that contribute to the development of chronic disease such as poor diet, exercise (Serdarevis & Lemke, 2013), and treatment adherence (Pinquart, Duberstein, & Lyness, 2007).

To date, though, research into the effectiveness of MI is largely confined to younger adults, and where it has been used with older adults there is limited evidence of success. In an early study, Delia Smith and her colleagues looked at the effectiveness of MI relative to a behavioural weight control program among older women with weight problems (Smith, Heckemeyer, Kratt, & Mason, 1997). Unfortunately, although the researchers found evidence of greater attention to recording food intake and blood glucose levels in those who were randomly assigned to the MI condition, there was no difference in weight loss outcomes between conditions. In line with current views about the status of MI as a vehicle to promote behaviour change, more needs to be done to investigate its efficacy in shaping health outcomes in older populations (Bennett et al., 2005; Bugelli & Crowther, 2008).

Nevertheless, an important feature of MI is its concern to promote a person's belief in his or her capacity to make healthy lifestyle changes. This is particularly important where the lifestyle changes may be perceived as physically demanding or more challenging, as is the case if someone is trying to change a lifetime of unhealthy behaviours and practices. In the domain of physical activity, for instance, self-efficacy is one of the more consistent predictors of positive health outcomes in older adults, both when it comes to initiating an exercise regimen and when it comes to maintaining it (van Stralen, Vries, Mudde, Bolman, & Lechner, 2009). Here, those who have higher self-efficacy tend to have greater capacity to overcome the barriers and concerns that typically accompany exercise (i.e., concerning fear of physical exertion, fatigue, and potential falls) and are likely to engage in more physical activity as a result (McAuley, Kramer, & Colcombe, 2004). Intriguingly, though, the common self-regulation approaches that have been successful in younger adults often appear to produce exactly the opposite effects in those who are older. For example, a systematic review of 24 studies led by David French found that approaches such as goal setting, self-monitoring, or receiving performance feedback all *lowered* self-efficacy and activity levels among seniors (French, Olander, Chisholm, & McSharry, 2014). In contrast, increased physical activity in older adults emerged in response to interventions that promoted vicarious modelling and collective brainstorming about overcoming barriers – factors that arguably all rely on the involvement of other people in an intervention. Taking this further, the involvement of others through group exercise may provide further opportunities to engage in such troubleshooting, whilst at the same time promoting this as a social activity that can further increase motivation to initiate and maintain exercise. Again, this is an observation that directs our attention towards the social identity processes that we will explore later in this chapter.

Social determinants of healthy ageing

One of the key points that we made in this book's opening chapters is that health is determined as much by our social, cultural, environmental, and economic circumstances as it is by our biological and psychological make-up. Indeed, it might be argued that because social determinants are modifiable, they are a better target for intervention than other factors which are inherently harder to change (e.g., personality variables or genetic make-up).

For older adults, as we intimated in Chapter 1 (e.g., Figure 1.2), the most important of these factors is probably *social isolation* (Cornwell & Waite, 2009). Indeed, in the United States close to one-third of people aged 65 and older lived alone in 2010 (West, Cole, Goodkind, & He, 2014), and figures are very similar for most other Western countries. And as people get older the risk of social disengagement and isolation increases. It has been known for some time that this is associated with reduced life expectancy (e.g., Berkman & Syme, 1979; see also Steptoe, Shankar, Demakakos, & Wardle, 2013), but it is clear too that it also affects the mental, physical, and cognitive health of older adults. In the case of cognitive health, for example, the work of Karen Ertel and her colleagues shows that memory decline among older people with the highest levels of social participation is half that experienced by those with the lowest levels (Ertel et al., 2008). Importantly, though, it is clear that isolation per se is not the critical factor here (Hawkley & Cacioppo, 2010). Rather, as illustrated in Figure 7.2, it is the subjective sense of *loneliness* that appears toxic for health (e.g., Tomaka, Thompson, & Palacios, 2006; Victor, Scambler, Bond, & Bowling, 2000).

Recognition of the growing cost of loneliness for individuals and for society has prompted the development and evaluation of a range of strategies to counter its negative health effects. In a meta-analytic review of these, Christopher Masi and colleagues explored the efficacy of four general strategies that are used in intervention across the lifespan, specifically, (1) providing social skills training, (2) facilitating more social contact and interaction, (3) increasing social support, and (4) challenging faulty cognitions (Masi, Chen, Hawkley, & Cacioppo, 2011). What these researchers found was that the more successful approaches to overcoming isolation involved raising awareness of maladaptive cognitions and challenging them through some form of reality testing. Interestingly, training to improve social skills – something that we might imagine isolated individuals tend to lack – had limited impact. Similarly, on their own, increased social contact and social support were not associated with improvement. As we know, not all contact and support is beneficial and, along the lines of the support hypothesis (H14), it matters that you identify with those who provide it. Accordingly, the fact that these latter approaches did not significantly reduce isolation may be more a reflection of the nature and quality

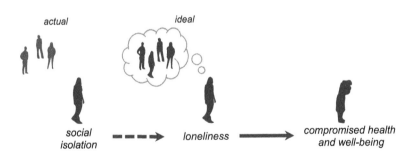

Figure 7.2 The distinction between social isolation and loneliness

Note: Loneliness is the psychological experience of unwanted social isolation, and it is one of the social factors that most compromises the health and well-being of older adults. This will often arise when a person is isolated from others, but note that isolation does not always lead to the experience of loneliness. This is because loneliness tends only to be experienced when the social relationships that a person has are at odds with those they would ideally like to have.

of the relationships between those on the giving and receiving ends of contact and support than of the strategy itself.

In this regard, it is worth noting that systematic reviews of interventions that are focused on managing social isolation in older adults tend to recommend approaches that are at least as much social as cognitive. In particular, two reviews by Mima Cattan and her colleagues directly compared the effectiveness of group and one-to-one health promotion interventions (Cattan & White, 1998; Cattan, White, Bond, & Learmouth, 2005). Both studies came to the same general conclusion – suggesting that successful interventions tend to have three distinctive features. Specifically, they tend (1) to be conducted over an extended period, (2) to be targeted at specific populations (e.g., people experiencing bereavement), and (3) to be delivered in groups.

In light of the methodological deficiencies of many studies in this area, Cattan and colleagues' later review is instructive as this focused on 11 studies that were identified as being higher in quality (Cattan et al., 2005). Among these, there were six effective interventions and all of these involved group delivery. In contrast, of the five ineffective interventions, four were delivered one on one. Notable, too, was the fact that successful group interventions tended to be very diverse – including those that focused on (1) providing support (e.g., for self-help and to overcome bereavement), (2) educational discussion, and (3) various forms of physical activity. This suggests that it is not the intervention strategy per se, but rather the mode of delivery (i.e., group vs. one on one) that may be the secret of intervention success. Of course, in systematic reviews such as these, it is difficult (if not impossible) to partial out the contribution of particular factors of this form. Accordingly, there is a need for more forensic experimental research, and this has been a focus for research efforts of our own that we will review later in the chapter.

Looking at existing research at a more general level, it would also appear that active social participation is another way of tackling social isolation. Consistent with this reasoning, another systematic review on the efficacy of interventions for social isolation shows that active engagement in group-delivered social activity achieves the best outcomes (Dickens, Richards, Greaves, & Campbell, 2011). In the wider literature on the social determinants of health there is also considerable evidence that such engagement has a positive impact on the health of older adults, especially in the cognitive domain. More specifically, those who are more engaged in their social network tend to have better cognitive integrity (Bassuk et al., 1999; Ertel et al., 2008) and to be less vulnerable to cognitive decline and progressive disease (Bennett, Schneider, Tang, Arnold, & Wilson, 2006; Fratiglioni, Wang, Ericsson, Maytan, & Winblad, 2000). The size of these effects also leaves no doubt about the importance of social connectedness for health. For example, Lisa Barnes and colleagues found that cognitive decline was reduced by 39% in people who had the largest social networks and by a massive 91% among those who were actively engaged in these networks (Barnes et al., 2004).

Nevertheless, beyond the eminently sensible recommendation to remain socially connected, the extant literature offers little in the way of practical advice for health practitioners. With whom should we connect to optimise our health? Is there a critical number of social connections that we should strive to achieve? And is a recommendation to 'connect more' actually going to help people to do this?

To answer these questions, we need a theory of social process that accounts for the benefits of social engagement and allows us to understand the mechanisms via which health enhancement occurs. This is especially important in the context of knowledge that not all social relationships are good for us. In particular, kith and kin who regularly engage in unhealthy behaviours (e.g., smoking, drinking) may not encourage or support the forms of behaviour change that are necessary for our health to improve (a point we will return to in Chapter 9). Clearly, then, health promotion is not simply a matter of encouraging social connections of any form. Instead, we need to establish which forms of connection are likely to be curative and which are likely to be damaging – and *why*. It is this theoretical gap that the social identity approach to health seeks to fill, and it is to this approach that we now turn.

The social identity approach to ageing

Many of the approaches described above recognise that social processes are implicated in the health of older adults. However, what they lack is a framework from which to understand and explain these social dimensions. In this regard, the framework that we presented in Chapter 2 appears broadly relevant to this task. Indeed, a number of the hypotheses that we spelled out there are particularly relevant to an understanding of health-related outcomes in the context of ageing. In what follows we will focus on those that speak to three aspects of health in the ageing process: (1) treatment, symptom perception, and underperformance in response to age stereotypes; (2) health deterioration following major age-related life transitions (e.g., retirement); and (3) the health benefits associated with interventions designed to enhance social identification.

Older adults' perceptions are shaped by age-based self-categorization and internalised age stereotypes

We noted in Chapter 2 that social identities are fluid. In particular, we define ourselves, or self-categorize, in different ways depending on the situations in which we find ourselves. At home a woman, Liz, may define herself as a mother, at work she may define herself as a manager, and when watching the Olympics she may define herself as Australian. In these different contexts, Liz's different self-categorizations will also have a powerful impact on her behaviour and her orientation to those around her: for example, whether she is sensitive and responsive, stern and directive, or excited and festive.

This is no less true for older adults. Nevertheless, for older people their age group is often a particularly salient basis for self-categorization. As Gail Wilson (2000, p. 8) notes: "at 60 or 65 in prosperous Western countries it has become very easy for large numbers of people to contest the boundary of old age, but at 80 it can be much more difficult". There are two key reasons for this. First, the abundance of activity groups and clubs, health messages, and concessions that target older people (e.g., labelling them as "pensioners") all reinforce the relevance of age as a meaningful basis for self-categorization (in line with the principle of *perceiver readiness*; Oakes, Turner, & Haslam, 1991, see Chapter 2). Second, a person's age is likely to be more salient when they are exposed to members of *other groups* (younger people, health professionals; Ward, 1984). In this context, as self-categorization theory would predict, age-based intergroup contexts thus often serve to make age-based self-categorization more *fitting* for older adults (Turner, Oakes, Haslam, & McGarty, 1994).

These categorization processes have positive and negative consequences. As noted in other chapters of this volume, strong group identification can be a basis for a range of psychological resources that protect people's health and buffer them against stress and adversity (e.g., see Chapter 5). However, such identification can also have damaging effects when it is informed by negative self-stereotypes.

Negative stereotypes about the competence and behaviour of older adults are pervasive. Across a range of modern societies, advertising messages in the media, ageist views about the older workforce, and evidence of weaker performance in older people all contribute to a view that older adults are "warm but incompetent" (Cuddy, Norton, & Fiske, 2005, p. 75). Although positive stereotypes do exist (e.g., that older people are wiser and more experienced), these tend to be eclipsed by negative images that are far more prevalent (Hummert, 2011; see Figure 7.3). So why is this relevant to the health of older adults? In line with arguments that we made in Chapter 4 – where we discussed the implications of stigma for health – the reason is simple: when they are internalised, negative age stereotypes and beliefs about ageing impact not only on the *treatment* of those who are older but also on the way they themselves *think and act*. And, as we will see, both of these processes can contribute to physical and cognitive decline.

When it comes to treatment, there is evidence that those who work in the health sector are no less likely to be ageist than members of the general public. For example, research has shown that negative

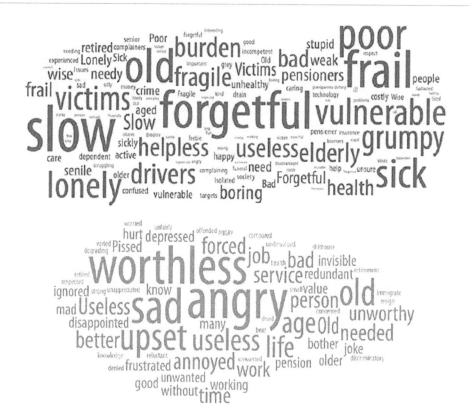

Figure 7.3 The negative content of the stereotype of older adults and older adults' responses to that content

Note: The blue word cloud includes terms that older adults in Australia see as being part of the stereotypic representation of older adults in the media; the red word cloud reflects the content of interviews which asked older adults how this stereotypic representation makes them feel. Larger words are more central to the stereotype and to older adults' responses to it.

Source: Australian Human Rights Commission (2013)

beliefs about, and attitudes towards older people, are not uncommon among nursing staff (Soderhamn, Lindencrona, & Gustavson, 2001; Wells, Foreman, Gething, & Petralia, 2004), students in health professional training (e.g., Taylor & Tovin, 2000), and other support staff providing care to older people (e.g., porters, see Gallagher, Bennett, & Halford, 2006). These centre around views that older adults are difficult to treat, that they respond poorly to treatment, and that they exaggerate their symptoms (Eymard & Douglas, 2012). Although early education during training that increases knowledge about working with older people can help to reduce these negative perceptions (e.g., Stewart, Giles, Paterson, & Butler, 2005), these efforts can sometimes backfire and lead some students to express a greater preference for working with *other* populations, including those with mental illness and psychiatric disturbance (Eymard & Douglas, 2012).

These attitudes often reflect the quality of *intergroup relations* (e.g., in the case of the relations between health professionals and older adults, the former might see themselves as intelligent and superior and older adults as slow witted and inferior; e.g., Allsop & Mulcahy, 1998). These are often difficult to modify without meaningful changes in the nature of these relations (Oakes et al., 1994; see also Sherif, 1956, 1966). They can also clearly impact on the nature of the service that health professionals deliver – for example, adversely affecting their sensitivity and responsiveness to older adults and the time they spend consulting with them (e.g., as reported by the UK's Care Quality Commission, 2011; see also Hummert, Shaner, Garstka, & Henry, 1998).

These age categorization processes also impact on older adults' own beliefs and behaviour – particularly, when it comes to symptom interpretation. Not least, this is because whether or not a person sees themselves as having a health problem and seeks professional help to address it, depends in large part on their experience and interpretation of health-related symptoms (Levine & Reicher, 1996). When symptoms are viewed as part of normal ageing ("we all experience a little forgetfulness as we age"), they might be overlooked. However, when these same symptoms are interpreted as indicative of a chronic condition ("I'm really worried that my memory lapses are a sign of some disease"), they are more likely to be seen to warrant professional investigation.

A key point here is that self-categorizing as an older person can actually affect which of these two courses a person pursues – a point confirmed in a programme of research by Lindsay St Claire and Yuequn He (2009). One of their studies focused on perceptions of hearing loss among older people. Participants in this study were encouraged to self-categorize as either an older person (achieved by highlighting "age" in the study questionnaire) or as an individual (achieved by highlighting "the self" in the study questionnaire). This simple manipulation resulted in those seeing themselves as older reporting greater hearing loss than those who were encouraged to see themselves as individuals, despite there being no difference between the groups on objective hearing tests (see Chapter 14 for a more detailed discussion of this study). As this shows, self-categorizing as older increases a person's sensitivity to age-related health concerns that can lead them to perceive symptoms to be present despite objective evidence to the contrary. This finding speaks to the norm enactment hypothesis (H8): that *when a person defines themselves in terms of a given social identity* – in this case, as an older person – *then they will enact the expectations associated with that category* – in this case, those related to hearing loss.

But why does this matter? In particular, why should we be concerned about symptom perception rather than just actual symptoms? One reason is that it is people's perceptions of their symptoms that lead them to seek (or not seek) support from health services, and this has implications for both their own treatment and for health care management in general. In particular, it can lead to people being either under-treated or over-treated, and, at a population level, it can lead to available services being either under- or over-used. In a world where it is ever more important for health care resources to be targeted appropriately (and how to do this is a focus for debate, especially in relation to age; e.g., Markle-Reid & Browne, 2003), insensitivity to the self-categorizations that inform older adults' engagement with health services thus has the capacity to be very costly on a range of levels.

Older adults' performance is shaped by age-based self-categorization and internalised age stereotypes

Clearly, though, hearing loss is just one of many symptoms that older adults commonly report. Other symptoms relate to various aspects of physical, mental, and cognitive health, and self-categorization processes are equally relevant to the way in which these are perceived and responded to. Moreover, work in some of these other health domains shows that self-categorization processes have an impact not only on perceptions but also on *performance*.

One phenomenon that is particularly relevant here is *social identity threat* or *stereotype threat* (Steele & Aronson, 1995; Steele, Spencer, & Aronson, 2002). This relates to the fact that when people are made aware of negative stereotypes associated with their social group membership (e.g., that older people are slow and incompetent), this tends to have a negative impact on performance in stereotype-relevant domains. In particular, evidence shows that when negative stereotypic expectations about an ingroup are salient, their internalisation can undermine performance in a way that confirms those expectations (e.g., Barber & Lee, 2015). For instance, an older person, who knows that older people as a group are believed to be poorer drivers than young people, will subsequently tend to perform less well on tests of driving performance (e.g., affecting brake rection time and crashes in driving simulation) than they would if their age, and the stereotypes associated with it, were not salient (Lambert, Watson, Stefanucci, Ward, Bakdash, & Strayer, 2016). This phenomenon is a particular concern in the context of a discussion of ageing and health because health settings often serve both to make older adults' age salient and to reinforce negative age stereotypes. For example, this can occur as a result of being targeted for health care because of one's age or because one is a member of a group of older people (e.g., retirees), or can arise from being exposed to information campaigns about age-related health conditions (e.g., dementia, stroke). In health contexts where assessment of ability is inevitable, cues such as these can clearly increase a person's awareness of their age and vulnerability and thereby reinforce their susceptibility to threat effects.

The domain in which these effects have been most commonly studied is *memory* (e.g., Abrams, Eller, & Bryant, 2006; Hess, Auman, Colombe, & Rahhal, 2003; Hess & Hinson, 2006; Kang & Chasteen, 2009; Rahhal, Hasher, & Colombe, 2001). For example, in laboratory settings, it has been found that simply emphasising the memory component of a task can lead older adults to perform the task less well (Rahhal et al., 2001). As self-categorization theory would predict (e.g., in line with H8), this effect is also more pronounced to the extent that participants identify strongly as an older person or place more value on their performance (Hess et al., 2003).

Nevertheless, because multiple cognitive abilities are prone to decline with ageing (e.g., decision making, problem solving, and reasoning) and any of these can be a focus for negative age stereotypes, it is also clear that these abilities can also be compromised by social identity threat. So what determines whether this is the case and, if so, which aspect of performance declines? In line with basic self-categorization principles (e.g., Turner et al., 1994), we would argue that this depends both (1) on whether or not a given individual self-categorizes as older and (2) on the specific *content* of this self-categorization – that is, what he or she understands being older to mean and entail. So, for example, we should see poorer memory performance when people expect ageing to be associated with memory decline; but where people expect other abilities (e.g., judgement and decision making), to decline then we should find greater underperformance on tasks that assess these specific abilities.

These hypotheses were tested directly in a study that two of us conducted with colleagues to investigate the effect of age-related expectations of cognitive decline on the clinical test performance of older adults (Haslam et al., 2012). All participants were between 60 and 70 years old with no known history of cognitive complaints or progressive decline. Half were primed to self-categorize as older. This was achieved by telling them that the study focused on people between the ages of 40 and 70 years and noting that they were at the older end of that age spectrum. The remainder were primed to see themselves as younger by informing them that the people taking part were between the ages of 60 and 90 years and hence that they were at the younger end of that range. As well as manipulating the nature of self-categorization (old vs. young), the study also independently manipulated the content of age related self-categorizations by telling half of the participants that ageing was associated with a specific decline in memory and the remainder that it was associated with generalised decline in cognitive ability.

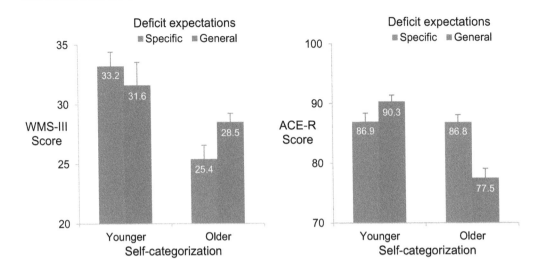

Figure 7.4 Scores on tests of specific memory and general cognitive ability as a function of self-categorization and expectations of the form of ageing decline

Note: Higher scores indicate superior performance. The key points to highlight here are that participants who are led to self-categorize as older tend to perform less well and that the nature of under-performance in this group of participants varies as a function of their expectations about the nature of the deficit that ageing entails. This means that (1) when older people expected aging to lead to a specific decline in memory, they performed particularly poorly on tests of memory (WMS-III as shown in the left-hand graph), but that (2) when they expected it to lead to general cognitive decline, they performed particularly poorly on tests of general cognitive ability (ACE-R as shown in the right-hand graph).

Here and in all other graphs, the error bars show standard error around the mean. This gives an indication of how precise the measurement of the mean is (with smaller error bars indicating more precise measurement). Around 95% of all observed values should lie within 2 standard errors of each mean.

Source: Adapted from Haslam et al. (2012)

Although there were no differences in cognitive ability at the start of the study, marked differences emerged as a result of these experimental manipulations. First, those participants who were led to self-categorize as older performed worse overall than those who self-categorized as younger. More interestingly, however, the pattern of performance decline among participants who self-categorized as older also varied as a function of their induced beliefs about the decline in ability expected with ageing. As can be seen in Figure 7.4, these participants performed worse on specific memory tests (but not general ability tests) when they had been led to believe that ageing produces a specific decline in memory. However, they performed worse on general ability tests (but not specific memory tests) when they had been led to believe that ageing compromises general ability.

The findings from the test of general ability – which was included because of its sensitivity and specificity in detecting risk of dementia – were especially striking in this study. For among those who had been led to self-categorize as older and to see ageing as associated with generalised decline, 72%

scored above the conservative criterion for dementia diagnosis, compared to an average of just 14% in the other three conditions. As with other research into the effects of age-based self-categorization (e.g., as reviewed by Giles & Reid, 2005, and Lamont, Swift, & Abrams, 2015), this study thus provides strong support for the group circumstance hypothesis (H3) in showing that *when a person defines themselves in terms of a given social identity, their health and well-being will be affected by the state and circumstances of the group with which that identity is associated* (in this case by ageism and negative age stereotypes). This point is further reinforced by Case study 7.1. This details the detrimental impact of these processes on one particular individual and suggests that the effects of social identity threat may contribute to progressive decline and therefore be more lasting than traditionally believed.

Case study 7.1 Alice

It is generally accepted that age stereotypes, when internalised, have only a temporary effect on our performance and behaviour. But is this always the case? A case reported by Merckelbach, Jelicic, and Jonker (2012), and highlighted in the British Psychological Society's *Research Digest*, suggests otherwise. In this, the authors describe the case of a 58-year old woman (who we will call Alice) who was incorrectly diagnosed as suffering from Alzheimer's disease. Alice had consulted a neurologist due to concerns about her deteriorating memory – something that was indicated by her increased reliance on external aids (e.g., calendars) to help her remember things. These concerns were further fuelled by the fact that Alice had a family history of Alzheimer's disease. The consultant's investigation led to Alice being diagnosed with dementia, and at this point she was reported to be "permanently in a state of confusion" (Merckelbach et al., 2012, p. 61). Some months later, however, a second opinion was sought, and this resulted in the diagnosis being revoked. However, it now proved almost impossible to convince Alice that she did not have a memory disturbance.

Clearly this case demonstrates the profound impact that misdiagnosis can have on people's lives. So what was the reason for Alice's progressive performance decline? The authors argue that her unshakeable belief that she had dementia resembled the development of false memories (Loftus & Pickerell, 1995) and proved intractable not only because the diagnosis made sense of her experience but also because it was provided by a trusted person. As an extension of this analysis, we would argue that Alice's convictions arose from her internalisation of the category "dementia sufferer" and that her continued decline reflected a *living out* of the meaning of this self-categorization. As this case illustrates, the effects of age stereotypes are not always transitory, and it is important to recognise the profound impact that diagnoses can have on health outcomes – especially when they are wrong.

Yet although it is clear that self-categorization in the context of ageing will often have negative consequences, it is apparent that this need not always be the case. Indeed, from the findings reported in Figure 7.4 (Haslam et al., 2013), one can see that whereas an older person's self-categorization as 'older' tends to compromise their performance, as a corollary, self-categorization as 'younger' tends to have positive consequences. This accords with a body of research into the phenomenon of *stereotype lift* which shows that self-categorizations which have positive content tend to boost performance (Walton & Cohen, 2003). Accordingly, beliefs and social comparisons that highlight positive aspects of ageing (e.g., as manifested in disagreement with the statement "as you get older, you are less useful") tend to have a positive impact on performance (e.g., Levy, Slade, Kunkel, & Jasl, 2002; see Dionigi, 2015, for a review). Indeed, merely highlighting the fact that older people are wiser and better at some tasks (e.g., on those that require word knowledge, such as crosswords) has been found to boost the performance of older (vs. younger) people (Swift, Abrams, & Marques, 2013).

One important practical question is thus how health contexts might be managed so as to minimise social identity threat and maximise stereotype lift. Some researchers have argued that this might be achieved by reducing references to performance during assessment, and this has been found to be somewhat effective (Hess et al., 2003, 2009). However, such strategies will often be impractical. For example, in a memory assessment clinic it will be hard to avoid making memory performance salient. Likewise, in a residential care home it will be hard to downplay the physical constraints that accompany old age altogether, not least for fear of neglecting one's duty of care.

Here, though, the social identity approach suggests several other ways in which the negative impact of self-categorizations can be counteracted. Along the lines of H5, a person can pursue *personal mobility strategies* that allow them to maintain a positive sense of self by distancing themselves from the stereotyped group. This was the approach that the comedian George Burns recommended when he observed that "you can't help getting older, but you don't have to get old" (Epstein, 2011, p. 174). Amongst other things, the growing market for cosmetic surgery and anti-ageing creams speaks to the allure of this strategy (as reflected in Figure 7.5), and it is one that becomes more viable if people perceive that they need not be tied to, or defined by, membership in an 'older' group – that is, when group boundaries are seen to be *permeable*. Indeed, such strategies are likely to help people avoid

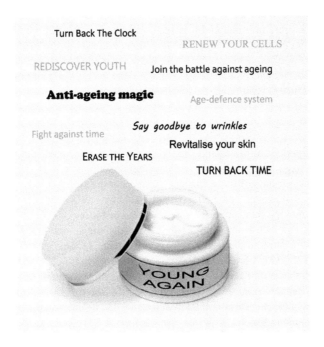

Figure 7.5 The appeal of personal mobility strategies in response to ageing

Note: If boundaries to age-based social categories are perceived to be permeable, people are more likely to be motivated to pursue strategies to avoid self-categorizing as older. A range of so-called cosmaceutical products appeal to this motivation. Interestingly, we were unable to find a cosmaceutical company that would allow us to reproduce an advert for one of their 'anti-ageing' products and so this image simply reproduces some of the slogans that adverts for such products contain.

Source: Pixabay and the authors

the disabling impact of negative age stereotypes of the form that an older person might encounter in routine interactions, as those stereotypes will have little impact if they do not self-categorize as older (Hess et al., 2003). Again, though, it appears that avoidant strategies of this form become less viable the older people become (Wilson, 2000).

In contrast to a strategy that involves dealing with the threats of ageing by denying their personal relevance, a more collective strategy involves challenging the status quo and, more particularly, questioning the legitimacy of age stereotypes and trying to root out ageism. One way to achieve this is by directly challenging the belief that cognitive decline is inevitable. This approach promotes group-based opposition and active resistance to ageism and tends to be used when the boundaries of the group are seen to be fixed and impermeable – that is, in contexts where it is hard for people to see themselves as anything other than an older person (e.g., when using an age pension card, attending a memory clinic, or a seniors' meeting).

Collective action strategies have certainly been adopted by a range of advocacy groups who lobby on behalf of older adults. As we saw in Chapter 4, challenging the legitimacy of stigmatising stereotypes is one effective way of counteracting both discrimination and prejudice (although this possibility is generally explored in domains other than ageism, e.g., those relating to mental health, gender, and race; Crabtree, Haslam, Postmes, & Haslam, 2010; Jetten, Branscombe, Iyer, & Asai, 2013; Smith & Postmes, 2011; Stewart, Latu, Branscombe, & Denney, 2010). We can also challenge beliefs and assumptions about what ageing entails, and this also tends to be more effective when undertaken collectively. At the formal end of the spectrum we see this in the World Health Organization's "#YearsAhead" campaign. At the more informal end it is seen in Portugal's "Graffiti Grannies" who actively challenge age stereotypes through their engagement in street art (see Figure 7.6).

In the ageing context, where a range of negative stereotypes can be entrenched, strategies such as these should help to reduce their impact on performance. However, the extent to which they actually achieve this goal in practice is something that awaits clarification.

Group memberships are protective in the context of age-related life transition

We all go through periods of life change, and these are often associated with significant forms of *social identity change* (e.g., losing some old and developing some new work group networks in the context of changing jobs). Some of these changes are more impactful than others, and a number of these arise in the process of ageing – including transitions such as retirement, bereavement, losing the capacity to drive, and moving into supported care, to name just a few. These are major life changes known to affect health and well-being, and the evidence now shows that group and social identity processes are here pretty central to successful adjustment (Jetten, Haslam, Iyer, & Haslam, 2010a).

Of these transitions, giving up paid work is one of the most significant, and, for those who are employed, it is an inevitable part of ageing. Yet successful adjustment to retirement is far from straightforward. About 25% of people in the United States find the transition stressful (Bosse, Spiro, & Kreslin, 1996) and experience a marked reduction in their well-being and health status (Wang, 2007; although these figures are lower among European retirees; see Pinquart & Schindler, 2007). Preparation for the change is widely recognised as key to successful adjustment, but its main focus is typically on financial planning. The major social upheavals that people experience – for example, losing a valued work identity and networks of supportive colleagues – tend to take a backseat in such planning, if they are considered at all. Alongside this, retirement itself signals to people that they are older and, for some, this is associated with the feeling that others no longer see them as productive members of society as they are now "on the scrap heap" (Klehe, Koen, & Pater, 2012, p. 313). In light of the foregoing discussion about the impact that others' beliefs have on one's own state of mind, it is therefore not surprising that this can also have a detrimental impact on health outcomes.

To date, most research that has examined the impact of retirement on health has focused on the impact of changes in individual relationships with a significant other (i.e., the loss of particular work

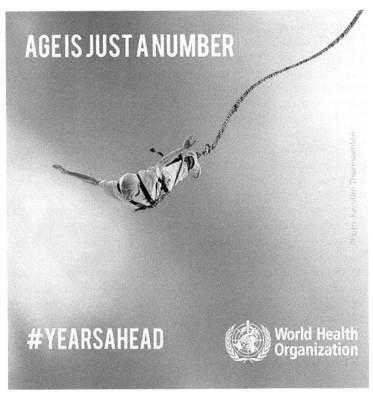

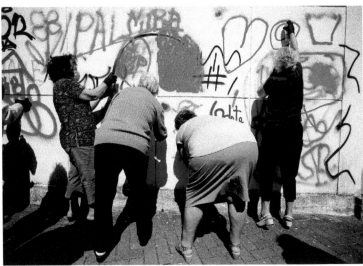

Figure 7.6 Challenging age stereotypes through collective action

Note: In different ways, the two forms of collective action seen here question assumptions associated with beliefs of the form captured by Figure 7.3.

Source: www.ifa-fiv.org/yearsahead-challenging-ageism/; Rafael Marchante, Reuters Pictures

friendships or changes that retirement brings to spousal relationships). However, our own research is starting to broaden this focus to investigate the impact of changes in group-based relationships on health outcomes. In particular, work that we conducted with Nik Steffens has investigated the contribution of social group ties to mortality in the 6-year period after retirement – with one key study looking at data from over 400 Britons who were going through retirement and being tracked within the English Longitudinal Study of Ageing (ELSA; Steffens, Cruwys, Haslam, Jetten, & Haslam, 2016). One of this study's most striking findings was that retirees who maintained group ties during this transition were far less likely to die prematurely. For example, among people with an average of two group memberships prior to retirement, those who kept both had only a 2% risk of early death; yet this increased markedly if they lost one or both groups – with the risk of mortality here increasing to 5% and 12%, respectively. Importantly, these results controlled for factors such as physical health and age that might otherwise be expected to restrict a person's ability to maintain group memberships. Significantly too, the study also found that life satisfaction 6 years post-retirement reduced by 10% with every group membership that people lost and did not replace.

Interestingly, Steffens and colleagues also compared these outcomes to those associated with changes in physical activity levels over the same post-retirement period. This analysis suggested that these changes were associated with a comparable level of risk. For example, maintaining weekly vigorous activity was associated with a 3% risk of premature death, but this increased to 6% if people exercised less than once a week, and to 11% if they stopped exercising altogether. Of course, as we noted earlier in this chapter, the effects of exercise on health are well understood and well documented (e.g., Berchicci et al., 2013; Kramer et al., 2006). Yet these findings – which are consistent with a number of hypotheses that are central to this book as a whole (e.g., H1, H11) – suggest that social group ties are no less important for health. Their importance, though, is far more commonly overlooked. Accordingly, it would appear that much is to be gained by drawing attention to the benefits of group life for retirees, not as a substitute for exercise but as something that might augment it (e.g., emphasising the value of exercising collectively) and that might offset health risks if exercise is not possible.

A second domain of ageing-related life change that has been investigated from a social identity perspective focuses on people's experience of giving up driving. Driving can be a sensitive topic for older adults, particularly as questions start to be raised about their ability to do this safely. It is often the case too that losing the ability to drive constitutes a major threat to older adults' independence and one which triggers a significant reduction in their self-efficacy and sense of control (Windsor, Anstey, Butterworth, Luszcz, & Andrews, 2007). Driving cessation is also associated with increased isolation because it tends to limit people's ability to stay involved in social activities that they value (Fonda, Wallace, & Herzog, 2001; Mezuk & Rebok, 2008; Ragland, Satariano, & MacLeod, 2005).

Along these lines, it has been argued that driving cessation is a potent marker of ageing, and that for many it signals a process of irreversible social identity change – from being a "younger old person" to an "older old person" (Jetten & Pachana, 2012). Moreover, when a person can no longer self-categorize as a driver, they have the sense of losing a valued identity and all that it entails (i.e., freedom, mobility, and independence). This was highlighted in qualitative research asking older people to imagine what giving up driving would mean for them:

> My independence would be horribly compromised. I would be severely restricted in contact
> with my children and grandchildren, with my religious faith community, and all my friends.
> (Jetten & Pachana, 2012, p. 108)

When it comes to managing this and other age-related life transitions, it is customary for practitioners and researchers alike to focus on practical matters. So, in the case of giving up driving, there is a focus on the challenges of finding alternative forms of transportation, whereas in the case of retirement, the focus is typically on ways of managing a limited budget. These are unquestionably important issues. Again, however, this focus ignores what can be seen as the core psychological issue that arises in these contexts – namely the challenge of *social identity loss*. As we have seen in a number of domains (and will explore further in the chapters that follow), this loss has very significant health implications that need to be tackled head on.

So how precisely can we manage the life and identity changes that are bound up with ageing in order to protect against mortality, morbidity, and misery? A good place to start is by recognising, rather than ignoring, the importance of group-based connections and by striving to kerb the negative impact that life changes can have on these. In particular, it is important to help people reframe age-related identities in positive ways and to maintain and build meaningful social connections – particularly in contexts where age and associated vulnerability is highly salient. How exactly this might be done is something we start to explore in the next section. It is also something that we will return to in Chapter 15, where we describe an intervention – GROUPS 4 HEALTH – that focuses on working with people to strengthen and maintain positive social identities with a view to improving their access to social support and to a range of other social psychological resources that sustain healthy adjustment.

Meaningful group identification improves health outcomes

One evening, when three of us were walking though the busy city streets of Nanchang in central China, we came across several groups of older women dancing in the streets (see Figure 7.7). The size of the groups varied, as did the music and the steps, but all were engaged in coordinated dance that they clearly enjoyed. Investigating this further, we discovered that we had stumbled across square dancing – a daily activity originally intended for older women living in the local area, but that is now engaged in by women of all ages. So what is it that encourages older women to take part in this activity – particularly in the suboptimal environment of a busy city street full of traffic noise, pollution, and congestion?

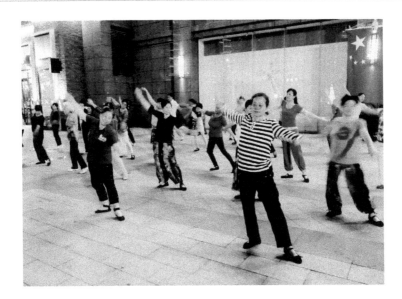

Figure 7.7 Square dancing in China

Note: This popular activity involves large numbers of women coming together in communal spaces in cities (e.g., outside shopping malls and public squares) to perform slow rhythmical dancing.

Source: The authors

On the basis of the points that we have already discussed, there would appear to be several reasons why older adults might participate in activity of this form. The value of physical activity is one, and this is certainly consistent with the emphasis on the importance of exercise for older adults' cognitive and physical health (e.g., Berchicci et al., 2013; Kramer et al., 2006). But square dancing is not just about exercise. It is also a good vehicle for group engagement and one that provides easily accessed opportunities for social identification. Consistent with this, it is apparent that women do not dance indiscriminately with just any group. Despite the fact that several different groups can be found in the same street, they dance with the same group every day, and most have done so for many years. Often too they wear similar outfits as a sign of their shared identity and of their unity and common purpose. As one participant told us (via a translator) "these are my sisters; this is my family".

Participants' level of engagement in these sorts of activities, and their overall level of enthusiasm, raises three further questions. Is group activity of this form good for older adults' health? If so, is it any better for health than engaging in the same alone? And if the answer to both of these questions is 'yes', then what is the key ingredient here: the group, the activity, or their combination? These are questions that we have sought to answer in an extended programme of research that we have conducted over the course of the past decade.

An initial line of research focused on the first two questions and involved investigating the degree to which (1) interpersonal social contact and (2) group-based contact were beneficial in protecting older adults' health. The reason for looking at this was to understand whether particular *types* of social relationships are advantageous for health – noting that most previous research has tended not to differentiate between these two types, but that this distinction is obviously of central theoretical interest to us (for reasons discussed in Chapter 2). For this purpose, we drew on longitudinal survey data from over 3,000 older British adults using the same ELSA database as our retirement research (Steffens et al., 2016). Our goal was to clarify the impact that changes in older adults' social connections with a significant other and with social groups had on changes in their cognitive health over a 4-year period (Haslam, Cruwys, & Haslam, 2014a).

The study's findings told a very clear story. First, they showed that group-based social connection – including membership of various clubs and societies, group activities in the local community, and church groups – was very beneficial to cognitive, or brain, health. Second, these benefits were far more pronounced than those associated with interpersonal connections (whose benefits tended to be statistically non-significant). Third, and most striking though, was the fact that the benefits of social group engagement increased markedly with age. As Figure 7.8 shows, above-average group engagement was associated with limited cognitive benefits for 50-year-old respondents (who, on average, functioned cognitively at the level of a 46-year-old). However, functional benefits were much more pronounced at the older end of the age spectrum. Here, 80-year-olds who were more socially connected performed cognitively at the same level as a 70-year-old. Of course, correlational studies of this form cannot conclusively rule out reverse causality (i.e., that people with better brain function are more socially connected, rather than the other way around). To try and deal with this, the same analysis was repeated, but only with older people whose cognitive abilities were likely to be preserved at the first time point, and the same pattern of results emerged. This suggests that if we want to stay mentally active for longer (and most of us do), then ensuring that we belong to more social groups would be a prudent investment.

More rigorous evidence of the distinctive benefits that flow from group-based ties is provided by experimental studies that allow us to manipulate (rather than just measure) variables of theoretical interest. The first of these was a randomised controlled trial that compared the efficacy of reminiscence therapy that was delivered individually (one on one) with that of the same intervention undertaken within groups (Haslam et al., 2010). The activity is commonly used to engage older people in the process of recollecting their past experiences and memories, and it is popular because these memories tend to be accessible even among those who have progressive disease (e.g., Alzheimer's dementia). In this context, the therapy is typically delivered with a view to improving both cognitive health (via cognitive

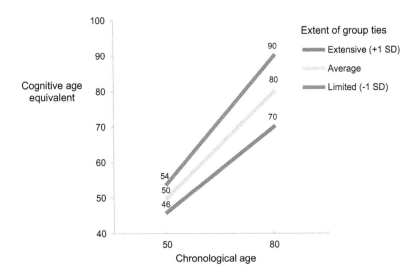

Figure 7.8 People's cognitive age as a function of their chronological age and the extent of their social group ties

Note: The chart shows results of simple slopes analysis illustrating the interaction between social group membership and age reported in Haslam et al. (2014a). The benefits of group ties (associated with lower cognitive age) become more apparent as people get older – so that those with extensive and limited group ties have a difference in cognitive health equivalent to 8 years when they are 50, but this difference increases to 20 years when they are 80.

Source: Haslam et al. (2014a)

stimulation) and well-being, although evidence of its effectiveness is decidedly mixed (Woods, Spector, Jones, Orrell, & Davies, 2005).

In our study we were interested in the role that group delivery might have on health outcomes and in whether this might occur through its capacity to build a meaningful new social identity among members of a reminiscence group. Relevant to the second and third questions that we posed earlier in this section, we reasoned that if it were simply the reminiscence activity that were important for health, then it should not matter how it is delivered. However, if it is something about meaningful group activity that promotes health, then we should see evidence of enhancement only when the intervention is delivered in groups.

The study recruited older people living in residential care who took part in reminiscence therapy over a period of 6 weeks, either with one other person or in a small facilitated group. The content of sessions and the time spent engaging in reminiscence was kept constant across conditions, as were the materials used to facilitate discussion, which comprised tangible props (e.g., objects, photographs) from particular time periods. Importantly too, the study also included a control condition in which groups of people came together to play skittles every week over the same period.

The findings were in line with hypotheses derived from social identity theorising (e.g., H11 to H15). First, they showed that only group reminiscence (not individual reminiscence) led to enhanced memory performance. Second, among those who reminisced together, these benefits were associated with a greater sense of shared social identity (and a reduced sense of isolation; in line with the connection hypothesis, H12). In contrast, those who reminisced one on one only felt more different and disconnected from their fellow care home residents after the intervention. Third, shared reminiscence also led to improved well-being, but so, too, did participation in other forms of group activity (playing skittles) that did not involve reminiscence. The key conclusions here, then, were (1) that reminiscence produced cognitive benefits when it was performed in groups, but (2) that *any* form of group activity had the capacity to unlock the benefits of increased social identification for well-being.

Nevertheless, some evidence which at first glance appears to challenge these conclusions emerges from a more recent randomised trial of the effects of joint reminiscence for dyads consisting of a person with dementia and their carer (Woods et al., 2012). The participants in this study were 488 people with mild to moderate dementia who were randomly assigned either to participate in reminiscence therapy (in groups containing up to 12 dyads) or to a control condition involving care as usual. The intervention itself was manualised, led by trained facilitators, and delivered weekly over a period of 3 months and then monthly for a further 7 months. Despite all this effort, no difference was found between the conditions on measures of life quality, mood, anxiety, or activities of daily living. Clearly this raises questions about the utility of this form of intervention for vulnerable older adults. Nevertheless, as the study did not directly compare group with individual delivery or measure group identification, the conclusions that can be drawn from it are limited to the value of reminiscence in general (relative to care as usual) and do not speak specifically to the value of group delivery as a means of building social identification in ways that promote well-being. Indeed, because the primary focus of the intervention was dyads rather than groups, it might be argued that the null results here reflect the fact that in this case reminiscence did little to help build social identification.

These were questions that we endeavoured to address directly ourselves in a second study with residents in care. Here, though, the focal activity involved older adults learning about the ways in which dehydration can be managed through appropriate water consumption (Gleibs, Haslam, Haslam, & Jones, 2011a). Our interest in this question had initially been stimulated by a news article (BBC News, 2008, see Figure 7.9) that discussed evidence which showed that if care home residents were encouraged to join "water clubs", this could counteract the serious and well-documented health problems caused by dehydration in older adults (e.g., Armstrong-Esther, Browne, Armstrong-Esther, & Sander, 1996; Gaspar, 1999). Although water clubs might help to alleviate these problems, our theoretical sensibilities led us to wonder whether it was the water that was delivering health benefits or the club.

To answer this question, residents were randomly assigned to one of four experimental conditions. Two of these involved an intervention in which participants learned about the pros and cons of drinking water, but in one condition they did this in a group (i.e., a water club) and in the other they did it on their own with a facilitator. There were also two control conditions in which people learned about current affairs either as part of a group (a news club) or on their own. Contrary to the idea that water is a uniquely powerful vehicle for health improvement (the thrust of the original news article), it was only residents who took part in group activities who showed post-intervention improvement on measures of health and well-being. Moreover, although some benefits were specific to the water club, the news club led to significant health benefits too – in particular, evidenced by a reduced need for visits from a general practitioner. Further analysis also showed that benefits to well-being in both types of clubs were achieved through residents' perceptions of improved social support, which itself arose from their strengthened sense of social identification (as suggested by H14).

Yet although these, and other, data provide evidence of the positive effect that social group connectedness has for the health of older adults, it is also important to stress that not just any group will do. For health benefits only emerged when interventions led residents to feel a strong sense of connectedness and identification with others. It is on this point that the social identity approach is informative by providing a theoretical framework to explain why some group relationships are curative and others are not. To this end, the theorising that we outlined in Chapter 2 makes a number of very clear predictions about which types of group membership will be most likely to provide a health-enhancing psychological resource. Specifically, they must (1) be a source of positive influence and support (as proposed in

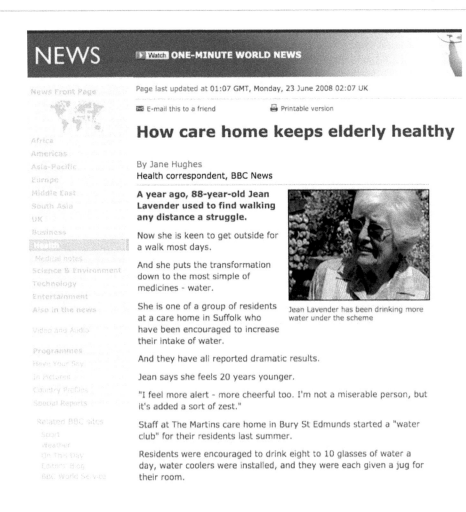

Figure 7.9 The activity or the group? Identifying the critical ingredient in group interventions

Note: This BBC News story pointed to the positive impact that water clubs can have on older adults' health and attributed this to the beneficial effects of the water while overlooking the importance of the club. This is emblematic of a widespread tendency to overlook the role of social group memberships in promoting health.

Source: http://news.bbc.co.uk/1/hi/7466457.stm

H9 and H14) and (2) provide a meaningful basis for social identification and belonging (as proposed in H1 and H2; for evidence that increased social identification through meaningful group engagement is associated with health improvement, see also Gleibs et al., 2011b; Haslam et al., 2014b, 2014c). This means that group intervention will tend to fail if people do not see themselves as 'fitting in' to a group. This sense of oneself as an 'outsider' can have multiple causes – including perceptions that the group does not meet one's needs or the experience of having limited input into its structure and activities (Haslam et al., 2014c).

There are also some clear lessons that the social identity approach provides in guiding group-based interventions of the form that we have examined in this section. First, identification with others is pivotal – for without it there is no reason either to engage in any group activity or to seek or provide health-enhancing support to other group members. Second, groups need to be meaningful to, and valued by, their members – for this increases the potential for the group to be integrated as an important part of self. Third, although a single positive group membership (e.g., a reminiscence group, a water club, or a design team) can be health enhancing, one of the benefits of encouraging people to join an initial group is that this can provide an impetus for them to go on and join more. And because better health outcomes tend to be achieved by those who belong to multiple groups (in line with H11; Haslam, Holme et al., 2008; Jetten et al., 2015), this is a very useful form of *social scaffolding* (Haslam, Cruwys, Haslam, Dingle, Chang, 2016c). Significantly too, although these points provide clear guidance as to how one might unlock the curative potential of social identities in older adults, they are not only relevant to this particular group. This point will be confirmed in the next chapter, and it is one that we will interrogate much more forensically in Chapter 15 where we translate these various insights into a structured intervention – GROUPS 4 HEALTH.

Conclusion

As the Rolling Stones – who know a thing or two about the topic – observe in their song "Mother's Little Helper", it's a drag getting old (Rolling Stones, 1966). As the song also suggests, people's primary response to the challenges of ageing is often pharmaceutical ("mother's little helper" being a reference to the medicines that are commonly used to treat anxiety and depression). And although there is some recognition among practitioners and researchers that social factors have a bearing on this process, attention to these is generally cursory at best.

As we argued at the very start of this book, to a large extent this negligence is due to the absence of an appropriate framework to account for social processes. The social identity approach helps to fill this gap, but importantly it does so in a way that accounts for both the positive and the negative effects of identifying as an older person. It also raises our awareness of other factors that have been largely neglected in the health domain to the detriment of older adults' well-being – most notably, the underperformance that can result from negative age stereotypes, the effects of self-categorization on both symptom interpretation and adjustment to life change, and the protective effects of social group intervention.

Sensitivity to these various factors adds considerably to the richness of our understanding of the ageing process. Importantly too, it adds appreciably to the arsenal of tools with which we can tackle the challenges of ageing. Clearly these will not always constitute 'cures'. However, they have the proven capacity not only to extend life, but also to make an extended life more worth living.

Points for practice

A range of messages for practitioners working with older adults emerge from the social identity approach we have outlined in this chapter.

1. *Membership in social groups can be protective of health in older adults and help to arrest health decline.* We need not focus solely on biomedical factors in treatment, and where these offer limited prospect of improving health, practitioners can still draw on the psychological resources that existing and new group memberships offer.
2. *Membership in social groups can be a burden to health in particular contexts.* If social identities associated with negative age stereotypes are internalised, they can undermine

performance and well-being. It is important to be sensitive to this possibility – especially in assessment contexts.

3. *Belonging to multiple positive groups, or having multiple positive social identities, can help to reduce the impact of negative age stereotypes*. If people have access to positive social identities, these can be used to counter the effects of underperformance highlighted in Point 2. More generally too, membership in multiple groups facilitates adjustment in the context of the challenging life transitions that often accompany ageing.

Resources

Further reading

The following publications provide a good introduction to the key issues explored in this chapter – showing clearly how the social identity approach to ageing can inform both theory and practice.

①   Knight, C., Haslam, S. A., & Haslam, C. (2010). In home or at home? Evidence that collective decision making enhances older adults' social identification, well-being and use of communal space when moving to a new care facility. *Aging and Society*, *30*, 1393–1418.

   This paper provides an early example of the way in which social group interventions can be introduced and tested in applied ageing contexts.

②   St Claire, L., & He, Y. (2009). How do I know if I need a hearing aid? Further support for the self-categorization approach to symptom perception. *Applied Psychology: An International Review*, *58*, 24–41.

   In this paper on hearing loss in older adults, the authors show clearly how the salience of age affects the process of symptom perception.

③   Haslam, C., Haslam, S. A., & Jetten, J. (2014). The social determinants of cognitive change: Identity processes as the source of both enhancement and decline. In K. J. Reynolds & N. R. Branscombe (Eds.) *The Psychology of Change: Life Contexts, Experiences, and Identities* (p. 133–150). New York: Psychology Press.

   This chapter provides an analysis of the curative and harmful health effects of group identification and self-categorization in older adults. It explores in some detail the group processes that contribute to these outcomes.

Video

①   Search for "Waldinger good life" to watch an excellent TEDx talk about the importance of social relationships for healthy ageing. www.youtube.com/watch?v=q-7zAkwAOYg   (15 minutes)
②   Search for "Catherine Haslam changemakers" and watch a talk about a number of experimental and intervention studies that are discussed in this chapter and which explore the importance of social identification for healthy ageing. www.youtube.com/watch?v=k_ zX2ktaYj4   (30 minutes)

Websites

① www.ifa-fiv.org/yearsahead-challenging-ageism/. This site provides details of the World Health Organization's #YearsAhead campaign to challenge ageism "by illustrating the important role that older people play in their families and communities around the world".

② www.boredpal.com/article.php?id=1491. This site provides a fascinating insight into the activities of Portugal's "Graffiti Grannies" and has some great photographs of their work.

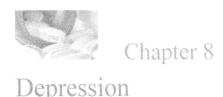

Chapter 8

Depression

Case study 8.1 Leo

Leo is a 28-year-old man who has been depressed for many years. The symptoms that bother him the most are his low energy and lack of motivation. This feels like a huge weight that needs to be overcome if he is to do even simple things, like grocery shopping. Leo feels ashamed and angry at himself for having accomplished little in the past ten years – he is about halfway through a bachelor's degree at university, does not work, and lives with his mother. Leo has little hope for the future and struggles to think of things he would enjoy doing. When asked to reflect on when things started going downhill, Leo felt that things took a turn for the worse when he moved interstate at age 17 following his parents' divorce. He left his networks behind and struggled to fit in at his new school and has had few social ties at all since starting university.

Unfortunately, Leo's experience is not uncommon. Depression affects people from all walks of life, and many people live with symptoms similar to his. Indeed, the prevalence of depression is higher than for any other mental illness, with at least 20% of people affected at some point in their lives (Kruijshaar et al., 2005). People with depression are more likely to be socio-economically disadvantaged (as we noted in Chapter 3), to be in conflict-affected or developing countries, to be women, and to be aged between 15 and 25 years.

Depression typically follows a chronic remitting-relapsing course which can severely limit a person's functioning for many months at a time. Although people sometimes use the term "depressed" to describe low mood, clinical depression describes a cluster of symptoms that includes feeling sad, but also *anhedonia*, which for many people causes more distress and impairment. Anhedonia is the inability to experience pleasure or satisfaction from activities that were once enjoyable. Depression is further characterised by cognitive symptoms (hopelessness, rumination, and suicidal thoughts), emotional symptoms (anger, guilt), physiological symptoms (changes to sleep, appetite, and energy levels), and behavioural symptoms, particularly withdrawal from normal activities (American Psychiatric Association, 2013).

On a more positive note, evidence-based treatments for depression do exist and have been shown to be of some benefit for about two-thirds of the people who undergo treatment for the condition (Hollon et al., 2014). Unfortunately, however, these treatments have not been able to reduce the burden of depression on society more generally, which has remained stable over the last two decades despite significant investment in treatment research and provision (Baxter et al., 2014).

Several factors have contributed to this lack of progress. The first is that evidence-based treatments are often expensive, and the mental health professionals that provide them are concentrated in more affluent areas (Saxena, Thornicroft, Knapp, & Whiteford, 2007). Consequently, effective treatment is mostly accessible to people in urban areas of developed countries who have considerable financial and social capital (Thomas, Ellis, Konrad, Holzer, & Morrissey, 2009) and who, as a group, tend to experience mild to moderate symptoms. Furthermore, among those who have access to appropriate health care, many either do not seek treatment or do not comply with recommended treatments (Goldman, Nielsen, & Champion, 1999; Sawada et al., 2009). This is often due to the stigma of mental illness or to the unpleasant side effects of antidepressant medication – which include sexual dysfunction, weight gain, and drowsiness (Dwight-Johnson, Sherbourne, Liao, & Wells, 2000).

A final concern with existing treatments is that their demonstrated effectiveness is in reducing acute symptoms, not in achieving long-term remission. That is, they may alleviate depression in the short term, but generally do not stop it from coming back. Speaking to this point, follow-up studies have suggested that even after receiving evidence-based treatment, 25 to 50% of people will experience depression relapse within 18 months (Fava, Rafanelli, Grandi, Conti, & Belluardo, 1998; Tracie et al., 1992). Moreover, 80% of the people diagnosed with depression will relapse at some point. The average person who has experienced depression will have four depressive episodes across their lifespan, each of about 5 months' duration (Judd, 1997).

These sobering realities about the availability and staying power of current treatments give some sense of the size of the global disease burden that depression currently poses. Indeed, depression is one of the top causes of disability in the world today (Vos et al., 2015), second only to back pain. This makes efforts to understand the condition, and to do something about it, a pressing concern for all health professionals.

Current approaches to depression

The biochemical model

An important theoretical foundation for the biochemical model is the medical principle that disease is caused by physical pathology. That is, if ill health is observed, it is assumed that its origin must lie in some form of internal dysfunction. Traditionally, mental illnesses (along with many complex and chronic health conditions) were considered beyond the scope of this medical model (Engel, 1977). However, in the 1950s, two medications were discovered to affect psychiatric symptoms: chlorpromazine in the case of psychoses and lithium in the case of bipolar disorder. These discoveries heralded an era of biological psychiatry in which treatment for mental health problems has become dominated by medical approaches, in particular, medication (Shorter, 1997). Underpinning the action of most antidepressant medications is the monoamine theory of depression, which argues that the psychological and physiological symptoms of depression are secondary to neurochemical phenomena (McNeal & Cimbolic, 1986; Singh & Gotlib, 2014).

This model is best known in its oversimplified form, in which depression is characterised as a "brain chemistry imbalance" – introduced in television commercials for the antidepressant drug Zoloft in the 1990s (Barber, 2009; see Figure 8.1). Testament to the continued dominance of this model, a study by Pamela Pilkington and her colleagues suggested that this conceptualisation is endorsed by 88% of the general public (Pilkington, Reavley, & Jorm, 2013). This is a problem because a number of experimental studies have found that belief in the biochemical model, either among people with depression or among health professionals, is associated with increased stigma as well as increased pessimism about the likelihood of recovery (Haslam & Kvaale, 2015; Kemp, Lickel, & Deacon, 2014; Leowitz & Ahn, 2015).

Measuring the dynamics of neurotransmitters is not easy because it requires invasive procedures such as radiolabelled injections or sampling of cerebrospinal fluid. As a consequence, research investigating the biochemical model typically relies on animal models of depression, genetic markers for depression, or responses to medication in clinical trials (Hollon et al., 2014). Of these sources, the strongest evidence for the biochemical model of depression is provided by studies showing the effectiveness of antidepressant medication, particularly selective serotonin reuptake inhibitors (SSRIs), the most commonly prescribed drug for depression. These medications increase the presence of the neurotransmitter *serotonin* in the brain by reducing its reabsorption (Andrews, 2015). Proponents of the biochemical model have suggested that SSRIs work because they correct low levels of serotonin in the brain that are caused by genetic vulnerability (McNeal & Cimbolic, 1986).

Chemical imbalance

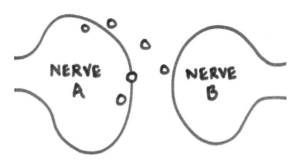

Figure 8.1 Re-creation of an image from the 1990s Zoloft commercial

Note: The "brain chemistry imbalance" model of depression is an oversimplification of the biochemical model and not supported by strong evidence. The advert portrayed depression as caused by "an imbalance of natural chemicals between nerve cells in the brain". It went on to say that because Zoloft could correct this imbalance, "you just shouldn't have to feel this way any more".

Source: The authors, based on www.youtube.com/watch?v=twhvtzd6gXA

Hundreds of studies have examined the brain chemistry and genetic profile of people with depression in an effort to establish an evidence base for biochemical models. However, meta-analyses which summarise and integrate the findings from these studies suggest that the case for the biochemical model is inconclusive and unconvincing (Anguelova, Benkelfat, & Turecki, 2003; Lasky-Su, Faraone, Glatt, & Tsuang, 2005; Wray et al., 2012). In particular, evidence suggests that those differences that do exist between depressed versus non-depressed people in terms of brain function, chemistry, or structure are more likely to *arise from* and *reflect* depression than to be its cause.

This is all well and good, but one might ask how it is possible that antidepressant medications can be effective in treating depression symptoms if there is not some pre-existing neurotransmitter dysfunction that needs correcting. One possibility is that antidepressants work through some other route. Again, meta-analyses drawing on unpublished trials of antidepressant medication registered in the United States under the Food and Drug Administration using Freedom of Information legislation are informative here (Fournier et al., 2010; Kirsch et al., 2008). Reviews of these data indicate that the clinical effectiveness of antidepressants, at least in mild and moderately severe cases, is no greater than that of a placebo (i.e., a sugar pill). This is not to say that these medications have no benefit. However, it suggests that, like placebos, their benefit may be primarily attributable to the very powerful forces of hope and expectancy, rather than to the active ingredients in the drugs themselves. Nevertheless, among people with more severe depression, the benefit of antidepressants over placebo were found to be significant, although this was at least partly because placebos are *less* effective.

Another possibility is that antidepressants work by dulling painful emotional experiences rather than by correcting dysfunctional brain chemistry. This is consistent with many patient accounts of their subjective experience of an "emotional numbing" effect of antidepressant medication (Price, Cole, & Goodwin, 2009). A relevant analogy here is that of ibuprofen or other painkilling medications: although these might be effective in dulling the experience of physical pain, few people would suggest that they work because they correct an 'ibuprofen deficit' that caused the pain. In this way, antidepressants may be helpful in treating symptoms and remain a beneficial tool in the treatment arsenal even if the biochemical model of depression is, by itself, insufficient.

Due to the mixed support for the biochemical model, recent characterisations of this framework are more modest in their scope than those promoted several decades ago. They state that although there are biological bases for all human behaviours and experiences, health conditions such as depression arise from a complex interplay of genes and the environment. Accordingly, researchers argue that neurochemical phenomena may be better understood as correlates or manifestations of depression, rather than as its primary cause (for an expanded critique of the biochemical approach, see Deacon, 2013).

The cognitive-behavioural model

The cognitive-behavioural model of depression is the dominant approach in psychology. This model is an integration of two influential bodies of psychological theorising: (a) *behavioural theories* that were developed in the first half of the 20th century and were first applied to depression in the 1960s and 1970s (e.g. Lazarus, 1968; Lewinsohn, 1975; Seligman, 1975) and (b) *cognitive theory* that emerged during the same period (Beck, 1964, 1970). The model is represented schematically in Figure 8.2 and emphasises the primacy of *depressive cognitions* – that is, negative thoughts about the self, others, and the future (A. T. Beck, 1979; J. S. Beck, 2011). These thoughts are argued to trigger the emotional symptoms of depression, specifically low mood, low energy, hopelessness, and guilt. These emotions then play a key role in motivating depressive behaviours, including reduced activity, social withdrawal, and suicidality. In turn, these behaviours are believed to reinforce and maintain depressive thoughts and a negative self-concept – resulting in a downward spiral of depression symptoms over time. When it comes to identifying the initial cause of these cognitions, cognitive-behaviour theorising

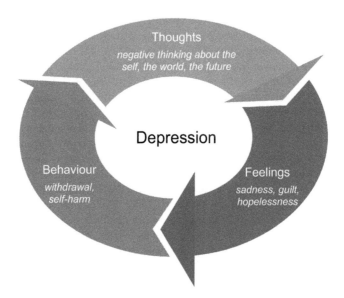

Figure 8.2 A schematic representation of central features of the cognitive-behavioural model of depression

Note: Cognition (thoughts), affect (feelings), and behaviour are inter-related aspects of experience that all bear upon the psychology of depression.

posits that stressful early-life events lead to the development of *maladaptive core beliefs* (e.g., that one is unlovable or defective) and that these make people vulnerable to depression (Eberhart, Auerbach, Bigda-Peyton, & Abela, 2011; Shah & Waller, 2000).

The cognitive-behavioural model is important because it underpins what has come to be seen as the "gold-standard" evidence-based psychological treatment for depression: cognitive behavioural therapy (CBT). Typically delivered in sessions that range in number from 12 to 20, this therapy consists of two primary intervention strategies (A. T. Beck, 1967; J. S. Beck, 2011). The first involves identifying and challenging depressive cognitions; the second involves introducing behaviours that are more likely to be rewarding and reinforcing.

The evidence base for the effectiveness of CBT is extremely strong. Meta-analyses have found that at least 60% of people treated with CBT experience substantial benefits (Butler, Chapman, Forman, & Beck, 2006). Nevertheless, support for the cognitive-behavioural model that underpins CBT has been less consistent. For instance, component analyses of CBT have suggested that cognitive challenging does not account for the effectiveness of the therapy (Longmore & Worrell, 2007). Improvement in symptoms and quality of life also appear to *precede*, rather than follow, change in cognitions (Fayers & Machin, 2007; Oei, McAlinden, & Cruwys, 2014). Indeed, the most effective component of CBT treatment itself appears to be the behavioural activation component (Cuijpers, van Straten, & Warmerdam, 2007), particularly when the behaviours that are activated promote social engagement (Scott et al., 2012; Veale, 2008). More generally, though, CBT effectiveness, like that of other psychological therapies, appears to be driven primarily by what are referred to as *common factors* (Ahn & Wampold, 2001; Honyashiki et al., 2014). These are elements of the therapeutic process that are common to a range of different treatments. Chief among these is the quality of the relationship between the therapist and patient (e.g., the amount of rapport they are able to establish; Grencavage & Norcross, 1990; Messer & Wampold, 2002), often conceptualised as the *therapeutic alliance* (see also Chapter 2).

In summary, then, the current state of evidence indicates that the cognitive-behavioural model has been crucial to the development of what is probably the most effective – and certainly the most influential – psychological treatment for depression. At the same time, though, it has been argued that the importance of altering cognitions may have been overstated (Jacobson et al., 1996; Longmore & Worrell, 2007). Furthermore, the cognitive-behavioural model is unable to account for the powerful role of social relationships in shaping the onset and prognosis of depression – an issue we will turn to now.

The interpersonal stress model

Both the biochemical and cognitive-behavioural models acknowledge the role of environmental stress in contributing to the onset of depression. Yet neither model offers a coherent framework to understand the kind or degree of stress that is likely to precipitate or prolong a depressive episode. This is something that is explored by a collection of related theories and models that point to the role of life events in the trajectory of the condition (e.g., of the form discussed in Chapter 5; see Table 5.1).

The first and most well-established line of research in this area draws on *attachment theory*. The fundamental tenet of this is that early-life interactions with caregivers are internalised and can go on to influence social interactions (particularly in family and intimate relationships) throughout the lifespan (Rothbard & Shaver, 1994). More specifically, researchers in this tradition have argued that interpersonal trauma (e.g., violence, emotional abuse) plays an important role in the development of depression, specifically by undermining social trust and hindering the development of appropriate social relationships and interaction styles (Anderson, Beach, & Kaslow, 1999; Cukor & McGinn, 2006; Styron & Janoff-Bulman, 1997).

A body of evidence has emerged to support this claim. For example, population-level data suggest that gender differences in rates of psychopathology (whereby women experience rates of depression and anxiety almost twice as high as those of men, a difference which emerges in adolescence) are at least partially accounted for by women's heightened exposure to interpersonal trauma (e.g., domestic violence, sexual assault, predatory harassment; Moore et al., 2015; Rees et al., 2014). It therefore appears that life stressors of this form can have a "downstream" impact on a person's depression risk – not least because such stressors can result in social networks that are less supportive and less accessible.

A related line of research has suggested that life stressors need not be traumatic or experienced early in life to affect one's risk of developing depression. Indeed, researchers have noted that key life events such as divorce, bereavement, and retirement commonly precede depression (Kendler, Hettema, Butera, Gardner, & Prescott, 2003; Paykel, 1994; Tennant, 2002). More particularly, it has been argued that any life event that is experienced as a form of loss can be an important trigger for the onset of a first depressive episode (Monroe, Rohde, Seeley, & Lewinsohn, 1999). This research is informative in two ways. First, it helps us to identify periods in life when people might be particularly vulnerable and where intervention might be appropriately targeted. Second, it provides evidence that the experience of depression is best conceptualised not as something that happens to *a certain type of person*, but rather as a state that may be relatively common – or even typical – given *a certain set of life circumstances*.

Importantly, though, the impact of life stress will not be the same for everyone, and one long-standing theory – the *stress-buffering hypothesis* – argues that some individuals might be less vulnerable to developing depression as a consequence of their access to social support. In ways alluded to in our discussion of stress in Chapter 5, this model highlights the protective benefit of social support in the context of stressful life events (Cohen & Wills, 1985). Specifically, it proposes that life stressors have the capacity to compromise mental health and, most pertinent for our present purposes, can lead to depression. However, people who have more social support are believed to be buffered against these effects. In line with this suggestion, evidence has consistently identified positive associations between perceived stress, social isolation, and mental illness (Ezquiaga, Garcia, Pallarés, Bravo, & García, 1999; Fiore, Becker, & Coppel, 1983; Paykel, 1994). There is also evidence that people who are more socially connected have a reduced physiological response to acute stressors (Cohen, Doyle, Turner, Alper, & Skoner, 2003).

Nevertheless, the stress-buffering hypothesis itself has received limited support. Most problematic is the fact that there is only limited evidence that the specific interaction between social support and stress predicts mental health outcomes. For example, results from meta-analysis indicate that a statistically significant interaction of the form predicted by the stress-buffering hypothesis was present in only 3 out of 58 longitudinal studies (Burton, Stice, & Seeley, 2004). Instead, research has consistently found direct relationships between social support, perceived stress, and mental health. These three variables are perhaps best conceptualised as related *outcomes* of social identity loss in the context of life transition, in ways described in more detail in the social identity model of identity change (Praharso, Tear, & Cruwys, 2017; see Chapter 3, Figure 3.6). It is clear, though, that social relationships do not simply moderate the dangers of stress exposure. Rather, their absence is *at the very heart* of the depressive condition.

Consistent with this insight, in the last ten years, there has been an increased focus on the *direct* relationship between social connectedness and depression. In particular, social isolation has emerged as a key risk factor for the development of depression (Hawkley & Cacioppo, 2003). Thus people who feel socially isolated have been found to experience a long-term elevated risk of depression, over and above any effect of gender, age, or socio-economic status (Cacioppo, Hawkley, & Thisted, 2010; Cacioppo, Grippo, London, Goossens, & Cacioppo, 2015). Furthermore, evidence suggests that an increase in loneliness – and accompanying social withdrawal – *precedes*, rather than follows, the development of depression (Cacioppo & Cacioppo, 2014; Glass, De Leon, Bassuk, & Berkman, 2006; Handley et al., 2012). Note, though, that this evidence is at odds with biochemical and cognitive-behavioural models, which typically conceptualise social withdrawal as merely a symptom or maintenance factor in depression (e.g., Kovacs & Beck, 1978). Nevertheless, loneliness is now well established as one of the major causes of depression. What is less clear, however, is what life conditions might conspire to make a person feel lonely. To date, theoretical analyses have focused primarily on deficits in *social skills* (Hawkley & Cacioppo, 2010) but they have not engaged with the social and structural realities that might lead a person to experience such deficits.

Speaking to a number of these issues, one form of psychological intervention that targets many of these social factors in depression – including social skills deficits, social loss, and trauma – is *interpersonal psychotherapy* (IPT; Klerman, Weissman, Rounsaville, & Chevron, 1984). IPT has been shown to be as effective as CBT in many well-controlled clinical trials (Cuipers et al., 2011; De Mello, Mari, Bacaltchuk, Verdeli, & Neugebauer, 2005). However, for all its strengths, IPT has two fundamental limitations. The first is that it focuses primarily on *interpersonal* processes, and as a result fails to capture the role of wider social *group* processes in depression outcomes. As we will expand upon later (and also in later chapters; e.g., Chapter 15), the social identity approach posits that it is social group relationships that are particularly critical for depression outcomes, due to their unique capacity to structure collective aspects of the self-concept (e.g., Turner et al., 1994). Furthermore, the empirical evidence base confirms the importance of groups, with recent evidence suggesting that it is psychological group membership, rather than interpersonal friendships (Haslam, Cruwys, & Haslam, 2014a) or social contact (Sani, Herrera, Wakefield, Boroch, & Gulyas, 2012), that does the heavy lifting when it comes to protecting mental and cognitive health.

The second and most important limitation of IPT is that although it targets some of the social factors that have been linked to depression, it is not aligned with any particular analytic framework that might explain social relationships or their role in depression. This is a curious legacy of the way in which IPT was actually developed, which was as an active control-therapy condition in randomised controlled trials of CBT. More specifically, IPT was intended to offer the social support and interpersonal contact components of CBT, but without the "active ingredients" – which were believed to be cognitive (Elkin et al., 1995; Klerman et al., 1984). So although IPT drew upon attachment and other interpersonal stress models in its development (Weissman, 2006), the expectation was that it would be less effective. But, instead, IPT turned out to be just as effective as CBT. Accordingly, although the unexpected effectiveness of IPT speaks to the importance of social factors, it is something of a blunt instrument when it comes to effectively targeting the social processes that the theoretical and empirical literature would suggest are vital to the development, remission, and relapse of depression.

If this were a murder mystery, we might observe that IPT tells us where the body is buried (which is very important), but not why or how it got there. To discover this, we need to take a more forensic theoretical approach which does justice not only to the interpersonal but also to the *group-based* social psychological dimensions of depression. This, of course, is precisely what social identity theorising affords.

The social identity approach to depression

In light of the strengths and limitations of the models discussed above, there are several goals that a *new psychology of depression* might seek to achieve. First, it should provide a parsimonious theoretical model of depression that advances understanding while simultaneously integrating both (1) a clinical account of depression symptoms and (2) a social psychological account of the nature of social relationships. Second, it should explain how and why stressful life events – especially social loss, trauma, and social isolation – appear to be particularly important triggers for depression onset and relapse. Third, it should be able to account for the effectiveness of the leading psychotherapies, CBT and IPT. Next, we outline how a social identity approach to depression achieves all of these goals.

Social relationships counteract depression when they inform the self-concept

When it comes to shaping psychological experience and mental health, not all social relationships are equal. Indeed, a core social identity principle is that the world, including the social world, is interpreted through the lens of self-categorization. That is, we understand ourselves not only on the basis of what makes us unique and different from others, but critically, on the basis of what we have in common with others (Turner, 1982). Moreover, as we noted in a number of previous chapters, when social rela- tionships are self-defining – such that they inform our collective sense of self – they have distinctive implications for mental health. Therefore, the social identity approach has a different understanding of *when* relationships, either group or interpersonal, will be protective and when they will not. Specifically, we argue that it is only when people derive a sense of social identity from their social relationships that they have profound implications for their well-being. Indeed, this is related to the core hypothesis (H1) that *because it is the basis for meaningful group life, social identity is central to both good and ill health.*

In support of this basic point, a large study that we published in *Social Science and Medicine* investigated the specific benefits of social group membership in a representative sample of English people aged over 50 (Cruwys et al., 2013b). The study modelled the long-term effects of joining a social group among people with and without a history of depression. Because of the large sample size, it was possible to statistically control for the effects of age, gender, socio-economic status, relation- ship status, ethnicity, and subjective health status, as well as initial depression severity and a person's initial number of group memberships. The study found that joining social groups (e.g., a choir, a neighbourhood club, an organisational association) reduced the likelihood of individuals experiencing a first episode of depression. However, the benefit of joining groups was three times more pronounced among those with a history of depression. Specifically, as Figure 8.3 shows, those people who joined one group reduced their risk of depression relapse from 41 to 31%. Those joining three groups reduced their risk of relapse to only 15%. These observations support previous claims that we have made on the basis of the social identity approach to health (e.g., H11, that *providing they are compatible with*

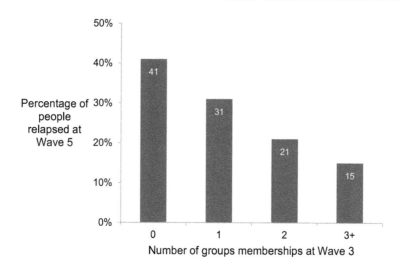

Figure 8.3 Group memberships predict the likelihood of depression relapse

Note: This graph plots the likelihood of depression relapse among a sample of people with a history of depression (*N* = 339) as a function of the number of social group memberships that they gained 2 years following their depres- sive episode. This analysis refers to the predicted probability of relapse after 6 years when controlling for Wave 1 age, sex, socio-economic status, subjective health status, relationship status, ethnicity, severity of initial depression, and initial number of group memberships.

Source: Based on Cruwys et al. (2013b)

each other, important to them, and positive, the more social identities a person has access to, the more psychological resources they can draw upon and the more beneficial this will be for their health). These findings also speak to the close relationship between social reality (i.e., one's "objective" membership of social categories) and individual well-being. And one of their important implications is that interventions which focus purely on improving interpersonal relationships (e.g., IPT) may be even more effective if they are expanded to focus on building shared social identities and shared group memberships.

Although these findings about the benefits of group membership are important, the social identity approach is particularly concerned with the subjective psychological representation of such group membership; that is, *social identification*. In other words, we would expect that group membership alone is not sufficient to protect against depression. Rather, it is only those groups which are psychologically important and self-defining that will provide these benefits (as suggested by H2: that *a person will experience the health-related benefits or costs of a given group membership only to the extent that they identify with that group*). For example, not every card-carrying member of a gym will strongly identify as a gym-goer. Moreover, it is easy to imagine that those who do not identify as gym-goers do not necessarily visit the gym very often.

This principle has been empirically tested in a number of studies that explore the social dimensions of the psychology of depression. First, Fabio Sani and his colleagues (2012) found that social identification with one's family (among Polish people) or one's army unit (among Eastern European troops) was a stronger predictor of depression symptoms than the amount of social contact that a person reported with the relevant group. Moreover, a major review that we conducted of all of the published studies that had measured social identification (with any group) and depression symptoms revealed a consistent, negative, and moderately strong relationship between these variables ($r = -.26$; Cruwys, Haslam, Dingle, Haslam, & Jetten, 2014b). In other words, the more a person identified with a given group (school, family, colleagues, support group, etc.), the less likely they were to feel depressed.

Most recently, a large representative study of 1,824 Scottish adults also found that these effects are cumulative with membership of multiple groups. Specifically, the number of social groups with which a person highly identified (between zero and three) proved to be a strong predictor of their self-reported depression symptoms (Sani, Madhok, Norbury, Dugard, & Wakefield, 2015). Generally speaking, then, social identifications appear to counteract depression, and the more of these one has, the merrier one tends to be.

Social identities counteract depression because they are a basis for meaning, agency, purpose, and support

The means by which social identification delivers strong protective and curative benefits for depression is a topic of ongoing investigation. To date, however, a number of mechanisms have been identified that are either (1) generally implicated in well-being or (2) specific to depression. In this section, we first review those general mechanisms. Before we do so, though, it is worth noting that – unlike some other theories of depression, in particular, the biochemical model – the social identity approach to health does not reify depression as a categorical disease state. Instead, the approach is more consonant with the notion of depression as one pole of a continuum of hedonic and effective psychological functioning (Cox, Enns, Borger, & Parker, 1999; Vredenburg, Flett, & Krames, 1993). And because social identities are a necessary component of a healthy and effectively functioning psychological system, many of the reasons why social identities benefit well-being in general also apply to depression in particular. As outlined in more detail in Chapter 2, these include the capacity for social identity (1) to provide a sense of *meaning* and purpose (H13), (2) to underpin various forms of *social support* (H14), and (3) to enhance one's sense of *collective efficacy* or power (H15).

In the context of depression, there is substantial evidence for H15, which relates to what is variously termed agency, control, or efficacy. In particular, Katharine Greenaway and her colleagues

(2015) report five studies, ranging from correlational studies with over 62,000 participants from 47 countries to experimental studies with American community members, all of which show that social identification fosters not just collective efficacy, but also a *personal* sense of control over life.

Evidence that supports H14 was reviewed in some detail in Chapters 5 (on stress), 6 (on trauma), and 7 (on ageing). However, to recap briefly here, a range of studies show that social support is a psychological resource that primarily emerges in the context of shared group membership (e.g., Haslam, Reicher, & Levine, 2012). Because of this, we might expect that the close link that has been found in many studies between social support and depression is broadly consistent with the predictions of the social identity approach. More specifically, we can hypothesise that social support and other resources (e.g., social participation, social contact, social trust) are the "fruits" or products of social identification. Not only are people more likely to receive such resources from other ingroup members, but they are also more likely to provide such resources to others, as subjectively and reciprocally perceived shared group membership provides a platform for effective and meaningful forms of social solidarity (Reicher & Haslam, 2010).

In this regard, an important recent development has involved a focus not so much on identifying the particular variables that are implicated in the social cure, as on exploring how these constructs fit together and relate to one another. Specifically, we have argued that variables such as self-esteem, belonging, meaning, and support should not be viewed as competitors for the status of the "true" mechanism through which social identity protects against depression, but rather as components of a broader suite of *social psychological needs* whose fulfilment proves beneficial to mental health. Supporting this idea, in three studies, Greenaway and her colleagues (2016) found that gaining a social identity led to concomitant increases in the satisfaction of these four psychological needs (i.e., esteem, belonging, meaning, and support). This in turn was reflected in reduced levels of depression symptoms, even when identity gain or loss was manipulated experimentally. Crucially, these studies also found that no single variable could explain these effects on its own. Instead, it was the combined effect of all four that constituted the critical psychological resource that social identity provided.

An important point to take away from this analysis, then, is that although depression of a clinically severe form is serious and potentially life threatening, it is not so qualitatively different from low well-being that the general protective benefits conferred by social identity are irrelevant. Instead, social identification is a source of psychological need satisfaction, whose precise nature is likely to vary as a function of the specific content of a person's group memberships (e.g., their norms, values, and practices) and of the social context in which they are imbedded. Indeed, it is the richness and versatility of the resources provided by social identity that render its protective benefit so adaptive and robust.

Social identities structure depression-related thoughts and perception

It may at times be tempting to view social identifications as either fixed structural features – Leo is a man, Leo is a South African – or as fixed aspects of personality – as a man, or as a South African, Leo is a 'high identifier'. However, both of these characterisations of social identification are an oversimplification. Instead, social realities fluidly shape the way in which social categorization occurs. In other words, our social identities have the capacity to change in response to moment-to-moment shifts in social context. If we want to understand how Leo defines himself, we need to know whether he is at a football match, at a funeral, or at university.

This seemingly straightforward point is, in fact, quite radical from the standpoint of many approaches to psychology, as it departs from the standard conceptualisation of the self as something that is individualistic, coherent, unified, and, above all, static. However, it is well supported by decades of social identity research which shows, amongst other things, that a person's likelihood of defining themselves in terms of a particular group membership is determined by the context-specific *fit* and *accessibility* of a given social categorization (e.g., in ways suggested by Figures 2.3, 2.4, and 2.5; Blanz, 1999; Doosje, Haslam, Spears, Oakes, & Koomen, 1998; Oakes, Turner, & Haslam, 1991). Thus Leo is more likely to self-categorize in terms of his national identity while watching the Olympics than while sitting in biology class, where he would be more likely to self-categorize as a student. These differences in the way we see ourselves – which correspond to our social identification with various groups – have important downstream implications for our thoughts, feelings, and behaviour in ways suggested by Figure 8.4. This is because thoughts, feelings, and behaviour depend in critical ways on processes of self-perception. We know, too, that, in the context of depression, negative thoughts about the self are a core feature of the condition. In light of this, we can revisit aspects of the cognitive-behavioural model outlined earlier in order to ask: How might social identities influence depressive thoughts, depressed mood, and depressed behaviours? More particularly, we can answer this question with reference to evidence that social identities are important determinants of maladaptive schemas and negative attributions in particular.

In line with this point, there is evidence that both self-blaming attribution styles and maladaptive core beliefs are shaped by social identity. Speaking to the first point, some of our recent research investigated the relationship between social identity and depressive attribution style (Cruwys, South, Greenaway, & Haslam, 2015). In a first study, 139 students in their final undergraduate year completed

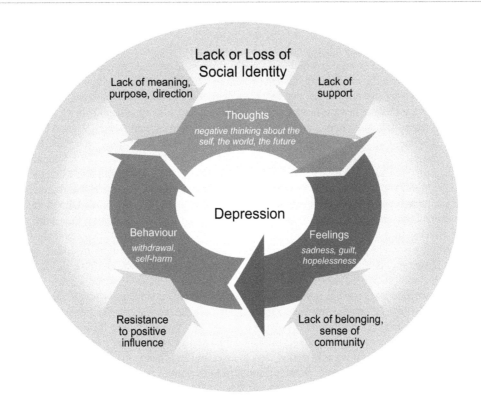

Figure 8.4 Social identities as a basis for thoughts, feelings, and actions

Note: Social identity is a major determinant of cognition, affect, and behaviour – aspects of experience that all bear upon the psychology of depression (as suggested by the cognitive-behavioural model; see Figure 8.2).

Source: Based on Cruwys et al. (2014b)

a questionnaire in which, amongst other things, they reported the number of groups they were members of and completed a measure of their attribution style. In line with predictions, it was found that those students who reported having the highest number of social group memberships were least likely to attribute negative events to internal, stable, and global causes (e.g., "I failed because I'm stupid"). This, in turn, was associated with these students reporting lower levels of depression symptoms than those who reported having fewer social group memberships.

A follow-up experiment with 88 people investigated whether simply reminding people of their social identities in an experiment was sufficient to buffer them from depressive cognitions in the face of failure. This involved providing all participants with false feedback that they had failed on a problem-solving task. However, compared to participants who were not reminded of their social identities, those participants who had first been asked to recall either one or three social identities were *less likely* (1) to attribute this failure to internal, stable, and global causes (the so-called depressive attribution style; Alloy, Peterson, Abramson, & Seligman, 1984) and (2) to experience negative mood following failure. These results highlight the role that social identity – and, more particularly, a lack or loss of social identity – plays in the development of those cognitions that maintain depression symptoms and are explicitly targeted in CBT. It also suggests that modification of such cognitions might be achieved through indirect social (e.g., family or school group interactions), as well as direct cognitive (e.g., psychotherapy), means. In short, healthy cognitions can be promoted by attending to people's outer worlds not just their inner ones.

These studies also indicate that cognitive-behavioural theorising might benefit from being elaborated to take stock of the way in which a person's moment-to-moment cognitions are shaped by social experiences and the availability of social resources. Note here that cognitive-behavioural and attachment models traditionally argue that early life experiences induce an *underlying vulnerability* to depression, manifesting in maladaptive core beliefs such as "I am unloveable" or "I will always be alone". Such beliefs have been thought to be relatively enduring and stable (Wang, Halvorsen, Eisemann, & Waterloo, 2010; Young, Klosko, & Weishaar, 2003). Accordingly, they are believed to change only in response to extensive therapeutic intervention (Nadort et al., 2009; Sempértegui, Karreman, Arntz, & Bekker, 2013). However, a social identity framework would argue that they are, in principle, fluid, social, and self-relevant throughout the lifespan. Indeed, CBT and attachment theorists would agree that such beliefs are adaptive responses to social reality in childhood. A social identity framework also recognises that certain experiences are more formative than others; for example, because they determine perceiver readiness (as explained in Chapter 2; Oakes et al., 1994). Consequently, we might posit that such beliefs are best challenged not through extensive self-examination in therapy, but rather through social experiences that contradict, and directly challenge, these beliefs.

This proposition was tested in further research that we recently conducted (Cruwys, Dingle et al., 2014a). In one study, 76 people who were experiencing homelessness were asked about their experience with a charitable association (the Salvation Army) that was providing them with short-term accommodation services. These individuals were then followed up 3 months later, by which time many of them were living in the community, with a view to assessing any change in maladaptive core beliefs that might have occurred over time. What we found was that those people who identified with the service most strongly were more likely to have extended their social networks by joining new groups in the interim, and that this is turn predicted lower endorsement of maladaptive core beliefs (here, measured as a 'social isolation schema' (i.e., the belief that one is different from others, isolated, and on the outside of groups)).

In other words, for members of this very vulnerable sample, positive social experiences associated with their encounter with the residential accommodation service were sufficient to initiate a virtuous cycle in which they were more likely (1) to have further positive social experiences and (2) to change their beliefs about the world in positive (i.e., counter-depressive) ways. In this way, the central point that the research makes is that those self-related constructs that have been established as relevant to depression in previous research – namely, attributions, schemas, and negative thinking – are actually structured by social identity, and hence can be responsive to social intervention.

A further consequence of the fluidity and responsiveness of self-categorization is that the experience of depression *itself* can be reified and come to define one's self-concept. That is, particularly when biochemical conceptualisations of mental illness hold sway, a person can come to see their experience of depression as reflecting some deeper truth about the kind of person they are. Here the term 'depression' is not just a description but also an *explanation* – with the person's reasoning reflecting a belief that "I am feeling depressed because I am a depressive person". Although such reasoning is fundamentally circular, it is nevertheless characteristic of the kind of deceptive (and potentially quite destructive) determinism provided by genetic and biochemical explanations for human experience (Dar-Nimrod & Heine, 2011).

As we outlined in Chapter 4, a substantial body of evidence now indicates that a person is more likely to define themselves in terms of a particular social category when they are subject to discrimination on the basis of that social group membership. Confirming the relevance of this point to the analysis of depression, Cruwys and Gunaseelan (2016) ran a study with 250 people with depression who were either experiencing current symptoms of at least moderate severity or had received a formal diagnosis from a health practitioner. As expected, participants reported high levels of discrimination directed at them due to their depression (see also Crabtree, Haslam, Postmes, & Haslam, 2010). The experience of discrimination in turn predicted higher levels of identification as a depressed person, with many participants reporting that depression was a central component of their self-definition. For instance, one person stated:

> Unfortunately depression is now so firmly rooted with me that it is an indelible part of my persona. I wouldn't know how to act without depression.

Furthermore, self-identifying as depressed was associated with *poorer* well-being, not only in terms of depression symptoms but also in terms of anxiety, stress, and life satisfaction more generally. Importantly, this contrasts with the more typical finding (again, see Chapter 4) that identification with a stigmatised group *protects* people from the generally deleterious effects that discrimination has on well-being (see also Dingle, Stark, Cruwys, & Best, 2015; Walter, Jetten, Parsell, & Dingle, 2015b).

So why might it be that identifying as a depressed person is so harmful for well-being, when identifying as a member of other stigmatised groups, such as an ethnic minority, is protective? There are potentially several reasons. First, unlike many social categories, being a "depressed person" is a *concealable* group membership. As a result, most people choose not to disclose their depression in a broad range of social contexts. However, previous studies have suggested that concealing stigmatised identities is, in itself, potentially harmful to well-being (Ellemers & Barreto, 2006; Jones, Jetten, Haslam, & Williams, 2012; Quinn & Earnshaw, 2013). Second, "depressed person" is an identity for which stigma is legitimised by the broader society, and often by sufferers themselves, in a way that is no longer acceptable for many other stigmatised groups (Corrigan & Watson, 2006; Rüsch, Zlati, Black, & Thornicroft, 2014). Third, and perhaps most importantly, the *content* of the identity "depressed person" explicitly includes lack of well-being as a defining characteristic. Accordingly, because people's well-being is shaped by the norms, values, and beliefs of their ingroup (following H8: *that when and to the extent that a person defines themselves in terms of a given social identity, they will enact – or at least strive to enact – the norms and values associated with that identity*), then when this identity content is negative, it will prove detrimental to their well-being. Indeed, this is exactly what Cruwys and Gunaseelan (2016) found. For identifying as a depressed person only predicted poorer well-being if (and to the extent that) participants believed that negative thoughts, guilt, hopelessness, and self-harm were *characteristic* of people with depression. If those participants had a more positive view of what being a depressed person meant and entailed (e.g., being more creative; Andreasen, 1987), then this identity proved far less deleterious to their mental health.

Depression interventions are effective to the extent that they modify social identities or the social realities that inform them

Psychological interventions are something of a "black box", and this is no less true in the area of depression than in any other. That is to say, an abundance of empirical evidence speaks to the effectiveness of various different kinds of interventions, but many studies also show no difference in effectiveness between different types of therapies. On this basis, some researchers have controversially concluded that all therapies are equally effective – a position known as the *dodo bird verdict* (after Lewis Carroll's dodo bird, who proclaimed "Everyone has won, and all must have prizes", Carroll, 1916; see Luborsky et al., 2002, for an example). However, a less controversial conclusion is that factors that are *common* across therapies are responsible for much of their effectiveness, and that in this respect the therapeutic alliance is a particularly critical ingredient (Budd & Hughes, 2009; Messer & Wampold, 2002). This is consistent with the evidence we reviewed earlier in this chapter that the effectiveness of CBT cannot be attributed straightforwardly to theorised mechanisms, particularly those of cognitive change.

With these issues in mind, several studies have investigated whether the effectiveness of existing psychotherapies (particularly CBT) is in part attributable to their social components. Of particular relevance are two studies that we published in the *Journal of Affective Disorders* (Cruwys, Haslam, Dingle, Jetten, et al., 2014c). In line with the broad thrust of this chapter, these showed that people who joined a new social group were likely to experience improvement in depression symptoms 3 months later. In Study 1, 52 people in the community who were experiencing disadvantage (e.g., at risk of homelessness, discharged from psychiatric hospital, unemployed) were facilitated to join a recreational group of their choice. These encompassed a wide range of activities, including soccer, yoga, sewing, or playing drums (see Figure 8.5). Participants were surveyed when they began attending the group and again approximately 3 months later. Among this disadvantaged sample (over half of whom had a formal psychiatric diagnosis), the study found that joining a recreational group led to symptom improvement in most participants (this is also consistent with other research on the benefits of social participation; e.g. Santini, Koyanagi, Tyrovola, Donovan, Nielsen, & Kouchede, 2017). However, the best predictor of who benefited from the groups was *not* participants' initial symptom severity, the frequency with which they attended the group, or which group they chose to take part in. Instead, over and above all these factors, it was *social identification* with the group in question that predicted reduced depression symptoms. Indeed, on average, participants who identified with their new group experienced a reduction in their symptoms that took them below the clinical cut-off for depression. Moreover, as we would expect (e.g., on the basis of H2, that *a person will experience the health-related benefits or costs of a given group membership only to the extent that they identify with that group*), participants who did not feel strongly connected to their recreational group were less likely to recover relative to those participants who felt highly identified with their group.

A follow-up study explored these same principles with a sample of 92 outpatients with diagnosed depression or anxiety who were undergoing group-based cognitive-behavioural therapy (GCBT). These participants were surveyed at commencement of treatment and completion of the intensive programme approximately 1 month later. The pattern of results was remarkably similar to those of the previous study. Again, initial symptom severity, frequency of attendance, and the type of group programme (depression versus anxiety focused) did not predict symptom improvement. Instead, and over and above the effects of all these factors, it was social identification with the psychotherapy group that facilitated symptom improvement. That is, those people who did not feel a sense of psychological connection to their therapy group did not reap the benefits of the evidence-based CBT that

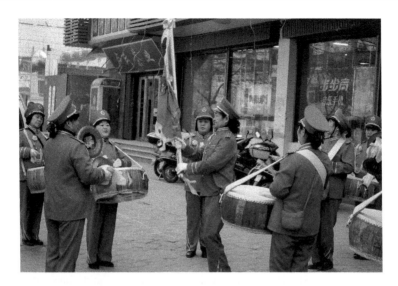

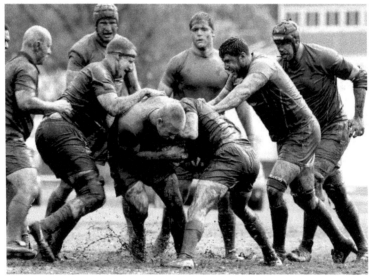

Figure 8.5 Meaningful group activity counteracts depression

Note: Vulnerable participants in Cruwys et al.'s (2014c) study were helped to join a range of social groups. For those who identified with the groups, this led to a marked reduction in their depression.

Source: Pixabay

was delivered within the group. In contrast, those participants who highly identified with the therapy group experienced a reduction in their depression and anxiety symptoms, as well as improved quality of life. In short, it appears that it was the group context – the 'G' in GCBT, at least as much as the 'C' – that achieved benefits for mental health (for a related analysis see Cruwys, Haslam,

Fox, & McMahon, 2015; Gleibs, Haslam, Haslam, & Jones, 2011a). This is an issue that we will return to in Chapter 15, where we flesh out precisely how we might structure psychological intervention to directly target this 'G'.

However, the social identity approach to depression differs from existing cognitive psychotherapies in a more fundamental way than merely focusing our attention on different intervention components or strategies. More generally, as we noted in Chapter 1, as an approach that seeks to engage with the psychological reality of social groups, it is compatible with the public health movement that strives to recognise and address the social determinants of health (e.g., Marmot & Wilkinson, 2005). In the case of depression, this means that the constellation of thoughts, feelings, and behaviours that manifest at an individual level are seen to reflect pathology that resides not *within the person* but rather within their social environment. The condition can thus be seen less as a problem of the mind and more as a problem of the social world by which that mind is structured (Turner & Oakes, 1997) – a world which includes such things as unemployment, poverty, isolation, and stigma (see Chapters 3 and 4). Indeed, here, it can be seen primarily as a problem of social disadvantage rather than of maladaptive cognition.

It follows from this that effective interventions for depression need not necessarily occur or be focused at an individual level and may in fact be more effective to the extent that they target the condition's *social determinants*. At the same time, though, we need to recognise that preventative interventions that improve a person's life circumstances and social reality *prior* to the onset of depression do not look like traditional health care. Instead, they will often involve policy change and will frequently be realised in educational or occupational settings rather than health care ones (Mrazek & Haggerty, 1994). Nevertheless, if we are interested in improving mental health at a population level, these are the interventions that are likely to have the greatest effectiveness *and* cost-effectiveness. This suggests that the most profound "social cure" involves creating social realities that empower individuals to restructure their own social worlds in ways that are optimal for their health (as suggested by the competition hypothesis, H7).

Conclusion

The new psychology of depression that we have outlined in this chapter provides a framework not only for *understanding* the social and structural factors that shape depression, but also for *intervening* to facilitate its prevention and treatment. This analysis flows from the realisation that depression is not merely low mood, but rather a cluster of symptoms that characterise what it is to lack the very things that make human life meaningful – belonging, connection, and purpose.

Other models of depression, including the biochemical model, the cognitive-behavioural model, and the interpersonal stress model, were reviewed, and we have seen that each offers useful inputs into a comprehensive biopsychosocial approach to complex multifaceted phenomena. Nevertheless, it is our contention that, in both the conceptualisation and the treatment of depression, the social elements of this model are all too often relegated to the fringe – as afterthoughts and optional extras. The rapidly growing evidence clearly indicates that we can no longer get away with paying lip service to these social factors. In short, in order to get to the bottom of depression, it is time that we take the 'social' as seriously as the 'bio' and the 'psycho'.

In this regard, the social identity approach is unique in offering not just a list of social factors that influence depression, but also a comprehensive theory of how these factors interplay both within and across levels of analysis. Ultimately, we argue that what it means to be an effective, functioning human being is to be embedded in social groups. This means that if, for a particular person, this is not the case, then depression is a likely consequence. And in these terms, the "cure" to depression necessarily involves not only the restructuring of people's brain chemistry and cognitions but also, and more fundamentally, improvements to their social life and associated social-psychological realities. The core issue, then, is not that people "shouldn't have to feel this way" (as the Zoloft advert put it), but rather that they shouldn't have to live in a world where feeling this way makes sense.

Points for practice

On the basis of the ideas and arguments presented in this chapter, it is possible to abstract three key points that are relevant to practitioners working with people suffering from depression:

1. *Depression often has social origins.* Depressive thoughts (such as attribution style and maladaptive schema), feelings (such as meaning and belongingness), and behaviours (such as self-harm and withdrawal) are predicated on social beliefs and circumstances, not just personality or biology.
2. *Depression often arises from either a lack of or a loss of social identities.* Accordingly, there is value to interventions that seek to increase people's social connectedness, particularly to meaningful social groups (see also Chapter 15 on GROUPS 4 HEALTH).
3. *Depressive symptomatology can be modified both within and outside traditional therapeutic settings.* For example, it is possible (and often recommended) to treat depression in community social and recreation groups and through structural and policy changes to social environments that place people at risk.

Resources

Further reading

The following readings provide a good introduction to the social identity approach to depression as well as to some of the data that support it.

① Deacon, B. J. (2013). The biomedical model of mental disorder: A critical analysis of its validity, utility, and effects on psychotherapy research. *Clinical Psychology Review, 33,* 846–861.

This article provides a very good evidence-based critique of the biochemical approach to depression.

② Cruwys, T., Haslam, S. A., Dingle, G. A., Haslam, C., & Jetten, J. (2014a). Depression and social identity: an integrative review. *Personality and Social Psychology Review, 18,* 215–238.

This review article provides a detailed discussion of the relationship between social identity and depression and provides a platform for many of the ideas presented in this chapter.

③ Sani, F., Madhok, V., Norbury, M., Dugard, P., & Wakefield, J. R. H. (2015). Greater number of group identifications is associated with lower odds of being depressed: evidence from a Scottish community sample. *Social Psychiatry and Psychiatric Epidemiology, 50,* 1389–1397.

This paper presents compelling evidence of the role that important group memberships play in buffering people against depression.

Video

①   Search for "Damien Scarf anxiety" to watch a TEDx talk in which Damien Scarf from the University of Otago presents a succinct overview of the implications of social identity and group belonging for depression (and health more generally) – with insights from his own personal experience: www.youtube.com/watch?v=cbHBZWbEk8A   (10 minutes)

②   Search for "Frances overdiagnosis" and watch a talk in which Psychiatrist Dr Allen J Frances reflects on the overdiagnosis of mental illness: https://youtu.be/yuCwVnzSjWA
(58 minutes)

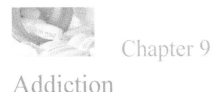

Chapter 9

Addiction

Case study 9.1 Peter

Peter is a 38-year-old father of two who works as a truck driver for a long-distance transport company. He grew up in a working-class suburb of a metropolitan city. Both of his parents worked long hours, often leaving young Peter and his three siblings to fend for themselves. Peter started drinking alcohol and smoking cannabis in his early teens along with two older brothers and other young neighbours. He did not view this as anything unusual or problematic, although he was aware that his parents and teachers did not approve of it. Peter recognised that his substance use had become problematic in his early 30s when he was using amphetamines to stay awake for long periods driving his truck. By that time, two of his brothers had also been treated for substance use disorders. They had recommended that Peter get some help – in particular, because, more and more, his substance use was affecting him negatively. His temper was frayed, he suffered severe agitation and insomnia, and he sometimes "crashed" and was unable to move for several days at a time. Peter entered a residential rehabilitation centre after his wife Tania decided to move out with her children, claiming that she "no longer recognised the man that she married".

Peter's case illustrates one of many trajectories into addiction – in his case, an early age of first substance use, and despite the negative consequences of use, a long-term reliance on substances. Within the story are some clues about how addiction may have developed. Some would attribute the emergence of substance abuse not only in Peter but also in two of his brothers to a genetic vulnerability for addiction in their family. Others might focus on his teenage experiences, arguing that Peter's repeated early exposure to alcohol and cannabis started him on the path to substance abuse.

Both explanations are consistent with theoretical models of addiction that gained currency in the 1970s. These theories were strongly influenced by animal experiments with laboratory rats which showed that when given a choice between saline water or water containing morphine, the rat would choose the morphine drink (Badawy & Evans, 1975), and would keep drinking the morphine in increasing doses over time (Badawy, Evans, & Evans, 1982). According to the researchers, these findings supported an "exposure" account of addiction – specifically, that when humans and other animals are exposed to opiates that are readily accessible over time, addiction is inevitable. As we will discuss in this chapter, there is more to addiction than exposure, but it is nevertheless striking that many health practitioners today still subscribe to a view that is not all that different from these early accounts. This approach views addiction as a biological condition (or disease) caused by a genetic vulnerability that is triggered by the "chemical hooks" in the substance itself. Exposure theory is also seen to be supported by evidence that the availability of alcohol – measured in terms of the density of alcohol outlets within a geographical location – is a longitudinal risk factor for adolescent alcohol use (Rowland et al., 2016).

Yet although exposure certainly plays a role in triggering a biological response, the problem with this disease model of addiction is that it does not account for social and psychological influences that contribute to the onset and continuation of substance misuse. In Peter's case, social and environmental factors relating to poverty, early neglect, substance use norms in peer groups, sibling substance using behaviour, and more recently his difficulty in coping with the demands of a stressful occupation and marital discord also need to be taken into account in understanding the origins of his substance use and continued abuse.

Consistent with this argument, there is evidence that sustained abstinence following treatment for substance abuse is negatively associated with ethnic minority status and economic hardship when controlling for baseline alcohol and drug addiction severity, age, and referral to treatment by the court system (Wahler & Otis, 2014). There is also growing recognition of the importance of social context in determining substance use. This insight emerged in the 1980s when Canadian psychologist Bruce Alexander and colleagues questioned whether the rats in the morphine studies described above might be taking the morphine because they had been isolated in cages. These researchers suggested that the morphine water may have been consumed as a way of adapting to an aversive and boring environment. Alexander tested this "adaptive model" of addiction by building "Rat Park", a large enclosure that contained interesting surfaces to explore and other rats to socialise with (see Figure 9.1). In Rat Park, the animals were offered the same choice of saline water or morphine water. Interestingly, in this socially and contextually rich environment, they were more likely to choose the saline over the morphine-infused water (Alexander & Hadaway, 1982).

By bringing into focus the important role of social stimulation and context, the adaptive theory of addiction was able to account for the other behaviours associated with addiction that are hard to explain from a purely biological perspective. For example, this theory may explain why patients who have been prescribed opiate analgesics in hospital for several weeks following an injury or operation typically do not develop a long-term addiction when they return home. Conversely, the adaptive theory of addiction may help to explain why addicted individuals often relapse after apparently successful treatment in controlled environments (e.g., jails, rehabilitation centres) when they are returned to their home environment where wider stressors are often present.

Many researchers in the field now embrace the notion that social factors are powerful predictors of one's risk of developing addiction, and this insight is supported by empirical evidence. For example, at the societal or community level, prevalence rates of substance misuse are substantially higher in socially disadvantaged neighbourhoods (e.g., Handley, Rogosch, Guild, & Cicchetti, 2015). At the more personal level, people in addiction treatment often connect the onset of their addiction to their engagement in particular social groups – "I moved into a share house with this group of party girls and we just drank all the time!" This insight has also affected the way that researchers and practitioners in the field think about, and try to promote, recovery. For example, the notion that 'buddying', mentoring, and other sources of social support are important for recovery is a key element of treatment both in therapeutic communities (that use what is known as a "*community-as-method*" approach to rehabilitation) and in mutual support groups (such as Alcoholics Anonymous).

Yet despite this tacit recognition of the importance of social factors in developing and recovering from addiction, it is most often the case that people seeking help for addiction will be offered an *individualised approach* such as counselling or medication. There may be little, if any, involvement of their family, friends, and colleagues in either the conceptualisation or treatment of their problems. In a sense, this is not surprising because it is only recently that more rigorous interrogations of the role of social factors – and social identities in particular – has been undertaken in addiction research. On the basis of this work, a more in-depth analysis of social factors has developed to understand both how they influence addiction trajectories and how they might be better leveraged in treatment.

In this chapter, we present an overview of the best-practice approaches that are currently advocated for addiction treatment. This reflects the fact that challenges of treatment are the primary focus of current approaches to understanding addiction. We then consider the social identity approach to addiction – looking first at how it advances our understanding of the social factors that drive addiction and then at how we can work with social identity processes to motivate behavioural change and recovery.

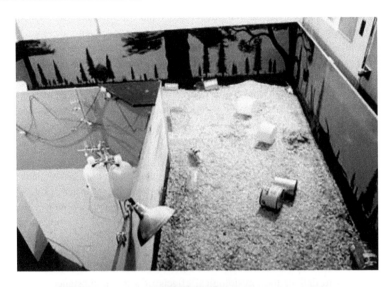

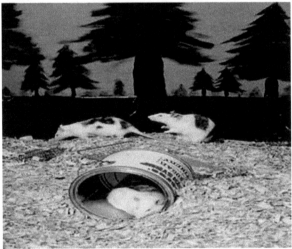

Figure 9.1 Images from Alexander's "Rat Park" study

Note: Bruce Alexander led work that questioned the conclusions reached by earlier researchers about how irresistibly addictive drugs were by revealing the role of solitary confinement in addiction. As we discuss later, his more recent book *The Globalization of Addiction* (2008) develops this idea to show that the dislocation of people from social life lies at the heart of addiction.

Source: Alexander, B. K. (2010). *Addiction: The view from Rat Park*

Current approaches to addiction treatment

Peter Miller's (2013) influential three-volume text *Interventions for Addiction: Comprehensive Addictive Behaviours and Disorders* includes 34 chapters that deal exclusively with approaches to treatment. Of these, the majority focus on individual factors that contribute to addiction, among which motivational interviewing, cognitive-behavioural therapy, and relapse prevention are key. There is also a chapter on adjunctive pharmacotherapies designed to replace the addictive substance and thereby decrease the cravings and harm associated with its use. Eight chapters, which constitute about one in four of the treatments on offer, could be considered more social in focus. These include three forms of family therapy, behavioural couple therapy, community reinforcement, and social network support. In the section that follows, we briefly review the most common of these evidence-based approaches to addiction management.

Biological and pharmacotherapy approaches

The biological approach sees addiction primarily as a manifestation of genetic and neurochemical factors. These include carrying a specific subtype of dopamine receptor gene (e.g., Connor et al., 2007) and changes in the dopaminergic and opioid systems that make a person more vulnerable to the rewarding effects of substances, thereby heightening their risk of misuse. The biological solution to addiction is to target and correct these neurochemical conditions with medication or pharmacotherapy.

As this approach has developed, however, researchers have focused less on finding a cure for addiction and more on developing substitutes for addictive substances. As currently applied, pharmacotherapy thus aims to deliver the physiological effects of a given substance while avoiding or minimising the harms associated with obtaining and using it. For example, smoking can be reduced by substituting nicotine patches for cigarettes; injecting, prostitution, and criminal activity can be reduced by substituting synthetic opioids for 'street' heroin.

Pharmacotherapy was first introduced by Vincent Dole and Marie Nyswander in New York in the early 1960s and involved prescribing the synthetic opioid methadone. Their model of *methadone maintenance treatment* (MMT) prescribed high doses of methadone to be taken by mouth rather than injected (Dole & Nyswander, 1965). Speaking to its efficacy, a number of randomised controlled trials of MMT have shown that methadone maintenance is more effective than detoxification, no treatment, or placebo in keeping people in treatment for longer and in reducing opioid use (Hall, Ward, & Mattick, 1998).

Unfortunately, though, these benefits do not seem to outweigh the problems that people experience when they use this synthetic opioid. First, there is evidence that people tend to relapse into heroin use once they stop taking methadone. Second, MMT is restrictive due to the need to take supervised doses every day. Indeed at times it can be experienced as punitive, with reports that treatment services sometimes punish 'failing' individuals by lowering their dose or discharging them from the methadone program (Degenhardt, Mattick, & Gibson, 2009). Third, methadone itself can be addictive with the result that it can take years to wean people off the drug that is intended to treat them.

In light of these and other limitations of MMT, there have been attempts to develop new forms of opiate pharmacotherapy. Buprenorphine – a partial agonist of the μ opioid receptors – is one drug used for this purpose. This has been found to be safer to use because it is harder to fatally overdose. It is also less restrictive than MMT because it does not always have to be administered daily. However, findings from clinical trials comparing buprenorphine with MMT have produced mixed findings. For although buprenorphine was as effective as methadone in reducing illicit opioid use, it was not as effective in retaining patients in treatment (Mattick, Breen, & Gibson, 2009).

Naltrexone is another type of pharmacotherapy that acts in a different way to the aforementioned drugs. Rather than being an opiate substitute, naltrexone blocks the opiate receptors and thereby stops the euphoric or rewarding effects of several drugs, including opioids and also alcohol. Unsurprisingly, this pharmacotherapy regimen is not particularly attractive to most substance users and, as a result, it suffers from a high rate of early dropout and poor compliance (Degenhardt et al., 2009). Nevertheless, despite limited evidence of its efficacy (Work Group on Substance Use Disorders *et al.*, 2006), naltrexone is one of three currently approved medications for the treatment of alcohol dependence (along with disulfiram and acamprosate).

Another major problem for advocates of the pharmacotherapy approach is that there are no efficacious or recommended medication options available for some of the most widely used drugs, such as cannabis and amphetamines. The approach would therefore not be appropriate for someone like Peter (Case study 9.1), as there are no pharmacotherapies that could replace amphetamines while he undergoes treatment (Shearer & Gowing, 2004). For this reason pharmacotherapies are generally ill suited as stand-alone options in treatment and, where they are used, they are primarily recommended as a supplement to other treatments. However, nicotine replacement therapy (known as 'methadone for smokers') and varenicline (known as 'buprenorphine for smokers') both show very effective increases in successful quit rates.

In line with this observation, clinical treatment guidelines in both Australia (Gowing, Ali, Dunlop, Farrell, & Lintzeris, 2014) and the UK (e.g., the National Treatment Agency for Substance Misuse, 2006) recommend that pharmacotherapy which merely manages the physical symptoms of addiction should be integrated with other systems of care and social support. This is because it is these latter forms of treatment – which provide people with opportunities for appropriate housing, social support, education, and employment – that are needed to help reintegrate people into their local communities. Interestingly, these guidelines also draw attention to the importance of social factors in managing the physiological symptoms of addiction. Before exploring these social factors in greater detail, we will first review three behavioural approaches and treatments to substance abuse that focus on individual factors: motivational interviewing, cognitive behavioural therapy, and relapse prevention.

Psychotherapeutic approaches

Developed by Bill Miller and Stephen Rollnick (1991), *motivational interviewing* (MI) is a counselling approach that draws heavily on Carl Rogers' person-centred therapy. As such, its core principles encourage (1) an accepting and non-judgmental attitude toward clients and (2) empathic understanding of their experiences, which support (3) their own ability to bring about change. This approach views motivation for change not as a stable characteristic of the client (i.e., "she relapsed because she is not motivated enough for treatment"), but as a dynamic process that can be enhanced through careful interaction between the therapist and the client (i.e., "we need to revisit her reasons for wanting change so that she renews her commitment after this relapse"). Motivational interviewing has been applied to clients with addiction to a wide range of substances (e.g., of a form suggested in Figure 9.2). The aim is to increase their motivation and commitment to change by using techniques of directive interviewing that explore the discrepancy between a client's stated goals and values, on the one hand, and their addictive behaviour, on the other, and then helping them to map out a future course of action to resolve this discrepancy.

Despite being quite popular, evidence for the effectiveness of MI as a treatment for substance abuse is mixed. Thus an early meta-analysis of 72 studies indicated that the technique was "highly variable" in its effectiveness (Hettema, Steele, & Miller, 2005, p. 91). This was especially true for the 32 studies that involved treatment for alcohol abuse (where effect sizes ranged from −0.08 to 3.07, with means of 0.41 up to 3 months post-treatment and 0.26 across all follow-up points, indicating small-to-medium effects). For 13 studies that focused on the effectiveness of MI in the management of illicit drug use, the range in effect sizes was again large (from 0 to 1.81, with corresponding means of 0.51 and 0.29). However, evidence of the capacity of MI to encourage smoking cessation was weaker, with the researchers concluding that it was not successful in treating this form of addiction (Hettema et al., 2005).

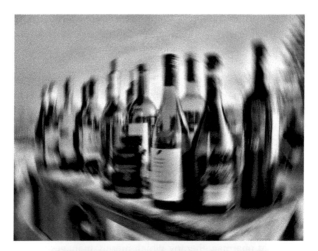

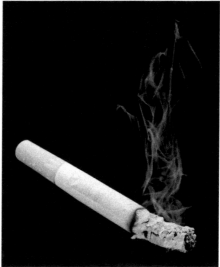

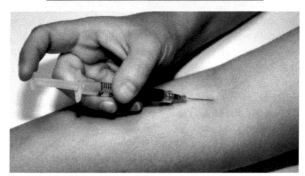

Figure 9.2 Some different forms of substance (ab)use commonly treated using behavioural approaches

Note: Commonly used substance abuse therapies include motivational interviewing; cognitive behavioural therapy; and family, group, and community therapies.

Source: Pixabay

A second, more extensive, meta-analysis of 119 studies also failed to find consistent evidence that MI has anything more than moderate-sized effects in treating addiction (Lundahl, Kunz, Brownell, Tollefson, & Burke, 2010). However, when compared with weak comparison groups (such as a wait-list control, or treatment as usual with no specific program), MI produced relatively lasting results (e.g., greater engagement in treatment up to a year post-treatment). Interestingly, this meta-analysis provided stronger evidence of the value of MI as a treatment for smoking cessation, with several studies reporting small but significant effects. Overall, though, when compared against specific treatments (such as cognitive behavioural therapy [CBT] or a 12-step program), MI was associated with weaker treatment effects (average $g = 0.09$, which indicates a small effect size).

Despite its varied impact, findings from these meta-analyses suggest that there are some contexts in which MI can be useful in counselling for addiction. In particular, this seems more likely to be the case when a treatment program is tailored to the individual client, when people receive feedback, and when MI is used in combination with other active therapies (e.g., CBT, as discussed later; see Baker et al., 2005). However, as with pharmacotherapy, it appears that MI is not particularly effective as a stand-alone therapy. It is also unclear what an optimal "dose" of MI should entail (Lundahl et al., 2010).

Behavioural theories of addiction identify three learning principles that support the development and maintenance of substance misuse. First, through *classical conditioning*, an association develops between contextual cues (e.g., meeting friends at a local bar on a Friday evening) and a behaviour (drinking alcohol). The second process is *operant conditioning*, in which the consequences of substance use (e.g., feelings of euphoria or reduced worry) reinforce the behaviour to make it more likely to recur. A third process of *vicarious learning* is also involved in which people engage in substance use behaviour after seeing it modelled by others such as their parents, siblings, or peers. Applying these principles to our case study, behavioural theory would suggest that Peter's early alcohol and cannabis use may have been learned through modelling from his older siblings and friends and positively reinforced through the relaxing and pleasant effects of the substances themselves and the sense of social inclusion with the substance-using peer group. Later on, his amphetamine abuse may have been negatively reinforced through the reduction of fatigue during his long work shifts.

As these learning principles highlight, there are triggers and reinforcers in addictive behaviour that, when identified, can be used to manage substance misuse. To this end, behavioural interventions aim to avoid or minimise the triggers for the addictive behaviour and to develop alternative (less harmful) behaviours that achieve similar positive consequences (e.g., relaxing through breathing or meditation rather than by drinking alcohol).

Contingency reinforcement treatment is one such intervention. It draws on operant learning principles by giving clients a reward (e.g., a gift voucher) contingent on their achievement of a relevant addiction-reducing goal (e.g., returning a clean urine drug test). Meta-analytic studies have concluded that contingency reinforcement is an effective approach across a range of substances (with studies producing moderate to high effect sizes; Dutra et al., 2008; Prendergast, Podus, Finney, Greenwell, & Roll, 2006). However, there is also evidence that the magnitude of this effect declines following treatment completion (Prendergast et al., 2006). In other words, once the contingent rewards for abstinence are removed, the intervention ceases to be so effective. Clearly, there is a need to find more naturalistic and sustainable reinforcers for abstinence in a person's daily life, and, as we will outline later, this is where social relationships may be particularly helpful.

These behavioural techniques are often integrated with cognitive techniques that increase a person's self-efficacy when it comes to refusing substances by identifying and addressing thoughts, expectancies, motives, and cravings associated with their use. For instance, these expectancies may relate to beliefs about the effects of using a particular substance – beliefs such as "drinking before a work function will give me social confidence" or "smoking marijuana helps me relax" (Li & Dingle, 2012). Moreover, cognitions underlying people's motives for using a given substance (e.g., "drinking is what most of your friends do when you get together" to achieve conformity or "as a way to celebrate" to experience enhancement) not only mediate behaviour, but can also be a suitable target for intervention (Cooper, Russell, Skinner, & Windle, 1992).

Consistent with this claim, research shows that challenging unhelpful expectancies can reduce substance use (e.g. Darkes & Goldman, 1998; Geisner et al., 2017). Substance-related expectancies and motives are also related to treatment seeking. This point is supported by a study of 195 individuals entering treatment for cannabis dependence conducted by Zoe Papinczak and her colleagues. This found that, compared to a control group of 269 non-treatment-seeking cannabis users, these treatment seekers had significantly more negative cannabis outcome expectancies and significantly lower levels of emotional relief and cannabis refusal self-efficacy (Papinczak, Connor, Feeney, Young, & Gullo, 2017). In other words, those who sought treatment expected their substance abuse to be more harmful and they were less confident that they could resist using the substance if they found themselves under emotional strain.

Nevertheless, cognitive change is only one component of substance abuse treatment and other components appear necessary to avoid relapse and promote ongoing recovery. This point is central to the *relapse prevention model* developed and refined by Alan Marlatt and colleagues (Marlatt & Gordon, 1985; Witkiewitz & Marlatt, 2004). Here, clients identify the situations that would place them at high risk for relapse, and after this they work with a therapist to put coping strategies in place to prevent relapse occurring. During treatment sessions, they might then use self-talk to identify the negative consequences of using substances, rehearse the reasons for staying abstinent, and/or practice substance refusal skills.

Yet although there are clear grounds for engaging in these strategies, a meta-analysis of cognitive behavioural therapy alone and cognitive behavioural therapy with relapse prevention shows that they have only small to moderate effects (ranging from $d = 0.28$ to 0.32, respectively, aggregated across diverse measures such as mean days abstinent, proportion of the sample abstinent, and scores on measures of substance dependence; Dutra et al., 2008). It has been suggested that these modest effects might be explained by limitations in people's capacity to use cognitive behavioural strategies effectively when they are faced with cravings and other negative affective states, family influences, and social pressure (Zywiak et al., 2006). Indeed, in light of these, more recent conceptualisations of relapse prevention have incorporated strategies to help people tolerate and better manage these negative affective states through meditation (see Figure 9.3).

As one example of this approach, Vipassana meditation was introduced by Alan Marlatt and his colleagues as an addiction rehabilitation strategy for inmates of King County Prison in Seattle (Bowen et al., 2006). Of the 173 inmates who completed both the baseline and 3-month post-discharge assessments, 57 completed the Vipassana meditation course and 116 received treatment as usual (TAU; i.e., the control group). In post-discharge assessments, those who took part in the meditation subsequently had significantly lower use of marijuana, crack cocaine, and alcohol than the controls. Furthermore, course participation was associated with significant improvements in psychiatric symptoms, drinking-related locus of control, and optimism.

A Westernised version of this approach, *mindfulness-based relapse prevention* (MBRP), is designed to decrease the conditioned response of craving in the presence of negative affective states. By teaching meditation strategies, MBRP aims to raise people's awareness of relapse triggers and help them monitor their internal reactions and develop more effective behavioural responses to counter the urge to use substances in response to emotional discomfort. To test the effectiveness of MBRP, an efficacy trial assigned 168 adults who had recently been treated for substance use disorders to receive either MBRP or TAU. Post-intervention, the trial found a significant decrease in days of substance use among participants in the MBRP group relative to those in TAU group. Moreover, the MBRP program was found to enhance participants' ability to tolerate cravings and negative emotions (Witkiewitz & Bowen, 2010). This is particularly important in light of the fact that many individuals with addiction experience co-occurring disorders such as anxiety and depression.

Unfortunately, though, gains were not sustained 4 months post-intervention, as at this point the MBRP and TAU groups were indistinguishable (Bowen et al., 2009). Clearly then, other factors are at

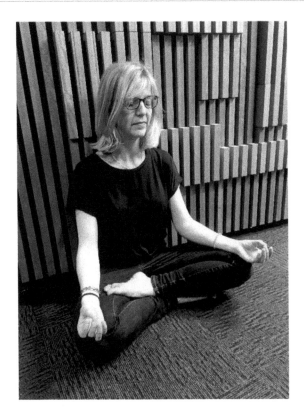

Figure 9.3 Practicing meditation

Note: Meditation is increasingly used within cognitive behavioural therapy (CBT) to help people deal with the negative
   affective states that can lead those with a history of addiction to relapse.

Source: The authors

play that mindfulness does not address. The most obvious of these are external processes such as interpersonal conflict or social pressure from substance-using peer groups. Again, this highlights the need
for theoretical models and interventions that recognise and engage with these social factors.

Psychosocial approaches

Interventions that target social, not just cognitive and behavioural, factors have developed in
the face of increasing recognition of the important role that these play in addiction trajectories (see
Frings, Albery, & Monk, 2017). Psychosocial approaches consider the psychological factors involved
in substance misuse but view the individual as a component of a system that involves themselves, other
people (both substance users and non-users), and a constellation of social norms and attitudes, all of
which interact with each other. In ways that we will also discuss when we look at eating behaviour in
the next chapter, these interactions occur within environments which contain an array of behaviourally

and psychologically relevant cues for substance use. This can be seen in research by Erin Westgate and her colleagues (2017). These researchers argued that, rather than being simply an individual response to attentional biases, alcohol consumption among students may also be predicted by the way those students cope with external pressures such as academic requirements. Consistent with this point, these researchers found that procrastinating around the production of academic work was linked to students' alcohol-related problems, craving, risk of alcohol use disorders, and lower academic attainment (Westgate, Wormington, Oleson, & Lindgren, 2017).

In contrast to the approaches we have discussed in previous sections, these psychosocial approaches all share an interest in involving people other than the addicted person themselves in treatment. This is in recognition of the fact that addiction neither affects, nor resides solely within, individuals. Instead, it typically affects many other people around them – families, friends, colleagues, and communities. Where psychosocial approaches differ is in the kind of social relationships they target. In what follows, we will review examples of different types of intervention that focus on the involvement of family, community, and mutual support groups.

Couple and family therapies

Behavioural couples therapy (BCT) for alcoholism and drug abuse (e.g., O'Farrell, & Clements, 2012; O'Farrell & Fals-Stewart, 2006) involves the partner of the person with an alcohol or other drug problem in all aspects of treatment. The purpose is to address and repair some of the damage that chronic substance misuse has done to the relationship – recognising that this damage can become a driving factor in ongoing substance misuse. Both partners engage with the treatment and with the notion of support for abstinence, with sessions dedicated to improving the couple relationship and examining how best to maintain abstinence and avoid relapse into substance misuse.

The utility of this approach is supported by evidence from a meta-analysis of 12 randomised controlled trials conducted with a total of 754 participants (Powers, Vedel, & Emmelkamp, 2008). Overall, the findings indicated that BCT was superior to individual-focused treatments and had moderate-sized effects ($d = 0.54$). Moreover, positive outcomes were observed across outcome domains particularly at follow-up (also with moderate effects on measures of frequency of use, consequences of use, and relationship satisfaction).

A key element of such interventions is their extended focus on helping family members process their own emotional distress rather than solely addressing the addicted individual's change process. Al-Anon – an organisation that runs recovery programs for families and friends affected by drug and alcohol addiction – provides one example of this approach. It suggests that family members should "detach themselves from the alcoholic's drinking in a loving way, accept that they are powerless to control the alcoholic, and seek support from other Al-Anon members" (Al-Anon Family Groups, 1981). Speaking to the potential efficacy of such an approach, an early correlational study with 77 family members aged between 12 and 68 years attending three Al-Anon programs in the United States found that length of membership was correlated with enhanced self-esteem and, that among the 60 who were spouses, length of membership was correlated with marital adjustment (Keinz, Schwartz, Trench, & Houlihan, 1995).

Recognising the wider social context within which addiction occurs is certainly a positive step, but a major challenge with this form of intervention is that the person with the addiction often refuses to engage with treatment. This means that whereas their partner may benefit from the treatment, the person who is the primary focus for intervention and the quality of the couple's relationship may remain unchanged (Halford, Price, Kelly, Bouma, & Young, 2001). In ways that we will elaborate in the second half of this chapter when we discuss the importance of social identity processes in recovery, this speaks to the need for participant family members to build a shared sense of engagement with any treatment and to develop common goals that are related both to substance use behaviour and to desired relationship outcomes.

Another common intervention for addiction involves residential treatment, typically in dedicated facilities such as hospitals or therapeutic communities, that promote and support abstinence through the delivery of rehabilitation and other residential services. These environments allow the person with addiction to take time away from their usual surroundings for a lengthy period (typically 3 to 6 months) so that they can engage in intensive treatment alongside others with addiction in a social context that advocates a drug-free way of life.

Seeking to assess the efficacy of this approach relative to some of the pharmacotherapy treatments that we discussed earlier, Maree Teesson and her colleagues conducted the Australian Treatment Outcome Study to examine outcomes for 745 heroin users entering treatment (1) as part of residential rehabilitation, (2) in methadone or buprenorphine maintenance therapy, or (3) in detoxification therapy (Teesson et al., 2006). Outcomes in these groups were also compared to those in a control group of heroin users who were not seeking treatment. The retention rate of participants was high, and 80% of participants in the study were interviewed again a year later. After that 1 year, a significant reduction in heroin and other drug use was observed across all three treatments. At this point, unlike those in the non-treatment control, the majority of those who had entered treatment were abstinent from heroin (65% in maintenance therapy, 52% in detoxification, and 63% in residential rehabilitation vs. 25% in the control). So although residential rehabilitation was clearly effective for heroin treatment, it appeared to be no more effective than outpatient maintenance treatment and only marginally more effective than detoxification (Teesson et al., 2006).

Another more recent Australian study by Rebecca McKetin and colleagues aimed to identify the factors that predicted abstinence among people attending residential rehabilitation units in Brisbane and Sydney (McKetin et al., 2017). Among the 176 methamphetamine users who received treatment, the median length of stay was 8 weeks, and 23% of participants were abstinent a year later. Interestingly, individual-level factors, including standard demographics, drug use history, or co-occurring mental disorders, did not significantly predict abstinence after a year of residential treatment. Instead, it was *social factors* – including living with other residents in treatment and establishing rapport with counsellors – that proved to have more of a bearing on positive outcomes.

To understand why residential treatment produces these beneficial effects, it is instructive to take a closer look at what it typically entails. *Therapeutic communities* (TCs) generally emphasise the role played by the community itself in promoting and maintaining change among residents. Individuals who reside in TCs usually also agree to subscribe to a set of community rules, including not using relevant substances for the duration of their stay and participating in a structured program of group activities that aim to facilitate recovery. In contrast to the medical model – in which doctors are the experts and their patients are the recipients of health care – this community-as-method strategy thus adopts a social cure approach. It aims to promote recovery from addiction by drawing on positive peer influence and building commitment to the community in ways that are underpinned by a belief in the potential for personal and collective growth and an ethos of strong mutual help (Best et al., 2016; De Leon, 2000).

The general effectiveness of TC treatment was confirmed by the findings of a systematic review by Malivert, Fatseas, Denis, Langlois, and Auriacombe (2012). Their review comprised 12 studies that together included 3,271 participants from 61 TCs. Treatment completion ranged from 9% to 56% with all studies showing a decrease in patients' substance use during their stay in a TC, but relapse was a common outcome after discharge. Treatment completion and retention were the most predictive factors of abstinence at follow-up. Nevertheless, although it is clear that these outcomes are generally positive, a lot more needs to be understood about the TC model.

For example, a lack of research using multiple time points precludes any firm conclusions regarding the optimal length of treatment in a TC (Perryman & Dingle, 2015). It is also unclear how individual-level factors interact with community-level factors to enhance or detract from treatment outcomes. It is well known, for instance, that TC residents often present with other disorders (e.g., posttraumatic stress disorder and depression) alongside their addiction, and some preliminary evidence suggests that, unsurprisingly, co-occurring disorders impede retention and result in poorer outcomes (Dermatis, Salke, Galanter, & Bunt, 2001; Herington, Dingle, & Perryman, 2017; Perryman, Dingle, & Clark, 2016; Ravndal & Vaglum, 1994). It also seems likely that entry into TCs has psychological and material impact beyond the person who received treatment, but the extent to which this is the case (and how it can best be managed) is unclear.

Mutual support groups

There is now a well-established body of evidence which shows that mutual support groups, such as Alcoholics Anonymous (AA) and Narcotics Anonymous (NA), help to promote long-term abstinence. Famously, these programmes or approaches follow a well-defined set of 12 steps (described in the chapters of the AA "Big Book", see Figure 9.4) that relate to clearly defined norms about abstinence as well as values of honesty and integrity. Moreover, a comprehensive analysis of mutual support groups by Rudolf Moos (2008) found that bonding and support, obtaining an abstinence-focused role model, and doing service work within the group were all vital ingredients to successful outcomes. These conclusions were echoed in a review of 24 studies that investigated the value of AA membership for people with alcohol dependence (Groh, Jason, & Keys, 2008).

Additional evidence about the mechanisms of action associated with AA membership comes from an analysis of data from 1,726 adults in the Project Match study (Project Match Research Group, 1998). This found that the extent to which individuals had made adaptive changes to their social network and increased social abstinence self-efficacy directly predicted recovery (Kelly, Hoeppner, Stout, & Pagano, 2012). Quantifying this effect, it was found that social network variables – specifically, the number of friends that an AA participant had and those friends' support for abstinence – uniquely predicted between 5% and 12% of the variance in drinking outcomes over the course of 3 years.

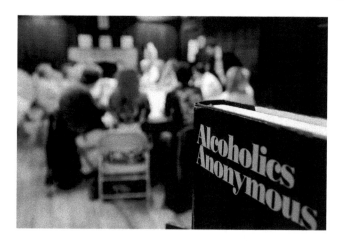

Figure 9.4 A meeting of Alcoholics Anonymous, with the 'Big Book' in the foreground

Note: Alcoholics Anonymous is a good example of a mutual support model in that it aims not only to build social support for those that attend the meetings, but also encourages attendees to help others.

Source: Getty images www.gettyimages.fr/license/542408898

The extent of a person's AA attendance following treatment accounted for a further 1% to 6% of the variance in drinking outcomes (Stout, Kelly, Magill, & Pagano, 2012).

Yet due to their religious ethos, these mutual support groups do not suit everyone. Fortunately, though, there is evidence that other mutual support groups that promote sober norms without such an ethos appear to be equally effective. For example, Self-Management and Recovery Training (SMART) groups are mutual support groups whose activities are informed by a cognitive behavioural framework. A study of 124 members of these groups in Australia found that participants' use of the cognitive behavioural skills that they learned in the program were predicted both by group cohesion and by development of an achievable homework plan (Kelly, Deane, & Baker, 2015). Unfortunately, though, the study did not assess longitudinal outcomes for substance use or the effect of psychosocial variables on outcomes, and so the longer-term outcomes of SMART group membership remain unclear.

The British programme *Jobs, Friends, Houses* (JFH) which operates in the northwest of England, is another interesting example of a mutual support initiative. This programme focuses on developing professional skills in individuals recovering from addiction (Best, 2016). More specifically, participants are supported by trained professionals (joiners, plumbers, electricians, plasterers, bricklayers, and a project manager) while undertaking the task of renovating business premises and community housing. The participants start as volunteers and, if they prove suitable, they then enrol in an initial 12-week building course with a local further education college (Blackpool and Fylde College) which is a key partner in the JFH social enterprise. The JFH project has attracted numerous building contracts due to the quality and efficiency of its work. Benefits to the participants include the adoption of a new valued work identity, as well as access to a range of social activities. Aside from attending mutual aid meetings, they can also enter photography courses, join a football team, and take part in a series of recreational activities.

An early report stated that relapse into substance use for those taking part in the programme have been negligible and there have been no reported instances of involvement in crime by participants of the programme (Best, 2016). So how has this been achieved? David Best argues that it results from the fact that the programme offers former substance users membership in a new work-oriented group that promotes norms around sobriety, clean living, skills development, and making a contribution to society in a supportive group context (Best, 2016). In ways that anticipate points we will return to later, these resources can all be seen to flow from being part of a meaningful and valued social group.

Before unpacking this point through the lens of social identity theorising, it is useful to try to draw together the various strands of research on existing approaches to understanding and managing addiction that we have reviewed thus far. One point that emerges clearly from this research is that treatments tend generally to have mixed results. Thus pharmacotherapies can be effective for some substances, but only when used in conjunction with other psychosocial supports. Among the psychotherapies, the combination of motivational interviewing and cognitive behavioural therapies appears most effective, and these therapies yield successful outcomes for a range of substances. Nevertheless, it is clear that their effectiveness is moderate at best and that individuals who go through them often relapse.

In contrast, there is evidence that treatment which involves residential rehabilitation, therapeutic communities, and mutual support groups tends to be associated with more sustained recovery. Indeed, although research methods and findings have been somewhat inconsistent across studies, it seems generally to be the case that sustained abstinence and recovery is associated with participants staying longer in residential treatment, having a positive therapeutic relationship with a counsellor, and contributing personally to the group or community.

In all this, one emergent theme is that social factors are key determinants not only of treatment engagement, retention, and outcomes, but also of relapse following apparently successful intervention. What the field lacks, though, is an empirically validated and theoretically coherent framework which would allow us to understand how these social factors influence outcomes at various stages from addiction onset to full recovery. As we aim to show in the remainder of this chapter, it is precisely such a framework that the social identity approach provides.

The social identity approach to addiction

Since his early Rat Park studies, Bruce Alexander has developed his analysis of society's influence on addiction by drawing on a large body of historical, anthropological, sociological, economic, biographical, clinical, and medical research (see Alexander, 2008). His *social dislocation theory of addiction* attributes the rapid spread of addiction, over a period of 500 years since Columbus' voyages, to an emerging global society (Alexander, 2017). Put simply, Alexander argues that addictive behaviours are a manifestation of the social atomisation that is endemic in modern forms of society. Dislocation theory applies not only to drug and alcohol misuse, but also to behavioural addictions such as sex, work, gambling, eating, shopping, Internet gaming, social media, and exercise. The theory regards the causes and consequences of these various behavioural addictions as essentially the same as those associated with substance misuse. From this historical and cultural perspective on the fragmentation of society, addiction is seen to be associated with the weakening of traditionally strong identifications with groups such as family, friends, occupational groups, religious communities, and so on.

The social identity approach is consistent with – and in many ways complements – the analysis provided by social dislocation theory. However, it focuses in more detail on the role that social identity processes play in the development of, and recovery from, addiction. For example, it does this by examining how addiction presents obstacles to the establishment and maintenance of positive social identities, but also how recovery can be encouraged by working to overcome such obstacles. In this, the approach places particular emphasis on the role that social group relationships play in addiction-related dynamics. Its perspective also differs from that in much of the addiction literature which has considered *interpersonal* relationships to be key facilitators in addiction treatment and focused largely on a person's therapeutic alliance with a counsellor (Meier, Barrowclough, & Donmall, 2005) or their relationship with another important person (e.g., as in the Important People Drug and Alcohol interview, IPDA, Zywiak et al, 2009). In the sections that follow, we spell out more fully a social identity analysis of addiction trajectories. In particular, we discuss in turn (1) the role of group identification, social influence, and social norms in predicting addiction; (2) the impact of stigma on intentions to quit; and (c) the way that the groups we belong to may facilitate, but also hinder, recovery from addiction. Recognising that more needs to be done to fully understand addiction trajectories, in the final part of this chapter, we examine recovery from addiction as a process of identity change. Specifically, we focus on the ways in which social identification contributes to the onset of addiction while also showing how social identity change is key to recovery.

Addiction trajectories are shaped by social identification, group norms, and social influence

When it comes to substance use, social influence is a potent force and it can take many forms. Behaviour relevant to substance use is modelled by parents; siblings; and friends at home, work, and school. This can affect our own behaviour in those contexts, as can wider media and cultural representations of substance use. For these behaviours and representations form the basis of group and societal norms which – by telling us what is normal and appropriate – have the capacity to influence us in positive or negative ways.

In line with this claim there is considerable empirical evidence of the effects that social norms have on health behaviour in general, and similar evidence is accruing on substance use. One study that speaks clearly to this issue was conducted by Marla Eisenberg and colleagues and involved 2,248 Grade 7 students (51.2 % female) attending 121 schools in the United States and Australia (Eisenberg, Toumbourou, Catalano, & Hemphill, 2014). The researchers were interested in the influence of ingroup norms on student use of alcohol, tobacco, and cannabis two years down the track. More specifically, they focused on the impact of two types of norms: *injunctive* (i.e., the behaviours approved by other members of their peer group, such as "drinking is cool") and *descriptive* (i.e., perceptions of how other members of their peer group behave, irrespective of whether their actions are approved of or not; e.g., "all of my friends smoke"). The results showed that injunctive ingroup norms had little influence on later substance use, but that descriptive norms were significantly associated with later tobacco and cannabis use. More specifically, students who perceived that their peers' substance use was higher were more likely to be using more tobacco and cannabis themselves two years later. In line with the influence hypothesis (H9), it thus appears that it is those people with whom a person perceives themselves as sharing social identity (in this case other members of their self-identified student peer group) who play the primary role in shaping their substance use (or non-use).

Interestingly, it is not necessary for people to come together formally as a group (e.g., as a support group) for shared identity to have this impact. For example, simply identifying with other users of the same brand of cigarettes or alcohol can affect people's substance misuse and health. This point was demonstrated in a study by Hugh Webb and his colleagues that investigated the effectiveness of plain tobacco packaging legislation (Webb et al., 2017). This legislative change was introduced in Australia in December 2012 in an attempt to reduce cigarette smoking. Webb and colleagues surveyed 178 smokers before and seven months after the plain packaging policy came into effect. Participants were asked to report their sense of identification with fellow smokers of their brand, positive brand stereotypes, quitting behaviours and intentions, and smoking intensity. Analyses showed that smokers, especially those who initially identified strongly with their brand, experienced a significant decrease in their brand identification following the introduction of plain packaging. More importantly, though, this was associated with lower subsequent smoking levels and increased intentions to quit (Webb et al., 2017).

Consistent with the identification hypothesis (H2) and the influence hypothesis (H9), it thus appears that the positive impact of addiction treatment is most pronounced for individuals who identify strongly with groups that promote responsible substance use or recovery (e.g., Best, et al., 2016; Buckingham, Frings, & Albery, 2013). This makes sense as these individuals should be more motivated to embrace norms that support recovery (e.g., to abstain from use of addictive substances) and therefore, as the norm enactment hypothesis (H8) would predict, they should also be more likely to behave in a manner that accords with those norms (e.g., seeking support when at risk of relapse).

As a corollary of this, though, if people do not socially identify with those who are trying to put them on a path to recovery, they are unlikely to follow it. As Amy Winehouse lyrically observed, when "they tried to make me go to rehab, I said no, no, no" (Winehouse, 2006). From a theoretical perspective, then, the key word here is "they".

Stigma affects intentions to quit

The stigma associated with problematic substance use can be an important factor that deters some people from going down the addiction path (Stuber, Meyer, & Link, 2008). This does not hold for everyone, though, and for those who do experience addiction stigma, it typically has negative consequences (along lines that we discussed in Chapter 4). In particular, this is because it often leads to the marginalisation and devaluation of substance-using groups and the creation of unhelpful 'us–them' divisions between those who need help and other members of society who might be well placed to provide it.

In line with this point, several studies have found that people with substance use disorders are more highly stigmatised than people who experience other health conditions (Corrigan et al., 2005; Room, 2005). Stigmatising attitudes regarding certain behaviours (e.g., substance use during pregnancy) and groups (e.g., injecting drug users) are widely accepted, culturally endorsed, and enshrined in policy (e.g., criminal law). This often means that, in addition to the many challenges that people with substance abuse problems confront when they go into treatment, they must deal with the fact that they belong to a highly stigmatised social group. This, for example, is a point that Russell Brand reflected on when discussing Amy Winehouse's treatment at the hands of the press as she descended into the addiction that would ultimately lead to her death (see Brand, 2011).

Furthermore, stigma (and the discrimination and social exclusion that are associated with it) can be so pervasive within mainstream society that substance users themselves consider widespread discrimination against them to be warranted and legitimate. How, then, does the perceived legitimacy of discrimination affect substance users' interpretation of group-based exclusion? To investigate this issue, Jetten, Schmitt, Branscombe, Garza, and Mewse (2011) conducted a study with 95 smokers in 2007 just after the UK had introduced a ban on smoking in public places. Perceptions of the legitimacy of discrimination were manipulated by presenting the participants with statements from other ingroup members arguing for or against the legitimacy of discriminatory treatment of smokers by non-smokers. So, for example, in the legitimate discrimination condition, a smoker stated, "I think it is understandable when smokers are not hired for jobs where being healthy and looking fit is important. I'm thinking of instructor jobs in health-clubs or something like that" (21-year-old, male smoker). On the other hand, in a condition where discrimination was represented as being illegitimate, a smoker had ostensibly said, "I don't think it is justifiable when smokers are not hired for certain jobs. I just think you should judge people on their qualities and not on whether they smoke or not" (21-year old, male smoker).

The researchers found that when pervasive discrimination was represented as being legitimate by the smoker ingroup, this undermined participants' willingness to engage in collective action to counter that discrimination. For example, here they were less likely to complain about the smoking ban to anti-discrimination organisations. More interesting for our present purposes, though, was the fact that smokers' willingness to quit smoking was higher when discrimination was appraised as legitimate than when it was appraised as illegitimate. In line with the mobility hypothesis (H5), it thus appears that the perception that stigma was legitimate increased smokers' motivation to try to cross group boundaries and become a non-smoker. By contrast, and in line with the competition hypothesis (H7), when smokers experienced discrimination against them as illegitimate, they were more likely to dig their heels in and express a desire to continue smoking. In other words, when the treatment of a substance-using ingroup is perceived to be unfair, members of that group are less likely to want to restore a sense of positive identity by leaving the group and more inclined instead to fight for the protection of the group's interests.

This finding is important from an applied perspective because it suggests that the way that policies relating to substance use are perceived will have an impact on the way that the targets of those policies behave. If the policies are understood to be fair and legitimate, they will encourage people to reduce their use of the substance (see Menzies, 2011; Orbell et al., 2009). At the same time, though, if they are perceived to be unfair, they may only stimulate resistance and thereby entrench the behaviour that they are intended to reduce.

Addiction trajectories are shaped by multiple group memberships

A person's social group memberships are critical to their addiction trajectories. Testament to this point, a study by Fabio Sani and his colleagues of 1824 patients from five general practitioner (GP) clinics in Scotland found that the greater the number of groups that participants belonged to and identified with (e.g., family and community groups), the less likely it was that they smoked cigarettes or drank heavily, and the more likely it was that they exercised and ate a healthy diet (Sani, Madhok, Norbury, Dugard, & Wakefield, 2015). Moreover, these effects were significant even after taking into account a range of other factors – including the number of groups with which people had regular contact, their relationship status, level of education, gender, and age. In line with the multiple identities hypothesis (H11), it thus appears that belonging to more social groups had a positive effect on health and well-being.

Clearly though, positive outcomes of this form are dependent on group norms about healthy behaviour and responsible substance use. This means that if a person identifies most strongly with a group whose members misuse alcohol and other drugs, then their own attitudes and behaviours are also likely to support misuse. Yet aside from the negative health effects of continued substance abuse that such groups might encourage, they can also make it difficult for a person to recover from alcohol and drug addiction. The challenge that people often face in this situation is that the using group still functions as an important psychological resource. In particular, despite hindering recovery, other members of user groups might still be a valuable source of social support – for example, offering shelter when living rough or providing emotional support and companionship when other relationships breakdown as a result of addiction. In line with points that we made in Chapter 2 (e.g., see Figure 2.8), such groups may also provide substance users with an important source of social connection, meaning, and control. As Shirley, a former user in Amy Reed's book *Clean* observes: "Getting rid of the drugs doesn't get rid of all the other ways you learned to deal with the world. It's not that easy" (Reed, 2012, p. 61). For this reason, users will often be reluctant to change their using behaviour because that would also mean turning their back on the (often limited) social resources that they have to draw on.

The multiple identities hypothesis (H11) can also help to explain why many people in addiction recovery find joining certain types of support groups difficult, even if those groups are, in principle, easily accessible. In particular, this is because it may be stressful or challenging for people to belong to multiple groups whose norms are incompatible. For example, groups such as AA explicitly promote abstinence, whereas the person's family and friendship groups may hold a heavy drinking norm.

This raises the question of what happens when a person belongs to multiple groups which differ markedly in their substance use norms. More specifically, which groups take precedence in shaping addictive behaviour? Our case study of Peter illustrates these dynamics well. Peter was a member of a number of groups that influenced his behaviour, but some groups seemed more influential than others. In particular, he was influenced in his drinking and marijuana use by a social group that included his older siblings and neighbours. At the time he started drinking, Peter was also part of a wider family group and a school group, and individuals in both groups (e.g., parents and teachers) did not approve of his substance-using behaviour. However, because Peter identified more strongly with his using group of siblings and friends, norms associated with family and school groups were not sufficiently influential to reduce his using behaviour and to stop it from becoming problematic. This is not an uncommon pattern among people who misuse substances and are part of multiple social groups (e.g., see Buckingham & Best, 2017; Mawson, Best, Beckwith, Dingle, & Lubman, 2015).

The social identity approach helps us understand the basis of these dynamics and explains how membership in groups can both facilitate and hinder recovery. In this regard, social identity mapping (Cruwys et al., 2016) provides a useful visual method for understanding the influence of a person's group networks and their substance use norms (see Appendix for details and Chapter 15 for a discussion of its use in an intervention context). The method has been adapted for use in drug and alcohol treatment contexts (Beckwith, et al., 2017; Best et al., 2014; Haslam, Dingle, Best, Mackenzie, & Beckwith, 2017), and Figure 9.5 provides an example of how one member of a therapeutic community, "Matt", mapped the groups that were important to him.

Social identity maps provide a visual representation of a person's social group memberships that can capture not only current networks but also those that have an impact during periods of significant life change (e.g., when transitioning from social substance use into problematic use, or when entering into treatment). Importantly, this allows them to be used as a basis for the development of social network change goals to support recovery. These goals might include renewing ties with groups that are supportive of abstinence, decreasing or modifying the nature of activities with groups whose norms support heavy substance use, or developing new group memberships that represent important aspects of the individual's identity but which are not associated with substance use.

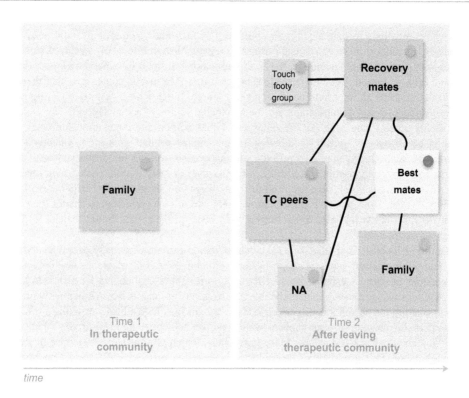

Figure 9.5 Social identity map for "Matt"

Note: To develop social identity maps, participants are asked to list their social groups and then write group names on separate Post-it notes of different sizes as a function of their importance (Cruwys et al., 2016). These Post-it notes are then placed on a larger A3 sheet after which participants can then add ratings on each Post-it note for various features of each group. The compatibility of groups is then indicated by straight, wavy, or jagged lines (see Appendix for details). The first of these two maps was produced by "Matt" when he was in a therapeutic community (TC); the second was produced after he left the TC. In this case, group norms for substance use are also shown with dots (red indicating heavy use and green indicating non-use).

Source: Adapted from Haslam, Dingle, Best, Mackenzie, & Beckwith (2017)

To explore the potential for social identity mapping to support intervention in this way, David Best and his colleagues (2014) used the method in their work with six TC residents. In their maps, these residents reported an average of five groups. The most common groups that they identified were family (26% of groups), followed by the therapeutic community group and mutual aid groups (13% each). Less frequently mentioned groups included extended family, friends, substance users, other services, religious groups, and leisure groups. Four of the six participants rated their identification with the TC as quite strong (with a mean score of 6 out of 7) and identification with mutual support groups such as AA was also high (mean = 6), whereas identification with family and other groups was lower (means = 5.6 and 5.5, respectively).

The maps also highlighted compatibility – or a lack of compatibility – between the groups that were part of participants' social worlds. For example, one participant's map pointed to incompatibility between friendship groups among whom substance use was high and family groups who were low users or non-users. In therapeutic terms, this split between the two social worlds and the perceived risk it entailed had clear implications for the participant when she reflected on the map. Accordingly, when planning for her departure from the TC, she identified two key goals that needed to be pursued upon her return home: first, to move away from a social network of users who would be a major trigger to relapse; second, to develop new social group networks that supported abstinence, which would mean that sober activity would not be confined to her family alone.

This mapping exercise points to the fact that in an addiction context where groups can be both helpful and harmful to health, it is important to take stock of all people's social group networks and the norms that are bound up in this. In this regard the mapping process serves as a practical tool for bringing these networks to light. Importantly too, the process also empowers participants by giving them insight into the possible sources of risk and also refuge within their social networks so that they can take more control of them.

Addiction trajectories centre on processes of social identity change

There is growing evidence that addiction trajectories not only involve identity change but also that recovery can be understood as a process of identity change – more specifically one which centres on changes to social group memberships. Addiction onset, for example, involves a change from seeing oneself as a non-user to seeing oneself as a user that occurs in the context of increasing involvement and perceived importance of using groups relative to non-using groups. Similarly, attempts at recovery typically involve leaving substance using groups and affiliating more strongly with either new or pre-existing non-using groups which support a new identity as a person in recovery. The latter transition becomes possible when people come to see that membership of a using group need not define them and that by leaving this group they can regain a positive identity (along the lines of the mobility hypothesis, H5).

Such observations highlight the ways in which a social identity analysis can help us understand not only how people develop an addict identity that reinforces their substance misuse, but also how they can transition away from this into recovery. Speaking to this point, this section explores a range of closely related models that have been developed to account for the role of social identity processes in this journey. As we will discuss further, in the case of AA it also espouses the idea of a stable alcoholic identity – "once an alcoholic, always an alcoholic" – which may restrict the process of identity transition (from a using to a non-using identity, see the next section).

Social identity pathways are implicated in addiction onset and recovery

In line with the earlier points, two of us recently collaborated with Dan Frings on a qualitative study with 21 adults residing in a drug and alcohol therapeutic community to explore how social identity processes played out in addiction onset and recovery (Dingle, Cruwys, & Frings, 2015). As Figure 9.6 illustrates, this identified two distinct pathways into and out of addiction. On the one hand, the experience of participants who lost valued identities as a consequence of addiction onset was characterised by an *identity loss* pathway. As the following comment illustrates, these individuals described their identity as a substance user in negative and stigmatised terms:

> In my good bits, I excel, really excel. I was playing basketball too, got drafted for the Northern Tigers in the under 16s, I was like 15 and competing for the Olympics. I had a really beautiful girlfriend when I was 16. And then everything just went 'poof'.
>
> (Male, 1 week in treatment for amphetamines)

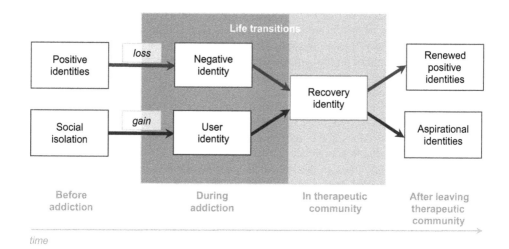

Figure 9.6 Social identity pathways into and out of addiction

Note: This model draws together findings from thematic analysis of interviews with 21 adults in a drug and alcohol therapeutic community showing two social identity–related pathways into and out of addiction. The upper blue pathway
   describes individuals who experienced a loss of positive social identities with the onset of their addiction and who
   saw their addicted self in terms of a negative identity. These people tended to view their membership of the therapeutic community as a transitional identity that facilitated development of a non-user identity to support restoration
   of previous positive identities (e.g., related to family and work). The lower red pathway describes individuals who
   were socially disconnected and who saw the onset of their addiction and membership of a substance-using group as
   gaining a new valued social identity. For these individuals, membership in the therapeutic community was also seen
   as a transitional identity from which they were able to scaffold the development of new positive social identities
   supported by family, study, work, and other interest groups.

Source: Adapted from Dingle, Cruwys, & Frings (2015)

On the other hand, though, some participants reported experiencing the onset of their addiction
quite differently and in ways that were characterised by an *identity gain* pathway. This was especially
true for individuals who had been socially isolated prior to addiction and who found that the onset of
their addiction provided them with new group memberships, albeit associated with substance use, that
filled the gap in their social lives. In the words of one participant:

> All I cared about was fitting in with some people and I found that through bad kids and
> gangs, and sort of the crime, and all that kind of lifted. Obviously drinking, my older sister
> introduced me to drinking when I was 12, by the age of 13 I was pretty much binge drinking
> every day at school.
>
> (Male, 1 week in treatment for amphetamine misuse)

But after a person has become addicted, what is it about therapeutic groups and communities that
might foster their development of a recovery identity? This research highlighted two factors. First,
Dingle and colleagues suggest that it is critical for people with addictions and their health professionals
to understand the pathways that led to their addiction onset. This is because sustained recovery after

leaving the TC was found to be associated with developing new positive and aspirational identities while in treatment, yet this was only possible when residents recognised which identities they needed to relinquish or move away from. Specifically, after leaving TC treatment, participants who had been on the identity loss pathway looked to restore positive identities that they had prior to the onset of their addiction (e.g., those associated with work, sporting, or family groups) and that would support their ongoing recovery. In this vein, one participant observed:

> I really value education. I need to [finish] my education, I need to get somewhere good. Coz I don't want to be a bum the rest of my life, I'm better than that.
> (Female resident, 26 weeks in treatment for poly-substance use)

Individuals on the identity gain pathway, however, aspired to develop new positive identities to support their ongoing recovery. For some, this aspirational identity was associated with finding a partner and perhaps starting a family. For others, it was related to an occupational or career identity:

> I think all of my self-esteem was just crushed that I had none left, but slowly bit by bit it is coming back. But I want a lot more. Now I am aspiring to write a book.
> (Female resident, 6 weeks in treatment for poly-substance use)

Second, regardless of their pathway into addiction, all participants indicated that their addiction became increasingly problematic over time. However, entering a therapeutic community for abstinence-based treatment and rehabilitation was seen as a turning point primarily because it allowed those with addictions to develop a new social identity as a member of the TC. In line with the theoretical analysis set out in Chapter 2, there are two features of a person's identity as a member of a TC that support recovery. In line with the connection hypothesis (H12), the first is that within these communities of former substance users in recovery, people report feeling a sense of acceptance and freedom from being judged and discriminated against. Indeed, this goes some way to explaining why those seeking treatment for addiction problems may prefer help that is provided by others who have experienced addiction themselves, such as the case in AA and NA groups and often in TCs. Second, in line with the support hypothesis (H14), this sense of connection to others in turn increases members' willingness to engage with treatment and accept support within the TC.

In sum, it appears that TCs promote recovery by providing the basis for a shared identity among their members associated with norms that centre on abstinence and "right living" (e.g., embracing values such as honesty and respect for self and others, and adoption of a healthy lifestyle). In this way too, the recovery or TC identity serves as a transitional identity between an "addict" identity and a "clean" or "non-user" identity. As one participant in our study put it:

> It's like building the foundation of a house, and all the community and staff have had input into building that foundation for me. The foundation isn't ready yet and has to be rooted in firm strong ground otherwise I'll just sink in the sand. I want to be strong and I don't want to quit.
> (Female, 6 weeks in treatment for poly-substance misuse)

Therapy groups facilitate social identity change

A second identity change model of addiction – the *social identity model of cessation maintenance* (SIMCM) – has been developed by Dan Frings and Ian Albery (2015, 2017). This highlights the central role that group therapy plays in providing the basis for a person with addiction problems to identify as someone in recovery.

A schematic representation of this model is provided in Figure 9.7. The model starts by noting that, in ways suggested in Chapter 2 (Oakes et al., 1994; see Figure 2.6), taking part in group therapy (e.g., AA) itself tends to make a recovery identity more meaningful and thereby more salient. However, Frings and Albery (2017) argue that salience of a recovery identity is not in and of itself sufficient for recovery. Instead they argue that the strength of a recovery identity is dependent upon several social cognitive processes that trigger and facilitate the transition from no longer self-identifying as a user to seeing oneself instead as a non-user (e.g., as an 'ex-smoker').

The key *social cognitive moderators* that the model identifies relate to the fact that a person's identity as a recovering addict identity will tend to become more complex and more accessible as a result of being activated in a diverse range of contexts. In line with self-categorization theory's principle of perceiver readiness (Oakes et al., 1994), this means that over time there will be a broader range of social situations in which people can define themselves as a person in recovery. Moreover, in line with the norm enactment hypothesis (H8), as this happens, they will be more motivated to act in ways that are consistent with this recovery identity. For example, they are more likely to refuse a friend's offer of a cigarette and to avoid places where the temptation to smoke is likely to be strong.

SIMCM also proposes that group treatment has positive effects via other *social identity mediators*. In particular, group therapy exposes people to social influence from other group members who can thereby exert control in ways that support cessation. This control could involve reinforcing positive behaviour but also challenging people's violation of group norms. Therapy groups can also help to contextualise what it means to lapse and relapse and help people to understand the perceived costs of such behaviours. Consistent with the identity restoration hypothesis (H4), there is also evidence that when the treatment group acts as a resource in this way, it helps to increase group members' self-esteem and that this is another important contributor to their recovery (Frings & Albery, 2015).

To test SIMCM, Frings et al (2016) conducted a study of 44 people who were members of mutual support recovery groups (AA/NA/CA) or SMART recovery groups (a CBT-based alternative). These participants were asked to list behaviours they saw as normative and deviant within their group and to rate a

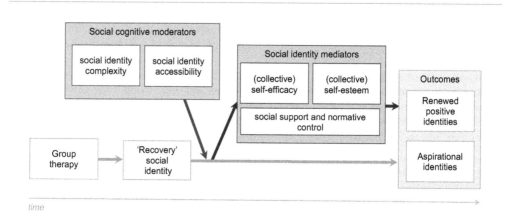

Figure 9.7 The social identity model of cessation maintenance (SIMCM)

Note: This model illustrates how group therapy supports the emerging recovery identity which is related to treatment engagement and cessation maintenance through several social cognitive moderators and social identity mediators.

Source: Adapted from Frings & Albery (2015)

variety of responses to deviant behaviours. They also measured participants' perceptions of the negative consequences of relapse for both themselves and other members of their group, as well their self-efficacy in relation to cessation and their endorsement of both an addict identity and a self-help group identity. Consistent with their model, the results showed that participants who identified more highly with their self-help group perceived themselves to have more social control over substance-related behaviour. There was also evidence that recovery groups used social support and control both to help individual group members maintain their cessation and to regulate group behaviour in ways that ensured the group could continue to function (Frings et al, 2016). Thus the group tended to respond constructively to deviant behaviours (e.g., by explaining that the behaviour is undesirable and describing clearly what behaviour is expected by the group). Challenges to deviant behaviour (e.g., avoiding or 'freezing out' a group member after a deviant behaviour) were also mediated by the perceived costs of an individual's relapse for the group.

SIMCM has broad relevance to addiction contexts in which the development of a new "recovery group" identity is central to success. As such, it is relevant to a wide variety of treatment contexts, including both outpatient and residential therapeutic community programmes. At the same time, though, it is clearly the case that, as we saw in the previous section, recovery does not depend on recovery identity alone, but rather is shaped by the dynamic constellation of other identities within which this one identity plays out. This point is central to the third and final model of identity change that we consider next.

Recovery involves shifting identification from using to non-using groups

The *social identity model of recovery* (SIMOR; Best et al., 2016) describes the recovery journey as a socially negotiated process that centres on changes in the balance of a person's social identities that serve to support either substance use or abstinence. As can be seen from Figure 9.8, this balance can be represented as a see-saw on which the relative influence of groups that hinder or encourage recovery changes over time.

At the start of the recovery journey, a person's using groups will tend to be more salient and influential. Early recovery involves increased exposure to groups that support recovery (in ways suggested by SIMCM) and a commensurate shift in social influence such that these groups begin to have greater sway than those which support using. Finally, as a person enters a phase of stable recovery, recovery-friendly groups become even more meaningful in their life. Here group norms which support recovery maintenance exert a strong influence, and abstinence becomes embedded as part of a person's self-concept. What this model recognises, then, is that a person's recovery trajectory is not only contingent on their membership of a recovery group, but is also shaped by their membership of a wider array of groups that support (or do not support) recovery and abstinence. In these terms, recovery maintenance and relapse hinge on the relative influence of these countervailing social psychological forces.

Consistent with this model, work by Sarah Buckingham and colleagues provides evidence that over the course of treatment people's social identity typically shifts from that of an 'addict' to that of a 'person in recovery' or a 'non-user' (Buckingham, et al., 2013). Moreover, it is clear that this shift is predictive of improved health outcomes. More specifically, this research identifies two processes that are linked to higher abstinence self-efficacy and good health. The first process, *evaluative differentiation*, involves participants in treatment coming to evaluate the addict identity increasingly negatively at the same time that they evaluate the recovery identity more positively. The second process, *identity preference*, is one which leads a person to identify more strongly with the recovery identity at the same time that they identify less strongly with the addict identity and, through this, gaining a more positive sense of self.

Buckingham and her colleagues (2013) conducted two studies to explore these two processes. The first involved 61 members attending AA and NA in the UK. The study showed that greater evaluative differentiation was significantly related to lower relapse rates and reduced substance use. Furthermore, greater preference for a recovery identity was associated with higher levels of self-efficacy, and this

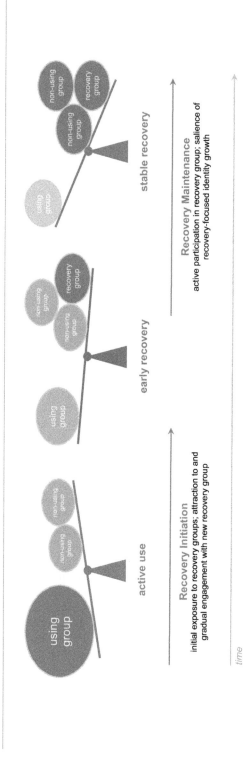

Figure 9.8 The social identity model of recovery (SIMOR)

Note: This model illustrates how the salience and influence of an individual's substance-using groups is higher than their other groups at the start of their recovery process. The salience and influence of using groups decreases over time as non-using and recovery group memberships become more important and influential.

Source: Adapted from Best et al. (2016)

predicted both the number of months that a participant was drug-free and reduction in their substance use behaviour. The second study involved 81 ex-smokers accessed via an online site. Again, identity preference was related to higher self-efficacy, and this in turn was related to lower relapse (i.e., less likelihood that a person would start smoking again). Together, these findings suggest that – regardless of whether they are delivered face to face or online – group programs achieve lower relapse rates and better health outcomes to the extent that they succeed in encouraging participants to relinquish an addict identity and instead embrace one that centres on recovery.

Further evidence that identity shift of this form is implicated in recovery comes from a study that two of us conducted with 132 adults in a residential therapeutic community for drug and alcohol treatment (Dingle, Stark, Cruwys, & Best, 2015). As can be seen from the results presented in Figure 9.9, at the beginning of treatment most participants identified quite highly with their substance-using social groups. However, for those who stayed in treatment, this changed markedly over time. In particular, during the first month of treatment, 76% of the participants reported a decrease in their sense of identification with substance-using social groups. Meanwhile, their identification with other members of the therapeutic community increased steadily across fortnightly measurement intervals.

Importantly too, follow-up assessments were conducted with a representative subsample of 60 of the participants around seven months after they had left the TC. Here the degree of identity change – measured by the difference between user identity and recovery identity ratings over the treatment period – accounted for 34% of the variance in drinking quantity, 41% of the variance in drinking frequency, 5% of the variance in other drug use frequency, and 49% of the variance in life satisfaction.

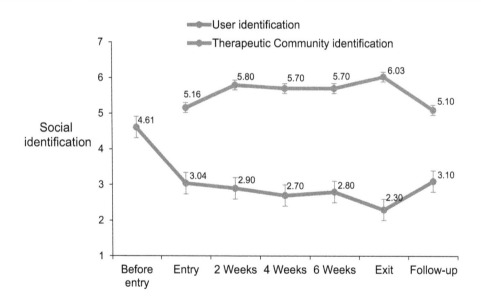

Figure 9.9 Identification with substance-using peers and with the therapeutic community as a function of time in treatment

Note: Participants in this study were residents of a drug and alcohol therapeutic community (TC). Importantly, a shift in the relative strength of identification with other members of the TC rather than with users predicted reduced substance use at follow-up an average of 7 months after leaving the TC.

Source: Adapted from Dingle, Stark, Cruwys, & Best (2015)

Note as well that these analyses controlled for initial substance abuse severity and social identity ratings at entry to the TC. In ways suggested by the social identity approach more generally, it thus appears that identity change is not simply a correlate of addiction-related behaviour but one of its important drivers.

The addiction trajectory of Peter, our case study, serves clearly to illustrate the processes of identity change captured by SIMOR. Specifically, although his substance-using siblings and neighbours initially held great sway over his behaviour, during and after treatment, his recovery peer group, his abstinent family, and his writing group gained greater influence. The behavioural norms and attitudes espoused by these groups were supportive of abstinence from substance use and, in line with the above research findings, should provide a basis to sustain Peter's efforts towards abstinence. There is no guarantee of this, of course. Nevertheless, the positive family identity that he has reacquired and his acquisition of a new identity as a writer have furnished him with a more positive sense of self and, as a result, it is clear that he is now in a far better position to deal with life's challenges than he ever was before.

Case study 9.1 Peter (continued)

Peter completed a 3-month residential rehabilitation programme in which he learned numerous cognitive behavioural coping skills and became aware that his social network consisted mostly of other substance users. In the final month of his program, he started attending a creative writing group once a week and enjoyed writing about his experiences when he had spare time at the rehabilitation service. He developed a reputation for being a scribe, and other residents asked him to read his stories out loud for entertainment. His discharge plan included regular attendance at the rehabilitation follow-up group, ongoing attendance at the writing group, and appointments at the employment agency. Peter recognised that he needed to find a new job that would embody a sober way of life around others, rather than a solitary truck driver's life. He has started to spend time with his family again. Reflecting on the ways in which his life had changed for the better, he remarked: "my biggest motivation is to be a good husband and father again . . . Tania and I are taking it one day at a time . . ."

Conclusion

Strictly speaking, the question is not how to get cured, but how to live.

(Conrad, 1899/1999, p. 124)

This chapter highlights the fact that addiction to substances is complex and multifaceted. It is also clear that effective addiction management requires attention to a person's wider social environment. In particular, effective addiction management requires an understanding of the influence of people's group memberships upon their addiction trajectories and of the norms related to substance use that these groups promote. As well as arming people with individual-level skills such as substance refusal self-efficacy, it is therefore important to identify non-user social groups and activities that can support their recovery following treatment. Here both structured groups (e.g., outpatient services and mutual support groups) and unstructured groups (e.g., as developed through workforce participation and training) can have a role to play in contributing to sustainable long-term recovery. Moreover, over time, those individuals who increase the depth and breadth of their meaningful non-user group memberships are likely to rely less on substance-related groups and services and to sustain and embed their recovery. This analysis accords with George De Leon's (2000) observation that the success of the community-as-method approach that is used in therapeutic communities centres on a process of identity change, involving "dissipation of old identity elements, restructuring elements of new social and personal identities during treatment, and continued identity development beyond treatment in the real world" (De Leon, 2000, p. 345).

But in addition to understanding trajectories into and out of addiction, the social identity approach provides clear direction when it comes to both assessing social identities in a meaningful way and devising appropriate strategies for intervention. The former can involve asking participants to indicate how much they identify with their substance-using peers and with members of a recovery group (as in Buckingham et al., 2013; Dingle, Stark, et al., 2015). Alternatively, it can involve semi-structured interviews with questions about participants' group-related experiences of addiction and of treatment (as in Dingle, Cruwys et al., 2015). However, this approach can sometimes feel a little abstract to people who are not used to thinking about their social group relationships in this way (or to psychological assessments more generally), and here social identity mapping (Cruwys, Steffens, et al., 2016, see Figure 9.5) provides a more concrete way of understanding the impact of group networks on substance-using behaviour.

Having used a method of this form to assess the way in which addiction trajectories are being shaped by social identity dynamics, it is then possible to design interventions which promote positive forms of social identity change by orienting people to those social groups which are most likely to provide them with the resources they need to successfully tackle and overcome addiction. This can be a long and challenging path. Significantly too, even if it leads to success, it does not constitute a 'cure' for addiction. Instead, it is simply a recipe for a more positive social sense of self – and, with it, hopefully, a better life.

Points for practice

On the basis of the ideas and arguments presented in this chapter, it is possible to draw out four key points that are relevant for practitioners working with people experiencing addiction problems:

1. *Social factors influence a person's response to all forms of addiction treatment.* Because of this, we suggest that regardless of the treatment approach an individual seeks or receives for their addiction, attention should be paid to social factors so as both to measure their influence and harness their power with a view to optimising treatment and promoting ongoing recovery.

2. *The path from addiction onset to recovery is best understood as a process of social identity change.* Addiction onset may involve social identity loss or identity gain, and these two pathways have different implications for treatment. When it comes to addiction recovery, therapeutic intervention provides opportunities to transition from a 'user' identity to a 'recovery' identity, and the success of this will play an important role in shaping a person's outcomes.

3. *On the path to recovery, it is just as important to pay attention to ways in which one can break with using groups as it is to strengthen and build identification with non-using groups.* Informal groups (such as work or friendship groups) that hold abstinence norms can be every bit as helpful in supporting an individual's recovery as formal groups (e.g., therapeutic community groups).

4. *It is important to manage social identity loss well so that a person remains supported through their identity transition.* Moving away from using networks is an important part of treatment, but doing so results in loss of group memberships that may have been important sources of support in the past. In this context it is important to build new networks supportive of recovery to buffer that loss. As proposed in SIMOR, identity loss must be offset with identity gain.

Resources

Further reading

The publications listed here provide important pointers to the social dimensions of addiction and to the way that addiction recovery can be understood as successful identity change.

① S. A. Buckingham, & Best, D. (Eds.) (2017). *Addiction, behavioral change and social identity: The path to resilience and recovery.* Abingdon and New York: Routledge.

This book provides an expanded analysis of research that examines the relevance of social identity processes to addictive behaviours.

② Hari, J. (2016). *Chasing the scream: The first and last days of the war on drugs.* USA: Bloomsbury.

The journalist Johann Hari spent three years researching the War on Drugs and the nature of addiction. His findings, summarised in this book, provide compelling evidence for a social approach to addiction.

③ Alexander, B. (2017). *Dislocation theory of addiction: A hopeful prophecy from a time of despair.* Available from the website www.brucekalexander.com/articles-speeches/dislocation-theory-addiction

This is an expanded version of a presentation that Bruce Alexander gave to the "New Directions in the Study of Alcohol Group" in the UK.

Video

① "Hari Scream TED" to find a TED talk in which Johann Hari expands on his book *Chasing the Scream*. As the title suggests, this challenges widely held beliefs about the nature of addiction and the best way to treat it. www.ted.com/talks/johann_hari_everything_you_think_you_know_about_addiction_is_wrong   (14 minutes)

② "Bruce Alexander Addiction" to see an interview with Bruce Alexander which highlights the problems with conventional medical approaches to treating addiction and the importance of understanding the impact that social dislocation has on the development and maintenance of addiction. www.youtube.com/watch?v=XhK-6jSN3x8   (18 minutes)

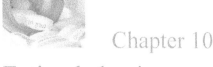

Chapter 10

Eating behaviour

Case study 10.1 Sandra

Sandra is a 45-year-old businesswoman who struggles with her weight, which has increased by 20 kilograms since having her first child at age 32. She often skips breakfast or lunch in her efforts to try to lose weight. Sandra feels helpless to try and change her eating at dinner times, because she cooks for her husband, who prefers meat-based meals, as well as her two children. One of her children has allergies to milk and eggs, and the other is a "picky" eater, who doesn't like to try new foods. Sandra tends to over-eat in specific situations, most often at parties or social events, where she feels unable to control her eating. She has tried almost a dozen different restrictive diets, sometimes losing as much as 10 kilograms – but she has always quickly regained this weight, and more. Sandra experiences shame and embarrassment about her body shape and size, which interferes with her life in a number of ways – it makes it hard for her to be intimate with her husband; she avoids beaches, pools, and gyms; and she finds reminders of appearance, like women's magazines or clothes shopping, distressing. Sandra fears people don't take her seriously at work because of her obesity.

Eating is a fundamental feature of our lives, and is often a source of great enjoyment. Yet this does not prevent it from presenting a problem for many people, often with serious health consequences. Indeed, the most common factors that contribute to preventable disease burden are both related to eating: (1) not eating enough fruit and vegetables, and (2) being overweight or obese (Australian Institute of Health and Welfare, 2016). In short, most people in the modern world eat too much of some things and not enough of others, so much so that eating is one of the biggest contributors to ill health.

Understanding eating behaviour is therefore a priority for health professionals and health researchers. In this chapter, we first explore the variety of ways in which eating can depart from those behaviours which support good health. Second, we summarise each of the dominant models that have been proposed to explain and predict unhealthy eating. Third and finally, we present a social identity approach to eating behaviour (the situated identity enactment model; Cruwys, Platow, Rieger, Byrne, & Haslam, 2016), along with evidence that speaks to its usefulness.

What do we mean by unhealthy eating? This is a domain in which misinformation abounds and where it is therefore easy to get on the wrong track. Indeed, several industries (e.g., companies selling diets and supplements) only thrive to the extent that people believe that there is something wrong with the way they eat and that they need to put it right. In this chapter, however, we use the term unhealthy eating broadly, to refer to any eating behaviour that is likely to have negative consequences for physical or mental health in the short or long term. This includes both over-eating behaviours (e.g., bingeing, overconsumption of energy-dense foods) and under-eating behaviours (e.g., fasting, purging, restrictive dieting). The serious consequences of such behaviours include obesity, diabetes, cancer, eating disorders, malnutrition, depression, and even early death. Rather than focusing on these disorder categories, however, in this chapter we focus on the specific eating behaviours that may ultimately lead to one of these diagnoses.

People sometimes mistakenly think that over-eating and under-eating behaviours, and the disorders they pre-empt, are so different from one another that they cannot be understood using the same theories or approaches. That is, if the problems of obesity and eating disorders (e.g., anorexia nervosa) are opposites, how can they have the same causes? In fact, disorders of under-eating and over-eating are not opposites but instead are best conceptualised as points on a spectrum of eating pathology, as shown in Figure 10.1. There are several ways in which this interrelationship is apparent. First, the most common type of eating disorder is actually binge-eating disorder, which often co-occurs with or precedes obesity (Stice, Marti, & Rohde, 2013). Research has shown that rates of comorbid obesity and eating disorders are increasing faster than either condition alone (Darby et al., 2009). Sandra's story is a typical example here: her eating is unhealthy both because it has led to weight gain with physical health consequences (obesity), but also because her associated distress compromises her mental health and functioning (meeting criteria for binge-eating disorder).

Second, certain thoughts, feelings, and behaviours tend to occur in both over-eating and under-eating. In terms of thoughts, unhealthy eating is often associated with people placing a particularly strong emphasis on body, weight, and appearance when it comes to evaluating their self-worth. In terms of feelings, people who struggle with unhealthy eating are often distressed and dissatisfied with their body, their weight, and their appearance. In terms of behaviours, attempts to lose weight (with varying degrees of success) are seen across the under- and over-eating spectrum. It is these psychological commonalities that underpin all forms of unhealthy eating that we will seek to understand in this chapter, as well as answering the broader question of how we can best intervene to change unhealthy eating behaviours at the population level in order to reduce the harm they do to health.

The incidence of unhealthy eating also varies across the spectrum of eating disorders presented in Figure 10.1. Some conditions are quite rare (e.g., between 0.6% and 4.3% of women experience anorexia nervosa across the course of their lives; Smink, van Hoeken, & Hoek, 2012) and others are almost ubiquitous (e.g., 94.5% of Australians consume less than the recommended amount of fruit and vegetables; Australian Bureau of Statistics, 2012). The likelihood of experiencing a particular kind of disordered eating also varies dramatically depending on demographic characteristics. Women aged 15 to 25 are at particular risk of under-eating pathologies, with the majority of this group having engaged in unhealthy dieting and almost 90% experiencing body dissatisfaction (Hay, Mond, Buttner, & Darby, 2008; Ricciardelli, & McCabe, 2002). Similarly, only 10% of people who experience an eating disorder are men (Smink et al., 2012), although the gender disparity is narrower for binge-eating disorder (Kessler et al., 2013). Gender ratios are also more equal for obesity (Kanter & Caballero, 2012). Nationality is a particularly powerful predictor of obesity risk, with its prevalence ranging from 1.1% of the adult population (in Bangladesh) to 71.1% (in Nauru; World Health Organization, 2017a). Indeed, this unequal distribution of unhealthy eating is one of key phenomena that the models we will discuss next have sought to explain.

Current models of eating behaviour

In this section, we review the five dominant models of unhealthy eating. These are associated with distinct forms of explanation that focus on biological, individual difference, social cognitive, socio-cultural, and interactionist determinants of the various conditions outlined earlier.

Biological models

The two biological variables that have received the most attention from researchers working in the unhealthy eating field are genetic makeup and metabolism. In the first instance, anorexia nervosa, bulimia nervosa, and obesity have all been suggested to have a genetic basis (Ramachandrappa & Farooqi,

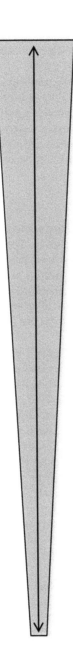

under-eating

over-eating

Anorexia nervosa   *Bulimia nervosa*   Purging   Unhealthy dieting   Body dissatisfaction   Bingeing   *Binge-eating disorder*   Obesity

Figure 10.1 The spectrum of over- and under-eating pathology

Note: Eating behaviour is best represented along a continuum reflecting the extent to which it involves under-eating or over-eating. Behaviours in *italics* are recognised psychiatric diagnoses.

Source: Based on Neumark-Sztainer (2003)

2011; Trace, Baker, Peñas-Lledó, & Bulik, 2013). Indeed, most of the research into obesity has focused on identifying genes or abnormalities in biological functioning that might explain an individual's weight gain (Hill & Melanson, 1999). Several genes that govern the expression and regulation of hormones, such as leptin and ghrelin, are implicated in the development of obesity (Kalra, Bagnasco, Otukonyong, Dube, & Kalra, 2003). In anorexia nervosa, abnormalities in neuroendocrine functioning (in particular, of serotonin) have been found to pre-date the development of an eating disorder and persist after treatment (Kaye, Frank, Bailer, & Henry, 2005).

The key benefit of biological models is that they can help identify those individuals in a given population who are most at risk of engaging in unhealthy eating behaviour. At the same time, though, genetic and metabolic factors cannot, on their own, provide a plausible explanation for the prevalence of obesity and other forms of unhealthy eating in modern society (Hill & Melanson, 1999). In particular, population-level changes in genes and metabolism occur over a very long timespan (e.g., over the course of many generations), whereas obesity has only become common at a societal level in the past 50 years.

Individual-difference models

In researching unhealthy eating, psychologists have primarily focused on the forms of unhealthy eating that fall into the category of psychiatric disorders. That is, they are concerned with those behaviours, as defined by psychiatrists and clinical psychologists, that (1) depart from what is culturally acceptable or expected and (2) cause significant distress or impairment to the individual (American Psychiatric Association, 2013). Given this classification system, it is perhaps unsurprising that efforts to understand the development and maintenance of unhealthy eating have focused on individual-level pathology – that is, on maladaptive characteristics that distinguish people who eat unhealthily from the general population.

Illustrative of such research, a wide range of personality features have been identified as increasing vulnerability to disordered eating. Some of the characteristics associated with under-eating pathology include perfectionism (Wade, Wiksch, Paxton, Byrne, & Austin, 2015), need for control (Vitousek & Manke, 1994), and low self-esteem (Shea & Pritchard, 2007). All of these individual differences are more prevalent among people with eating disorders, and some prospective research has suggested that they emerge prior to unhealthy eating (Paxton, Eisenberg, & Neumark-Sztainer, 2006; Tyrka, Waldron, Graber, & Brooks-Gunn, 2002). In this work, researchers have typically framed under-eating as a maladaptive strategy that is used to buffer the negative effects of these various personality characteristics. In other words, people are thought to engage in pathological eating as a way of keeping their personal shortcomings at bay. For example, a severely restricted eating regimen is hypothesised to satisfy, at least in the short term, the need for perfection or control, and in this way the behaviour is reinforced (Fairburn, Shafran, & Cooper, 1999). Moreover, subsequent weight loss may be met with approval from others and, if it is, this positive feedback will bolster the self-worth of individuals with low self-esteem (again, at least in the short term), and therefore be similarly reinforcing (Cockell et al., 2002).

For over-eating pathology, a separate set of psychological precursors has been proposed, including impulsivity (Dawe & Loxton, 2004; Yeomans, Leitch, & Mobini, 2008), poor self-monitoring (Baker & Kirschenbaum, 1993), and emotional dysregulation (Cassin & von Ranson, 2005; Vitousek & Manke, 1994). Interest in these various personality characteristics is premised upon an underlying belief that binge eating arises from deficits in self-control (Heilbrun & Bloomfield, 1986; Tangney, Baumeister, & Boone, 2004). According to these models, eating unhealthy food is rewarding in the short term, and individuals who over-eat lack the capacity to inhibit the urge to eat, particularly in the face of strong negative emotion (Whiteside, Chen, Neighbors, Hunter, Lo, & Larimer, 2007).

It is worth noting that individuals with bulimia nervosa typically present with personality features from both the "under-eating" and "over-eating" clusters of eating disorder, and, given the lack of stability in diagnoses over time (Fitcher & Quadflieg, 2007), it is not straightforward to link personality features to diagnostic categories (Vitousek & Manke, 1994). Nevertheless, this line of research has certainly demonstrated robust associations between specific eating behaviours and a variety of personality variables.

As with most biological models, one strength of the individual-difference approach is it allows researchers and practitioners to anticipate which individuals in a given population are most likely to exhibit unhealthy eating behaviour, potentially before this manifests itself as a problem. Indeed, individual-difference approaches have proven utility when it comes to predicting an individual's risk and prognosis, as well as in informing treatment planning. However, these approaches also share with biological models a central feature that limits their capacity to provide a comprehensive explanation of unhealthy eating. For in relying on a model of illness that locates pathology within the individual, they fail to explain the process through which population rates or types of pathology vary over time. Moreover, although individuals with eating disorders may have low self-esteem that predates the development of their particular condition, it does not follow that low self-esteem is the *cause* of their disorder. A further complication is that evidence suggests that in recent decades self-esteem has actually increased at a population level at the same time that disordered eating has become more widespread (Twenge & Campbell, 2001). So although self-esteem may help explain differences between *individuals* in unhealthy eating, it is unlikely to help us understand population trends.

In addition, and as we have noted in other chapters (e.g., Chapter 5), individual-difference models are often descriptive rather than explanatory (Dar-Nimrod & Heine, 2011). In this, they can be seen to constitute what Robert Wicklund (1990) refers to as zero-variable theories because the thing that does the explaining is also the thing that needs to be explained. For example, arguing that individuals develop binge-eating disorder because they lack self-control does not add a great deal of explanatory power because the fact that a person lacks control over their eating is how we know they have binge-eating disorder in the first place.

Social cognitive models

In a separate line of research, three influential health psychology models have been applied to unhealthy eating behaviour, particularly over-eating pathology. These models are often referred to collectively as social cognitive theories. This is because they share a focus on the putatively social and, particularly, cognitive determinants of health behaviour. These three models are represented schematically in Figure 10.2.

The first of these models is the *theory of planned behaviour* (TPB). This model suggests that eating intentions are the proximal psychological determinant of behaviour and that intentions have three distinct inputs: personal attitudes, social norms, and perceived behaviour control (Ajzen, 1991). For instance, people may value health (attitude), know lots of people who are healthy eaters (norm) and believe they have the psychological and financial resources to eat as they choose (control). The second model is the *health belief model*, which states that a behaviour (e.g., binge eating) is the outcome of a person's beliefs about (1) the perceived threat posed by the behaviour (including the severity of outcomes and their personal susceptibility); (2) specific cues to action (e.g., media campaigns); and (3) the perceived benefits of, and barriers to, engaging in behaviour change (Rosenstock, 1990). The third socio-cognitive model is the *transtheoretical* or *stages of change model* and this outlines a series of psychological states (or stages) that differ in their implications for a person's readiness, orientation towards, and commitment to change (Prochaska & Velicer, 1997). For example, it argues that individuals may be in a pre-contemplative or contemplative stage, where they have not yet engaged in

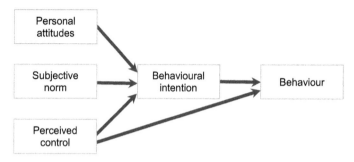

(a) The theory of planned behaviour

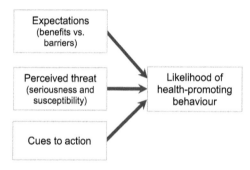

(b) The health belief model

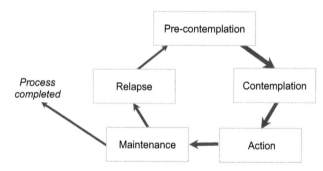

(c) The transtheoretical (or stages of change) model

Figure 10.2 Social cognitive models of health behaviour

Note: These three models of behaviour change are commonly used to understand and treat unhealthy eating behaviour. As shown here, each identifies different factors that are hypothesised to contribute to problematic health behaviour. However, it has been argued that these factors are so broad that they are hard to test empirically and that, as a result, the theories are hard to falsify.

Source: Based on (a) Azjen (1991); (b) Rosenstock, Strecher, and Becker (1994), (c) Prochaska and DiClemente (1982)

behaviour change (e.g., reducing their consumption of saturated fat) and are not committed to doing so; or alternatively, they may be in an action or maintenance stage, where motivation is high and behaviour change has commenced.

Each of these three models has been influential in its own right, generating hundreds of publications and several applied interventions that aim to harness the model to assist people with positive behaviour change (for reviews, see Armitage & Conner, 2001; Bridle et al., 2005; Harrison, Mullen, & Green, 1992). The stages of change model has also been particularly valuable in applied contexts – most specifically, in informing the development of motivational interviewing, an evidence-based psychological intervention that has been found to assist in weight loss (Armstrong et al., 2011; Rubak, Sandbaek, Lauritzen, & Christensen, 2005; see also Chapter 9). However, all three socio-cognitive models have also been quite widely criticised, and an array of cogent points have led many researchers and practitioners to question their continued dominance in the field. For instance, Jane Ogden (2003, p. 424) has argued that although the social cognitive models may have been helpful for directing research efforts, their constructs are so broadly specified as to be unfalsifiable. As she puts it:

> The models cannot be tested, they focus on analytic truths rather than synthetic ones, and they may create and change both cognitions and behavior rather than describe them and as such do not pass the criteria set for a good theory.

Along similar lines, Falko Sniehotta and his colleagues (Sniehotta, Presseau, and Araújo-Soares (2014, p. 1) argue that it is "time to retire" the TPB. These authors draw attention to the fact that despite hundreds – if not thousands – of published investigations of the TPB, few experimental tests of the model have been published, and those that do exist have typically shown limited support for the model (e.g., Sniehotta, 2009). Furthermore, the few intervention studies that have drawn upon the TPB have typically been ineffective, or have been effective but not via the mechanisms theorised in the model (e.g., Chatzisarantis & Hagger, 2005). For similar reasons, Robert West (2005) argues that the transtheoretical model should also be abandoned. He states that by providing the illusion of scientific rigour and suggesting inappropriate intervention strategies (i.e., with the goal of getting people to think about behaviour change rather than actually undertake it), it may have done more harm than good to health promotion.

Yet from the social identity perspective that informs the new psychology of health proposed in this volume, there is a further important reason why these social cognitive theories can be seen to provide an inadequate model of eating behaviour. This is because, much like the biopsychosocial model espoused in health psychology more generally, they are often "social" in name only. That is, although they allow for the possibility of contextual input and change over time, the models give primacy to cognitive states and processes (e.g., attitudes and intentions). The result is a model of behaviour change in which the critical ingredient is individual responsibility arising from individual virtues, such as perceptual accuracy, motivation, or self-control. As we will argue further below, this does not allow for the possibility that such individual differences (e.g., in self-control) are influenced by the same social determinants as eating behaviours themselves (Reynolds & Branscombe, 2015).

Moreover, a further problem with these models is that they prove unhelpful when it comes to changing the behaviour of the very people who struggle most with unhealthy eating. In particular, as Chris Crandall and his colleagues have argued, this is because by locating the cause of problems such as obesity primarily within *the individual as an individual*, such models imply that the stigma directed at such individuals is acceptable, or even justified (Crandall, 1994; Crandall, Nierman, & Hebl, 2009). And, as we saw in Chapter 4 (e.g., see Figure 4.3), rather than motivating healthy change, stigma and blame are often directly harmful for both physical and mental health. Speaking to this point, obesity is

Overweight Haters Ltd.

It's really not glandular, it's your gluttony ...

Our organization hates and resents fat people. We object to the enormous amount of food resources you consume while half the world starves. We disapprove of your wasting NHS money to treat your selfish greed. And we do not understand why you fail to grasp that by eating less you will be better off, slimmer, happy, and find a partner who is not a perverted chubby-lover, or even find a partner at all.

We also object that the (beautiful) pig is used as an insult. You are not a pig. You are a fat, ugly human.

Figure 10.3 An example of blatant anti-fat prejudice

Note: This card was given to a woman while she was travelling on the Underground in London by someone claiming to be from a group calling itself "Overweight Haters Ltd."

Source: Recreated by the authors

already ranked by members of the public as one of the most justifiable forms of discrimination (Puhl & Heuer, 2010), and so it is perhaps unsurprising that people who are obese face discrimination – often overt – across all areas of their life, such as employment, education, and even in health care (Puhl & Brownell, 2001; see Figure 10.3). In such contexts lay theory can also often rationalise such discrimination as something that is justified on the grounds that it motivates the people it targets to engage in behaviour change (and hence is "for their own good").

Prejudicial beliefs of this form may be legitimised by the social cognitive models in the sense that all would see prejudice as a potential driver of positive forms of cognitive change that are for the good of the individual. For instance, the theory of planned behaviour might posit that being stigmatised will influence personal attitudes towards one's eating behaviour (e.g., leading to intentions to lose weight); the health belief model predicts that stigma influences beliefs about the benefits of relevant behaviour (e.g., restrained eating); the stages of change model argues that stigma prompts contemplation of relevant forms of behaviour change (e.g., dieting). Here, though, the theories run into empirical difficulty because the evidence suggests that, in fact, what happens is the very opposite. Certainly, people who are subject to weight-based stigma or teasing experience a decrease in their body satisfaction (Paxton et al., 2006); however, low body satisfaction actually predicts weight *gain* over time, even after controlling for initial weight (Van den Berg & Neumark-Sztainer, 2007; Vartanian & Novak, 2011).

This is an important finding, with two implications for our understanding of eating behaviour. First, it suggests that the *desire* to change one's eating or appearance is neither necessary nor sufficient for actual behaviour change. In other words, *on their own*, cognitions may not be as powerful in initiating changes as the social cognitive models suggest. Second, it indicates that a more comprehensive understanding of eating behaviour needs to encompass its social, contextual, and environmental under-pinnings (including, for example, attention to the role of culture and discrimination), not just its cognitive ones, if we are to do justice to the "social" component of a biopsychosocial approach. Accordingly, it is to these factors that we now turn our attention.

Socio-cultural models

According to socio-cultural models, a number of features of the social environment make disordered eating more likely. To begin with obesity, a common line of reasoning is that the modern environment is *obesogenic*, in the sense that urban density and the hyper-availability of palatable food make weight gain almost inevitable (Swinburn, Egger, & Raza, 1999). By contrast, for most of human evolutionary history, nourishing food has been scarce and difficult to obtain (Ulijaszek, 2002). In such an environment, a preference for high-fat and high-sugar foods (historically, meat and fruit, respectively) may have been evolutionarily adaptive, as it ensured intake of these energy-dense foods when they were available (Milton, 1999, 2000). Additionally, a tendency toward over-consumption is observed in almost all mammals when they are placed in a food-rich environment (Ulijaszek & Lofink, 2006). This would have been advantageous prior to agriculture, when weight gain during plentiful times might have been protective during inevitable and imminent scarcities (Cordain et al., 2005). However, agricultural revolution and technological innovation have allowed humans to progress to a point where they can readily control food supply in many countries in the world. In the last century in particular, our capacity in the Western world to process food has facilitated the production of highly palatable food in great variety and quantity. Furthermore, advances in technology (particularly those which have led to the widespread ownership of cars) have reduced people's average calorie expenditure in developed countries to a point well below that required for weight maintenance (Saris et al., 2003). Putting these various developments together, the increase in obesity that has been observed over the course of the last century is thus broadly attributable to changes in the social environment that encourage higher calorie consumption while reducing the daily need for calorie expenditure (Dixon & Broom, 2007).

To provide one example of the obesogenic environment in action, consider rapid increases in food portion sizes. In one study, Robert Jeffery and his colleagues provided women with lunches for an 8-week period (Jeffery et al., 2007). Depending on study condition, these lunches contained an average of either 767 kilocalories (kcal) or 1528 kcal. Across the 8-week period, participants who received large portions consumed an average of 332 kcal more at lunch each day. Moreover, there was no evidence that they compensated for this increased consumption over time (e.g., by eating less at other meals; see also Marchiori, Waroquier, & Klein, 2012). As a result, participants in this large portion group gained an average of 0.64 kg over the course of the study, whereas those in the small portion group gained an average of just 0.06 kg. These findings are an important indication that cultural shifts in food availability can impact significantly on people's eating behaviour and weight at a population level.

Although the obesogenic environment can be invoked to explain increasing rates of over-eating, it is clear that a quite different explanation is needed to account for problems of under-eating – which, as noted earlier, primarily affect women (Hoek, 2006). In this regard, Western developed countries have been said to hold a *thin ideal*, in that almost all successful and attractive women are portrayed by the media as unrealistically thin (Cusamano & Thompson, 1999). Moreover, as Figure 10.4 illustrates, cultural ideals of what defines beauty have shifted slowly but drastically over the last century to endorse thinness as a necessary feature. Research has confirmed this gradual trend toward valuing thinness – for example, by tracking the physical dimensions and body mass index (BMI = kg/m^2) of centrefold models in *Playboy* magazine (Seifert, 2005) or contestants in the Miss America pageant (Wiseman, Gray, Mosimann, & Ahrens, 1992). The widespread use of digital alteration to make media images of

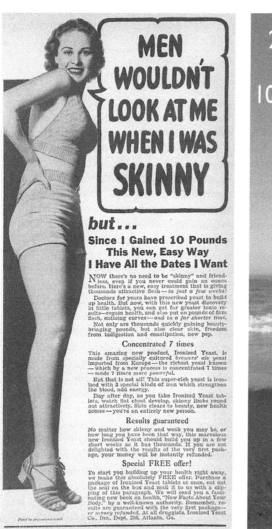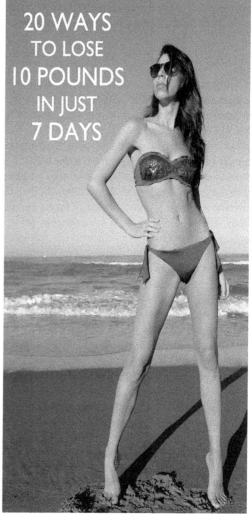

Figure 10.4 Illustrations of the way in which notions of ideal body size change over time

Note: As these adverts show, notions of ideal body weight have changed dramatically over time. Thus whereas in the 1940s being thin was portrayed as problematic, today it is represented as the ideal.

Source: (a) www.elephantjournal.com/2012/08/men-wouldnt-look-at-me-when-i-was-skinny-but-since-i-gained-ten-pounds-i-have-all-the-dates-i-want/ (b) Pixabay, http://www.recentfit.net/2016/09/20-simple-ways-to-lose-10-pounds-in-week.html

women appear thinner also illustrates and contributes to this unrealistic ideal (Reaves, Bush Hitchon, Park, & Woong Yun, 2004).

The argument here is that this shift has had a significant psychological impact on women by forcing them to engage in unfavourable social comparison. This then motivates them to reduce their weight in order to obtain this ideal. However, because ideal weights are often physiologically unattainable (Norton, Olds, Olive, & Dank, 1996) and dieting is a largely ineffective weight reduction strategy (Hill, 2004; Lowe & Timko, 2004), women may engage in increasingly harmful and extreme weight loss strategies over time. In this way, the central features of unhealthy eating (overvaluation of shape and weight, body dissatisfaction, and dieting) can, at least partly, be attributed to the discrepancy between ideals of female attractiveness and women's actual body shapes (Dittmar, Halliwell, & Stirling, 2009). As an aside, it is also worth noting that cultural ideals need not prescribe thinness, and there is recent evidence of an emerging "fit" ideal of athleticism in some Western cultures (Tiggemann & Zaccardo, 2015). Of course, the more general point is that any ideal can be unrealistic and hence provoke harmful body-change strategies (e.g., in the case of the fit ideal, leading to unhealthy forms of over-exercise; Tiggemann & Zaccardo, 2015).

A significant body of evidence supports the link between exposure to the thin ideal, increased body dissatisfaction, and under-eating pathology. For example, even in a brief laboratory manipulation, exposing women to adverts that contain very thin models has been shown to lead to an immediate decrease in their body satisfaction relative to women who were shown adverts containing healthy-weight models (Levine & Murnen, 2009). Interaction with a thin peer is also sufficient to reduce women's short-term body satisfaction (Krones, Stice, Batres, & Orjada, 2005). Research has also demonstrated that women rate celebrities as more attractive when they are digitally altered to look underweight, particularly if respondents' body satisfaction is already low (Willinge, Touyz, & Charles, 2006). This effect is not limited to adults: after being exposed to images of Barbie dolls (rather than to Emme, a doll with a more realistic body shape, or to images unrelated to body shape) girls as young as 5 to 8 years old have been shown to express more body dissatisfaction and to nominate a thinner ideal for themselves (Dittmar, Halliwell, & Ive, 2006).

Speaking to more long-term consequences, Patricia van den Berg and her colleagues conducted a longitudinal study to investigate the role that reading women's magazines played in reinforcing the thin ideal (van den Berg, Neumark-Sztainer, Hannan, & Haines, 2007). They found that, to the extent that women were more exposed to the thin ideal (i.e., as a result of reading more magazines), they had a higher rate of unhealthy dieting and eating disorders five years later, independent of their eating behaviour at baseline. Similar effects have been found for online and social media, where amount of exposure to body-focused content (especially "thinspiration") is associated with body dissatisfaction (Fardouly, Pinkus & Vartanian, 2017).

Evidence of the impact of these socio-cultural forces is also apparent at a societal level. Cross-cultural research indicates that under-eating pathology spreads to new nations as they become increasingly developed and globalised (Makino, Tsuboi, & Dennerstein, 2004). For instance, Fijian girls' risk of eating pathology more than doubled (from 12.7% in 1995 to 29.2% in 1998) following the widespread introduction of Western television programmes (Becker, Burwell, Gilman, Herzog, & Hamburg, 2002). Moreover, a girl's risk of eating pathology could be predicted not only from her own television-viewing habits, but also from those of her friends (Becker, 2004). In Hong Kong, the prevalence of body dissatisfaction and eating disorders have both increased, from negligible rates prior to 1990, to rates similar to those of other developed countries by 2000 (Nasser, Katzman, & Gordon, 2001). Ideals of female beauty in Western culture thus appear to play an important role in precipitating the rise in disordered eating behaviour.

In sum, socio-cultural explanations for unhealthy eating have proved useful in helping to identify variables responsible for macro-level differences in eating behaviour that have been observed across both time and demographic groups. For example, the socio-cultural approach can help explain why women are more prone than men to under-eating pathologies (because the thin-ideal primarily applies to women; Thompson & Stice, 2001), whereas both men and women are susceptible to over-eating pathologies (because men and women tend to be equally exposed to the obesogenic environment).

Interactionist models

Bearing in mind the strengths and limitations of each of these approaches, some researchers have attempted to integrate across multiple levels of analysis. One promising area of research examines the *interaction* between individual-level variables (e.g., genetics) and environmental factors. More specifically, *epigenetic* (or gene–environment interaction) models have the potential to identify the relationship between genetic and environmental risk factors (Plagemann et al., 2009; Qi & Cho, 2008). However, one concern with these models is that their 'environmental' components are often underspecified, with the research focus primarily on the genes that may be "switched" on and off in particular contexts. Furthermore, such models do not specify or theorise about the role of psychological factors (e.g., body dissatisfaction), and these are a key part of the cluster of features that comprise unhealthy eating.

Other researchers have attempted to integrate the individual-difference and socio-cultural approaches to unhealthy eating in order to come to grips with the *interaction* between these levels of analysis. In particular, these models attempt to account for the fact that, although all people are exposed to various influences from the society in which they live, only a subset of the population will develop disordered eating. This has led to a focus on variables that increase or decrease individual vulnerability to social influence, with the goal of bridging the gap between socio-cultural phenomena and individual behaviours.

Illustrative of this approach, a number of factors have been found to moderate the impact of the societal thin ideal. In particular, women who are high in self-determination (Pelletier & Dion, 2007) or self-concept clarity (Vartanian, 2009) have been observed to be less likely to have internalised societal standards of attractiveness. Other research has suggested that a tendency to resist pressures to conform to societal norms (measured as a stable individual characteristic) may also be protective for women (Twamley & Davis, 1999). Conversely, research has indicated that factors such as heightened sensitivity to food cues (relative to internal cues of hunger or satiety) may elevate the risk of binge eating (Burton, Smit, & Lightowler, 2007; Lowe & Kral, 2006). The feature that is common to all of these models is that they look to identify features of individuals – such as confidence in one's self-image – that have the capacity to protect them from, or else make them vulnerable to, being influenced by cultural or environmental realities, exposure to which is posited to be inherently damaging.

Thin-ideal internalisation is a particularly influential exemplar of this approach. This refers to the relative degree to which an individual endorses the idea that thinness is desirable for one self and for others (Thompson & Stice, 2001). This concept has informed the most comprehensive efforts to date to take account of *both* the sociocultural and individual-level determinants of disordered eating. Specifically, the thin-ideal internalisation model acknowledges that cultural standards and ideals regarding appearance do not influence all individuals equally. Instead, these standards must be *internalised*, that is, accepted psychologically as valid, before behaviour will be influenced. Lending support to this claim, individuals who show high thin-ideal internalisation have been found to be more vulnerable to negative social influence than those who internalise the thin-ideal less (Stice & Agras, 1998; Thompson, van den Berg, Roehrig, Guarda, & Heinberg, 2004). For instance, they are more likely to experience a reduction in body satisfaction following exposure to thin-ideal media (Dittmar et al., 2009) and they exhibit increased negative affect and disordered eating over time (Thompson & Stice, 2001).

A clear strength of these interactionist models is that they are more nuanced than single-factor frameworks in that they acknowledge the role that both individual-level factors and the social environment play in shaping behavioural outcomes. This is a theme that is developed further in the social identity approach to eating, which aims to provide a *dynamic* form of interactionist theorising which recognises the capacity for psychology and society to structure each other (Haslam, Jetten, Reynolds, & Reicher, 2013; Reynolds et al., 2010; Turner & Oakes, 1997).

The social identity approach to eating

With the exception of the interactionist model, the distinct foci of mainstream approaches to problematic eating behaviour have tended to pull different groups of researchers in very different directions. As a result, the literature in this area is something of a smorgasbord, which makes the task of developing an integrated theory of unhealthy eating behaviour quite challenging. Nevertheless, as we will see, there are a number of features of the foregoing review work that point to the unifying potential of a social identity approach to this topic (Cruwys et al., 2016).

Most importantly, a key strength of the social identity approach is that it has the capacity to integrate across the different levels of analysis that previous research has shown to be important. Moreover, it also has the potential to specify *how* these different levels of analysis interact. In particular, the social identity approach clarifies how abstract social phenomena such as societal norms, discrimination, or the food environment structure the psychology of a particular individual and hence how they come to shape their eating behaviour.

It is useful to illustrate this potential with reference to the issue of obesity. This condition is ultimately defined in biological terms: such that if a person has a BMI equal to or greater than 30 he or she can be considered obese. A wide range of variables predict the accumulation of excess body fat. Perhaps the most obvious are those that are biological – for example, the person's family history and the presence of particular genes (Barness, Opitz, & Gilbert-Barness, 2007). However, focusing only on these biological risk factors is problematic for a number of reasons. First, many of them are immutable and therefore do not provide opportunity for intervention. Second, biological risk factors are often expensive to monitor and consequently the risk of pathology may only become apparent at a late stage, when the disease process (e.g., obesity) is already apparent. Third, and perhaps most importantly, it has been observed that biological-level variables do not routinely account for the majority of variance in the condition (Hill & Melanson, 1999).

For these reasons, health professionals and researchers who are interested in obesity have embraced analysis at the individual (i.e., behavioural and psychological) level. Risk factors at this level include saturated fat intake and physical inactivity (Haslam & James, 2005; Saris et al., 2003), as well as personality characteristics akin to those we have already discussed such as poor self-control or emotional dysregulation (Hibscher & Herman, 1977; Tangney et al., 2004). Attention to such factors adds greatly to our capacity for intervention and prevention in the majority of health conditions, and this is a domain in which the work of clinical and health psychologists has been very influential.

Importantly, however, risk factors at the socio-cultural level are often at least as powerful as risk factors at the individual or biological levels. For example, obesity can be predicted from an individual's nationality, socio-economic status, or level of education (Dixon & Broom, 2007; Dykes, Brunner, Martikainen, & Wardle, 2004). Although a socio-cultural explanation for such differences is compelling, this tends to be articulated more in discussions of aetiology (e.g., when asking "Why are people obese?") than in discourse about treatment and intervention ("How can we help people lose weight?").

Perhaps the most important reason for the limited influence of socio-cultural models in the realm of intervention is the lack of an explanatory framework. When a health professional is faced with an individual whose risk of obesity is attributed to lack of exercise and poor diet, the approach to intervention is readily apparent (although not necessarily effective). In contrast, dealing with an individual who is at risk of obesity because they have low socio-economic status poses many more challenges. How might intervention proceed? Indeed, without knowing how and why socio-economic status and level of education modify obesity risk, it is near impossible to intervene in an informed way.

What we see here, then, is that there is a chasm between socio-cultural and individual-level models of health, both in their methods and in their ability to specify a mechanism of action. Nevertheless, from a social identity perspective, the socio-cultural approach to health is not fundamentally irreconcilable with the individual and biological approaches to health. Indeed, it is here that the value of the social identity approach becomes apparent because, as we saw in Chapter 2, its particular focus is on specifying the processes through which individuals represent and internalise features of their social environment (Turner & Oakes, 1997). And by providing such a model, the social identity approach articulates the mechanisms through which socio-cultural variables can shape individual behaviours. For example, a social identity model of obesity might propose that the norms and values of low socio-economic status groups are more likely to endorse behaviours known to increase obesity risk, such as high saturated fat intake. To the extent that an individual identifies with a relevant group (which could be a professional group, a family group, a community group, etc.), he or she is then more likely to act in accordance with these behavioural expectations (as suggested by the norm enactment hypothesis, H8) and, consequently, to be at increased risk of becoming obese.

One advantage of a social identity model is that within such formulations socio-cultural research has more utility and now *can* be used to inform health interventions. Such models also provide a framework within which to understand individual-level phenomena. For instance, in the obesity example outlined earlier, a high-fat diet is described as an individual risk factor. However, eating high-fat foods may also be a defining and valued feature of an individual's social group network (e.g., part of what it means to be a blue-collar worker). In this context, eating unhealthily can be understood as a manifestation of much more than simply a lack of individual self-control. Indeed, more generally, when social influence is conceptualised as a meaningful and *normal* psychological process (rather than one that is evidence of personal shortcoming or weakness), the behaviours that result from it can equally be seen as socially and contextually meaningful – and normal rather than aberrant.

Elaborating further on such ideas, *the situated identity enactment (SIE) model of eating* (Cruwys et al., 2016) gives primacy to three social-psychological determinants of behaviour: social context, social identity, and social norms. In addition to being important predictors in their own right, in tandem, these three variables have the potential to unify the socio-cultural and individual-difference predictors of eating behaviour within an integrated framework that allows us to explain unhealthy eating from a population perspective.

The SIE model is represented schematically in Figure 10.5. As this indicates, social context is a central input into the model (as indicated on the left-hand side of the figure). More particularly, this refers to specific features of the socio-cultural environment which cue particular social identities and particular social norms (on the right-hand side of the figure). Social identities then provide a basis for *social influence* (in line with H9 and H10) such that a person's identification with a particular social group moderates the predictive utility of that group's social norms. Finally, eating behaviour (at the bottom of the figure) is directly shaped by the specific content of social identity (social norms). In what follows, we will unpack the various components of this model and discuss some of the evidence that supports its key propositions.

Social context provides cues that shape eating norms and invoke eating-relevant identities

Identities do not emerge or evolve in a vacuum. Instead, as we argued in Chapter 2 (e.g., see Figures 2.3 and 2.4), the social context in which people find themselves has a powerful influence over the

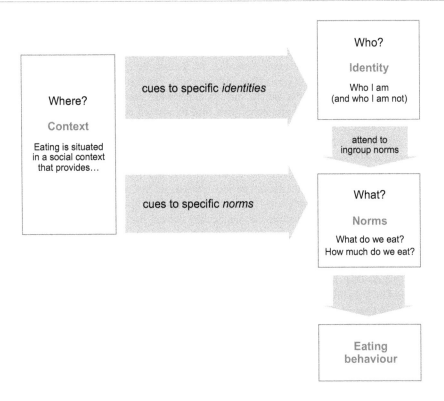

Figure 10.5 The situated identity enactment model

Note: In this model eating behaviour is predicted by three factors that are understood to be important from a social identity perspective. These are the *social context* that a person finds themselves in and its role in increasing the salience of particular *social identities* and the *norms* they promote.

Source: Based on Cruwys et al. (2016)

subjective social identities that form, become salient, and go on to shape their behaviour – including what and how much they eat. More specifically, the SIE model suggests that social context shapes eating via two inter-related psychological pathways: by cueing particular social norms and/or by cueing particular social identities.

Nevertheless, social context is such a broad construct that invoking this in any theoretical analysis risks being too vague and unspecified to contribute to meaningful scientific enquiry. The social identity approach addresses this issue through efforts to specify the key characteristics of the social context that determine identity salience and content, which can then be used to predict the influence of specific contextual variables on eating. As outlined in Chapter 2, these are the *fit* of a particular social identity (or self-categorization) and a person's *readiness* to use it (Oakes et al., 1994). Fit depends on the normative and comparative context in which people self-categorize; readiness depends on previous experiences that make some self-categorizations more likely to be primed than others.

Another important point to make about social context is that it includes both stable and dynamic elements. Social context is thus composed of both the broad, socio-structural realities that form the backdrop against which people live their lives and the more fluid, moment-to-moment changes in the frame of reference against which perceivers evaluate themselves, others, and the world. At the former end of the spectrum, we find the factors emphasised by the socio-cultural models previously discussed, such as the ideal of thinness and the obesogenic environment. The social identity approach does not eschew the critical importance of these factors. Instead, along with other features of the social context, they are conceptualised as the "raw ingredients" that feed into social norms (associated with specific social identities) that influence individual behaviour. Importantly, though, a central principle of the social identity approach is that all perception is relative, with contextual information providing cues to both social identities and social norms that are likely to be more or less relevant in any given situation (Smith, Louis, & Tarrant, 2016).

By way of example, imagine that Sandra (who we discussed in Case study 10.1) attends a party where the food that is available is primarily vegetable platters, fresh fruit, and dips. In this context, a cheese platter may be construed as a (relatively) unhealthy choice. By contrast, if the foods available were chocolates, chips, and other processed snacks, Sandra might construe a cheese platter as a (relatively) healthy choice. In this way, the *comparative context* in which individuals make their eating choices imbues particular food choices with particular meaning and provides information about what particular eating behaviour is appropriate. Similarly, if only children at the party had helped themselves to the food or if the event was defined as a children's party, Sandra, as an adult, might be less likely to construe it as acceptable to help herself. This *normative context*, or information about what is appropriate for one's group, shapes both identity salience (so that Sandra sees herself as an adult in this context, rather than as a woman, say) and the specific identity-relevant norms that are invoked in a particular context (as an adult, I should not eat the fairy cakes).

Speaking to this analysis, a variety of minor cues to social norms for consumption (what might be called 'nudges'; Thaler & Sunstein, 2008, but which can profitably be understood through a social identity lens; see Mols, Haslam, Steffens, & Jetten, 2015) actually account for a great deal of the variance in food choice and intake in many studies. For instance, serving sizes (Jeffery et al., 2007), the size of crockery (Raghubir & Krishna, 1999), music (Wansink & van Ittersum, 2012), and menu order (Dayan & Bar-Hillel, 2011) have all been shown to influence consumption. All of these studies provide participants with normative information – that is, a sense of what eating behaviour is appropriate – either directly (e.g., by providing 100 cookies and asking participants to "eat as much as you like") or indirectly (e.g., by cueing participants to social norms associated with takeaway food versus restaurant food).

Testing these ideas more directly, a study by Mark Tarrant and Kathryn Butler (2011) manipulated comparative context by asking British participants to judge the healthiness of their food choices compared either to Americans (Condition 1) or to Japanese people (Condition 2). Perhaps unsurprisingly, British people perceived their choices to be healthier when the context cued a comparison with Americans. However, participants in this study also expressed greater *motivation* to engage in healthy eating in the context of a "high performing" outgroup (in this case, Japan). This finding has particular relevance to the social cognitive theories reviewed earlier, and speaks to the way in which social context, and not just individual differences, can structure cognitive phenomena such as self-control, motivation, and attitudes, and through this, shape eating behaviour.

Social identity determines attention and conformity to eating norms

In another effort to update and improve upon social cognitive theorising, a number of researchers have focused specifically on augmenting the theory of planned behaviour to incorporate social identity principles (i.e., to make the "social" in social cognitive theories a more equal partner). In this, they have demonstrated that the social norm component of the model has improved power to predict eating behaviour when participants are not asked about social norms *in general*, but rather about norms within their valued and salient *social groups*. Put another way, a body of evidence now points to the interactive impact of social identification and social norms – such that people only conform to an eating norm when they identify with its source (Åstrosm & Rise, 2001; Louis, Davies, Smith, & Terry, 2007; White, Smith, Terry, Greenslade, & McKimmie, 2009). This important finding is specified in the SIE model.

One experimental study in this vein invited participants into the laboratory ostensibly to provide ratings of promotional videos for their university (The Australian National University, ANU; Cruwys et al., 2012). Participants were provided with a tub of popcorn upon arrival "to help them feel more relaxed". They were then randomly assigned to one of five experimental conditions. The first condition was a control, in which participants did not see or speak to another participant prior to completing the study. In the other conditions, participants encountered a previous participant (actually an actor following a script) who introduced themselves as a fellow ANU student or a student at a rival tertiary institution, Canberra Institute of Technology. The previous participant also mentioned in passing either that they had eaten all of the popcorn provided or that they eaten none of it (participants also saw this person's empty or full popcorn container). In line with social identity principles (specifically, the norm enactment hypothesis, H8), we predicted that the impact of the norm set by this previous participant would vary as a function of the extent to which they were seen as an ingroup (rather than an outgroup) member.

The results of the study are presented in Figure 10.6 and provided clear support for this hypothesis. Specifically, participants ate more or less popcorn in accordance with the previous participants' eating behaviour *only* when this person was a fellow ANU student. When the previous participant was an outgroup member, participants' popcorn consumption was no different from that of participants in the control condition – in other words, there was no evidence of any social influence.

A range of other studies have extended this theoretical logic to explore the relationship between social identity and obesity. In one of these, Maya Guendelman and her colleagues observed that recent immigrants to the United States are concerned with signalling their ingroup status to other Americans (Guendelman, Cheryan, and Monin, 2011). As a way of achieving this goal, they are more likely to enact behaviours they believe are consistent with the ingroup norm. In the context of eating behaviour, the authors found that behaviours seen to be consistent with the American identity included eating energy-dense, high-fat foods. The unfortunate consequence was that, among recent immigrants, identification with the new host country was associated with a greater risk of developing obesity. Here, then, as the authors put it, getting fat was a way of fitting in.

In another influential line of research, Daphna Oyserman and her colleagues (Oyserman, Fryberg, and Yoder, 2007) found that minority and disadvantaged groups in the United States often see healthy behaviours, such as going to the gym or eating salads, as outgroup behaviours – things that White middle-class people might do, but not "things *we* do". As a consequence, they found that when participants thought of themselves in terms of their minority group membership, they were less likely to choose such behaviours for themselves and instead were more likely to endorse unhealthy behaviours – such as eating take-away foods – that were more readily identified as "things we do". In a related finding, several studies by Jonah Berger and his colleagues have found that healthy eating can actually be encouraged by this tendency for people to avoid behaviours that are seen to be normative for an outgroup (Berger & Heath, 2008; Berger & Rand, 2008). Specifically, these researchers found that if unhealthy choices such as pizza and soft drink were portrayed as normative among a disliked outgroup (e.g., in their study, graduate students), people were less likely to choose these unhealthy foods themselves.

A central point that can be derived from these studies is that eating behaviour is often – in fact, probably *always* – a reflection and enactment of identity. Whether it is a family Christmas (Schmitt,

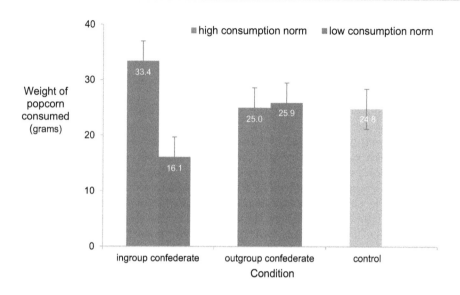

Figure 10.6 Popcorn consumption as a function of consumption norms and their source

Note: These results are from a study investigating the effects of shared group membership on eating behaviour. When participants were exposed to a fellow university student who ate more popcorn, they too ate more popcorn, and, when the fellow student ate less popcorn, so did they. Importantly, though, no such effects were observed when the student was from a rival institution. In other words, participants only conformed to eating norms when these were communicated by a member of their ingroup.

Source: Cruwys et al. (2012)

Davies, Hung, & Wright, 2010), a January detox diet, veganism, or a boycott of halal meat, it is not just that "we are what we eat" but also that *we eat what we are*. Not least, this is because a range of social identities *prescribe* and *proscribe* various forms of eating behaviour – eating fish on Fridays, not eating pork, loving grits, hating horsemeat (e.g., Hackel, Coppin, Wohl, & Van Bavel, 2015; Loughnan, Bastian, & Haslam, 2014). Moreover, it is clearly the case that the extent to which one does or does not do these various things is not so much a matter of personal taste as of social identification. There is also reason to believe that people who comply with a particular diet for ethical (e.g., vegan), religious (e.g. kosher), or health (e.g., gluten-free) reasons are typically more adherent than those who attempt to diet for weight loss reasons. Why might this be?

A hypothesis that we might derive from the SIE model is that it is not just moment-to-moment eating behaviour that can be predicted by contextually salient identities, but also that one's capacity to sustain a particularly pattern of eating behaviour over time relies upon the ongoing importance of a social identity with which such eating is consistent. In these terms, sticking to a particular diet is less about control and more about identity enactment. When it comes to dieting, "true discipline is really just self-remembering; no forcing or fighting is necessary" (Eisenstein, 2003). Thus in Case study 10.1 with which we began the chapter, Sandra might have had little problem sticking religiously to a low-fat diet when she self-defined in terms of her identity as a businesswoman, but in the home where she self-defines as a mother, a different set of priorities and relevant eating norms that this identity entails changes her behaviour in quite dramatic ways.

A recent review by Cruwys and colleagues (Cruwys, Bevelander, & Hermans, 2015) sought to examine the 69 experimental studies examining social influence and eating behaviour that have been published since 1974, with a view to understanding when and why social influence affects food intake and choice. Many studies have been conducted in an attempt to address this issue and establish moderators, or boundary conditions, of the impact of social norms on eating behaviour. However, one key conclusion drawn by this review was that norms generally exert a very powerful impact on eating behaviour, and most of the moderators that are considered important by established theorising are not supported by the evidence. Thus in only five of the studies was there no significant modelling effect (i.e., where participants did not conform to the social norm). Moreover, this modelling effect was robust across all conditions in most studies. For instance, the eating behaviour of participants who had fasted for 24 hours still conformed to social norms, and the same was true for participants who were dieting, obese, or seeking to create a positive impression or who were with familiar others (Conger, Conger, Costanzo, Wright, & Matter, 1980; Goldman, Herman, & Polivy, 1991; Herman, Koenig-Nobert, Peterson, & Polivy, 2005; Rosenthal & Marx, 1979). Accordingly, we can conclude that the power of social norms on eating is both consistent and generalisable.

Importantly, norms have been found not only to influence the eating behaviour of members of the general public but also that of young women who are at elevated risk of eating disorders. This, for example, was shown to be the case in a study conducted to explore factors that predicted the success of a group-based eating disorder prevention intervention (Cruwys, Haslam, Fox, & McMahon, 2015). Results showed that participants perceived there to be a significant shift in the norms of the group across the first two sessions of the programme such that, as the programme progressed, they were less likely to believe that fellow group members endorsed norms of dieting and thinness. In line with social identity theorising, the degree of change in these norms early on in the programme then predicted the degree of reduction in the correlates of disordered eating (thin ideal internalisation, dieting intentions, and body satisfaction) by the conclusion of the programme. In other words, social norms are important not just in shaping typical eating, but also in shaping pathological and uncommon eating. It may seem counterintuitive that *ab*normal behaviour could be influenced by what is normative. This again is where the social identity approach has particular utility, because it argues that it is the norms of the particular social group with which a person identifies – which may deviate dramatically from a societal average – that are critical in predicting a person's behaviour.

In another study that makes a similar point, young women participated in a study with a friend in which they believed they were communicating virtually via a messenger programme about images of celebrities (Cruwys, Leverington, & Sheldon, 2016). In fact, the messages that participants read were predetermined from a script such that they were (1) predominantly self-degrading, negative comments about one's body ("fat talk"; e.g., "She looks great after losing all that weight"); (2) positive, body-accepting comments ("positive body talk"; e.g., "It's great to see that she doesn't care about having her photo taken so soon after having a baby"); or (3) unrelated to appearance ("neutral talk"; e.g., "She's such a great actress"). What emerged was that participants were more likely to respond to their friend with the same kind of talk that they had read. This also had important consequences: participants who were exposed to fat talk and responded in kind were more likely to score highly on the correlates of disordered eating than those in the other conditions. That is, although all women in the study were exposed equally to the cultural thin ideal (in the form of a thin celebrity), it was the (ostensibly) expressed attitudes of a member of their friendship group that determined their risk of unhealthy eating. In line with this conclusion, the systematic review by Cruwys and colleagues (2015) concluded that shared social identity is one of the few confirmed moderators of the powerful influence of social norms on eating behaviour.

Nonetheless, it would be an oversimplification to say that eating is merely a function of an inter-action between social identification and norms that leads high identifiers to engage in whatever eating behaviours are normative for their ingroup. This overlooks complexity in the way norms emerge and are interpreted, as well as the importance of identity-based leadership in shaping group norms and the desire to act in the best interests of the group (Haslam, Reicher, & Platow, 2011; Steffens et al., 2014). In this regard, it is important to note that eating behaviour and body shapes have been not only idealised but also *moralised* within Western culture. That is, the very fact that eating and body shapes predict health outcomes has legitimised the societal value placed on particular kinds of eating and particular kinds of bodies (Saguy & Gruys, 2010; see also Chapter 4). Accordingly, various forms of eating behaviours are seen to signal not just health but also purity, goodness, and virtue – in part because they are seen as challenging and arduous to perform (Conrad, 1994; Rozin, 1996). A social consequence of this is that people may sometimes aim to present themselves as engaging in such behaviours (e.g., choosing salad over chips) more than they really do.

We have recently demonstrated that such reasoning can lead to a paradoxical form of count-er-normative influence in social groups whereby participants are *less* likely to engage in healthy eating behaviours when they are normative of a group with which they strongly identify. Specifically, in three studies results showed that when the eating behaviour of participants' ingroup was depicted in virtuous terms ("good", "healthy", "correct"), high identifiers engaged in vicarious licensing (see Kouchaki, 2011; Wilcox, Vallen, Block, & Fitzsimons, 2009). This vicarious effect enabled partici-pants to experience the healthy eating behaviour of the group as their own and, as a result, they were less likely to personally engage in healthy eating behaviours themselves (Banas, Cruwys et al., 2016). Lower identifiers, on the other hand, showed a more typical normative influence effect. Although these patterns were complex, the key point they confirm is that group norms exert a powerful influ-ence over eating behaviour, but this is contingent on eaters internalising the group membership with which those norms are associated as part of their sense of self. This speaks to the fact that food consumption is an important way of living out valued identities, but that, psychologically speaking, identity itself is a moveable feast.

Group-based stigma can fuel an epidemic of unhealthy eating

In addition to this paradoxical "backfiring" of healthy eating norms, the moralisation of eating behaviour has a variety of other negative consequences. Chief among these is that it exacerbates the low-status position of people who are obese, as well as marginalising those who deviate from the thin ideal. As an example, consider people who are considered medically 'overweight' (defined as having a body mass index between 25 and 30). A recent study of over 100,000 people corroborates previous findings that being in this overweight category does not predict worse health outcomes than having a lower BMI, and is, in fact, associated with longer life expectancy than a so-called "normal" BMI of between 18 and 25 (Afzal, Tybjærg-Hansen, Jensen, & Nordestgaard, 2016). However, the over-weight category is often lumped together with obesity (which can indeed compromise health), not only by media and other commentators, but also by health researchers. This is perhaps one example of how cultural standards of beauty permeate not just women's media, but also health care, thereby compounding the stigmatisation of those whose body shape does not conform to societal standards (in ways discussed in Chapter 4).

Indeed, the severity of discrimination against people who are obese is so severe it can be con-sidered a significant contributor to the cluster of eating pathology described earlier in the chapter (Polivy & Herman, 1985). Specifically, H5 states that when status differences between groups are perceived to be legitimate and boundaries between groups are perceived to be permeable, people will be most likely to seek to *leave* the low-status group via strategies of *individual mobility*. In the case of people who are obese, overweight, or even at a healthy weight, strategies such as dieting, purging, and exercise can be conceptualised as attempts at precisely such individual mobility. Moreover, much as the 'token' promotion of one or two women can create the perception of permeability in workplace leadership (Danaher & Branscombe, 2010), so successful weight loss stories that proliferate in mainstream women's entertainment and advertising mistakenly foster the belief that weight is controllable and one can readily transition from the low-status 'obese' group into the high-status 'thin' group via strategies such as dieting. In fact, this is not the case. Instead, we know from many years of research that the majority of people who diet achieve only a brief plateau in a longer trajectory of weight gain. Dieting is thus, at best, an ineffective, and at worst, an actively counterproductive strategy for achieving weight loss (Lowe & Timko, 2004; Presnell, Stice, & Tristan, 2008; Stice, Cameron, Killen, Hayward, & Taylor, 1999).

Beyond individual mobility (in the form of dieting), other identity-management strategies (*social creativity*, H6, and *social competition*, H7) are less commonly deployed by people with obesity (but see Figure 10.7 for an example). However, they are possible, and in line with social identity theorising (after Tajfel & Turner, 1979), they can be seen to afford more realistic prospects for social change. As evidence of this, in recent years a growing body acceptance movement has been met with increased enthusiasm by a range of public commentators (e.g., Health at Every Size – http://haescommunity. com/) and can be seen to have had a range of positive consequences. Not least this is because it allows people who are obese to draw upon a range of identity resources (including support from ingroup members) that gives them the confidence to escape a vicious cycle of body dissatisfaction and dieting. In line with the new psychology of health that we have advanced in this book as a whole, there is

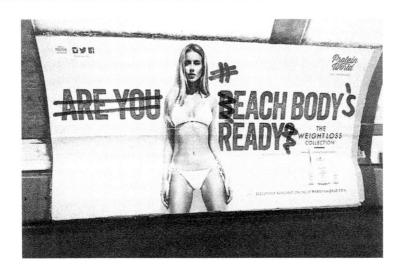

Figure 10.7 An example of a body image–related social change strategy

Note: This is an example of a challenge to prevailing cultural representations of approporiate body size. The original advert for a protein supplement asking "ARE YOU BEACH BODY READY?" was met with a storm of protest – both formal (e.g., through complaints to the Advertising Standards Authority) and informal (by defacing the poster, as here).

Source: Flickr, the authors

preliminary evidence too that this is beneficial for both the mental and physical health of the individuals involved (Lewis et al., 2011).

Conclusion

Tell me what you eat and I will tell you who you are.
Jean Anthelme Brillat-Savarin

To conclude, we can return to the example of Sandra with which we began this chapter (Case study 10.1). Sandra is typical of the modern reality of unhealthy eating – struggling with a combination of obesity, unhealthy weight loss strategies, body dissatisfaction, and discrimination. We have reviewed a variety of models that help us to understand eating. Because each of these models has important (and complementary) things to say and contribute to our understanding of disordered eating, we argued that the way forward for the field is not to plumb for one approach at the expense of another, but rather to find a non-trivial way of integrating their insights. The social identity perspective offers a dynamic model of multi-level integration in which the internalisation of group memberships is seen as the *mechanism* through which socio-cultural realities (which cue norms associated with specific social identities) come to have concrete consequences for eating behaviour and, ultimately, for health.

This analysis is spelled out concretely within the situated identity enactment model that recent work in the social identity tradition has sought to elaborate and test. By attending to context, identity, and norms, this makes specific predictions about social environments and social group memberships that may increase the risk of unhealthy eating and also makes some concrete recommendations about how to mitigate such risk.

A key message here is that eating, like all behaviour, is fundamentally a reflection and instantiation of our social beings. Indeed, it is worth noting that eating and social identity thus coalesce not only around pathology but also around festivology (e.g., Christmas, Thanksgiving, Ramadan; Fischler, 1988; Scholliers, 2001). The great French gastronome, Jean Brillat-Savarin, was thus correct to observe that what we eat determines who we are, but it is also the case that who we are determines what we eat. In these terms, unhealthy eating is not so much a sign of pathology in individuals as a sign of pathology in groups. Accordingly, it is to groups – and to group psychology – that we must turn if we wish to address the problems that unhealthy eating creates both for individuals and for society.

Points for practice

Arising from the discussion in this chapter, the following points are some of the most important for practitioners working in the area of unhealthy eating:

1. *Structural interventions that target the social context are likely to be most effective in achieving widespread improvement in unhealthy eating.* Examples of such interventions include regulating junk food advertising, eliminating taxes on fresh fruit and vegetables, and banning ultra-thin models from fashion shows. Because social context affects the content of social norms and the social identities that become salient, changes to this are likely

to have sustained and broad effects. Their efficacy is also well supported by empirical evidence (e.g., Brownwell & Frieden, 2009; Magnus, Haby, Carter, & Swinburn, 2009)

2. *Interventions which rely on individual self-control are likely to fail, as well as to increase discrimination directed at those who experience unhealthy eating.* Individual choices about health behaviour are strongly shaped by social context and social influence, and are therefore rarely successful in combating entrenched patterns of behaviour that stem from environments that are not conducive to healthy eating.

3. *Practitioners should support body acceptance as a means of improving the mental and physical health of people who struggle with unhealthy eating.* Body acceptance is not just an individual belief, but also a social change movement that challenges the moral value placed on thinness and resists the discrimination directed at people who experience unhealthy eating. Such a movement is likely to benefit mental health by reducing the shame associated with one's body shape and size, and to benefit physical health by reducing unhealthy, and ultimately unsuccessful, efforts at weight loss.

Resources

Further reading

To find out more about the social identity approach to eating, the following papers are a good place to start.

① Cruwys, T., Platow, M. J., Rieger, E., Byrne, D. G., & Haslam, S. A. (2016). The social psychology of disordered eating: The Situated Identity Enactment model. *European Review of Social Psychology, 27, 160–195.*

This article presents the social identity enactment model and supporting evidence in the context of eating disorders.

② Guendelman, M. D., Cheryan, S., & Monin, B. (2011). Fitting in but getting fat: Identity threat and dietary choices among U.S. immigrant groups. *Psychological Science*, 22, 959–967.

This paper uses the social identity approach to understand the distribution of obesity in migrant groups in the United States.

③ Cruwys, T., Bevelander, K. E., & Hermans, R. C. J. (2015). Social modeling of eating: A review of when and why social influence affects food intake and choice. *Appetite, 86,* 3–18.

This review article provides a comprehensive overview of experimental research that explores the role of social influence in eating.

④ Fardouly, J., Pinkus, R. T., & Vartanian, L. R. (2017). The impact of appearance comparisons made through social media, traditional media, and in person in women's everyday lives. Body Image, 20, 31–39. http://doi.org/10.1016/j.bodyim.2016.11.002

Video

① Search for "Kilbourne Lafayette ads" to watch a TEDx talk in which Joan Kilbourne explores how the advertising industry creates and promulgates misleading images of women's bodies and which explores the range of negative effects that this has on individuals and society. www.youtube.com/watch?v=Uy8yLaoWybk   (16 minutes)

Websites

①   http://haescommunity.com/. The Health at Any Size Movement aims to combat the discrimination targeted at people on the basis of their weight – promoting respect, awareness, and compassionate self-care. It offers resources for the general public and practitioners aiming to provide a supportive service for overweight and obese people.

②   www.nationaleatingdisorders.org/get-involved/the-body-project. This is the website of the National Eating Disorders Association (NEDA) in the United States. It provides useful information about these disorders as well as about ways to tackle them, including The Body Project.

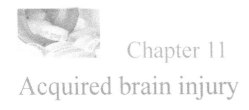

Chapter 11

Acquired brain injury

Probably the best-known case of acquired brain injury (ABI) is that of Phineas Gage (see Figure 11.1) who suffered a major injury after a 6-kg, 1.1-metre-long tamping iron was blown through his head while he was working as a blasting foreman on a railroad construction project in Vermont (Twomey, 2010). Gage is known to most students of neuroscience and psychology through textbooks that describe him as so radically and permanently changed after this injury that one might imagine he had little hope for recovery. However, recent interrogation of Gage's case by Malcolm Macmillan and Matthew Lena sheds a very different light on his story (Macmillan & Lena, 2010). For whereas many reports suggest that he lived out the rest of his life as the victim of his impulses and "animal propensities" (Harlow, 1868, p. 339; Macmillan, 2000), what these typically fail to note is that Gage actually adapted well to his injury and made a reasonable recovery (see Griggs, 2015, for a discussion of how Gage is represented in contemporary introductory psychology textbooks). Certainly, there is general agreement that Gage was 'no longer himself' after the accident, but it was clear too that he generally functioned quite well in society (Macmillan, 2008). Reports indicate that he was able to regain and maintain meaningful employment that engaged him physically, cognitively, and socially and also provided him with a means to support himself financially. Accordingly, instead of being seen as a classic case of the irreversible effects of brain injury, Gage should probably be held up as an example of the remarkable psychosocial adaptation that is possible even after devastating injury. But this then raises an important question: How does such psychosocial adaptation come about? It is on this question that we focus this chapter.

One feature of Gage's experience that is common in ABI is the need to adapt to a changed self. As the following quote illustrates, this involves coming to terms with the fact that one is no longer 'the same person' that one was before the injury (Ownsworth, 2014):

> I wasn't the way I used to [be] . . . 35 years builds you up dealing with everything to get you to that point, then one day this happens, you wake up with a totally different everything.
> (Muenchberger, Kendall, & Neal, 2008, p. 985)

Such change is not simply a consequence of the physical disability that arises from ABI, although this certainly contributes to outcomes. Instead, very often it is driven by cognitive and psychological changes (i.e., to social and emotional functioning) which are far more impactful in the longer term across the different forms of the condition (Wilson, 2008). These symptoms often present the greatest challenge to recovery and, because they are often not visible, they contribute to the characterisation of brain injury as a hidden disability. In this chapter we start by examining current understanding of the nature of such injury and approaches to its treatment, before considering how a social identity approach builds on this to provide new directions to assist in the management of ABI.

The nature and impact of ABI

Acquired brain injury (ABI) is a major cause of disability and death worldwide (WHO, 2008). It refers to any damage to the brain that occurs after birth and can either be *traumatic* where it is

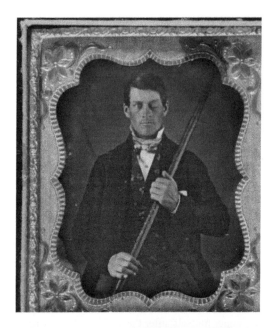

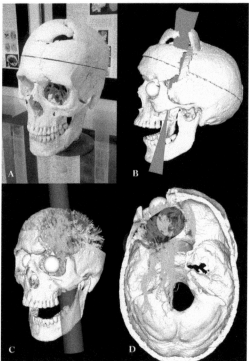

Figure 11.1 Phineas Gage

Note: The top photograph shows Gage holding the tamping iron that was the cause of his brain injury; the images in the figure below this are reconstructions of the brain damage caused by his accident.

Source: (a) Wilgus & Wilgus, 2009; (b) Van Horn et al. (2012)

Table 11.1 Mechanisms of injury and common causes of ABI

Nature of injury	Common causes
Traumatic	Motor vehicle accident
	Concussion
	Falls
	Assault
Non-traumatic	Brain haemorrhage (e.g., stroke, aneurysm)
	Reduced oxygen to the brain (e.g., cardiac arrest)
	Viral infection (e.g., encephalitis, meningitis)
	Progressive disease (e.g., multiple sclerosis, Parkinson's disease, Alzheimer's disease)
	Brain tumour
	Brain swelling (e.g., hydrocephalus)
	Drug and alcohol misuse
	Toxic exposure (e.g., to lead)

caused by an external physical force involving a blow to the head (as in the case of Phineas Gage), or *non-traumatic* where it can have multiple causes including disease, infection, toxic poisoning, tumour, and substance misuse. Some of its most common causes are presented in Table 11.1. Progressive diseases (such as vascular dementia, Alzheimer's disease, multiple sclerosis, and Parkinson's disease) are not always listed as examples of ABI, but because these are acquired and pose similar psychosocial challenges to those experienced by people with other recognised forms of ABI, they are sometimes included among the non-traumatic causes of the condition. The incidence of ABI varies across studies and countries. To take just one example, research conducted by the Australian Institute of Health and Welfare showed that just under 433,000 (or 1 in 45) Australians experience significant activity restrictions due to disability caused by ABI. Of these, three-quarters were of working age and a third experienced severe or profound activity limitations (AIHW, 2007). As Thomas McAllister (2008) argues, though, because these figures are based mainly on hospital records, they markedly underestimate the actual number of people affected by brain injury—which he suggests is likely to be three- to four times larger.

Case study 11.1 Amanda

Amanda was 28 when she fell from a balcony at a New Year's Eve party. She fractured some ribs and broke an arm and leg in the fall, but also suffered a head injury. Over time, her broken limbs healed, but the injury to her head continued to plague her, as it led to changes from which she could not fully recover. Since her fall, she has problems concentrating for any length of time, has trouble following conversation if more than one person is talking, and has become more forgetful. She needs a lot more rest than she used to, becoming physically and mentally exhausted very easily. It takes her much longer now to think things through and plan activities. These changes have made it impossible for Amanda to keep her job as a teacher, which she loved, and she is struggling to find other possible career paths to fill this gap in her life. She is less sociable than she used to be and doesn't feel like she has any real friends any more. The friends she had from before the accident find it difficult to understand why she repeats herself and why she lashes out when she can't follow what they're saying. As a result, she sees them less and less. Amanda also avoids going out in public. She finds that social situations and being in a noisy crowd just overloads her brain. She is also afraid of being "found out" – thinking that when people discover that her brain doesn't work properly, they'll see her as "damaged goods" and avoid her anyway.

As the experiences of Amanda in Case study 11.1 suggest, in the wake of brain injury, a person's life is often very different from the one they had previously lived (see also Wilson, Winegardner, & Ashforth, 2014, for personal accounts of recovery from brain injury). This reflects the fact that brain injury has a range of serious consequences. These commonly include physical changes in the form of scarring, pain, slurred speech, motor disability, fatigue, and sexual dysfunction. Equally common are cognitive changes, the nature and extent of which are typically identified through assessment (see Lezak, Howiesen, Bigler, & Tranel, 2012, for comprehensive coverage). These affect a person's ability to reason, plan, organise, make decisions, and remember – with more than 50% of survivors reporting these problems following injury (Tate et al., 2006). Nevertheless, the particular combination of physical and cognitive changes that a person experiences following ABI varies as a function of the brain regions that have been damaged. In the case of traumatic brain injury, for example, the acceleration and deceleration of the head tends to produce more diffuse and widespread lesions throughout the brain, affecting a range of abilities that often include mental speed, attention, memory, planning, problem solving, self-awareness, and self-monitoring (e.g., Smith, Meaney, & Shull, 2003; Kumar et al., 2009).

These same functions can also be affected when someone suffers from a stroke, which is another common form of ABI. Here though, because the pathology involves disruption to blood supply (affecting the flow of oxygen that brain cells need to function), damage tends to be more localised and is often isolated to a particular hemisphere or region. This often produces a more specific pattern of cognitive impairment, with preservation of some aspects of a particular function but disturbance to others. For example, a person may be able to learn and recall visual information, but struggle to remember information they hear. These localised effects may extend to physical damage, producing weakness, paralysis, or changes in sensation to one side of the body, but which can further vary in the extent to which they affect upper and lower limb function.

These examples of injury show that getting to grips with the physical and cognitive impact of ABI on a person's life requires some understanding of brain anatomy – as the brain regions affected provide clues about the kind of impairments a person might experience. However, anatomical knowledge is not always diagnostic when it comes to understanding the psychological consequences of ABI. A key reason for this is that psychological problems – related to mood, behaviour, personality, and social participation – can present in all forms of ABI. Where there is variation, it is mostly in terms of symptom severity and in the extent to which symptoms affect a person's life, and their impact is often considerable. Indeed, rates of depression in the region of 30% to 50% have been reported not only in the early stages of a person's recovery following brain injury (e.g., Bombardier et al., 2010; Ownsworth et al., 2011), but also many years later (e.g., Wolfe et al., 2011). Anxiety is common too, with high levels in up to 70% of those who experience traumatic brain injury (Chaudhury, Pande, Saini, & Rathee, 2005) – most often in the form of posttraumatic stress, generalised anxiety, and panic disorders (Hibbard, Uysal, Kipler, Bogdany, & Silver, 1998; Gould, Ponsford, & Spitz, 2014). Consistent with this, Richard Bryant and his colleagues found depression and anxiety to be among the most common psychiatric disorders that present following traumatic brain injury (Bryant et al., 2010).

As Amanda's case illustrates, very often brain injury disrupts people's ability to participate in meaningful social activity of the form necessary for work, recreation, and daily living. In particular, after ABI, people can find it difficult to maintain social relationships, and this can have a major impact on their adjustment to injury (e.g., Degeneffe, 2001; Temkin, Corrigan, Dikmen, Marchamer, 2009). This means not only that people struggle to sustain valued friendship networks, but also that they have problems developing new ones. As a young man taking part in a study by Christian Salas and colleagues put it:

> Yeah, well all my friends before my accident couldn't handle it so they all dumped me. They couldn't cope, so they dumped me. I mean I've got new friends since, but I haven't got loads.
> (Salas, Casassus, Rowlands, Pim, & Flanagan, 2016, p. 8)

Opportunities to engage socially with others can also be limited by altered roles and other consequences of the injury (e.g., fatigue, cognitive impairment). About 18% of people with brain injury experience a breakdown in key relationships with family members or partners (Nalder et al., 2012), and this also seems to extend to wider social engagement. For example, in a study of people with ABI by Bonnie Todis and colleagues, only a quarter of participants engaged in activities that brought them into contact with other people, with the remainder generally engaging in activities on their own (Todis, Sohlberg, Hood, & Fickas, 2005). To start to appreciate the significance of this finding, stop for a moment and think what it would mean if all the things that you enjoy doing you never did with anyone else. To say that this would make your life less meaningful and a whole lot less pleasant (in ways that we discussed in Chapter 2) is something of an understatement.

For these reasons there is general consensus that it is the psychosocial (i.e., social and emotional) consequences of ABI that have the greatest bearing on client outcomes. Not only do these hinder recovery and adjustment on their own, but they also exacerbate the effects of physical and cognitive disability. As a consequence, these psychological factors have become central to the way in which brain injury is understood and how recovery is managed in rehabilitation.

Current approaches to acquired brain injury

The cognitive behavioural approach

As the earlier overview highlights, brain injury makes a person especially vulnerable to psychological and emotional distress (Levin et al., 2005; Oddy, Coughlan, Tyerman, & Jenkins, 1985; Williams, Evans, & Fleminger, 2003). It is therefore not surprising that the combination of psychosocial problems that typically present in ABI has led to widespread adoption of models and approaches that are used to manage mood and emotional disorders more generally. Of these, the cognitive behavioural approach is particularly influential and now has the strongest evidence base for treatment of psychological disturbance following ABI.

As we discussed in some detail in Chapter 8, the cognitive behavioural approach draws attention to the way in which emotional distress and maladaptive behaviour can be exacerbated by biases and distortions in thinking (Beck, 2005; Beck, 2011). In light of these, efforts to promote recovery from ABI centre on strategies akin to those that are used in mainstream cognitive behavioural therapy (CBT) – including restructuring techniques to change thinking patterns, Socratic questioning to challenge negative beliefs, and cognitive rehearsal to practice ways of countering cognitive distortions.

At the same time, though, because cognitive dysfunction is symptomatic of ABI, it has proved necessary to adapt these techniques for use with this population. In particular, this is because problems with memory and executive function (e.g., problem solving, planning, and reasoning) can impact on a person's ability to initiate and follow through with restructuring techniques, to challenge thoughts, and generate more positive ways of thinking. Tamara Ownsworth (2014) summarises the various adaptations that have been trialled among people with ABI as including (1) simplified procedures, (2) more repetition, (3) greater use of visual cues and external aids to overcome any influence of memory problems, and (4) self-instruction techniques to encourage people to stop and check before they act so that they can better monitor and regulate their behaviour (e.g., Hodgson, McDonald, Tate, & Gertler, 2005; Hsieh et al., 2012; see also Khan-Bourne & Brown, 2003).

Results from studies that draw on this adapted approach have generally been positive, and many studies report improvement in clients' post-intervention emotional well-being (e.g., Bradbury et al., 2008; Williams et al., 2003). However, these cognitive behavioural approaches are often implemented alongside other strategies to manage cognitive impairment and, as a result, it is not entirely clear whether these improvements are due to the cognitive behavioural approach per se or instead to other factors (e.g., the specific strategies that are used to compensate for impairment or the social context in which it is delivered; Fann, Hart, & Schomer, 2009). There is certainly evidence of improved outcomes following use of cognitive behavioural therapy alone (Waldron, Casserly, & O'Sullivan, 2013), and although most studies tend to find that these gains are restricted to the particular aspect of psychosocial dysfunction that the therapy targets (e.g., depression, anxiety, coping, or anger management), there is some evidence of wider effects on psychosocial functioning (Ponsford et al., 2016).

As Brian Waldron and colleagues observe, one interesting question on which the literature is mute is whether the effectiveness of cognitive behavioural approaches differs as a function of whether they are delivered one on one or in a group (Waldron et al., 2013). These researchers speculate that group-based approaches may be particularly beneficial because, by allowing people with ABI to work with others who have similar experiences, they provide unique opportunities for support and learning. At the same time, the researchers recognise that group-based interventions also present particular challenges and risks as a result of the range of social and emotional problems that people with ABI experience. Nevertheless, it would appear that these can be managed by drawing on the knowledge of skilled practitioners who understand the nature of injury and its consequences. In this context too, it is important to understand the social psychological processes that are likely to affect the participation and interaction of people with ABI in group contexts (Walsh, Fortune, Gallagher, & Muldoon, 2014). And in this regard, as we will discuss further below, the social identity approach may be especially useful in helping practitioners both (1) to understand how best to work with these social influences and (2) to determine when group-based approaches are most likely to prove positive for those involved.

The self-concept approach

We noted earlier that ABI often has a devastating impact on a person's sense of self, to the point that it is common for them to report feeling themselves to be a very different person from the one they were before their injury. Indeed, mirroring work on stigma that we discussed in Chapter 4 (e.g., after Goffman, 1963), it is not uncommon for people with ABI to describe themselves as "damaged-goods" (Ylvisaker & Feeney, 2008, p. 717) and as being less capable, more dependent, and generally less valuable than they were before their injury (Carroll & Coetzer, 2011; Ellis-Hill & Horn, 2000). There is also evidence that this altered sense of self is tied to people's social interactions with others. This is seen in Jacinta Douglas's (2012) account of Michael, who, after ABI, was "lost because he doesn't interact with others" (p. 237). Reminiscent of Neil Ansell's experience of losing himself when he sought solitude (see Chapter 2), others in this qualitative study highlighted similar experiences of social loss. For example, they reported *"I have no friends anymore, only my family", "just photos, not people"* (p. 68). As Douglas (2012) observes, this sense of social loss is generally observed to result from, but also to feed into, limited opportunities for people to live out and realise important aspects of themselves (e.g., as a teacher in Amanda's case), and it makes it difficult for them to maintain some semblance of continuity with their pre-injury self.

Increasingly, researchers and practitioners are recognising the impact that ABI has on a person's self-concept (see Beadle, Ownsworth, Fleming, & Shum, 2016, Ownsworth, 2014). A recent review evaluated the effect of rehabilitation in general on changes in self-concept following traumatic brain injury (Ownsworth & Haslam, 2016). Looking specifically at the impact of psychotherapy, family-based support, cognitive rehabilitation, and activity-based interventions, the researchers found evidence of positive enhancement in self-concept in 10 of the 17 studies reviewed. Overall, though, the evidence base was small and limited and the findings mixed. Nevertheless, it was an instructive exercise in highlighting the need to focus on, and further improve, measurement of self-concept change in intervention.

On the measurement front, there have been a number of developments over the years in indexing the self-concept with a view to better understanding the nature of these changes in brain injury. In this regard, the Head Injury Semantic Differential Scale (Tyerman, 1987; Tyerman & Humphrey, 1984) is probably the tool that is most widely used for measuring changes in self-concept in brain injury populations. To index these changes in self, people are asked to make judgements about themselves before and after injury, but also to think about *who they aspire to be* through use of adjectives that are presented along a continuum (e.g., attractive-unattractive, active-inactive, irritable-calm, bored-interested; see Ownworth, 2014, for a description). The aim is to identify discrepancies in these aspects of self which are seen to undermine adjustment and then to use this information to help people develop a more positive and functional sense of self in light of the changes brought about by injury.

Closer interrogation of these changes has led to the development of a number of models of identity change following brain injury, each of which provides a framework to help resolve self-discrepancy. In one of these, Fergus Gracey and his colleagues propose the *Y-shaped model* that is represented schematically in Figure 11.2 (Gracey, Evans, & Malley, 2009). In this, people are encouraged by rehabilitation practitioners to develop a more coherent sense of self by learning to reconcile discrepancies between the post-injury self they experience and the self they aspire to. Here the left arm of the Y represents the current self and the right arm the aspired-to self, with each containing aspects of identity that are both personal (e.g., an individual's idiosyncratic roles, lost abilities, coping style) and social (e.g., relationships with others, forms of social participation, social stigma). As the model suggests, the experienced and the aspired-to selves are likely to be highly discrepant initially, as reflected by the distance between the two arms, but the aim of intervention is to work progressively towards their reconciliation within an integrated and coherent sense of self such that the two arms come together at the base of the Y.

Gracey and colleagues argue that such resolution is best achieved through a series of 'behavioural experiments' which help a person test and reflect upon their self-relevant beliefs with a view to producing a more realistic self-appraisal. For example, after ABI it is common for people to believe that they have become entirely dependent on others. But this belief can be tested behaviourally to determine the extent to which it is true – for instance, by setting the goal of completing a specified task and evaluating how many of its elements require support and how many can be performed independently. If a person proves capable of performing elements of the task on their own, additional experiments are then devised to help consolidate and embed the perception of a more independent and functional self in a range of different situations. Clearly this is a demanding process, but early data suggest that it can be an effective means of improving mood, self-esteem, and social participation (e.g., Cooper, Gracey, Malley, Deakins, & Prince, 2010; Gracey & Ownsworth, 2012).

Another model through which to achieve identity reconstruction involves a procedure known as *metaphoric identity mapping* (MIM; Ylvisaker et al., 2008). As with the Y-shaped model, this aims to help people with ABI develop a more realistic and valued sense of self after injury. Here, though, the process of self-reconstruction is promoted through the use of metaphor. This involves identifying a positive and personally meaningful metaphor – which can be a person, an animal, an image, or a symbol that embodies a quality the injured person aspires to have – whilst reflecting on the reasons for

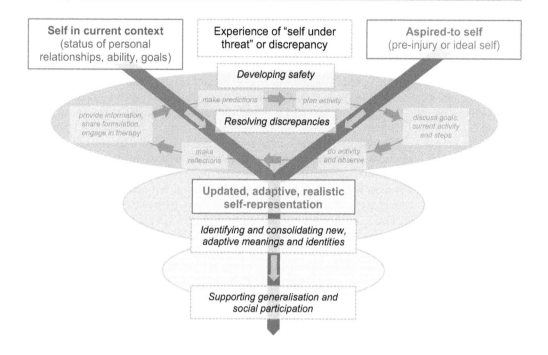

Figure 11.2 The Y-shaped model of rehabilitation

Note: Through a series of behavioural experiments (signified by ellipses in the figure) a person learns to resolve discrepancies between their experienced and aspired-to self. As a result their sense of self-discrepancy reduces (i.e., the arms of the Y converge) and they are thereby able to achieve a coherent sense of identity.

Source: Gracey, Evans, & Malley (2009), reproduced with permission

their choice (e.g., choosing Malcolm X as a metaphor because he is determined and fights against the odds, or a lion because it symbolises strength). To support identity change, people are then encouraged to internalise and strive to become the metaphor and to work strategically towards set goals in the way that the metaphor or symbol would.

Evidence from clients and practitioners suggests that this model is particularly useful in helping ABI sufferers to develop a more positive self-concept (Ylvisaker & Feeney, 2000; Ylvisaker et al., 2008). However, as with the cognitive behavioural approach, its efficacy can be limited by the nature of cognitive impairment itself. Specifically, Mark Ylvisaker and colleagues recognised that deficits in areas of memory and idea generation can present barriers to metaphor internalisation (Ylvisaker et al., 2008). More evidence is also needed to show (1) that the process of reflecting on the particular traits and behaviours of a metaphor actually does more than facilitate goal attainment (Playford, Siegert, Levack, & Freeman, 2009) and (2) that it actually promotes identity reconstruction (Caplan et al., 2016).

A third model that recognises, and seeks to overcome, the threat to a person's self-concept that results from brain injury has been developed by Caroline Ellis-Hill and her colleagues (Ellis-Hill, Payne, & Ward, 2008). Their *life thread model* emphasises the importance of striving to re-create a sense of self and identity through the development of a *life thread symbol*. This involves weaving together the different stories and memories of a person's life into a coherent overarching self-narrative. This process focuses on all those threads of a person's life that have been disrupted through injury – not only the physical and financial changes, but also those impacting on the roles a person has in life, their social relationships, and access to opportunities. When these threads are intact and integrated (as is typically the case before injury), they provide the basis for self-coherence and continuity. However, following ABI, the threads can be seen to become frayed and severed, and hence must be re-established or re-woven to make sense of one's life. Along the lines of narrative therapy that we discussed as an approach to the treatment of trauma more generally (see Chapter 6), this approach centres on the idea that by sharing stories with others it is possible for a person to regain a sense of self-coherence and stability.

In slightly different ways, these three models all highlight the importance of striving to reconstruct a sense of personal self following ABI. And although self-concept approaches have primarily informed the rehabilitation of specific populations (e.g., those with stroke or TBI, as seen in work by Ellis-Hill, Ylvisaker, and their colleagues) it is clear that they have broad relevance as a framework for conceptualising and responding to the changes that arise from all forms of ABI. In particular, all three models share an emphasis on the need for the process of self-reconstruction to involve collaboration with significant others (e.g., family members, work colleagues) and for it to take place in the broader social context within which the self is lived out (e.g., the home, the community). This is seen in the Y-shaped model's behavioural experiments, in the setting of the goals that metaphors help to achieve, and in the sharing of stories that serve to regain a sense of self-continuity.

In line with these ideas, it is apparent that the process of clarifying personal roles and identities is critical for recovery from ABI. What is less clear, however, is how these approaches can account for the particular role that loss of social group relationships appears to play in undermining a person's sense of self after brain injury (Haslam, Holme et al., 2008). As we have stressed throughout this volume, groups are not only an important source of support, but also inform our sense of who we are within our social world (Tajfel & Turner, 1979). It is through family, friendship, professional, and interest groups, for example, that we come to understand what is important to us in life and which principles and values we choose to live by (Postmes & Jetten, 2006). Group-based relationships – which are often changed dramatically following ABI – are therefore central not only to the nature of the self that emerges after injury but also to efforts to reshape that self. As we will see later in this chapter, refining self-concept models in ways that allow us to better understand and manage these changes to the social self has therefore been one of the main objectives of social identity research in this area.

The holistic approach

The holistic approach originated in the work of Yehuda Ben-Yishay (1978), Leonard Diller (1976), and George Prigatano (1986), who all argued for the importance of dealing with the social and emotional changes brought about by brain injury alongside efforts to deal with physical and cognitive change. As with similar responses to health challenges that we have discussed in other chapters (e.g., Chapter 8), the holistic approach is allied with the "biopsychosocial" model of health (Wright, Zeeman, & Biezaitis, 2016, p. 1) – which was developed to counter reductionist approaches that prioritise the medical aspects of disease and illness. In ABI the holistic approach provides a framework for engaging with the complex *interactive* effects that changes in a person's biology (e.g., brain swelling, haemorrhage, paralysis, seizures), psychology (e.g., cognitive impairment, behaviour change, mood disturbances), and social circumstances (e.g., relationship breakdown, recreational limitations, and changed employment prospects) have on their life after injury (Wilson, 2002; see also Wilson, Gracey, Evans, & Bateman, 2009). This understanding is then used to inform health care delivery. As Barbara Wilson (2008) argues, an understanding of each factor is essential, but on its own is insufficient. So, for example, we might implement a specific cognitive intervention to help a person compensate for memory problems (e.g., training them to use electronic aids to remember appointments and things they need to do; Kim, Burke, Dowds, & George, 1999; Kim, Burke, Dowds, Boone, & Park, 2000). But if we ignore the symptoms of depression that will often present alongside those memory problems (e.g., those that result from them feeling inadequate) or the impact that memory loss has on their social activity (e.g., their ability to continue to play bridge with their friends), then the treatment is likely to be suboptimal. Indeed, failure to attend to these other factors can sometimes make the problem worse.

Rather than dealing with different aspects of brain injury in isolation, interventions informed by the holistic approach strive to integrate insights from the multiple perspectives offered by an interdisciplinary team. These will often involve (1) psycho-education (to enhance understanding of disability), (2) cognitive assessment and intervention (e.g., to understand and treat deficiencies in attention, planning, and problem solving), (3) other psychological intervention (e.g., cognitive behavioural therapy to treat mood and behaviour problems, Y-shaped models to manage identity change), (4) physiotherapy for mobility problems, (5) training of functional skills to regain independence (e.g., in activities of daily living), and (6) vocational training. Group treatment is also a common feature of these programmes, and it is used to facilitate collaborative learning among individuals who confront similar challenges and to compensate for – and help to overcome – problems in thinking, mobility, communication, and social integration. Although the specific content varies across programmes, all share the same fundamental goal of enhancing functional outcomes. The key message here is that practitioners can only optimise ABI outcomes if they recognise and manage *all* of its sequelae.

This integrative approach to treatment has been found to improve participation in work and education (e.g., Klonoff, Lamb, Henderson, & Shepherd, 1998; Salazar, et al., 2000) and to increase participation in community activities (e.g., Malec, 2001; Sander, Roebuck, Sturchen, Sherer, & High, 2001). Furthermore, a systematic review by Keith Cicerone and colleagues underscores the utility of the approach as a means of improving community integration, independence, and productivity many years after injury (Cicerone et al., 2011). This utility has many different dimensions, including (1) the generally positive reactions of recipients, practitioners, and others involved in the rehabilitation process (Wilson, et al., 2014; Wright et al., 2016); (2) the value of learning with and from others; and (3) the delivery of sustained benefits. These elements have all contributed to the holistic approach being the preferred approach to brain injury rehabilitation today (Cicerone et al., 2011). Indeed, although concerns have been raised about the cost of multi-dimensional programmes, it has been argued that these are outweighed by the savings that are derived in the long-term (Prigatano & Pliskin, 2002).

Nevertheless, of all the components that contribute to holistic practices, the social are probably the least clearly specified – tending largely to be characterised in terms of participation (e.g., vocational, leisure; World Health Organization, 2001). Although participation and engagement are important, they cannot alone account for the broader impact of social processes on the course of ABI (Haslam, Holme et al., 2008). Take, for example, the impact that the stigma of brain injury has on a person's economic and social circumstances or the social disadvantage they can experience as a result of an inability to work. As we saw in Chapters 3 and 4, the impact of these factors on health is widely recognised, but they are not always a priority when it comes to helping people adjust to ABI. More generally too, theorising in the field of brain injury places little emphasis or value on the importance of understanding the processes through which such factors have an impact. This is unfortunate because this limits the potential for approaches to the management of brain injury to benefit from wider theorising that might integrate models of ABI outcomes and treatments with those seen in the management of other conditions (Haslam, Jetten, Haslam, & Knight, 2008). Looking at ways in which social identity research might redress this state of affairs will therefore be our main focus in the remainder of this chapter.

The social identity approach to acquired brain injury

Adjustment to acquired brain injury involves processes of social identity change

Throughout this volume we present theoretical arguments and empirical data that point to the powerful impact of group memberships on health. Amongst other things, we show that group membership has the capacity to impact positively on health when groups are internalised and thereby help to inform our sense of self, when they provide us with social support in periods of challenge and adversity, and when they encourage us to engage in positive health behaviours. However, it is not uncommon for people who experience ABI to lose their membership in groups, to experience problems maintaining group memberships, and to struggle to join new groups. As a consequence, people find they have access to fewer psychological resources to support their adjustment precisely at the time when they need those resources most.

In seeking to understand why this loss and change in social group relationships impacts so greatly on ABI outcomes, it is instructive to return to the social identity model of identity change (SIMIC) that we first introduced in Chapter 3. Not least this is because SIMIC was initially developed precisely to theorise about changes to identity of the form that ABI typically entails (Haslam, Holme et al., 2008).

As we discussed in Chapter 3 (e.g., Figure 3.5), SIMIC identifies key group processes that help protect people against the negative effects that significant life changes can have on well-being. Fundamental to the model is the idea that belonging to multiple social groups prior to a life-changing event is critical to a person's ability to negotiate change successfully. This is because those group memberships have the capacity to support well-being in two ways (Haslam, Holme et al., 2008; Iyer, Jetten, Tsivrikos, Postmes, & Haslam, 2009; Jetten, Haslam, Iyer, & Haslam, 2010a). First, SIMIC's *social identity gain pathway* suggests that belonging to multiple groups is important because it provides a platform from which to extend our social group ties by joining new groups. Joining new groups then adds to a person's resource base in ways that tend to protect well-being by promoting adjustment (e.g., as suggested by the hypotheses presented in Chapter 2). Second, SIMIC's *social identity continuity pathway* suggests that the more groups a person belongs to, the more likely it is that they will be able to retain at least some of those group memberships after the life change. And again, those existing groups will tend to protect well-being because they provide people with a stable resource base (and an associated sense of self-continuity; Sani, 2008) that helps them adjust to the various changes they confront.

However, as a counterforce to these positive effects, it is apparent that ABI tends to compromise both of the pathways that are specified in SIMIC (Haslam, Holme et al., 2008). This in turn means that people with ABI will typically have access to fewer of the resources they need to support successful adjustment. This occurs because problems that arise following ABI can undermine a person's ability either (1) to build upon existing social group networks (in ways that promote social identity continuity) or (2) to develop news ones (in ways that promote social identity gain). Speaking to this point, it is widely acknowledged that people with ABI, like Amanda, are prone to becoming socially isolated, and this is especially true for those with severe injury (Yates, 2003). Such isolation is also experienced by family carers, and there is evidence that experiences of disconnection become more embedded over time (e.g., Douglas & Spellacy, 2000).

Yet although ABI will generally tend to compromise social identity acquisition and continuity, it is also the case that where people *are* able to gain a sense of social identity by joining new groups, this will tend to have positive implications for their health and well-being. This point is confirmed by an intervention study in which Douglas and her colleagues attempted to break the pattern of isolation experienced by people with ABI by introducing them to a programme of new community group activities (e.g., art, lawn bowling, woodwork, cricket, drama, and computing groups; Douglas, Dyson, & Foreman, 2006). The goal here was to enrich the social worlds of people with severe injury whilst allowing their families time to engage with, and benefit from, their own social networks. As hypothesised – and in line with findings from group interventions that we discuss in other chapters (especially Chapters 8, 13, and 15) – the researchers found that those who engaged regularly in group activity for more than 6 months reported greater social participation in general and also improved mental health outcomes. On the other hand, there were negligible gains among those who did not participate in group activity or who only did so for a short time.

So how exactly does sustained participation in group activity contribute to these positive outcomes? It is hard to answer this question definitively, but some clues emerged from interviews that Douglas and colleagues conducted with those who participated in the activity programme. In these, participants indicated that they gained confidence from taking part in group activities and that this participation also made them feel better about themselves. Interestingly, participants' feelings were not so much about the activities themselves as about the sense of belonging they gained and the new identities that they fostered. This was reflected in comments such as "I like being a craft person", "[I like] meeting and being with other people", and "I'm in a group, us guys" (Douglas et al., 2006, p. 144). Consistent with the identification hypothesis (H2; see also Cruwys, Haslam et al., 2014c), it thus appears that the benefits of activity groups were predicated upon participants coming to identify with those groups.

Evidence of the importance of social identity continuity for recovery emerges from another qualitative investigation by Douglas (2013) – this time of people who had been living with a severe traumatic brain injury for more than 10 years. A prominent theme that emerged from these interviews was that it was important for those who had experienced ABI to feel that they were still 'part of society', something that hinged upon their sense of connection to social groups. As in Douglas and colleagues' previous study, this was partly achieved by joining new groups – for example, "Lots of friends at the farm, where I volunteer" and "A group of guys from rehab who have had ABIs"; Douglas, 2013, p. 68). However, it was also achieved through their capacity to maintain (and in some cases strengthen) membership of groups that they had belonged to prior to their injury – for example, "Friends I had since before the accident [who] stayed with me" and "Family [who are] just there, and I know they're there for me"; Douglas, 2013, p. 68). As summarised in Figure 11.3, it thus appears that the two SIMIC pathways are both important for the well-being of ABI sufferers because they provide them with access to social identity resources that allowed them to recover and maintain their sense of self after their injury.

Quantitative evidence of the importance of the social identity continuity pathway for ABI recovery also emerged clearly from the study of people recovering from stroke in which we first tested the

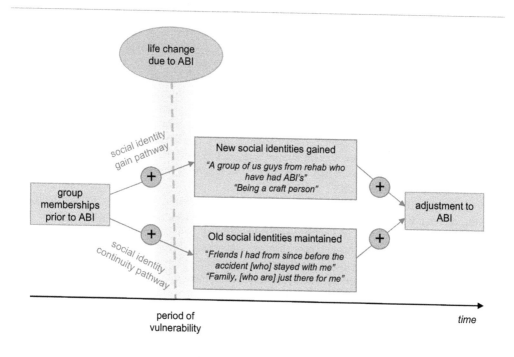

Figure 11.3 Pathways to successful social identity change in ABI

Note: As these quotes from qualitative research by Douglas (2013; Douglas et al., 2006) illustrate, successful adjustment results from social identity work that involves both (1) joining new groups and (2) maintaining old group networks.

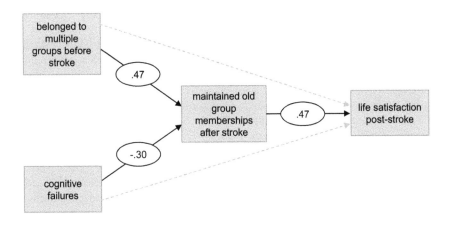

Figure 11.4 The importance of maintained group memberships for stroke recovery

Note: Analyses indicated that having multiple group memberships prior to a stroke and having cognitive problems as a result of a stroke both predicted post-stroke adjustment (i.e., life satisfaction). However, these direct pathways were non-significant when maintained old group memberships were also entered as a predictor. This suggests that belonging to multiple groups and experiencing cognitive problems are important for well-being because both determine a person's capacity to maintain group memberships after the stroke.

Source: Haslam, Holme et al. (2008)

continuity pathway of SIMIC (Haslam, Holme et al., 2008). This involved giving the participants surveys which, alongside questions about stress, cognitive functioning, and well-being, also asked them about the groups they were in before their stroke and the groups they were in after it. As Figure 11.4 shows, findings from the study indicated that having multiple group memberships before a stroke was associated with the maintenance of group memberships after that stroke ($r = .47$), and that this in turn predicted life satisfaction ($r = .47$). Speaking more directly to the underlying process here, mediation analysis showed that being in multiple groups before a stroke was important for life satisfaction after it *because* those people who were in more groups were more likely to hold on to at least some of them after their injury.

Interestingly too, further mediation analysis showed that although the cognitive difficulties associated with a stroke were predictive of reduced well-being (as previously shown by Clarke, Marshall, Black, & Colantonio, 2002; Starchina et al., 2007), this, too, was mediated by people's capacity to hold onto pre-existing group memberships after their stroke. Although, unsurprisingly, cognitive deficits were associated with compromised well-being ($r = -.36$), it thus appeared that this was primarily because they interfered with people's capacity to maintain valued group memberships ($r = .30$). This led us to the conclusion that:

> It is their implications for sustaining social life that make cognitive and physical damage particularly traumatic. Accordingly, the maintenance (and, if necessary, repair) of that social life should be treated as a primary focus of attention and intervention, rather than as a matter of only secondary concern.
>
> (Haslam, Holme et al., 2008, p. 687)

More generally, what these studies show is just how central the process of social identity change is to people's ability to lead fulfilling lives after brain injury. Notably, it appears that adjustment will typically be poor where injury reduces a person's access to a meaningful and valued group life – either by disrupting their membership of the social groups they belonged to before injury or by limiting their ability to join new groups after injury.

But just as SIMIC allows us to understand why this is the case, so too the model provides clear targets for *intervention*. For where effort is made to develop and strengthen the social group ties that are implicated in the two pathways that are specified in the model, it is clear that there is considerable potential for positive adjustment (Douglas, 2013; Haslam, Holme et al., 2008). This is a point we will unpack in much more detail in Chapter 15 where we describe an intervention that targets both social identity gain and social identity continuity pathways (GROUPS 4 HEALTH; Haslam, Cruwys, Haslam, Dingle, & Chang, 2016c). At this point, though, it is worth noting that this agenda is very much in line with the goals of self-concept and holistic approaches to rehabilitation (e.g., Gracey & Ownsworth, 2012; Wilson, 2008). Indeed, SIMIC provides a particularly useful framework for this work because it offers practitioners a wider perspective on the nature of self-concept change following ABI, whilst orienting them to the key ways in which holistic rehabilitation can encourage adaptive forms of identity change.

People with ABI can pursue a range of different self-enhancement strategies

One question that has particular relevance in an ABI context is how those who experience brain injury represent themselves to the world. In particular, is it better for them to self-categorize as someone with a brain injury or as a non-injured (i.e., 'normal') person?

On the one hand, defining oneself in terms of one's condition – for example, as a person with dementia, stroke, or head injury – can open up opportunities to access support from people who have similar experiences and who self-categorize in the same way. Along these lines, Linda Clare and colleagues drew on a social identity framework to explain how networks of people with ABI can promote positive identity and well-being (Clare, Rowlands, & Quin, 2008). In their research they interviewed people from an online mutual support and self-help group for people with dementia. What they found was that the network became like a family for its members – providing them with a platform for reciprocal support and a means to (re)gain a sense of pride, ongoing purpose, self-worth, and value in society despite their diagnosis (in ways suggested in Chapter 2).

On the other hand, though, as we saw when discussing stigma in Chapters 3 and 8, there are also contexts in which identification with injury groups can compromise one's self-worth, particularly where it signifies disability or a sense that a person is in some way "damaged goods". Yet regardless of the stigma associated with ABI and the challenge it creates in maintaining a positive self-concept, as the identity restoration hypothesis (H4) suggests, those with ABI are motivated to regain a positive sense of self. How, then, might this be achieved?

Along the lines of ideas that we set out in Chapter 2, the social identity approach highlights two ways in which people with ABI can try to restore a positive sense of self (after Tajfel & Turner, 1979). As illustrated in Figure 11.5, the particular path chosen depends on the extent to which a person's membership of a given group (e.g., people with stroke) is seen (1) as fixed (i.e., where group boundaries are impermeable and they cannot leave the group – for example, because there is no prospect of complete recovery) and (2) secure (i.e., so that the group is stable or legitimate – for example, because there is no suggestion of misdiagnosis).

When a person's injury is relatively mild, where the physical effects of ABI are less obvious so the condition can be hidden, and when there is no perceived benefit associated with belonging to an injury group, the mobility hypothesis (H5) suggests that individuals are likely to try to distance themselves from the ABI group and to seek to present themselves to the world as non-injured or "healthy". However, this mobility strategy is less viable when the injury or illness is more severe, and in this context another strategy must be pursued. Here, the creativity hypothesis (H6) suggests that one way

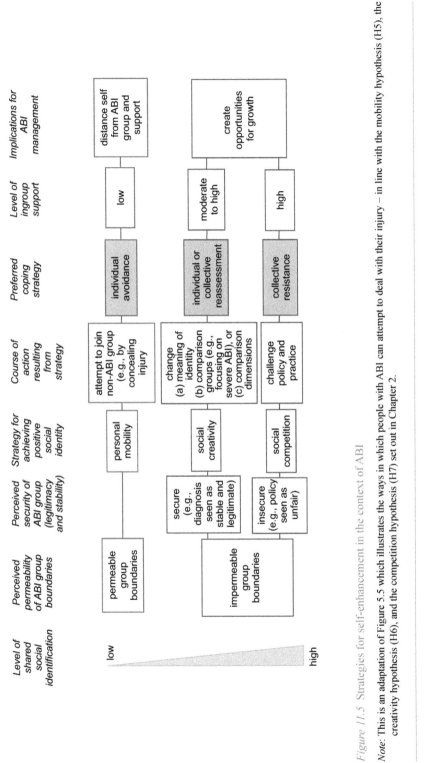

Figure 11.5 Strategies for self-enhancement in the context of ABI

Note: This is an adaptation of Figure 5.5 which illustrates the ways in which people with ABI can attempt to deal with their injury – in line with the mobility hypothesis (H5), the creativity hypothesis (H6), and the competition hypothesis (H7) set out in Chapter 2.

of striving to regain a sense of positive identity is by redefining what it means to have a brain injury. In ways suggested by Tajfel and Turner (1979), this may lead people to make downward social comparisons (e.g., with other people who have more severe injuries) and to avoid upward social comparisons (e.g., with people who do not have a brain injury). The idea here is that although a person with ABI may recognise that they are worse off than people without an injury, they can still appreciate that they are better off than those who are more severely affected. Indeed, as we will see later, this shift in social comparison may sometimes provide a basis for posttraumatic growth.

Social creativity strategies are more likely to be adopted when negative beliefs about people with ABI are seen to be legitimate. This occurs, for example, when those with ABI see themselves as disabled and as less entitled to participate fully in all aspects of life (e.g., employment, recreation). However, the social competition hypothesis (H7) suggests that the more people with ABI see such beliefs as unfair and as not adequately representing their abilities and rights, the more likely it is that they will

Here are a few of our issues.

We would like to see the doctors develop a "Post TBI Syndrome" classification.

We would like the definitions of ABI and TBI to be consistent in all of the medical organizations, associations, professional societies, governments, etc.

We would like people to understand that TBI is a form of ABI, but the two terms are not synonymous.

We would like politically correct terminology utilized to identify us. For example, change Persistent Vegetative State to Persistent Wakeful But Unaware State.

We would like organizations not to harvest patient data about us for profit, especially without our knowledge or consent.

We would like folks to pay attention to our survivor priorities. We put the safety net for survivors as the number one priority ahead of cognitive retraining by rehabilitation hospitals (although that is important also).

We would like helmets on children, and adults also, in activities such as bicycling, skiing, etc.

We would like every association operating in our name to have survivor board members or at least a brain injury survivor advisory council in operation.

We have so many, many concerns. As of 11–20–10 we have over 70 policies on these and other topics.

We invite you folks who have not had a brain injury but insist that you represent our concerns to read them.

That is our advocacy. Our ideas.

Figure 11.6 Pursuing social change in ABI management

Note: These extracts from the website of the Brain Injury Network in the United States are indicative of the ways in which it seeks to challenge prevailing policies and practices related to the management of ABI.

Source: www.braininjurynetwork.org/braininjuryadvocacy.html

push back against these beliefs and to work with others to collectively improve their situation (e.g., in ways discussed in Chapter 5). This strategy is rarely discussed or investigated explicitly in the ABI literature, so we do not elaborate on it further. Nonetheless, it is clear that in the world at large, groups that campaign for the rights of people with brain injury (e.g., Headway in the UK, Synapse in Australia, the Brain Injury Network in the United States; see Figure 11.6) are increasingly focused on the need to challenge – and *change* – assumptions, policies, and laws that are seen as unfair and discriminatory.

People with ABI can pursue a strategy of individual mobility
by choosing not to disclose their injury

As we noted earlier, when symptoms are not obvious and so can be concealed, people with ABI can choose not to disclose their condition to others. Indeed, under these circumstances, a person can choose whether to identify or not identify as someone with a head injury. A key good reason for adopting the latter, distancing, strategy is that it allows people to avoid any perceived stigma or discrimination, and this, in turn, may allow them to maintain a positive view of the self (see Figure 11.7). Along these lines, a person may refuse to seek out injury support groups because their members are not seen to reflect the way the person sees themselves. As one of the people with brain injury studied by Heidi Muenchberger and her colleagues put it, "I'm not like them . . . I didn't want to be a part of a group that had a disability . . . and my disability was quite invisible to look at" (Muenchberger et al., 2008, p. 987).

This pathway is described by Janelle Jones and colleagues in work which argues that non-disclosure can also be beneficial because it minimises the need for a person to present themselves publicly

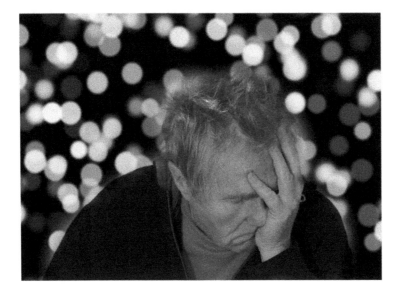

Figure 11.7 The stigma and concealment of acquired brain injury

Note: Negative perceptions of various forms of ABI can lead people to conceal their diagnosis if they can. However, because this personal mobility strategy cuts them off from social support, it can be problematic.

Source: Max Pixel

as in some way altered (Jones, Jetten, Haslam, & Williams, 2012). Even though non-disclosure is not always possible (e.g., with those one knows well and with whom one interacts frequently), where it is, it can reduce the likelihood that a person will have to deal with the uncomfortable social interactions that we saw earlier in Amanda's case – negative evaluations, discrimination, and even social exclusion. This can seem like an attractive option because people who have brain injury may have low self-esteem to start with (Andrews, Rose, & Johnson, 1998; Anson & Ponsford, 2006; Garske & Thomas, 1992), and, as we saw in Chapter 4, stigma and discrimination will generally tend only to lower it further (Link, Struening, Neese-Todd, Asmussen, & Phelan, 2001).

Importantly, though, the research of Jones and colleagues also shows that there are limits to the benefits of non-disclosure. In an initial study the researchers compared two groups of patients – one with ABI and the other with orthopaedic injury – to explore the impact that visibility and stigma surrounding brain injury have on well-being outcomes. The reason for choosing these patient groups was that both had experienced some form of injury that impacted on their long-term functional outcomes, but these differed in their visibility – with orthopaedic injuries being more obvious. Surprisingly perhaps, the study found that the ABI group (who were more inclined and able to conceal their injury), reported greater emotional distress and reduced well-being relative to the group with orthopaedic injury.

Looking to discover the reasons for this difference in well-being, the researchers went on to examine the role of anticipated discrimination (Jones et al., 2011). What they found was that among those people who were able to conceal their injury, a key reason for not disclosing it to others was that they expected to be discriminated against if they did. Their well-being was therefore compromised by the perceived need to keep their injury secret and by the fear of what would happen if they were unable to, putting a strain on them and their relationship with others.

The limitations of individual mobility and social distancing strategies are also brought to the fore by other research. For example, a qualitative study by Sophie Tabuteau-Harrison and colleagues looked at the ways in which people with multiple sclerosis (MS) adjusted to their diagnosis (Tabuteau-Harrison, Haslam, & Mewse, 2016). This found that if people perceived themselves to have adjusted well to their MS diagnosis, they were more likely to avoid and distance themselves from others with the condition. This was characterised by one 49-year-old MS sufferer, E, as a "lone wolf" strategy (p. 51) in which distancing from other people with MS protected her self-esteem. Another 59-year-old man, G, noted that a similar strategy helped him avoid "feeling a failure" and being "dispirited" (Tabuteau-Harrison et al., 2016; p. 51). Nevertheless, as in the research of Jones and colleagues, a cost was associated with using this strategy because it also had the effect of reducing the size of people's social networks and leading them to feel more cut off and socially isolated.

In this way, an individual mobility strategy limits a person's capacity for identifying and forming meaningful relationships with others who have ABI. As a consequence, it reduces opportunities for social support, both from those with ABI and from relevant support agencies (Jones et al., 2011). Indeed, Juliet Wakefield and her colleagues make the point that where social identification is low or absent, even if a person does seek out help from a relevant practitioner or agency, this may actually prove to be counter-productive because it will often lead them to have negative interactions with support providers (Wakefield, Bickley, & Sani, 2013; see also Tabuteau-Harrison et al., 2016).

People with ABI can pursue a strategy of social creativity that is a basis for posttraumatic growth

Clearly, though, when wanting to escape the threats to self-esteem that ABI presents, individual mobility is not a strategy that is open to everyone. This is especially true when the symptoms are highly visible and a person cannot reasonably pass themselves off as uninjured. As we argued earlier, under these conditions, individuals are more likely to resort to social creativity or social competition strategies to restore a positive sense of self.

The opportunities for this in the case of ABI may seem to be quite limited and hence rather unpromising. However, as we discovered when discussing various forms of trauma in Chapter 6, adversity can prove to have positive consequences if it is a catalyst for finding a strong sense of personal meaning and purpose. This is a possibility that is sometimes reflected in the experiences of people with ABI (Jones et al., 2011). For even in the face of the severe impairment that often follows brain injury, there are examples of people for whom it is an avenue to a greater appreciation of life, increased personal strength and resilience, as well as improvement in their relationships. Indeed, evidence of posttraumatic growth (PTG) suggests that it is possible to have a positive experience of change, despite – and sometimes because – one struggles to come to terms with a major negative life event. Moreover, PTG is not simply an expression of better coping or resilience, although both are part of the positive change that a person can experience in the context of struggling with a traumatic event. As Stephen Joseph argues, PTG involves a process of identity change that cuts "to the very core of our way of being in the world" (2011, p. 147).

There are several common experiences that people who report psychological growth following brain injury typically share and, interestingly, these are the very conditions that promote strategies of social creativity. First, PTG is more common among people who experience more severe ABI, limiting the extent to which individual mobility is possible. For example, there is evidence of greater growth among those who report higher levels of functional impairment in physical, cognitive, emotional, behavioural, and social domains (Jones et al., 2011; Silva, Ownsworth, Shields, & Fleming, 2011). For these individuals, hiding their condition is not an option because the symptoms of ABI are evident in much of their behaviour (e.g., high levels of forgetfulness, difficulty controlling emotions, extreme fatigue). Second, PTG is more common later in the recovery process when the possibility of shedding the negative identity and taking on another one has become more remote. This is evident from research by Joanna Collicutt-McGrath and Alex Linley (2006) which found significantly greater levels of growth among people who had suffered their injury an average of 10 years previously than among those who had done so more recently. After ten years, further significant improvement is unlikely, and the residual symptoms of ABI are more stable and harder to explain as simply a temporary aberration.

As Collicutt-McGrath and Linley (2006) observe, there are reasons to be sceptical about the possibility for such circumstances to be a gateway for growth. After all, one might expect that the more entrenched a person's difficulties are, the more these would preclude them from ever regaining a positive sense of self. Nevertheless, as the creativity hypothesis (H6) suggests, it is precisely the recognition that life change is a permanent consequence of injury that leads people to seek alternative ways to understand their place in the world. As social identity theory proposes, this is because the motivation for creativity is stimulated where a person cannot distance themselves from, or "exit", their group (i.e., where the group boundaries are impermeable; Ashforth & Kreiner, 1999; Ellemers & Haslam, 2012).

Theoretically, social creativity can take several forms (see Tajfel & Turner, 1979). However, one that is particularly common in reports of growth following ABI involves changes in *social comparison*. As we discussed in Chapters 2 and 3, social group comparisons can either lift us up or bring us down. For example, if an individual identifies as a nurse, then situations that encourage an upward social comparison with a group that is perceived to have higher professional standing (e.g., doctors) are likely to reduce their self-esteem because they highlight their lower status. Yet if the same person engages in a downward comparison (e.g., with a professional group that has lower status such as residential care workers), then this will generally lead them to see themselves as relatively fortunate and well off, and this will tend to enhance their self-esteem. In the case of ABI, downward comparisons of this form appear to play an important role in promoting

PTG. This can be seen in the following comments from a man, Stuart, who had sustained a brain injury in a car accident:

> [There are] so many people worse off that there is no point feeling sorry for yourself. I'm pretty lucky considering the others who were in rehab and you know, it could be worse – [I] could not be here.

> (Douglas, 2013, p. 69)

Providing further support for the importance of such comparisons, in a sample of 15 stroke survivors, Berit Gangstad and colleagues found that PTG was quite strongly associated with a tendency to make favourable comparisons with other stroke sufferers ($r = .41$; Gangstad, Norman, & Barton, 2009).

Related to this point, Jones and colleagues (2011) found that posttraumatic growth after ABI was underpinned by processes of both personal and social change. The specifics of their study, involving 630 people with brain injury, are summarised in Figure 11.8. Consistent with SIMIC, those who reported having adjusted successfully to the life changes brought about by their injury were more likely to report having taken on board a *new identity as a survivor* and thereby to have gained a strong sense of their personal identity (i.e., of who they were as individuals; Postmes & Jetten, 2006). In addition, they reported greater improvement in their social relationships post-injury and increased access to social support.

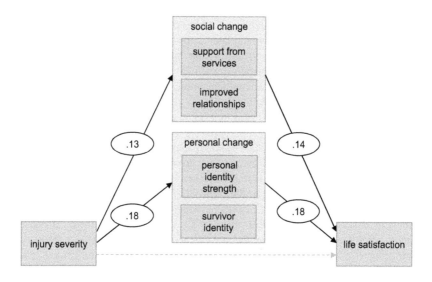

Figure 11.8 Change processes implicated in successful post-ABI adjustment

Note: Analysis indicated that people with more severe injuries tended to have better post-ABI adjustment (i.e., life satisfaction). However, this link was non-significant when personal and social change factors were also entered as predictors. This suggests that severe ABI can be associated with better outcomes because it is a basis for people to undergo such change. In particular, this is because they are more likely (1) to undergo personal change by taking on board a new identity as a survivor and thereby gain a strong sense of their personal identity and (2) to receive social support and have improved social relationships.

Source: Based on Jones et al. (2011)

Together with the work discussed in the previous section, these findings provide clear evidence that social identity processes have a central role to play in people's efforts to regain a positive sense of self after ABI. In particular, it appears social mobility and social creativity are two key strategies that people pursue, but that which is pursued depends on structural factors that shape their perceptions of their membership in an injury group (in particular, the perceived permeability and security of that group membership). This leads some people to reject an identity as a person with brain injury, but others to embrace it. Interestingly too, although the former strategy might appear to be more promising, it is the latter – which is typically pursued by those with more severe injury – that seem to offer better prospects of psychological recovery. This is often because it involves taking on a new identity as a survivor that gives people a renewed sense of meaning, purpose, and connection and thereby provides opportunity for posttraumatic growth.

Although much more work needs to be done to test these ideas fully and explore their practical implications, this would seem to be a very fruitful way of integrating and further developing our understanding of growth following injury. Importantly too, this integration also has the potential to provide new directions for practical intervention, not least by pointing to the ways in which collective identity management strategies which have previously been rather underexplored, might not only promote adjustment but also help to bring about productive forms of change (e.g., of the form proposed in Figure 11.6).

Cognitive deficits can interfere with self-categorization processes

Throughout this volume we have argued that social identification is necessary to unlock the psychological resources associated with group membership. This is often described in social terms, but in fact, as John Turner and colleagues argue, the processes involved are also inherently cognitive, and this becomes apparent when we start to disentangle how it is that people develop their connectedness with groups of other people (Turner, Oakes, Haslam, & McGarty, 1994). For example, for a person to see themselves, or self-categorize, as a teacher, they need (1) to recognise teachers as a meaningful social category; (2) to see themselves as more similar to than different from other teachers; and (3) to categorize themselves as part of a group of teachers, so that the person's thoughts and behaviour are shaped not by their idiosyncratic personal perspective on the world but by the shared perspective of the collective (in this case, "us teachers"; Oakes, Haslam, & Turner, 1994). All three processes involve cognitive operations, and therein lies the challenge for some people with brain injury. For if ABI produces cognitive impairment, then a person's capacity to fully engage in these self-categorization processes may be compromised.

This is an issue that Stephen Walsh and colleagues raise when interrogating the curative potential of social group membership following brain injury. In their work they rightly ask: What happens when people have limited cognitive ability to "do" self-categorization (Walsh et al., 2014)? For example, if Margaret has dementia and cannot remember that she is part of a lunch club, then she may not be in a position to seek out any of its members when she feels isolated. And if Mark has become more egocentric and prone to angry outbursts following a stroke, he may find that members of his pre-injury groups are less willing to engage with him and give him support when he needs it. As Walsh argues, such deficits and others can limit a person's capacity to derive health benefit from group membership precisely because the cognitive processes required to make the most of their curative resources are compromised.

A related point is made by Daniel Skorich in work which explores the relationship between self-categorization and autism (Bertschy, Skorich, & Haslam, 2017; Skorich et al., 2016; Skorich, Gash, Stalker, Zheng, & Haslam, 2017). This observes that some of the well-documented cognitive correlates of autism can be attributed to problems of social identification and self-categorization. In particular, weak central coherence (Frith & Happé, 1994) can be seen to reflect general difficulties in categorization, and theory of mind deficits (which make it hard to see the perspective of others; Baron-Cohen, 2005) can be seen to reflect difficulties in *self*-categorization which interfere with shared identification. Although autism is not a brain injury, the point of contact with our present considerations is that this work suggests that particular forms of cognitive deficit can interfere with a person's ability to see themselves as part of a wider group network in ways that have implications for both their behaviour and their treatment.

Yet although such impairments may diminish a person's capacity to make the most of group memberships, they do not rule out all potential for cure. Indeed, just as insulin can be used to manage diabetes, so neuro-rehabilitation can be used to manage cognitive impairment – by drawing on a person's strengths to help them develop and strengthen group ties despite cognitive limitations. Using the examples earlier, Margaret may benefit from a group reminiscence intervention that creates a sense of connection to social groups that she can remember being part of before the onset of her dementia (Haslam et al., 2010). And through rehabilitation, Mark may find ways to control his behaviour in ways that allow him to regain some of his old group ties and develop meaningful new ones.

Speaking to these possibilities, there is evidence that the perception of group belonging can be protective of health even in the face of severe cognitive impairment. For example, in a study with older people living with and without progressive dementia, we found that people with more severe impairment reported *better* quality of life than those with mild impairment and equivalent quality of life to that of people with no impairment (Jetten, Haslam, Pugliese, Tonks, & Haslam, 2010b). Statistical analysis indicated that this was attributable to the fact that those with severe dementia perceived themselves to belong to more groups than those with mild illness (and to belong to a similar number of groups to those with no illness) and had a stronger sense of personal identity as a result. This reflected the fact that the cognitive decline associated with more advanced dementia allowed people to believe that they were still strongly connected to people who they had socialised with before their illness took hold. The key point here, then, is that it was *perceived group belonging*, not poor memory or insight, that predicted individuals' overall well-being.

Clearly there is a need to better understand the various ways in which cognitive impairment can compromise a person's ability to develop and maintain a sense of social identity with others, and this requires more targeted research with ABI (and other) populations (for a discussion, see Skorich et al., 2017). In the meantime, though, our current knowledge of cognitive limitations can already help to inform interventions that help people build and maintain group ties where this is possible. For example, if there are gaps in a person's knowledge of their old group ties, these pre-existing social identities may be strengthened by incorporating various memory strategies that help people to remember the names of those who are part of a new group they have joined. In other cases, intervention may involve more strategic social identity construction and reconstruction of the form offered by the GROUPS 4 HEALTH programme that we discuss in the final chapter of this book. Indeed, these adaptations are not dissimilar to those proposed by cognitive behavioural approaches which are applied in holistic rehabilitation to help manage the psychosocial difficulties that arise following ABI. Thus, even though we recognise – and need to be sensitive to the fact – that cognitive impairment may limit a person's capacity to benefit from CBT, in an adapted and simplified form, it may still produce beneficial effects for those with ABI. This is especially true, we believe, when those adaptations are informed by awareness of the curative value of efforts to strengthen social identification.

Conclusion

There are many parallels between the social identity approach and other current approaches to managing the consequences of ABI. This is largely due to the importance that brain injury practitioners and researchers attach to the role of social factors and the self-concept in supporting recovery (e.g., see Douglas, 2012; Gracey & Ownsworth, 2012; Ownsworth, 2014). Irrespective of the type of ABI or its severity, changes to self-concept and social functioning are a common denominator in recovery across the injury spectrum. Importantly too, they are a key feature not only of the lives of those with ABI, but also of the lives of those who care for and support them. In focusing on these factors, the social identity approach is not at odds with current approaches but rather enriches them by specifying more clearly the nature of the 'social' in the biopsychosocial and holistic approaches that provide the dominant frameworks for practical intervention.

In this, the social identity approach also offers a new perspective from which to understand people's experience of recovery. As we have shown, working with people's social identities and understanding how they have changed in response to injury is critical to a person's adjustment. Equally vital is the recognition that growth following profound trauma is possible, but that the capacity for this is a function of how a person sees, or categorizes, themselves in relation to others. As with the contexts and conditions that we have discussed in other chapters (e.g., Chapters 6 and 7), the process of maintaining old social identities and building new ones is critical to outcomes. More specifically, though, it appears the capacity to develop an identity as an injury survivor can be particularly beneficial because this is a socially creative perspective on the self that allows people with ABI to make sense of their condition, to feel better about themselves (in comparison to others), and to work with others to find constructive ways forward (Jones, Williams et al., 2012).

Returning to the case of Phineas Gage with which we began this chapter, it is unclear how much social processes of this form played a role in his particular path to recovery. This is due in part to the fact that far greater attention is paid to the horrific nature of his injuries and to the unruly and socially dysfunctional man that Gage is said to have become than to the ways in which he was able to get on with his life (Griggs, 2015). Nevertheless, get on with his life he did. Not least, he did so by moving to Chile and taking on a new career as a stage-coach driver – a job which would have required considerable cognitive and social skill. This is a point upon which Richard Griggs embellishes in the context of a broader discussion of Gage's life at this time:

> Driving a six-horse stagecoach team in which each horse was controlled separately by differing movements of the reins over steep and rough terrain clearly required complex sensory – motor/cognitive skills, and dealing with the non-English-speaking passengers in a foreign country clearly required social skills. With respect to Gage's recovery, Kotowicz (2007) pointed out that a Harvard surgeon, Henry Bigelow, is the only person known to have observed Gage a good time (well over a year) after his accident and to have published his observations (Bigelow, 1850) . . . Bigelow described Gage as having "quite recovered in his faculties of body and mind" and does not mention anything strange or unusual about his behavior (Macmillan, 2000, p. 392). In addition, Macmillan and Lena found a statement from Dr. Henry Trevitt, a doctor who lived in Chile at the time Gage was there and knew Gage well. The doctor reported that Gage "was in the enjoyment of good health with no impairment whatever of his mental faculties" (p. 648).
>
> (Griggs, 2015, p. 197)

So although the specifics are unclear, it appears that adapting to injury by developing new roles and social relationships (e.g., as a stage-coach driver) was a very likely contributor to Gage's health and well-being after his injury. Moreover, his capacity to forge new social connections in the wake of this strikes us as no less interesting than any other part of his remarkable life. Indeed, although we know very little about it, when it comes to understanding Gage's brain injury, his pathway to recovery is probably the *most* interesting part of the story.

Points for practice

There are several key messages that the social identity approach offers for practitioners working in the area of ABI:

1. *Understanding social identity change is key to enhancing adjustment to ABI.* Brain injury often leads to loss and change in relationships with other individuals and important social

groups (e.g., friendship, family, work, and interest groups). This is central to the experience of social isolation, but goes deeper because this affects the way a person with ABI comes to understand who they are. Working with people to help them maintain identity-relevant relationships where possible and to gain new ones is therefore very important in promoting adjustment.

2. *Individual mobility strategies that involve injury concealment can offer some protection from the negative consequences of ABI.* It is common to feel stigmatised, of less value, and disabled are common following brain injury, and this may reduce people's sense of positive self-worth. Negative effects are limited when there is the possibility for people to not disclose injury (e.g., where the effects of ABI are more hidden). However, this strategy may only offer a short-term solution to regaining a positive identity, as distancing oneself from others with injury often also prevents people from seeking and accessing social support.

3. *Social creativity strategies that redefine injury groups through downward social comparison can promote posttraumatic growth.* Where it is not possible to conceal ABI, adjustment and growth can be promoted by making positive social comparisons – notably, by seeing oneself as a survivor of injury who is better off than others with brain injury. Evidence also suggests that this can provide a long-term solution to the challenge of regaining a positive identity.

4. *Cognitive impairment may compromise self-categorization and the extent to which a person can benefit from group membership.* Cognitive impairment can hinder the development of strong social bonds with groups, limiting the extent to which a person can use them as a social psychological resource (e.g., as a basis for social support). Recognising the impact of these deficits and adapting social interventions accordingly can therefore help to optimise a person's potential for adjustment to ABI.

Resources

Further reading

The following references provide a good basis for exploring identity change in ABI.

① Ownsworth, T. (2014). *Self-identity after brain injury*. London: Psychology Press.

This volume provides a broad perspective for understanding changes to the self-concept associated with brain injury. It provides an analysis of mechanism, ways to assess identity, and possible directions for intervention with brain injury populations.

② Jones, J. J., Jetten, J., Haslam, S. A., & Williams, W. H. (2012). Deciding to disclose: The importance of maintaining social relationships for well-being after acquired brain injury. In J. Jetten, C. Haslam, & S. A. Haslam (Eds.) *The social cure: Identity, health and well-being* (pp. 255–272). London: Psychology Press.

In this chapter Jones and colleagues provide a social identity analysis of the costs and benefits of self-disclosure as a strategy for regaining positive identity following ABI.

③ Walsh, R. S., Fortune, D. G., Gallagher, S., & Muldoon, O. T. (2014). Acquired brain injury: Combining social psychological and neuropsychological perspectives. *Health Psychology Review, 8,* 458–472.

This review paper is the first to integrate neurological and social psychological approaches in brain injury and to consider the consequences of cognitive impairment on a person's capacity to benefit from membership in groups and social connectedness.

Video

① Search for "Brain Trauma" to listen to a story on the ABC Catalyst programme that describes the physical, cognitive, and social consequences of brain injury. It does this by exploring the experiences of Sam Howe – a young man who was involved in a car accident – and those of the health professionals who work in brain injury rehabilitation. www.abc.net.au/catalyst/stories/3291518.htm   (9 minutes)

② Search for "Meaning, purpose and growth after head injury" to find another short video in which Dr Trevor Powell talks about posttraumatic growth as it is experienced by people who are coming to terms with the life changes that brain injury can produce. www.youtube.com/watch?v=3Zj8rnpFwu0   (9 minutes)

Websites

① www.slate.com/articles/health_and_science/science/2014/05/phineas_gage_neuroscience_case_true_story_of_famous_frontal_lobe_patient.html. This site provides extensive coverage of the history of Phineas Gage in ways that delve beneath the myths to explore his psychosocial adaptation in recovery.

② http://synapse.org.au/information-services/changes-in-relationships.aspx. This site describes some of the common relationship changes that people can experience in recovery from ABI and is one of many information sites provided by Synapse (an organisation that supports people with brain injury).

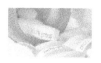

Chapter 12
Acute pain

Pain is an important human experience, and it can take many different forms. Pain can be sharp and stabbing when we burn our hand on the stove, throbbing when we experience a toothache or headache, or dull and aching following an injury that damages our back muscles. What all forms of pain have in common is that pain hurts. Aside from it being aversive, pain also blocks a person's ability to focus on anything else other than their pain. Consider hitting your thumb with a hammer. It is likely that you will ignore the task at hand for a little while (e.g., fixing a kitchen cupboard) and that all your attention will go to dealing with the pain – for example, by holding your thumb, shouting and cursing, and perhaps even by hopping around in some sort of pain dance. This shows that pain can be all absorbing. Indeed, one's normal life can often only resume – in the sense that one can only focus again on engaging with everyday demands – once the pain is controlled.

The duration of pain is key, and in the research literature, a distinction is made between chronic and acute pain. Whereas acute pain is characterised by recent onset, limited duration, and a clearly identifiable cause (e.g., a cavity in one's tooth that requires a visit to the dentist), chronic pain is long-term (lasting more than 3 months), is not clearly related to a specific injury, and may not even have a clear cause (see Day, 2017). Because acute and chronic pain differ in their presentation, how they are experienced, and how they are treated, it is important to consider them as completely different phenomena. This also becomes obvious when we examine the way that people talk about their pain. Whereas chronic pain is draining and debilitating, the response to acute pain can be quite different: such pain can (under certain conditions and in some contexts) be motivating and energising. Indeed, it may even enhance the perceived meaning and purpose of life. In this chapter, we focus solely on understanding acute pain, although chronic pain will be considered in Chapter 14 as part of our discussion of chronic physical health conditions.

Acute pain has received less attention in health contexts than chronic pain. Yet as we will argue here, it is no less important for health – not least because acute pain can turn into chronic pain. It is primarily for this reason that we believe it merits a chapter of its own. However, this decision also hinges on the fact that there is now considerable evidence of its unique psychological and social dimensions. As an illustration of this, reflect on the following apparent paradox: that even though acute pain hurts and we go to great lengths to alleviate it, it is not the case that we avoid it at all costs and at all times. Indeed, it is clear that despite its aversiveness, on occasion people engage voluntarily in behaviours that produce pain. This is true, for example, of people who take part in chilli-eating competitions or who engage in extreme sports or who dive into ice-cold water to celebrate the arrival of New Year (see Figure 12.1).

As we will outline in this chapter, the social identity approach can help us make sense of these behaviours and also explain how the pain experiences that they trigger affect our emotional and physical well-being in profound ways. As we will see, the way people relate to others around them and, in particular, the degree to which they perceive themselves as sharing identity, is key to understanding these health outcomes. But before we can make the case for this claim, we need to start by defining the phenomenon of acute pain and understanding how it has traditionally been examined.

Defining pain

The International Association for the Study of Pain Task Force on Taxonomy (1994) defines pain as "[a]n unpleasant sensory and emotional experience associated with actual or potential tissue damage

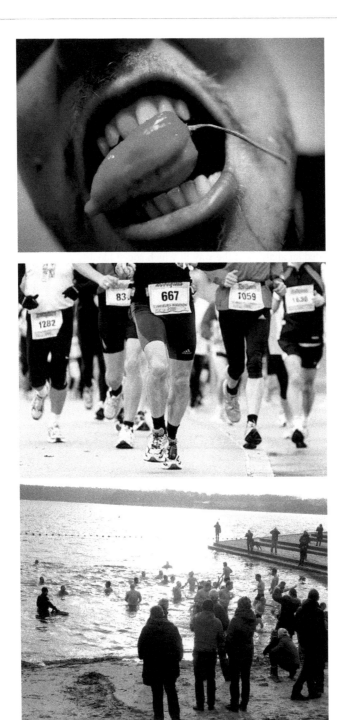

Figure 12.1 Sources of pain: eating a chilli, running a marathon, taking part in a New Year's dive ritual

Note: These examples demonstrate that we do not avoid pain at all costs. Rather, in circumstances such as these we deliberately engage in activities that produce pain.

Source: Lauri Rantala, flickr; Pixabay; the authors

or described in terms of such damage". A few points are important to note in this definition. First, it highlights the distinction between *nociception* and *pain*. Nociception refers to the stimulation of nerve fibres that convey information about potential tissue damage to the brain; pain is a subjective perception that arises when nociception reaches a particular threshold. This means that pain and nociception can be completely decoupled: pain can occur without nociception, and nociception may not trigger the subjective experience of pain (see Anisman, 2016; Moseley & Arntz, 2007).

Second, and following from the previous point, if we abandon the notion that pain equals nociception, we can consider other non-physical experiences that trigger a pain response. Pain is simply everything that hurts. For example, people report pain when they experience discrimination, ostracism, or social rejection (MacDonald & Leary, 2005) or when they experience a romantic break-up. Even though some evidence suggests that when a person experiences this so-called social pain there is similar neuronal activity in the brain regions associated with pain perception to that observed when they experience physical pain (Eisenberger, Lieberman, & Williams, 2003), it is nevertheless apparent that there are important differences between social pain and experiences such as hitting one's thumb with a hammer. Earlier chapters provided an analysis of the way in which social identity processes contribute to social pain associated with stigma and discrimination (Chapter 4) and trauma (Chapter 6), and in the second part of this chapter we will also consider social pain experienced in the context of ostracism and social rejection. Nevertheless, our main focus here is on the psychological and subjective experience of acute physical pain.

Importantly for our current purposes, increased recognition in recent decades that there is a significant psychological dimension to acute pain has led researchers to develop a *social psychological* analysis of this phenomenon. This growing interest in the social and psychological processes surrounding acute pain (e.g., concerning the appraisal of pain and the reasons for seeking it out) has important connections with, and draws heavily on, insights from social cure research. In particular, this is because, as we will argue below, the social identity approach to health and well-being helps us understand how acute pain is experienced and how it is affected by the process of *meaning making*. However, to understand how this and other approaches have developed, it is helpful first to explore acute pain from a broader historical perspective

Current approaches to acute pain

Physiological models: the role of sensory pathways

Pain has captured the attention of thinkers for centuries and, from the outset, attempts to understand its origin and function gave rise to very different conceptualisations of relevant phenomena. For example, Greek philosophers such as Hippocrates and Aristotle focused on the body to understand pain and attributed an important role to the heart as the central organ implicated in pain perception. In contrast, during the Renaissance, the cause of pain was believed to lie outside of the body and was thought to be a punishment from God. In these times, pain was considered to be a spiritual and mystical experience, and so it was not surprising that people believed the only way to treat it would be to reaffirm one's faith in God (e.g., through prayer and the endurance of suffering).

René Descartes is generally credited with being the first person to recognise the central role of the body and the brain in pain sensation. As Figure 12.2 illustrates, he believed that when pain is experienced (in this case, burning of the skin), the pain sensation travels via a tube (which can be thought of as an early conceptualisation of nerve fibres) to the brain where the pain message is received. Indeed, despite the rudimentary nature of Descartes' thinking, it was in this analysis that the contemporary focus on the physiology of pain originated.

Descartes' influence is evident in models that were developed in the late 19th century to describe the different pathways through which pain travelled to the brain (Melzack & Wall, 1965).

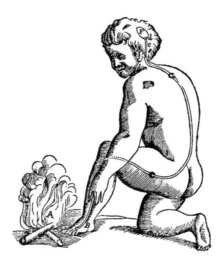

Figure 12.2 Descartes' representation of the experience of pain in *Traite de l'homme* [*Treatise of Man*]

Note: Descartes introduced the idea of brain–body interaction in the experience of pain. Illustrating this, he proposed that pain would travel from the activated area via a tube to the brain. Despite being rather simplistic, some of these ideas informed physiological approaches to pain development.

Source: Descartes (1664/1972)

On the one hand, proponents of *specificity theory* proposed that pain has its own dedicated nerves, pathways, and sensory modalities (e.g., of touch and vision that are only activated in pain contexts) to carry sensations to the brain (e.g., von Frey, 1894). On the other hand, advocates of *pattern theory* disputed this view and argued instead that receptors for pain are shared with other senses (e.g., Goldscheider, 1894). According to this alternative view, pain occurs following intense stimulation of various senses, which translates into specific signals that are detected and recognised as pain by the brain.

Even though there were significant differences in the way that these models saw pain as being transmitted to and registered in the brain, what they had in common was an assumption that the amount of pain that a person suffered was proportionate to the severity of the injury they had experienced. However, this focus on physiology meant that neither of these theories could explain experiences of pain that have no physiological cause. A good example of this is phantom limb pain. This refers to an experience reported by up to 80% of people who have undergone limb amputation in which they experience sensations in the limb that has been removed – sensations that in most cases are quite painful (Sherman, Sherman, & Parker, 1984). Moreover, as well as being unable to account for such phenomena, early theories which assumed that the experience of pain was simply a reflection of sensory insult could not explain cases – such as those of soldiers discussed in Case study 12.1 – in which people with severe injuries reported only minor pain or none at all. These indicate that there is more to pain than physiology alone and that other processes – notably those that are psychological and social – play an important role in determining a person's actual experience of pain.

Case study 12.1 Soldiers on the battlefield

One of the oldest and best documented examples of the difference between nociception and pain sensation comes from field work by the Harvard University researcher Henry Beecher. He was struck by the fact that many World War II soldiers with severe injuries reported no pain at all immediately after their injury (see Figure 12.3). Indeed, when asked, 25% of the soldiers treated for serious wounds and injuries in field hospitals reported only mild levels of pain and 32% reported no pain at all. What is more, 75% did not want any medication for their pain. Beecher believed that this mismatch between the severity of injury and pain was due to the soldiers' relief that their injury allowed them to leave the battlefield behind. As he put it:

> In this connection it is important to consider the position of the soldier: His wound suddenly releases him from an exceedingly dangerous environment, one filled with fatigue, discomfort, anxiety, fear and real danger of death, and gives him a ticket to the safety of the hospital. His troubles are about over, or he thinks they are.
>
> (Beecher, 1946, p. 99)

Yet while escaping the dangers of the battlefield must have been a positive experience for these soldiers, this analysis does not explain the *underreporting* of pain and injury. For if soldiers believed that being wounded would release them from battle, they should have been motivated to exaggerate their pain and injuries, not downplay them. But even though we can only speculate about the reasons for this discrepancy, it speaks to the fact (1) that pain is not simply a physical experience but also a deeply psychological one and (2) that the experienced intensity of pain is very much determined by the meaning that is given to it.

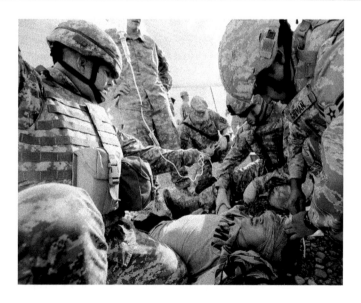

Figure 12.3 Pain on the battlefield

Note: Responses to pain on the battlefield vary as a function of the meaning that is attached to that pain.

Source: Tech. Sgt. Craig Lifton, 332nd Air Expeditionary Wing, US Air Force

In response to attempts to understand why the intensity of a pain source does not always correspond with a person's reported pain, theories needed to become more sophisticated. A particularly significant development in this regard was Ronald Melzack and Patrick Wall's (1965) *gate control theory* (Anisman, 2016). This holds that pain messages are modified by a gate mechanism located in the spinal cord. Here the opening and closing of the gate system (i.e., exacerbating or attenuating the pain experience, respectively) is believed to occur as a function of the interplay between three factors: (1) activity which stimulates pain fibres and leads to the gate being opened, (2) activity in peripheral fibres which leads to the gate being closed, and (3) messages from the brain (containing sensory, emotional, cognitive, and behavioural information) that can also open or close the gate.

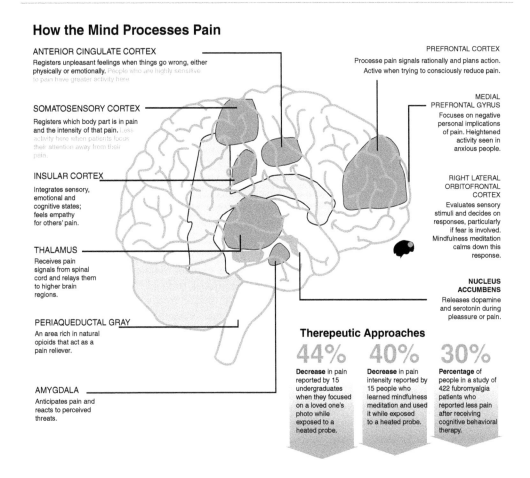

How the Mind Processes Pain

ANTERIOR CINGULATE CORTEX
Registers unpleasant feelings when things go wrong, either physically or emotionally. People who are highly sensitive to pain have greater activity here.

SOMATOSENSORY CORTEX
Registers which body part is in pain and the intensity of that pain. Less activity here when patients focus their attention away from their pain.

INSULAR CORTEX
Integrates sensory, emotional and cognitive states; feels empathy for others' pain.

THALAMUS
Receives pain signals from spinal cord and relays them to higher brain regions.

PERIAQUEDUCTAL GRAY
An area rich in natural opioids that act as a pain reliever.

AMYGDALA
Anticipates pain and reacts to perceived threats.

PREFRONTAL CORTEX
Processe pain signals rationally and plans action. Active when trying to consciously reduce pain.

MEDIAL PREFRONTAL GYRUS
Focuses on negative personal implications of pain. Heightened activity seen in anxious people.

RIGHT LATERAL ORBITOFRONTAL CORTEX
Evaluates sensory stimuli and decides on responses, particularly if fear is involved. Mindfulness meditation calms down this response.

NUCLEUS ACCUMBENS
Releases dopamine and serotonin during pleassure or pain.

Therepeutic Approaches

44%
Decrease in pain reported by 15 undergraduates when they focused on a loved one's photo while exposed to a heated probe.

40%
Decrease in pain intensity reported by 15 people who learned mindfulness meditation and used it while exposed to a heated probe.

30%
Percentage of people in a study of 422 fubromyalgia patients who reported less pain after receiving cognitive behavioral therapy.

Figure 12.4 Brain regions involved in registering and processing pain

Note: The areas in orange are areas in the brain that are involved in different forms of pain registration and processing. The statistics in the bottom right-hand corner provide an indication of the effectiveness of social support, mindfulness meditation, and cognitive behavioural therapy in decreasing pain. Interestingly, according to these data, merely thinking of social support from a loved one is a very effective way to ameliorate the experience of pain.

Source: www.tricitypsychology.com/how-the-mind-processes-pain/

By taking account of both the physiological and the psychological factors that determine pain perception, gate control theory – which has provided an important platform for contemporary physiological research – helps us start to understand why severity of injury does not necessarily map onto pain experience. For example, if an injured person manages to distract themselves, the gate may be closed and there will be little correlation between the stimulation of their pain fibres and the amount of pain they experience. In this way, the theory proved to be a harbinger of current approaches to acute pain which understand the experience of pain to be shaped not only by our evolutionary history and biology, but also by our psychology.

Psychological models: the role of cognitive appraisal and individual differences

Recent decades have witnessed a range of significant developments in our understanding of the psychological factors underlying pain (see Figure 12.4). For example, Kim Burton and colleagues found that psychological factors were the most potent predictors of repeat acute episodes of lower back pain, accounting for 69% of the variance in outcomes (Burton, Tilotson, Main, & Hollis, 1995). Relatedly, other researchers have found that people's fear of pain is generally more disabling than their actual experience of it (Crombez, Vlaeyen, Heuts, & Lysens, 1999). These findings are also consistent with evidence of the effect that placebos can have in pain management. For even though the effects of placebos vary, there is now considerable experimental evidence that the mere perception that one has received pain-reducing treatment can reduce the experience of pain relative to a control condition in which no placebo is administered (see Vase, Skyt, & Hall, 2016; see also Anisman, 2016). This suggests that pain expectancies and psychological processes more generally have an important role to play in understanding responses to acute pain.

So what are these psychological factors and how do they affect pain appraisals? In line with the transactional model of stress that we discussed in Chapter 5, one factor that research has homed in on is a person's *cognitive appraisal* of pain (after Lazarus, 1966). Here a range of studies have shown that people's perceptions of the meaning of pain can have a dramatic effect on their pain experience. For example, Kurt Gray and Daniel Wegner (2008) found that when electric shocks were seen as intentional (rather than unintentional), participants reported experiencing more pain.

Related research has shown that a person's control over pain can attenuate their neural response to it. As an example of this, an experimental study by Tim Salomons and his colleagues placed participants in a scanner and then exposed them to a painful heat stimulus (Salomons, Johnstone, Backonja, & Davidson, 2004). All participants were then given a joystick and told how to use it. However, those in one condition were told they that if they used the joystick correctly they could reduce their exposure to the heat from 5 seconds to 2 seconds, whereas those in another condition were told that their use of the joystick would have no effect. In reality, though, the participants in the control condition were only given the illusion of control and hence participants' actual exposure to the painful heat was the same in both controllable and uncontrollable conditions. Nevertheless, neuroimaging showed that the belief that pain was controllable led to attenuated activation in three neural areas known to be associated with pain: the anterior cingulate, insular, and secondary somatosensory cortices.

Other work has focused on individual differences between people in the extent to which they feel and experience pain. Of particular interest is the extent to which people *catastrophise* their pain experience (see Figure 12.5). Here Michael Sullivan and colleagues (Sullivan, Rogers, & Kirsch, 2001) argue that catastrophising is a key construct in understanding pain because high catastrophisers are more likely than low catastrophisers to ruminate about their pain ("I can't stop thinking about how much it hurts"), to feel helpless ("there is nothing I can do to reduce the intensity of the pain"), and to magnify the pain experience ("I'm afraid something serious may happen"). Not surprisingly too, high catastrophisers are more likely to experience pain intensely, to show emotional distress in response to pain, and to be fearful of future pain (Sullivan et al., 2001).

Also relevant to the psychology of pain is research which examines cultural differences in pain reporting (e.g., Rollman, 1998; Wolff, 1985). In particular, it has been observed that whereas people from Southern Asia are expected to suppress pain responses and show their stoicism, those in other

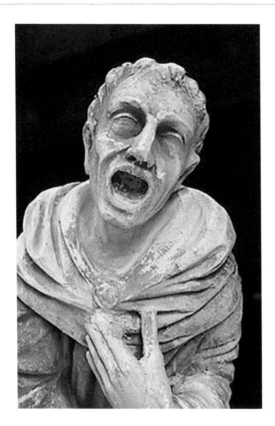

Figure 12.5 The expression of pain and suffering

Note: Individuals differ in the extent to which they catastrophise their pain – with high catastrophisers being more likely to let pain dominate their thoughts and expectations than low catastrophisers.

Source: Pixabay

cultures express their pain more freely. Along these lines, researchers have found that Chinese children report higher levels of pain than Italian children in response to having blood drawn from them. However, observational measures also showed that the Chinese children responded in a more controlled manner to their pain than the Italian children (Bisogni et al., 2014). It thus appears that there are profound cultural differences in pain expression and that these relate to different normative expectations that prevail within different groups (e.g., national, religious, ethnic).

Related to this point, there is also a large literature that explores gender differences in the experience and expression of pain (e.g., Greenspan et al., 2007). In particular, women generally report lower pain thresholds and tolerance than men (Unruh, 1996). However, against the idea that this is simply a reflection of physiological differences, there is evidence that this is mediated by gender differences in catastrophising cognitions (Sullivan, Tripp, & Santor, 2000) and also varies as a function of the context in which the pain is encountered (e.g., in clinical vs. community contexts; Dao & LeResche, 2000).

In summary, a growing body of work shows that an individual's response to painful stimuli depends not only on the severity and intensity of nociceptive input. Rather, responses to painful stimulation also depend in important ways on the cognitive and affective context in which pain is experienced and are at least partly determined by individual differences and cultural influences. These in turn suggest that *social learning* has an important role to play in the way that people experience and respond to pain. As we will see in the next section, this is a point that has been taken further within the framework of hedonic models of pain.

The hedonic model: pain as a basis for growth

Against the idea that all pain is aversive, recent psychological work has started to explore the ways in which pain can also come to be understood as a source of pleasure. As we intimated earlier, this is important when it comes to understanding why it is that people often go out of their way to experience pain – for example, by taking part in painful rituals (Xygalatas et al., 2013), by exposing themselves to painful stimuli (Ferris, Jetten, & Bastian, 2017), or by immersing themselves in painful environments (Hopkins & Reicher, 2017).

To explain these various behaviours, one clearly has to appreciate that pain can have benefits as well as costs. Seeking to document these, Brock Bastian and his colleagues provide an overview of the different psychological benefits of pain (Bastian, Jetten, Hornsey, & Lekes, 2014c). These are summarised in Table 12.1.

Table 12.1 Three classes of psychological benefit that flow from acute pain

1. Pain facilitates pleasure

Pain enhances subsequent pleasure	Pain provides a contrast for pleasure, and this increases the relative pleasantness of subsequent experiences.
Pain heightens sensory sensitivity	Pain heightens arousal and focuses attention on sensory experience, thereby increasing sensory receptivity.
Pain facilitates pleasure seeking	Pain provides a justification for indulgence in pleasures that might otherwise arouse a sense of guilt.

2. Pain strengthens the self

Pain increases self-regulation	Pain captures attention and brings cognitive resources on-line for effective problem solving in response to the threat of pain.
Pain enables identity management	Pain promotes a physical experience of the self, thereby reducing aversive high-level self-awareness and enabling identity change.
Pain demonstrates virtue	Pain may be interpreted as providing a symbolic test of a range of personal virtues.

3. Pain promotes affiliation

Pain arouses empathy in others	Pain expression increases empathy and arouses care and concern in others.
Pain increases relational focus	Pain may lead people to seek social support. Pain therefore provides a novel source of social connection with others.
Pain increases solidarity	Pain may be used to increase the value of relational ties with others, and shared pain may increase bonding.

Source: Based on Bastian et al. (2014c). Reprinted by permission of SAGE Publications

---

The first broad class of processes relate to the observation that *pain is closely related to pleasure* (as argued by Morris, 1991). More specifically, Bastian and colleagues identified three reasons why pain and pleasure are not always opposing constructs and why pain, under some conditions, may even induce pleasure or evoke a positive and rewarding response. First, pain triggers pleasure when it provides an important contrast for subsequent pleasurable experiences. Consistent with this idea, and in line with their *opponent process theory*, Siri Leknes and colleagues showed that the termination of pain is often followed by a sensation of pleasure (Leknes, Brooks, Wiech, & Tracey, 2008). As Allison Moorer's (2014) song puts it "It's gonna feel good when it stops hurting".

Second, pain may arouse pleasure because, under some conditions, it increases sensitivity to subsequent sensory input (e.g., a cold drink might taste better after a long run). In these contexts pain can increase positive outcomes such as attentiveness and awareness (Bastian, Jetten, & Hornsey, 2014b). Bastian and colleagues argue that this may explain why pain is often induced when people want to draw attention to their sensory experiences (e.g., during yoga).

Third, pain facilitates pleasure because it triggers self-rewarding behaviour. For example, Bastian and colleagues (Bastian, Jetten, & Stewart, 2013) showed that because pain is associated with punishment, once the pain has subsided, people are more likely to feel justified indulging in 'guilty pleasures'. These researchers provide evidence for these justice-related processes in two studies. In the first of these they found that participants who experienced physical pain were more likely to reward themselves by taking sweets from a bowl than those who did not experience pain. This effect, however, was evident only when pain was preceded by recollection of previous moral behaviour, not when it followed recall of an immoral past behaviour. The authors argued that this was because self-rewarding behaviour was only seen as justified in the context of reminders of one's own goodness. In the researchers' second study, after they had performed a number of tasks, participants were asked to choose a gift from a bowl containing either highlighters or chocolates. Consistent with predictions that physical pain promotes indulgence in guilty pleasures (in this case eating the chocolate), participants who experienced physical pain were more likely to take the chocolate than the highlighter. However, this effect was only evident for people who were sensitive to their being the victims of injustice. Together, then, these two studies show that physical pain leads to self-indulgence – especially in the context of a sense of personal morality or entitlement.

Bastian and his colleagues also identified a second class of benefits whereby through increasing perceptions of cognitive control and reducing rumination, pain can serve to strengthen the self (Bastian et al., 2014c). Indeed, in line with this logic, it has been suggested that the desire to reduce rumination is one motive that underpins people's willingness to experience pain by engaging in self-harm. Here, then, self-harm is thought to promote greater self-regulation which enables distraction from traumatic thoughts (Nock, 2010).

Other positive outcomes that boost the strength of the self relate to the capacity for pain to facilitate identity change. This process can clearly be observed during initiation rites in which individuals take part in painful ceremonies to mark the transition from one identity to the next (e.g., from child to adult; see Atkinson & Whitehouse, 2010). Painful ceremonies also test the individual and provide an opportunity for them to display their strength and virtue to others (see Figure 12.6). More specifically, by withstanding the pain that various rites of passage contain, a person is able to signal their self-control, maturity, strength, and perseverance in ways that attest to their suitability for the group they want to join (e.g., adults). In line with this point, there is also evidence that if people are able to withstand pain then they are more likely to be seen as virtuous. Indeed, this is seen in Aristotle's (340bc/2014, III-9) claim that "death and wounds will be painful to a courageous person and he will suffer them involuntarily but he will endure them because it is noble to do so or shameful not to".

There is also evidence of a connection between pain endurance and guilt reduction. That is, people are more likely to endure pain if they feel guilty. This is exactly what Bastian, Jetten, and Fasoli (2011) found in a study where participants were made to feel guilty by reflecting on their past

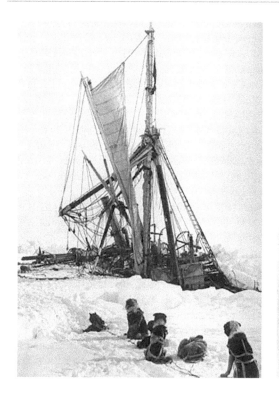

MEN WANTED

for hazardous journey, small wages, bitter cold, long months of complete darkness, constant danger, safe return doubtful, honor and recognition in case of success.

Ernest Shackleton
4 Burlington Street, London W1

Figure 12.6 Pain as a vehicle for self-affirmation

Note: This advert was intended to recruit volunteers to go on an expedition with Ernest Shackleton to the South Pole. It promised pain but also glory, and the expedition ultimately provided plenty of both (for detailed accounts, see Lansing, 2002; Shackleton, 1920). It is worth noting, however, that researchers have never been able to locate a copy of the original advert (Discerning History, 2013).

Source: The authors; Wikipedia

moral transgressions. These participants were more likely than those who did not go through this reflection process to inflict pain on themselves by holding their hand in ice-cold water (a so-called cold-pressor task) for longer. Moreover, interestingly, enduring greater pain appeared to be functional for those who were made to feel guilty because it was only in this condition that perceived guilt declined significantly after the painful experience (i.e., guilt was not reduced for participants in a control condition who were also made to feel guilty but completed a non-painful physical task). In this way, seeking out pain can help people to reduce feelings of guilt and to restore their sense of integrity and virtue.

The third class of pain benefit that Bastian and colleagues identify speaks directly to the matters of social identity that we will discuss further in the following sections (Bastian et al., 2014c). The argument here is that pain provides an important basis for seeking out support from others and that *pain promotes affiliation*. This is a two-way street in the sense that just as pain can lead a person to seek support from others, so witnessing the pain of others can trigger an immediate visceral or gut-level empathic response in observers (Goubert et al., 2005).

Moreover, in line with points that we discussed in Chapter 5, not only does pain increase the likelihood of receiving social support, but so too the process of drawing on that social support is generally associated with more effective pain management (Zhou & Gao, 2008). Illustrative of this point, the presence of a supportive companion during childbirth has been found to be associated with a reduced need for medication to manage pain (Cogan & Spinnato, 1988), and significantly shorter duration of labour and fewer complications (Klaus, Kennel, Robertson, & Sosa, 1986). Likewise, experimental studies show that participants who receive support from a friend during a cold-pressor task report less pain than participants who complete the task alone or only have non-supportive interactions with someone else (Brown, Sheffield, Leary, & Robinson, 2003). Other research also shows that this pain-ameliorating effect of social support can emerge even when participants only have a picture of a partner while in pain (Master et al., 2009).

Yet although such work is suggestive of the way in which group processes are relevant to the experience of pain, it is nevertheless generally the case that when it addresses the role of social factors, most of the work in this area focuses either on individual or on interpersonal relationships (e.g., see Dunkel Schetter, 2017; Pietromonaco & Collins, 2017). An obvious question that this raises for us is whether there is also a role for pain-related theorising which attends to the *group-based relationships* that inform a person's sense of social identity. In the next section we argue that there is and, moreover, that many of the earlier findings can be understood through the lens of social cure theorising of the form that we have advanced in this book as a whole. In particular, as we have highlighted in other chapters, this is because it is only when people share identity with others (e.g., as partners and close friends) that those others have the power to improve their ability to cope effectively with pain.

The social identity approach to acute pain

One observation that Bastian and colleagues make in the process of outlining the various benefits of pain is that these benefits are often experienced in the company of others (Bastian et al., 2014c). For example, by definition, pain can only serve the function of displaying one's virtue and strength when other people are able to witness this. Moreover, it makes sense that people should be more likely to want to display their virtue by undergoing pain when they share identity with those who witness it. Likewise, it is primarily when people want to manage their social identity in particular ways that pain serves the important function of forging group bonds or expressing important aspects of identity. It is in such contexts, then, that we see how acute pain functions to bring people together and, through this, to shape health and well-being in powerful ways.

In the following sections, we build first on the analysis of Bastian and colleagues to demonstrate how pain can promote group cohesion and facilitate group formation. Here we show that pain can act as a "social glue" that turns individuals who have no previous basis for connection into a meaningful social group. In line with the connection, meaning, support, and agency hypotheses that we set out in Chapter 2 (H12 to H15), this then allows the socially curative properties of the group to be unlocked. Building on this, we will then review research which reveals an important group dimension to the experience of witnessing other people's pain. In this context, it is apparent that people are more likely to "feel" the pain of ingroup members than that of outgroup members and that ingroup members' pain is more likely to trigger an empathic response. Finally, we explore the role that social identity processes play in determining how people appraise their own pain and how group memberships – and the social identities that are derived from those groups – helps them to cope with pain. In these sections, we will not only look at the relationship between social identities and physical pain, but also touch on the ways in which social identities affect the appraisal and coping response to social pain in the form of ostracism and rejection.

Pain is a social glue that binds people to the group

Even though pain can be experienced alone and in isolation, more often than not, it is shared with others. Moreover, there is good evidence that pain is a particularly powerful way of drawing people together. In particular, this claim is supported by work which shows that people appear to value their group memberships more after they have undergone painful initiation rites to become part of the group (see Figure 12.7).

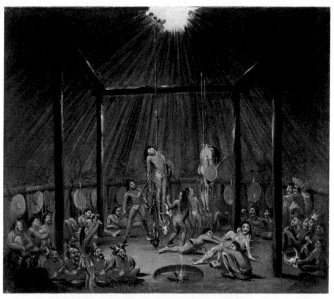

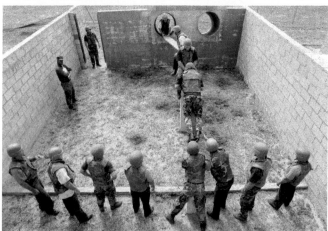

Figure 12.7 Pain as part of group initiation

Note: It is common for pain of one form or another to be a prominent feature of group initiation. As a result, prospective groups members are able to prove that they value membership of the group. These scenes show men being initiated as warriors into the Mandan tribe of Native Americans and as leaders in the U.S. Marines.

Source: Wikipedia

This point was demonstrated in a classic study by Harold Gerard and Grover Mathewson (1966) who subjected women to either a mild or a painful electric shock prior to joining a group discussion. In some conditions the shock was described as a necessary pre-requisite to joining the group, whereas in other conditions it was unrelated to the discussion group. When pain was said to be unrelated to group membership, there was no difference in participants' ratings of the attractiveness of the group in the mild and severe shock conditions. However, when people were led to believe that pain was a necessary part of joining the group, the severity of shock had a significant impact on the perceived attractiveness ratings – with participants who had received a severe shock rating the group as much more attractive than those who only received a mild shock. In line with the earlier work of Elliot Aronson and Judson Mills (1959), this finding was explained with reference to Leon Festinger's (1957) *cognitive dissonance theory*: when people know that pain is the only way to gain access to the group, enduring more of it needs to be rationalised with reference to the outcome. Here, then, this rationalisation takes the form of an attribution that "this must be a really great group for me to endure this amount of suffering to get accepted into it". Indeed, this process of cognitive dissonance has been used not only to account for ratings of group attractiveness after pain, but also to explain why entry into many groups and communities is marked by both a requirement and a willingness to endure pain and suffering. This means, on the one hand, that entry to groups is deliberately made painful so that people will value their membership of them and, on the other hand, that prospective group members are willing to undergo pain as a way of proving that they do indeed value the group.

However, beyond the context of group initiation, there are also other accounts of this capacity for pain to bring people together. In this vein, Brian Turner and Steven Wainwright (2003) describe how the experience of pain is commonly associated with increased solidarity and social bonding that helps strengthen a sense of "us". More specifically, these researchers studied ballet dancers and found that the experience of injury and tolerance of pain were so intrinsically bound up with their profession that the experience of pain became a core element of dancers' social identity. This is seen in one female dancer's response to an interviewer's question about injury:

> I don't think of them as injuries. You know that what you're doing are things you can do and positions that other people can get into, so somehow you realise that it's not quite normal. And so you always have aches and pains, which is part and parcel, and if you don't get aches and pains then you are not performing, you're not pushing yourself far enough. So to some extent it's built into the discipline of ballet. Part of the discipline is to have pain.
>
> (Turner & Wainwright, 2003, p. 282)

Because for these professional dancers, ballet is "not just something that you do – it is something that you are" (Turner & Wainwright, 2003, p. 284), the combination of dancing, injury, and pain becomes the embodiment of what it means to be a dancer and, as the researchers argue, this experience also increases their solidarity with other dancers. Here, then, it is not just a case of 'no pain, no gain', but also of 'no pain, no us'.

Other researchers have also argued that taking part in intense and painful rituals enhances group cohesion and promotes cooperative behaviour (Atran & Henrich, 2010; Durkheim, 1912). Evidence to support this reasoning is provided by the work by Dimitris Xygalatas and colleagues (2013) who studied charitable giving in the context of two different forms of mass religious ritual during the Hindu festival of Thaipusam in Mauritius. Although both rituals represent ways to express commitment to the group, one ritual involves a much more painful method of demonstrating devotion in so far as participants are required to pierce their skin with large skewers and hooks. This high-ordeal ritual contrasts starkly with a low-ordeal ritual which involves individuals taking part in religious prayer and meditation sessions. Here the researchers found that the more pain people experienced during the high-ordeal ritual, the more they subsequently donated to the temple (i.e., their ingroup). In fact, participants donated nearly twice as much money after taking part in the high-ordeal rather than the low-ordeal ritual. Interestingly too, identification as a Mauritian was significantly higher after taking part in the high-ordeal ritual. What we see here, then, is how pain can bring people together by strengthening their commitment to the group and their willingness to make personal sacrifices on its behalf.

Similar patterns were observed in the context of a collective mid-winter swim in Tasmania (Ferris et al., 2017). Swimmers were invited to participate in the study on the morning of the winter solstice both before and immediately after the swim was completed. Comparing these ratings, it was clear that after their swim participants in these painful group experiences not only felt more identified with other

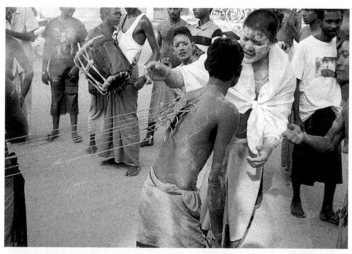

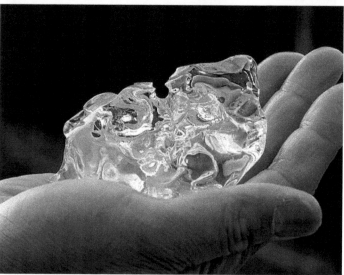

Figure 12.8 High-ordeal experiences in the field and the laboratory

Note: These are images of a piercing ritual in India (top) and an ice-immersion ordeal in the laboratory (bottom). Both these contexts are ones in which pain is found to enhance commitment to the group and group cohesion.

Source: Pixabay

swimmers but also with the broader festival as a whole. It thus appeared that the painful experience enhanced swimmers' sense of shared identity not just with those who underwent the same painful experience, but also with others who were part of the broader identity within which the activity was embedded.

The capacity for pain to bring people together has also been observed in laboratory studies. In particular, this is seen in studies by Bastian, Jetten, and Ferris (2014a) which invited participants to a lab and assigned them to groups comprising between three and five people who were not previously known to each other. These groups were randomly assigned to complete painful tasks together (e.g., holding their hand in ice-cold water, eating hot chilies, doing wall squats), or non-painful tasks (e.g., holding their hand in water that was room temperature, eating a hard-boiled sweet, or standing on one foot; see Figure 12.8). After these tasks group cohesion and trust were measured, and trust was also examined behaviourally by asking participants to play an economic game with their fellow participants in which outcomes depended on their willingness to cooperate with each other.

In line with the connection hypothesis that we discussed in Chapter 2 (H12), results showed that, relative to participants in the non-painful condition, those who had endured painful tasks together rated their groups as more cohesive and had significantly more trust in other group members. Moreover, this elevated trust was shown not just in ratings but also in the choices that participants made in the economic game. More specifically, when they had shared the experience of pain, participants showed that they were more likely to trust their partner to cooperate by cooperating more themselves from the game's outset.

But the benefits of collective suffering do more than enhance feelings of cohesion and unity. In a study of the Hajj in Mecca, David Clingingsmith, Asim Khwaja, and Michael Kremer (2009) showed that the pilgrims' endurance of extreme living conditions and exposure to extreme weather serves to create a sense of connection among people of different ethnicities, nationalities, sects, and genders – groups that are typically divided in day-to-day life. In their research, Clingingsmith and colleagues (2009) compared the responses of those who were able to attend the Hajj because they had won a ticket in the Hajj lottery with those who were not successful in the lottery and so unable to attend. What they found was that those who attended the Hajj reported a greater sense of shared identity than those who had to stay at home, despite the fact that the Hajj attendees reported lower levels of emotional and physical well-being as a result of the physically taxing nature of their experience.

Again, then, it appears that collectively enduring harsh conditions draws people towards others who have undergone similar forms of suffering. More specifically, what the earlier research shows is that enduring pain collectively serves an identity function by connecting us to others, and that this feeling of connectedness is linked to a range of positive psychosocial outcomes such as greater cooperation and pro-social behaviour. Indeed, although the studies provide no evidence that shared identity made pain more bearable (something we will explore more later), their findings suggest that shared pain can facilitate group formation and that, as set out in Hypotheses 12 to 15, this can bring people together in powerful ways – in particular, by imbuing them with a sense of connection, meaning, support, and agency.

"Our" pain is more real than "their" pain

According to the first line of Peter Gabriel's song, "Not One of Us", "It's only water in a stranger's tear". In line with this observation, there is good evidence of an 'us' versus 'them' effect when it comes to the experience of pain. In short, the pain that 'we', the ingroup, experience is appraised differently – and typically seen to be more real, severe, and harmful – than the pain that 'they', the outgroup, experience. This point is brought home by the findings of a minimal group study in which participants were randomly assigned to one of two arbitrary groups (Montalan, Lelard, Godefroy, & Mouras, 2012; for more details of this paradigm see Chapter 2). In this participants were all shown the same pictures of people who had their hands and feet in painful situations. However, when it came to rating the pain of the people in the pictures, if they were in the participants' ingroup, those people were thought to be experiencing greater pain than was the case if they were in an outgroup. Along similar lines, neuroscientific studies have also found that electroencephalogram (EEG) activity associated with mirror neuron activity (which is seen to be indicative of greater empathy) is more pronounced when participants watch videos of a needle syringe piercing the hands of someone who is in their ethnic ingroup rather than in an ethnic outgroup (Riecansky, Paul, Kölble, Stieger, & Lamm, 2015; see also Avenanti, Sirigu, & Aglioti, 2010).

Research examining the neural underpinnings of empathy supports similar conclusions (for a review see Cikara & Van Bavel, 2014). For example, a study found that there was greater activation of the anterior insula (a brain region typically activated during the experience of pain) when participants viewed members of an ingroup soccer team suffering pain than when they viewed outgroup members experiencing the same pain (Hein, Silani, Preuschoff, Batson, & Singer, 2010). Likewise, another study found that when Chinese and Caucasian participants viewed videos of people's cheeks being given painful (needle penetration) or non-painful (cotton swab) stimulation, there was relatively more activation in brain regions associated with the experience of pain when exposed to the painful stimulus only if the recipient was a member of the participants' cultural ingroup (Xu, Zuo, Wang, & Han, 2009). Thus whereas we find 'our' pain engrossing, 'their' pain is much more likely to leave us cold.

Similar findings have been reported when we observe the emotional pain of others. In particular, a study by Jenifer Gutsell and Michael Inzlicht (2012) found that people show similar brain responses when they are sad *themselves* as they do when they *observe* sad ingroup members (in this case other people who shared their ethnic identity); however, the same responses were not evident when participants observed sad outgroup members (those with a different ethnic identity). Indeed, on the contrary, Mina Cikara and Susan Fiske (2011) found that when people see an outgroup member suffer, brain regions associated with *positive* affect are activated. In other words, this research provides neural evidence of *schadenfreude* (literally 'harm joy') – the state of taking pleasure in others' pain (Leach, Spears, Branscombe, & Doosje, 2003; Spears & Leach, 2004)

In sum, the appraisal of others' pain is shaped in no small way by the degree to which those others are perceived to share social identity by those who witness it. When they do (i.e., so that they are members of a psychological ingroup), their social and/or physical pain becomes 'our' pain and we feel the same hurt that we expect them to. This then facilitates support provision and, in line with the support hypothesis (H14), ingroup members can expect to give each other more support and to construe that support more positively in ways that help to unlock a social cure. But because outgroup members do not share identity with us, their suffering is much more likely to be overlooked or, alternatively, the seriousness of their pain will tend to be downplayed. And because this fails to unlock the curative powers of empathy and support, it is much more likely to have deleterious effects on their health and well-being.

Social identity affects the appraisal of pain

But what happens in situations when, rather than witnessing others' pain, we experience it ourselves? In particular, do social identity processes also have a bearing on whether we appraise our own experience as more or less painful? Well, yes they do. In particular, and in line with some of the evidence that we presented when discussing stress in Chapter 5, there is good evidence that social identification with other group members plays a significant role in determining how painful we find the suffering that results from challenging circumstances.

This point emerges clearly from research conducted by Kavita Pandey and colleagues at the Magh Mela in northern India (a Hindu religious festival that we previously discussed in Chapter 2; Pandey, Stevenson, Shankar, Hopkins, & Reicher, 2014). Here the researchers found that all the pilgrims they interviewed agreed that the conditions were extreme and that the cold was painful. However, they generally agreed too that the cold made their experience as pilgrims more meaningful. In other words, because the cold was perceived as identity affirming, it was not construed as being especially painful.

As one female pilgrim put it, "people are saying that it is so cold, but it is this cold that we like here" (Pandey et al., 2014, p. 680).

The question this raises is whether the pilgrims did not feel the cold or else felt it but just did not experience it as painful. This is not easy to answer, as the experiences themselves are variable and complex. Nevertheless, Shail Shankar and colleagues (2013) provide experimental evidence which suggests that experiences one would normally associate with severe pain were not registered as painful by the Magh Mela pilgrims. In their study they presented pilgrims with some of the intense noises of the Mela through headphones and, in different conditions, told them either that these had been generated at this religious festival or in the city outside. When pilgrims believed the noise had been generated in the city, they rated it as quite unpleasant and even painful. However, when they believed that the noise was from the Mela, they found it blissful and serene and were prepared to listen to it for almost twice as long. Again, the reason for this is that when the cacophony was thought to be generated at the Mela, it was understood to be identity affirming – and hence was experienced as a source of joy rather than pain.

This point was confirmed in a subsequent qualitative study that Shankar and colleagues undertook to explore participants' own reflections on their experiences at the Mela. In line with the conclusions that they drew from their experimental evidence, the nature of these is exemplified by the following exchange between an interviewer and two pilgrims:

Interviewer: Like there is this noise all the time, there is this crowd, people are coming.
Pilgrim 22a: No. No disturbance.
Pilgrim 22b: It feels so nice.
Interviewer: It feels so nice?
Pilgrim 22a: It is pure joy.
Pilgrim 22b: You get darshan [a Hindu term for divine visions]. There are discourses from morning to evening. This is pure joy. This is what we have come for, no?
(Shankar et al., 2013, p. 92)

Along similar lines, other research also indicates that group memberships and intergroup comparisons can affect pain appraisal. In particular, a classic study (Lambert, Libman, & Poser, 1960, Experiment 2) found that intergroup comparisons which pose a threat to ingroup identity affect people's capacity to tolerate pain. This brought Jewish and Protestant participants into a laboratory and tested their pain tolerance before making their religious identity salient. They were then told about scientific findings purportedly showing that members of their religious group were able to withstand pain to a lesser or greater extent than members of the other religious group. Rising to the occasion when provoked, both religious groups increased their pain tolerance when they had been told that their religious ingroup was less able to tolerate pain than the outgroup. And whereas Jewish participants showed no change in tolerance when they had been told their group had superior pain tolerance, Protestant participants showed superior tolerance under these conditions.

Findings such as these accord with the proverbial wisdom that pain is a lot easier to bear when it has meaning. In this they suggest that people's capacity to suffer pain is not fixed but rather varies as a function of the significance that this suffering acquires through the lens of a salient identity. Above all else, this means that pain proves far easier to endure to the extent that it is understood to promote ingroup interests – so that here pain *is* gain.

Social identity can help people cope with physical pain

All in all, then, there is considerable evidence that group membership (and the social identity associated with it) affects people's primary appraisal of pain. But does social identity also affect secondary appraisal – that is, how well equipped we feel to respond to the pain? For example, does it matter whether it is an ingroup member or an outgroup member who tries to support us through the painful experience?

Research by Michael Platow and his colleagues (2007) suggests that shared identity does indeed matter when it comes to benefitting from the social support that might help people cope with pain. In their study, participants were invited to come to the laboratory and, when they were there, asked to perform a cold-pressor task (in which, as discussed earlier, they were asked to keep their hand in freezing cold water until they could no longer tolerate the pain). After they had completed this procedure participants were informed that this first task merely served the purpose of allowing them to experience how painful the task could get and that they would now complete it again in what was actually the critical trial. As well as unobtrusively measuring the time participants held their hand in the water, the experimenter measured galvanic skin responses (GSR, a measure of physiological arousal) as well as subjective experiences of stress after both trials.

Importantly for the present purposes, after the first trial had been completed, the experimenter left the room for a short while and during this period another person entered who introduced themselves as someone who had taken part in the same study previously. In actual fact, and unknown to participants, this person was a confederate working for the experimenter. The confederate identified themselves as either sharing (e.g., by saying they were a science student if the participant was a science student) or not sharing group membership with the participants (e.g., by saying they were an arts student if the participant was a science student). What is more, the confederate told the participant how they should appraise the upcoming cold-pressor task by saying, "Well, don't worry, the second time is much easier". There was also a control condition in which no confederate entered the room between the two trials.

What the researchers found was that although the amount of time that participants held their hand in the ice-cold water in the second trial did not differ across the three conditions, subjective ratings of stress and physiological arousal (i.e., GSR) were both significantly lower when they had been reassured about the second trial by an ingroup member than when they had been reassured by an outgroup member or when they had received no reassurance at all. Along the lines of our previous discussion in Chapter 5, Platow and colleagues (2007) explained these findings with reference to the processes of social influence that structure secondary appraisal (e.g., "Can I cope?"; see Figure 5.2). More specifically, in line with the influence hypothesis (H9), they reasoned that social support was more effective in moderating appraisals of pain when it came from an ingroup member because this person was seen as more qualified to inform participants about the meaning of their experience (in ways argued by Haslam, Jetten, O'Brien, & Jacobs, 2004; Turner, 1991). In this case, then, when the ingroup member indicated that the ingroup norm was that "we are able to tolerate pain", those experiencing pain were more likely to internalise this as an appropriate way of orienting to and interpreting their sensory experience.

Jones and Jetten (2011) took this logic further by examining whether the beneficial effects of ingroup support require ingroup members to be physically present when a person undergoes a painful experience. Might merely thinking about important groups that one belongs to be sufficient to unlock the beneficial effects of group membership? Moreover, might this be further enhanced if people think about not just one group that they belong to, but about multiple ingroups? As suggested by the multiple identities hypothesis (H11), Jones and Jetten reasoned that if membership in social groups has beneficial effects for health and well-being, then it follows that the more of these group memberships that a person has psychological access to, the more protected they will be when confronted with a painful stressor. This is because, as we suggested in Chapter 2, feeling that one is connected to others and embedded in a larger social network should contribute to a sense of existential security (Durkheim, 1951) and a feeling that one has "ground to stand upon" (Lewin, 1935, p. 175), and this secure sense of self should make the person stronger and more resilient in the face of potentially painful challenges.

Jones and Jetten (2011) tested these predictions in a laboratory-based study. This involved randomly assigning participants to one of three conditions in which they were asked to think about

(1) one group, (2) three groups, or (3) five groups to which they belonged. For each of these groups participants were then asked to consider what membership meant to them and to rate how important membership in this group was for them. Then, in an ostensibly unrelated second part of the study, they were asked to complete a cold-pressor task (as in Platow et al., 2007). They were told that when the physical pain of the task became too intense to bear, they should take their hand out of the water.

The results of the study are presented in Figure 12.9. From this it can be seen that, in line with H11, participants who had been asked to think about more groups that they belonged to were able to endure pain for longer. Indeed, those who thought about five groups were able to keep their hand in the freezing water for about twice as long as those who only thought about one group. The significance of this study is that it shows very clearly that it is social group membership, and not just social support, that produces greater resilience in the face of pain. The study also shows that ingroup members do not need to be physically present in order for the benefits of group membership to manifest themselves. Overcoming pain is therefore not just a question of receiving tangible support from ingroup members; sometimes mere awareness of one's group memberships can be a source of solace in the face of life's slings and arrows.

Extending this line of reasoning, other research using neuro-scientific techniques (specifically, functional magnetic resonance imaging; fMRI) shows that multiple group memberships can play a somewhat different role when it comes to responding to pain. This is a point that emerges from a study conducted by Laura Ferris and her colleagues (Ferris, Jetten, Molenberghs, Bastian, & Karnadewi, 2016). In this, participants were presented with cues that alerted them to either one or four group memberships that they had identified as being important to them in a previous session by having the names of those groups shown on a screen for a few seconds. At the same time, though, there was a subset of trials in which they simultaneously received either painful or non-painful stimulation of their hand

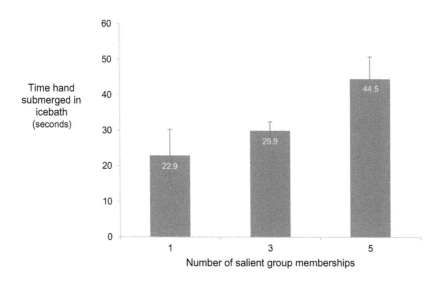

Figure 12.9 Exposure to pain as a function of the number of groups made salient

Note: When more groups were made salient, the amount of time that people kept their non-dominant hand submerged in the ice bath increased. Consistent with the multiple identities hypothesis (H11), this suggests that simply thinking about important group memberships can help to enhance physical resilience.

Source: Based on Jones and Jetten (2011)

(being either pricked with a toothpick or touched with a cotton bud). The experimenters then asked participants to rate their pain and observed the activation of pain regions in the brain (specifically, the dorsal anterior cingulate cortex and anterior insula activation).

Results from the study showed that participants in the four-group condition rated their pain as more severe than those in the one-group condition. This had not been predicted, but they can be seen to indicate that people are more motivated to *express* their pain when multiple group memberships are salient. What was particularly interesting, though, was the relationship between this expression of pain and participants' pain-related brain activation. For although their subjective ratings of pain increased when more group memberships were made salient, this manipulation led to a corresponding *decrease* of activity in the pain regions of their brains. Although these findings are complex, one way of making sense of them is to see that multiple group memberships are a psychological resource that provides the basis for an adaptive coping response to pain (in line with H11) in which pain expression mitigates against pain experience. That is, by motivating us to articulate our pain, social identities can thereby also help us deal with it (in ways also suggested by our discussion of trauma and resilience in Chapter 6).

Support for this analysis can also be gleaned by returning to the case of the Magh Mela. For here, too, it is apparent that social identities structured pilgrims' secondary appraisal processes in ways that helped them cope with pain. In particular, Pandey and her colleagues (2014) found that a strong sense of shared social identity with others at the festival was the basis for mutual support that allowed pilgrims to endure intense physical hardship (especially that which resulted from freezing temperatures). As an illustration of this, the researchers describe an exchange in which two pilgrims, R and V, provide support to a young girl who is afraid of the bitter cold:

> The cold wind is blowing strong. It is really feeling chilled. R asks the kid to go and take dip. She is a girl around 9 years of age. She was feeling cold. As R told her to go and take dip, she replied "I do not feel like taking bath in this cold".

> R: Oh, so you do not want to take dip.
> V: Come on, take off your sweater and go and take dip. Be fast.
> Girl: It is very cold.

> We hear a voice – "it is not cold dear". We turn around and see that he is an adult of around 45–55 years. He continues "It is just now. Once you go there, it is not cold". I notice he has just come out of the water and is changing clothes. I also encourage/try to motivate the child "It is not that cold. The sun is also there, it would not be cold". The girl finally starts taking off her sweater. She is shivering. Slowly she moves towards the water.

> Man: Do not be scared. When you are scared of anything it will get over you. Do not let your fear dominate on you. Say to mother Ganga, "Oh mother, I am coming. I am not fearful of the cold I am coming to take dip".
>   (Pandey et al., 2014, p. 685)

As Pandey and colleagues note, the key point here is that just as it is the group that ultimately makes pain meaningful, so, too, it is the group that encourages pain to be confronted.

Social identity can help people cope with social pain

There is an increased recognition that social identity not only affects the way that acute physical pain is appraised and responded to, but also the way that people respond to social pain – for example, the pain that results from being ostracised or rejected by others. Social rejection is distressing and, as we suggested earlier, there is a growing body of work which shows that even the pain and hurt from minor forms of rejection or exclusion (and even single instances of it) can be observed at the physiological level (McQuaid, McInnis, Matheson, & Anisman, 2015). For example, people report an increase in negative emotions even when they are rejected by a computer or scripted confederate (Zadro, Williams, & Richardson, 2004), when they simply imagine a negative reaction from people (Leary, Haupt, Strausser, & Chokel, 1998), or when they vicariously experience others' ostracism (Coyne, Nelson, Robinson, & Gundersen, 2011).

Responses to rejection are not limited to feeling hurt, but are also evident in the aggression levels of those who are rejected. And even though aggression is not directly tied to a person's own health, it is clear that it can negatively affect the health of others. In this regard, a number of studies have reported an increase in participants' aggression or anger following rejection (e.g., DeWall, Twenge, Bushman, Im, & Williams, 2010). For example, research showed that participants who had been made to feel excluded by others were more critical (e.g., they provided more negative evaluations of unknown job applicants) and more behaviourally aggressive (e.g., exposing others to higher levels of aversive noise) than those who had been included or were in a control condition (Twenge, Baumeister, Tice, & Stucke, 2001).

But although these findings make sense, one issue to keep in mind is that when people are rejected in a laboratory context, they typically face the rejection on their own. In that sense, they are cut off from the type of supports that they would normally draw on to help them deal with rejection – most notably, input from other people and groups that are important to them.

Again, the social identity approach explains why and how group membership might be an important social resource to help counteract the experience of social pain in such contexts (Haslam, Jetten, Postmes, & Haslam, 2009; Jetten, Haslam, & Haslam, 2012; Tajfel & Turner, 1986). In particular, as we have seen in a number of earlier chapters (e.g., Chapters 2 through 5), salient group memberships can enhance people's sense of connectedness to others, and this can be just as important for well-being as the physical presence of others that offer support. Indeed, sometimes it will be more important.

This is a hypothesis that two of us tested in a study which we conducted together with Morgana Lizzio-Wilson to see whether the mere salience of group membership might be enough to diminish the extent to which rejection subsequently enhances aggression (Cruwys, Lizzio-Wilson, & Jetten, 2017). We also examined whether the effects of group membership salience were cumulative – that is, whether, as the multiple identities hypothesis (H11) would suggest, thinking about more group memberships results in an incrementally weaker relationship between rejection and aggression. To test this prediction, the study experimentally manipulated the psychological availability of group memberships (none, one, three, or five) prior to an experience of rejection that involved participants being left out of a group. The results are presented in Figure 12.10, and from this it can be seen that, as predicted, individuals who experienced rejection were less likely to retaliate aggressively when they were psychologically conscious of their social group memberships. In this case, though, the buffering provided by group membership did not appear to be cumulative – instead the salience of *any* number of group memberships (one, three, or five) served to reduce aggression. This pattern clearly contrasts with the linear effect observed in other studies of physical resilience (e.g., Jones & Jetten, 2011; see Figure 12.9) and suggests that all reminders of group membership help people cope with the pain of rejection.

Returning to issues that we first raised in Chapter 2, it is also the case that Cruwys and colleagues' (2017) study has important implications for our conceptualisation of the nature of the psychological resource that is provided by group memberships. This is because, in contrast to "the more, the merrier" message (as specified by H11; Iyer, Jetten, Tsivrikos, Postmes, & Haslam, 2009), its results suggest that the salience of one group membership alone can be protective when it comes to buffering the effects of rejection. Nevertheless, this does not necessarily undermine the multiple resource message, as having access to multiple group memberships might be important in different contexts. In particular, although *in the moment* the key thing might be that a person has access to a single meaningful group

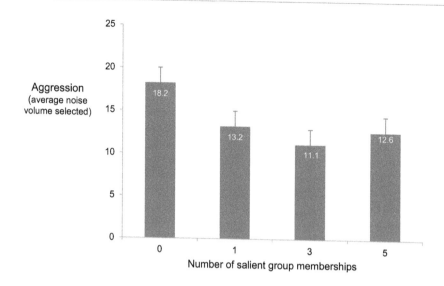

Figure 12.10 Aggression as a function of available group memberships following social rejection

Note: Results show that participants in conditions where one or more group memberships were made salient were less
likely to aggress than those in the condition where no groups were made salient. No differences in aggression were
found between the one-, three-, and five-group conditions, suggesting that effects of multiple salient group memberships are not cumulative. These results imply that reminding oneself of one's social resources can help people
cope with the experience of rejection.

Source: Cruwys et al (2017)

membership, over a period of time (e.g., while going through a life transition) having a greater number
of meaningful group memberships nevertheless increases the chances that, *at any given moment*, a
person will have an appropriate social identity to draw upon when they need it (e.g. Iyer, et al., 2009;
Jones & Jetten, 2011).

Although much more research needs to be done to explore these issues, it seems plausible that
social identity resources also have an important role in helping individuals manage their negative
reactions to social rejection effectively outside the laboratory. This is important because such rejection
is a common experience – whether it centres on major events such as missing out on a new job or the
breakdown of a relationship, or more minor incidents such as being ignored by a shop assistant or
having a colleague forget your birthday. The point to note here is that, by and large, individuals manage such rejection without feeling the need to retaliate aggressively. Social identity research helps us
understand why this is the case, suggesting too that meaningful group memberships are an antidote to
the multiple sources of pain that punctuate everyday life.

Conclusion

Pain is commonly associated with illness, injury, and harm, but it is also commonly experienced
in a range of normal, enjoyable, and healthy pursuits. Our knowledge regarding the role of pain within
these domains in reinforcing behaviour, providing for a sense of goal achievement, or facilitating

social bonding is limited. It is clear, however, that a social identity approach to pain adds substantially to this understanding. In particular, this is because through this lens we are able to understand how pain can act as social glue, to bind us to others, how it underpins pain maintenance behaviours, and when it can be used strategically for benefit. It is also clear that social identity processes affect both primary and secondary appraisal of pain – that is, our sense that pain is harmful as well as our belief that we can cope effectively with it.

More generally, the social identity approach helps shed light on the ways in which pain is given meaning through social interaction – most critically, through group memberships that make enduring pain seem noble, worthwhile, and character building. It also suggests that a failure to engage with relevant group processes (e.g., of valorisation and support) will often reduce our ability to treat and manage pain effectively. Not least this is because when it comes to coping with pain, social identity theorising shows how the *psychological availability* of group memberships can buffer us from the negative impact of pain and rejection. This in turn speaks to the importance of the psychological representation of social relationships and contributes to a substantial evidence base which indicates that psychological group membership is more important for health than more concrete social resources such as contact (Sani, Herrera, Wakefield, Boroch, & Gulyas, 2012) or company (Teng & Chen, 2012).

Importantly too, the social identity approach also opens up new strategies that individuals can deploy to understand and deal with the different kinds of pain that they encounter in their day-to-day lives – most notably by pointing to the palliative power of meaningful group memberships. Indeed, the capacity to draw on group-based social relationships even when others are *not* physically present would seem to be critical to people's capacity to cope with the multiple sources of pain that are the stuff of a life well lived.

Points for practice

The focus in this chapter has been on the way in which social identities and group memberships affect primary appraisals (i.e., "is this painful?") as well as secondary appraisals (i.e., "can I cope?") associated with acute pain. Given this, the following three points are important to bear in mind when working with people who are experiencing acute pain.

1. *Be aware that the expression of pain is not just determined by actual tissue damage and physiological responses, but also by psychological and social factors.* In particular, social context has a significant bearing on people's appraisals of pain, and the extent to which they can draw on effective social support from those around them (members of various groups) will impact significantly on their pain experience and pain tolerance.

2. *Do not assume that because social identity factors affect a person's pain experience or tolerance that their pain is any less real.* With greater recognition that psychological and social factors affect the experience of, and coping with, pain, it becomes all the more important to think about how to support those who experience it. In this regard it is a serious mistake to regard someone who presents with pain simply as someone who has failed to access effective social support.

3. *It is essential to recognise the ways in which identity-related resources can be mobilised when it comes to helping people cope with their pain.* This point speaks to the fact that there are important new challenges ahead for practitioners: for the more it is understood that pain is not just a neural experience in the brain, the more it becomes important to effectively manage the social environments of those who experience pain. At the same time, this is also good news, as it highlights that there are things we can do to help those who experience pain and that there are solutions other than simply prescribing pain medication.

Resources

Further reading

The following publications provide a good introduction to work that explores the psychological and social dimensions of pain.

① Bastian, B., Jetten, J., Hornsey, M. J., & Leknes, S. (2014). The positive consequences of pain: A biopsychosocial approach. *Personality and Social Psychology Review, 18,* 256–279.

This review paper maps out the positive biological, psychological, and social consequences of physical pain. It explains how pain can be identity affirming and how social group membership affects pain appraisal and coping.

② MacDonald, G., & Leary, M. R. (2005). Why does social exclusion hurt? The relationship between social and physical pain. *Psychological Bulletin, 131,* 202–223.

This review brings together research on social and physical pain and shows that the two forms of pain have much in common when it comes to how they are experienced by sufferers.

③ Platow, M. J., Voudouris, N. J., Gilford, N., Jamieson, R., Najdovski, L., Papaleo, N., . . . & Terry, L. (2007). In-group reassurance in a pain setting produces lower levels of physiological arousal: direct support for a self-categorization analysis of social influence. *European Journal of Social Psychology, 37,* 649–660.

This paper reports a study which provides evidence that pain appraisals and pain experience are affected by social influence processes in ways hypothesised by self-categorization theory (as set out in H9).

Video

① Search for "Why we need pain to feel happiness" to watch a TEDx talk by Dr. Brock Bastian: www.youtube.com/watch?v=W_x9cbrdgnw. This discusses the relationship between pain and pleasure and the way in which the two are often part and parcel of the same experience.   (15 minutes)

② Search for "Mackey Pain and Brain" to see a 20-minute YouTube video by Professor Sean Mackey (www.youtube.com/watch?v=otUVzK4hToM). This provides an overview of the way that the brain is involved in pain perception and pain regulation. In particular, he discusses studies which show that pain is not just in the brain and explains how psychological factors affect pain perception.   (20 minutes)

Websites

In recent years *The Conversation* has published a series of pieces on pain. The following are particularly worth reading:

① https://theconversation.com/explainer-what-is-pain-and-what-is-happening-when-we-feel-it-49040. In this piece Professor Lorimer Moseley gives a brief account of what pain is and what happens when we experience it.

② https://theconversation.com/how-different-cultures-experience-and-talk-about-pain-49046. Professor Roland Sussex discusses cultural differences in the way people talk about pain and experience it.

③ https://theconversation.com/not-helping-a-partner-with-chronic-pain-may-be-the-quick-est-road-to-recovery-48978. Dr. Toby Newton-John explains the way that social support can both help and hinder recovery for those suffering from chronic pain.

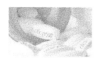

Chapter 13
Chronic mental health conditions

In his 2015 memoir *On the Move*, the much-loved physician and author Oliver Sacks recalls his brother Michael's schizophrenia and its treatment in the mid-1950s (see Figure 13.1). Michael was prescribed Largactil, the first available medication in a class of major tranquillisers. Sacks observed that although the medication helped with the positive symptoms of schizophrenia (hallucinations and delusions), it offered little assistance with the negative symptoms (social withdrawal, reduced capacity to experience pleasure, lack of motivation). Sacks saw his brother struggle with social and everyday living skills and, to deal with these, he thought he needed a social and "existential" approach – not simply medication – in order to restore a meaningful and enjoyable life (Sacks, 2015, p. 63).

Fast-forward 60 years, and the options for people with schizophrenia and other enduring and persistent mental health conditions (hereafter referred to as *chronic mental health conditions*, CMHC) have not kept pace with the breakthroughs seen in other areas of health. Major tranquillisers and combinations of medications continue to be prescribed – often with distressing side effects. The negative symptoms and the task of living a meaningful and enjoyable life remain a challenge for individuals, their families, and health care providers. In this chapter, we will explore current understandings and treatments of CMHC and then turn to explore how a social identity approach can provide a way forward for practice and policy related to the management of these conditions.

The nature and impact of CMHC

The term CMHC typically includes such conditions as schizophrenia, schizoaffective disorder, bipolar disorders, recurrent depression, posttraumatic stress disorder, personality disorders, and addiction (Woods, Willison, Kington, & Gavin, 2008). The topics of trauma, depression, and addiction have already been covered in some detail (in Chapters 6, 8, and 9) and so in this chapter we will focus primarily on schizophrenia, schizoaffective disorder, and bipolar disorders (as set out in Table 13.1). These conditions – also collectively referred to as the *psychoses* – occur in approximately 3% of the population. As we will explain in more detail later, a combination of genetic and environmental factors are recognised to be involved in their aetiology (Perälä et al., 2007).

A person with schizophrenia experiences distortions in thinking that can affect their language, perceptions, attention, and sense of self. The symptoms are often referred to in two classes: *positive symptoms* are those that occur when something is 'added on' to normal functioning, and *negative symptoms* are when aspects of normal functioning are reduced. The positive symptoms of psychosis include visual, auditory, or other sensory hallucinations (e.g., hearing voices that others can't hear) or delusional thoughts (e.g., believing that one is a deity, or a paranoid sense that one is being persecuted by others – the latter symptom being experienced by about 90% of first-episode psychotic patients; Bentall et al., 2008; Moutoussis, Williams, Dayan, & Bentall, 2007). In this, they generally reflect the person's inability to tell what is real from what is imagined. Some individuals experience these distortions episodically, with intermittent periods of healthy perceptions and thinking, whereas others experience ongoing perceptual and thinking disturbances. Closely related to this condition is schizoaffective disorder, in which an individual experiences severe changes in mood alongside some of the psychotic symptoms of hallucinations, delusions, and disorganised thinking that characterise schizophrenia. Psychotic symptoms in schizoaffective disorder may also present even in the absence of mood symptoms.

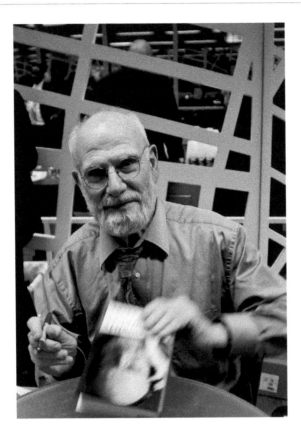

Figure 13.1 Oliver Sacks signing a copy of his book *Musicophilia*

Note: Sachs was a British neurologist who argued that in order for intervention for CMHC to be effective attention needs to be paid to their social dimensions.

Source: Dan Lurie, Flickr

In bipolar disorder, a person experiences periods of depression (with symptoms described in Chapter 8) and periods of mania that can last weeks (bipolar I) or days (bipolar II) or rapidly cycle. A diagrammatic representation of the time and intensity of fluctuations associated with various types of bipolar disorder is presented in Figure 13.2. During manic episodes, energy and activity levels are heightened and accompanied by a rush of creative ideas and speech with little sleep as well as elevated, or sometimes irritable, mood (Angst, 2012). In periods of mania, people may lose touch with reality and experience delusional beliefs or hallucinations. Their judgment and decision making may be impaired, and this can lead them to do such things as take on tasks they cannot manage, abandon responsibilities, engage in promiscuous sexual behaviour, or go on spending sprees that mean they accumulate sizeable gambling or credit debts. When manic individuals are so impaired as to threaten their own safety or that of others, hospitalisation is usually required. Moreover, it is often in the recovery phase from mania that

Table 13.1 Positive and negative symptoms of chronic mental health conditions

	Condition		
Symptoms	*Schizophrenia*	*Schizoaffective disorder*	*Bipolar disorders*
Positive			
delusions	g	g	s
hallucinations	g	g	s
thought disorders	g	g	s
mania		s	g
Negative			
low motivation	g	s	s
social withdrawal	g	g	s
social isolation	g	g	s
slow movement	s	s	s
little facial expression	s	g	s
anhedonia	s	s	s
low self-esteem	s	s	s
depressed mood	s	s	s

Notes: g = symptom generally present; s = symptom sometimes present (i.e., in particular periods of illness).

Positive symptoms are 'added on' to normal functioning; negative symptoms are 'taken away' or reduced. Positive symptoms also relate to aspects of CMHC that are condition specific (and tend to respond to drug treatment); negative symptoms are less specific and are more social in nature.

the patient is at significant risk from suicide – their depression being compounded by guilt and shame relating to the socially deprecating behaviour that they engaged in during the manic phase.

Although diagnostic classification systems such as the DSM5 and the ICD10 characterise the psychoses as separate disorders, other researchers argue for a single psychosis dimension (Crow, 1986; Reininghaus, Priebe, & Bentall, 2013). In fact the notion of a unitary psychosis has a long history. For example, in his 1859 text *Lehrbuch der Psychiatrie* Heinrich Neumann rejected the idea of separable disorders. In this regard, schizophrenia can be seen as a prototypical CMHC, and indeed, most of the evidence referred to in the following sections comes from research into this condition. This unitary approach to CMHC also seems warranted, given the strong overlap among symptoms of the conditions, such as perceptual and thought disturbances and their marked impact on the individual's social, emotional, and occupational functioning as well as on the activities involved in daily living.

CMHC typically begin in late adolescence or early adulthood – coinciding with the developmental phase in which most young people are establishing their identity, social networks, and intimate relationships and are either studying or starting their working life. It is not difficult, therefore, to imagine the wide-ranging impact that losing touch with reality has on the lives of individuals with CMHC and on their family and friends. Indeed, these consequences are readily apparent in

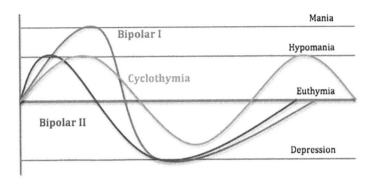

Figure 13.2 Mood fluctuations in subtypes of bipolar disorder

Note: In bipolar disorders people experience symptoms of depression and mania that fluctuate over time. In bipolar I the periods of mania last for weeks, whereas in bipolar II these symptoms usually last a number of days. In cyclothymia, people also experience emotional ups and downs, but these are not as extreme as those seen in bipolar I and II.

Source: http://neurowiki2013.wikidot.com/individual:cyclothymia

the so-called *negative symptoms* of schizophrenia (see Table 13.1). As a result of these, relative to other members of the population, people with CMHC tend to have fewer social contacts and supports, are likely to receive less income, and are at increased risk of unstable housing (Dingle, Cruwys, Jetten, Johnstone, & Walter, 2014; SANE Australia, 2010; see Figure 13.2). One example of this risk emerges from a report commissioned by the Queensland Mental Health Commission into the nature and causes of antisocial behaviour among tenants of social housing. In this, the authors observe that those tenants who are most at risk of eviction for antisocial behaviour have invariably experienced chronic mental health problems (Jones, Phillips, Parsell, & Dingle, 2014; QLD Mental Health Commission, 2015).

Compared to the general population, people who experience CMHC are less likely to engage in full-time work, post-secondary education, couple relationships, and childrearing (although cultural differences exist in relation to rates of marriage and children; Hutchinson, Bhugra, Mallett, Burnett, Corridan, & Leff, 1999; Prabha, Kommu, & Rudhran, 2012). They are also much more vulnerable to social isolation – which is perhaps unsurprising, given that the social networks and leisure activities that flow naturally from study, work, and family life are not so readily available to them (Morgan et al., 2011).

Furthermore, negative beliefs about oneself and one's condition tend to be widespread among people with CMHC, with half of this population reporting moderate to high levels of self-stigma (Brohan, Elgie, Sartorius, & Thornicroft, 2010). This in turn leads to low self-esteem and self-efficacy (Corrigan, Rafacz, & Rüsch, 2011). As we discussed in Chapter 4, stigma can adversely affect health and well-being via several pathways (e.g., see Figure 4.3) and is particularly damaging when a person perceives their stigma to be justified. Amongst other things, this is because stigma that is thought to be justified stands in the way of people identifying with others who share that stigma. Speaking to this point, Rusch, Angermeyer, and Corrigan (2005) found that self-prejudice can exacerbate the effects of CMHC because self-discrimination means that people fail to pursue work or independent living

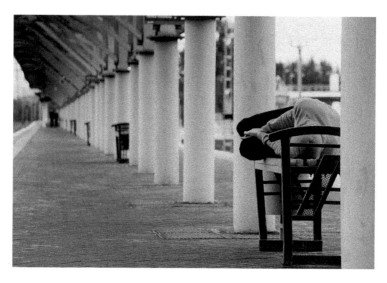

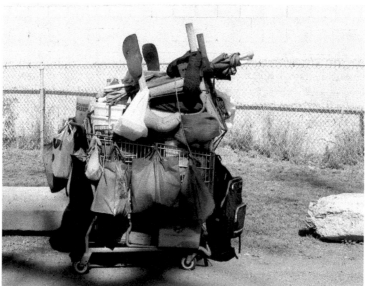

Figure 13.3 Living with schizophrenia

Note: Individuals experiencing schizophrenia and other chronic mental health conditions are much more likely than members of the general population to experience barriers to paid employment, housing, and other social resources.

Source: Pixabay

opportunities. In this way, a vicious cycle often emerges in which the symptoms of CMHC reinforce social exclusion, and this in turn reinforces those symptoms.

Not only are people with CMHC likely to be marginalised, but they are also likely to feel the negative effects of social exclusion especially keenly. This point emerges from a study by Yael Perry and her colleagues which compared the effects of ostracism on a group of individuals with CMHC to its effects on a group of matched controls (Perry, Henry, Sethi, & Grisham, 2011). Here participants were asked to play a computer game – Cyberball (Williams & Jarvis, 2006) – in which a (virtual) ball is thrown between themselves and two other (virtual) characters. The game simulates the experience of ostracism because, as it evolves, the two other characters start to pass the ball only between themselves, thereby making the participant feel left out (Williams, Cheung, & Choi, 2000). What the researchers found was that this social exclusion elicited an automatic, reflexive response in participants with CMHC such that the negative impact of ostracism on symptoms of depression, anxiety, and stress lasted significantly longer for them than it did for the controls. So although all participants found social isolation painful, for those with CMHC the pain was much more likely to persist.

Current approaches to CMHC

Environmental risk factors

Research into the combination of genetic and environmental factors that increase the risk of schizophrenia shows that family history is an important predictor of the condition in association with urban birth, cannabis use, and trauma exposure (see McGrath, Mortensen, Visscher, & Wray, 2013, for an overview). However, a recent review of the first decade of research into these risk factors concluded that the field has also been dogged by failure to replicate findings, diminishing effect sizes over time, and publication biases (Duncan & Keller, 2011).

Although a range of stressors – including housing, finances, work, inadequate nutrition, and negative life events – may trigger a psychotic illness in someone who is vulnerable (Falloon, Kydd, Coverdale, & Laidlaw, 1996), research also indicates that *social stress* can play an especially pivotal role. An example is the stress arising from ongoing demanding or critical social dynamics (e.g., as discussed in Chapter 5; Nuechterlein & Dawson, 1984). In the case of CMHC, this has been examined predominately within the family context, and here researchers have paid particular attention to evidence that *high expressed emotion* is especially common among individuals with CMHC as well as their family members.

Expressed emotion is a term coined by George Brown (1985) to describe family environments that have five key characteristics: critical comments, hostility, emotional over-involvement, (low) positive remarks, and (low) warmth (Wearden, Tarrier, Barrowclough, Zastowny, & Rahill, 2000). Work by Dingle and colleagues has found that although individuals with CMHC engage in emotion-improving strategies in much the same way as healthy adults, they engage with others in significantly more *emotion-worsening* actions (e.g., being more likely to respond with annoyance and to identify problems with their current situation; Dingle, Williams, Jetten, & Welch, 2017). As a result of such patterns, in high-expressed emotion environments the median relapse rate of people with CMHC over 9 to 12 months is 48%, but this is only 21% in a low-expressed emotion environment (Kavanagh, 1992; see Figure 13.4). Rarely, though, are these social and emotional issues adequately addressed or resolved within treatment.

Genetic and biomedical approaches

Family and twin studies indicate that the psychoses have the highest heritability of the mental disorders (see Figure 13.5). Speaking to this point, Paul Lichtenstein and his colleagues (2009) identified over 9 million individuals from 2 million nuclear families in the Multi-Generation Register of

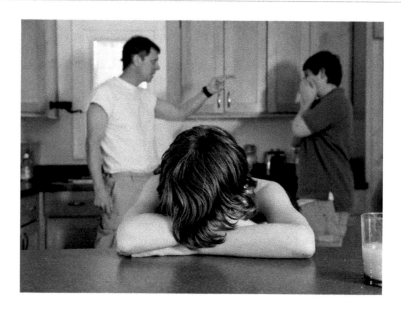

Figure 13.4 Expressed emotion in families

Note: Individuals with CMHC who live in environments where there is high expressed emotion have higher relapse rates after treatment (Kavanagh, 1992).

Source: Shutterstock

Sweden and used statistical modelling to estimate genetic and environmental contributions to liability for schizophrenia, bipolar disorder, and their comorbidity. They reported that schizophrenia was 64% heritable, bipolar disorder was 59% heritable, and comorbidity between the disorders was primarily due to additive genetic effects common to both disorders. Nonshared environmental effects on comorbidity were found to be around 30%. That said, research to establish that specific mental disorders can be explained by specific single nucleotide polymorphisms (DNA variations at a single nucleotide) still has a long way to go (Agerbo et al., 2012). Despite this lack of conclusive evidence, medical approaches have dominated the treatment of CMHC since the 1950s. One reason for this is that during a frank psychotic episode, individuals lose touch with reality, and it may be difficult for family members and friends to hold a coherent conversation with them. People experiencing psychosis may also be agitated and behave in odd or erratic ways in response to voices or delusional thoughts. Given the prominence of these positive symptoms, the most common approach to managing this presentation involves admitting the person to a psychiatric hospital where first-line treatment typically involves medication. This treatment approach is also common when managing people with bipolar disorder who are experiencing a manic episode.

The first-generation antipsychotic medications, such as chlorpromazine (marketed as Thorazine or Largactil and that was prescribed to Oliver Sacks's brother Michael; see Figure 13.5), have a strong affinity for dopamine D2 receptors as well as actions at a variety of serotonergic, adrenergic, and other receptor subtypes. The neurotransmitter dopamine is involved in the perceptual disturbances seen in the psychoses, so the function of blocking the dopamine receptors is to alleviate the positive symptoms of psychosis that present as hallucinations and delusions (Miyamoto, Duncan, Marx, & Lieberman, 2005). However, dopamine is also involved in motor and hormonal functions, so blocking dopamine

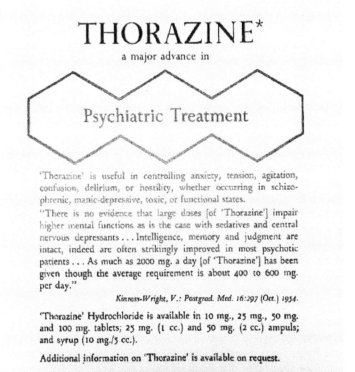

Figure 13.5 An 1950s advertisement for Thorazine

Note: Marketed by Smith, Kline, & French laboratories, Thorazine is a brand name for chlorpromazine (also marketed as Largactil). It is a first-generation antipsychotic medication which was at the forefront of the "psychopharmacological revolution" in psychiatry in the 1950s and is still widely used in the treatment of schizophrenia today (López-Muñoz et al., 2005).

Source: http://whale.to/a/chlorpromazine_ads.html

receptors can result in a range of distressing side effects such as tremor or uncontrollable movements of the face, arms, and legs, as well as weight gain, impotence, dysphoria, and emotional indifference (Gerlach & Larsen, 1999).

The second-generation antipsychotics, including the drugs Clozaril (clozapine) and Zyprexa (olanzapine), are marketed as having fewer side effects and greater effectiveness for the negative symptoms of CMHC. It is worth noting that these medications may produce diabetes and are often associated with weight gain. Clozaril also requires careful ongoing monitoring due to a significant association with lowered neutrophil (a type of white blood cell) count that could prove fatal if left undetected.

One of the most important studies that has examined patient response to antipsychotic medication was the European First Episode Schizophrenia Trial (Kahn et al., 2008). This was an open randomised controlled trial (RCT) conducted at 50 sites in 14 countries, and it found that the average improvement in symptoms (reflected in the change in total score on the Positive and Negative Syndrome Scale) was 60%, and neither symptom change nor rates of admission to hospital differed significantly between those on haloperidol (a first-generation medication) and those taking second-generation antipsychotic medications. At around the same time, Martin Lambert and his colleagues (2008) assessed remission and recovery over 3 years in a cohort of 392 patients with schizophrenia who had never previously been treated. In this study, over 90% of participants were prescribed a second-generation antipsychotic medication. Results showed that around 60% of the cohort achieved remission for at least 6 months and 52% experienced symptomatic recovery for at least 2 years. Only a minority (14%) did not reach any of the remission criteria.

Medication options for people who have bipolar disorder include lithium carbonate, the first mood stabiliser approved by the United States Food and Drug Administration (FDA) in the 1970s for treating both manic and depressive episodes. An estimated 60 to 80% of people with bipolar disorder respond to lithium treatment (Calabrese, Fatemi, Kujawa, & Woyshville, 1996; Harrow, Goldberg, Grossman, & Meltzer, 1990). However, patients often report dysphoria – in particular, a numbing of emotional experience – whilst being treated with lithium salts, and this affects their adherence to medication. Anticonvulsant medications that were originally developed for the treatment of epilepsy are also commonly used. This class of medications includes valproic acid (Depakote), lamotrigine (Lamictal), gabapentin (Neurontin), topiramate (Topamax), and oxcarbazepine (Trileptal; Leo & Narendran, 1999). Put simply, the mode of action of the anticonvulsant medications is to slow or block the flow of calcium ions across the neuronal membranes, thus dampening their electrical responsiveness and thereby preventing seizures. Some of these medications also have effects on potassium and sodium channels and on neurotransmitters such as serotonin and GABA – also resulting in a slowing of electrical responsiveness (Grunze, Schlösser, Amann, & Walden, 1999). Yet despite their stabilising effect on mood, there are also costs of using anticonvulsant medications, with the FDA in the United States warning that they may increase the risk of suicidal thoughts and behaviours (Leo & Narendran, 1999).

Overall, then, although it appears that medication can help to stabilise and improve positive symptoms in the majority of people, there is also a significant risk of experiencing a range of distressing side effects, as well as lingering negative symptoms. Some patients with schizophrenia report experiencing subjective sensations of change after only a few doses of antipsychotic medications. They often complain of "extrapyramidal" symptoms such as dystonia (abnormal muscle tone resulting in muscular spasm and abnormal posture), akathisia (restlessness and a compelling need for movement), parkinsonism, and dyskinesia (impaired voluntary muscle movement), as well as more diffuse experiences such as "not feeling like themselves", being sedated, apathetic, or "incapable of thinking straight" (Hogan, Awad, & Eastwood, 1983, p. 177; García-Cabeza, Gómez, Sacristán, Edgell, & González de Chavez, 2001). Moreover, such effects are a common cause of non-adherence to medication, which research has shown is an issue for between 15 and 30% of newly medicated patients (García-Cabeza, et al., 2001).

These various problems with medication are further compounded by difficulty in accurately diagnosing CMHC, possible trauma associated with hospital admission, and ethical issues around consent and treating people against their will (however necessary this may be). Aside from this, medical treatments are limited in their focus on biomedical factors, leaving untreated the impact of psychosis on the individuals' social, emotional, and vocational functioning. Accordingly, it is now widely recognised that other psychotherapeutic and community supports are required to deal with these consequences.

Cognitive behavioural therapy

The cognitive behavioural approach to psychosis contends that a person's interpretation of an unusual experience influences how they feel and behave in everyday contexts and is therefore vital to treatment (see Figure 13.6). Cognitive behavioural therapy (CBT) programmes to treat CMHC typically provide participants with psychoeducation about symptoms and their triggers, as well as coping strategies that help them examine and modify their beliefs about voices and better manage those voices when they are intense (e.g., through distraction).

Evidence suggests that CBT is a modestly effective intervention for psychosis. In particular, a review of 34 CBT schizophrenia treatment trials by Til Wykes and colleagues revealed that, overall, there were beneficial effects for the target symptom (which differed for each trial across 33 studies; effect size $d = 0.40$; Wykes, Steel, Everitt, & Tarrier, 2008). In addition, there were significant effects for positive symptoms (32 studies), negative symptoms (23 studies), global functioning (15 studies), mood (13 studies), and social anxiety (2 studies), with moderate effect sizes ranging from 0.35 to 0.44.

CBT for psychosis can also be delivered in a group format to patients in hospital or community mental health services. Speaking to the efficacy of this, a prospective trial compared 113 inpatients who received either a 4-week group CBT programme (GCBT) or treatment as usual (TAU; Owen, Sellwood, Kan, Murray, & Sarsam, 2015). The researchers measured participants' distress, mental health confidence, and symptoms of psychosis at baseline, post-intervention, and 1-month follow-up. Analyses showed that, compared with the TAU participants, those who received GCBT were significantly less distressed at follow-up and showed significantly increased mental health confidence (optimism, coping, and advocacy in management of mental health) across the study and follow-up periods. However, due to a high attrition rate (62.8% from Time 1 to Time 3), distinct treatment effects were

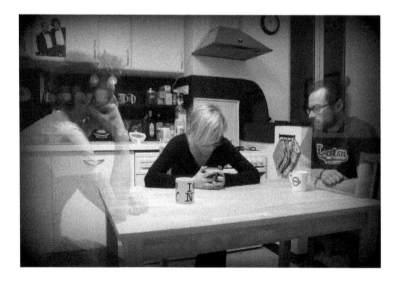

Figure 13.6 Addressing the cognitive aspects of schizophrenia

Note: Cognitive behavioural therapy (CBT) can be used to give people insight into the symptoms of schizophrenia (such as hearing voices) and to provide them with strategies for coping with these. CBT can be delivered one on one or in groups, but both forms of intervention appear to have only modest benefits – not least due to high attrition rates.

Source: Marco Castellani, Flickr

not demonstrated using a more conservative intention-to-treat analysis, which found that reductions in experiences of distress, hearing voices, and unusual beliefs occurred in both conditions over time.

These studies and others have contributed to guidelines for professionals that recommend individual CBT in the treatment of schizophrenia (e.g., American Psychological Association, 2004; Canadian Psychiatric Association, 2005). Some also recommend that this should start in the acute hospital phase (e.g., Royal Australian and New Zealand College of Psychiatrists, Galletly et al., 2016; National Institute for Health and Clinical Excellence, 2014). It is noteworthy, however, that the studies on which these recommendations are based do not provide an analysis of effective reach – that is, of the proportion of each sample who responded to the CBT intervention. It is likely that a proportion did not respond to CBT and, moreover, that this proportion was quite high. In addition, the review by Wykes and colleagues found that there was no effect of CBT on hopelessness, which is an important issue to address given that the lifetime suicide rate among people with schizophrenia has been estimated at 5% (compared to suicide rate estimates of around 0.01% to 0.03% in the general population; CDC, 2015; Hor & Taylor, 2010). On top of this, the findings reported by Mary Owen and colleagues (2015) indicate that participant engagement in GCBT is low and that the advantages of this treatment are modest at best. Indeed, this low engagement may reflect the fact that the positive and negative symptoms of schizophrenia – as well as the sedating effects of medication – can interfere with participants' capacity to engage effectively with CBT.

Importantly too, apart from the two studies in Wykes and colleagues' (2008) review that measured social anxiety, few CBT studies have measured social engagement or quality of relationships as an outcome of treatment. Accordingly, it is unclear how effective CBT is in addressing these important aspects of the condition.

Interpersonal and social rhythm therapy

Although interpersonal functioning is not addressed in CBT, it is more central to *interpersonal and social rhythm therapy* (IPSRT). While it has only been trialled in relation to bipolar disorders, this approach tackles deficiencies in social engagement head on – and hence is potentially relevant to the treatment of all CMHC. Like the original interpersonal psychotherapy for depression (Klerman, Weissman, Rounsaville, & Chevron, 1984; see Chapter 8), IPSRT focuses on trying to resolve participants' current interpersonal problems (e.g., unresolved grief, interpersonal disputes, role transitions, and interpersonal deficits) and preventing future problems in these areas. This approach draws on the principles of interpersonal therapy and has been adapted for bipolar disorder by including modules such as "grief for the lost healthy self," which aim to help mourn the life that a person might have lived were it not for the onset and impact of the disorder. The social rhythm component of IPSRT focuses on helping people with bipolar disorder to understand (1) the links between their mood and the quality of their social relationships and social roles, (2) the importance of maintaining regularity in their daily routines and sleep–wake cycle, and (3) the need to address factors that disrupt their social rhythms (Frank, Kupfer, Thase et al., 2005).

To test the efficacy of this treatment, Ellen Frank and her colleagues examined 2-year outcomes after randomly assigning 175 patients with bipolar I disorder to IPSRT or intensive clinical management (Frank et al., 2005). This found that although there were no differences between conditions in the time taken to achieve mood stabilisation, the IPSRT participants had more regular social rhythms at the end of acute treatment. This was also associated with reduced likelihood of relapse over the 2-year period.

Subsequent to this, a major study funded by the National Institute for Mental Health – the Systematic Treatment Enhancement Programme for Bipolar Disorder (STEP-BD) – sought to assess the effectiveness of three types of standardised, intensive, 9-month-long psychotherapy relative to a control condition in which people received a three-session, psychoeducational programme called collaborative care (Miklowitz et al., 2007). The intensive therapies that the researchers examined were

(1) family-focused therapy, (2) CBT, and (3) IPSRT, with only family-focused therapy involving group-based intervention. Nearly 300 people took part in their study, and all of them were already taking medication for their bipolar disorder.

The study found that over the course of the year, 64% of those in the intensive psychotherapy groups had remitted compared to 52% of those in collaborative care therapy. Moreover, although the drop-out rates of the groups were similar (36% of participants in the intensive programmes and 31% of those in collaborative care discontinued), patients in intensive psychotherapy became well an average of 110 days faster than those in collaborative care. All three of the intensive psychotherapies appeared to be quite effective. Nevertheless, rates of recovery were higher among those in family-focused therapy than in the other two therapies. This meant that after 1 year, 76.9% of the patients who received family-focused therapy had recovered compared to 56.7% of those who received CBT and 59.0% of those who received IPSRT. It seems possible that the superiority of family-focused therapy on this index reflects the fact that individual-focused treatments such as CBT and IPSRT tend to overlook the importance of social group factors (e.g., family and occupational group dynamics) or address these at the individual rather than at the group level. Because, as we have seen, these social factors are key to both aetiology and recovery in CMHC, there would thus appear to be value in treatments that take these factors more seriously.

Family environment and family-focused therapy

Individuals with CMHC often rely on their families to provide the emotional and practical resources they need to survive (Glynn, 2012). In this regard, a well-informed family that provides non-invasive support to a person who is suffering from CMHC can play a very important role in minimising the negative impact of the condition (Acero, Cano-Prous, Castellanos, Martín-Lanas, & Canga, 2017). Conversely, as we have already observed, high levels of tension within a family (e.g., as indicated by a high degree of "expressed emotion") can negatively affect the course of CMHC.

Building on research findings which point to the important of family influences on CMHC, a number of interventions have been developed to target the core issue of family disconnection and mal-adaptive communication patterns. These include *behavioural family therapy* (BFT; Falloon, McGill, & Boyd, 1984) and *family-focused therapy* (FFT; Miklowitz, 2008; Rea et al., 2003). Due to the high rates of comorbidity between the psychoses and substance use disorders (see Chapter 9), BFT has also been modified to include substance misuse components. For example, this can involve treatment being augmented through the inclusion of (1) routine assessment of substance use levels, (2) motivational enhancement to increase the participants' desire to change their substance use behaviour, and (3) training that models effective communication strategies in relatives so as to promote more positive discussion of substance use within the family (Mueser, et al., 2013).

Consistent with the findings of the study conducted by David Miklowitz and his colleagues, research generally indicates that these family-focused therapies are effective ways of treating CMHC (Miklowitz et al., 2007). For example, in a study that followed up 36 non-substance-abusing individuals with schizophrenia over a 2-year period, BFT was found to be superior to individual therapy in reducing relapse, symptoms, and hospital admissions (Falloon et al., 1985). More recently, a Cochrane review of family interventions for schizophrenia found that these were much more effective than customary care in reducing relapse 12 months after study entry (Pharoah, Mari, Rathbone, & Wong, 2010). This was reflected in an odds ratio of 0.55 – meaning that patients given family interventions were about half as likely to relapse into a psychotic episode within 12 months as those who received customary care.

When it is used to treat bipolar disorders, FFT commences with a psychoeducation component that focuses on providing information about the causes, symptoms, course, and treatment of bipolar disorder. Family members are then trained in communication skills through use of in-session role-play, and these are then practiced further in homework assignments. Again, research suggests this is quite an effective treatment. This, for example, was the conclusion of an RCT conducted by Margaret Rea and colleagues in which 53 recently hospitalised bipolar patients received either 9 months of FFT or an individually focused treatment (and where all patients received concurrent treatment with mood-stabilising medications; Rea et al., 2003). Here, compared to patients in individual therapy, fewer of those who received FFT were re-admitted to hospital and they experienced fewer relapses over the course of a 2-year follow-up period.

More recently, FFT was evaluated in a study of 129 adolescents and young adults at high risk of psychosis (Miklowitz et al., 2014). Here negative symptoms improved independently of treatment type, and results were also independent of concurrent medication. Importantly, though, participants who received FFT showed much greater improvement in positive symptoms than those in the comparison condition (where they and their families were merely helped to devise a personalised prevention plan). Consistent with the idea that group dynamics play a key role in the trajectory of CMHC, these findings suggest that having well-informed family members who are able to provide social support and communicate with minimal conflict contributes substantially to recovery over and above the effects of medication or individualised therapy.

In summary, family psychotherapies appear to be effective for around two thirds of participants, with the remainder either discontinuing therapy or not responding to it. On the other hand, when psychotherapies are only designed to address individual-level factors (e.g., in the form of unhelpful cognitions, behaviours, and communication styles), they often fail to tackle problems of social engagement and social functioning. Yet as Oliver Sacks observed in relation to his brother's treatment, these social dimensions of CMHC are critical. Accordingly, it is because they engage with these that therapies which are delivered in groups or with family involvement appear to have particular value.

At the same time, though, research in this area has largely been silent about the psychosocial mechanisms via which group and family dynamics influence either therapy delivery or outcomes. Not least, this is because research rarely includes direct measures of family group cohesion, connectedness, identification, or support (e.g., akin to those included in the Appendix). And on the rare occasions where these are assessed, there is little or no analysis of the role that they play in the prediction of patient engagement and outcomes. This, then, is an aspect of CMHC to which a social identity approach would appear to have a lot to offer. But before we can flesh this point out, we need to consider another more social approach to mental health care – one which is community based.

Community approaches to mental health

Doctor Eric Cunningham Dax moved to Australia from England to take up a position as the inaugural chairman of the Mental Hygiene Authority of Victoria in 1951 (see Figure 13.7). During his time in this role, Dax directed the mental health services for Victoria and implemented extensive reforms that saw the services change dramatically. Specifically, where previously they generally involved custodial confinement in poor conditions, his leadership led to the implementation of a much more modern system – one that was characterised by humane treatment of mentally ill individuals within their communities. Amongst other things, this was exemplified by his support for a range of group-based arts activities that gave patients a means of expressing themselves and their inner worlds to others. His book *From Asylum to Community* documented this 15-year reform process (Dax, 1961). Today, the Dax Centre at the University of Melbourne displays patients' artwork that was supported and collected by Dax and provides educational programmes that aim to increase understanding of mental illness and psychological trauma in the wider community.

Mental health service reforms – of which those directed by Dax are a good example – are part of a rich legacy that is evidenced in the activities of a range of charitable and non-government organisations that provide care, community activities, and/or vocational support for people with CMHC around the world today. In the United States they include organisations such as the National Alliance on Mental Illness and Intervoice; in the UK they include the mental health charity MIND and the support network

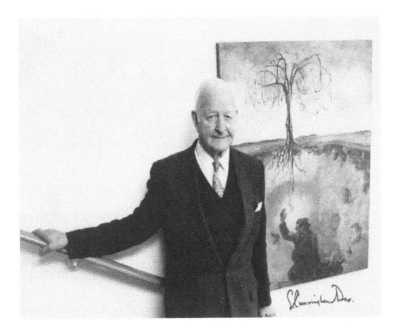

Figure 13.7 Dr Eric Cunningham Dax AO

Note: Cunningham Dax spearheaded reforms to mental health policy in Victoria and promoted arts engagement and other community approaches for patients with CMHC.

Source: www.daxcentre.org/the-dax-centre-about-us/

Hearing Voices; and in Australia they include church-affiliated organisations such as Anglicare, Salvos Care, Ozcare, and Centacare and other community agencies such as Richmond Fellowship (RFQ, 2015), Stepping Stones Club House, and Open Minds.

One interesting example of an Australian community agency that seeks to help people who are suffering from CMHC is Reclink. This is an inter-agency networking organisation located in numerous locations across urban, regional, and remote Australia. We discussed some of the Reclink programmes that try to tackle depression in Chapter 8 (Cruwys et al., 2014c) and noted that these involve coordinators liaising with local services (in areas of mental health, disability, drug and alcohol, homelessness, domestic violence, immigrant support services, and so on) to give their clients access to a range of group recreational activities that have varying levels of intensity and support. These activities include choirs, artist collectives, Australian Rules Football (see Figure 13.8), bowling, and yoga. Participants' existing health workers or agencies refer them to a Reclink activity, and those who require support to engage in this can access this from their home agency or via a Reclink support worker.

To explore the efficacy of the work that Reclink does to help people with CMHC, three of us collaborated with Melissa Johnstone and Zoe Walter to conduct a longitudinal study of 101 members of one of its networks in southeast Queensland (Dingle et al., 2014). Of these participants, 45% indicated in an initial survey that they had a formal diagnosis of mental illness – most commonly schizophrenia (14%), schizoaffective disorder (4%), bipolar disorder (4%), depression (8%), and anxiety disorders (7%). We then obtained surveys from 49 of these participants at a second time point 3 months later,

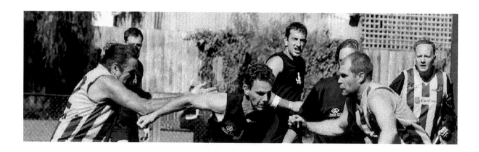

Figure 13.8 Players in a game of Australian Rules Football organised by Reclink

Note: Reclink is an Australian community agency that aims to improve the lives of people who are disadvantaged by providing them with opportunities to participate in sports and arts programmes.

Source: Reclink Australia

with analysis indicating that there were no differences at baseline between participants who dropped out and those who returned the second survey in terms of their gender, employment status, housing status, or mental health diagnosis. The results showed that after these 3 months there was a significant decrease both in respondents' social isolation and in the number of visits they had made to a general practitioner, as well as a marked increase in their overall life satisfaction. Indeed, 80% of those who had taken part in Reclink activities felt that their life had been improved by joining one or more recreational groups, 61% reported that their physical health and fitness had improved, and 82% indicated their mental health and well-being had improved.

Individuals with CMHC (as well as those health professionals who manage them) regard returning to work as a core element of recovery (McQuilken, et al., 2003; Tsang & Chen, 2007). Accordingly, some services aim to give people who suffer from these conditions access to community-based vocational skills training and supported work placements with a view to facilitating their return to work. Speaking to the potential utility of these efforts, in a review of 62 studies of factors that predict vocational success for people with CMHC, Hector Tsang and his colleagues found that positive symptoms, substance abuse, gender, and hospitalisation history were *not* significant predictors of work performance (Tsang, Leung, Chung, Bell, & Cheung, 2010). However, negative symptoms, cognitive functioning, education, social support and skills, age, previous history of successful employment, and rehabilitation with allied health professionals were all significant predictors of work performance. As the authors note, this suggests that efforts to address negative symptoms of CMHC (e.g., social isolation and social cognitive functioning) may be particularly useful in promoting successful recovery and "deserve the attention they are beginning to get as targets for novel medications and remediation strategies" (Tsang et al., 2010, p. 501).

An indication of what these efforts can look like is provided by a study in which 44 adults with CMHC and a history of job failure were randomly assigned to receive either (1) a vocational team-facilitated cognitive training programme (the Thinking Skills for Work Programme) together with supported employment (CT+SE) or (2) supported employment alone (SE Only; McGurk, Meuser, & Pascaris, 2005). This found that retention in the CT+SE programme was high (91%) and that over a 3-month period those who took part in this showed significantly greater improvements in neurocognitive functioning, depression, and autistic preoccupation on the Positive and Negative Syndrome

Scale than those in the SE Only group. Employment outcomes over 1 year also indicated that those who received CT+SE were significantly more likely to work (69.6 versus 4.8%, respectively), to work more hours, and to earn more wages (McGurk et al., 2005). Together, then, these results suggest that team-based community support which provides specialised skills training can make a real difference to whether people with CMHC successfully gain and sustain employment.

The foregoing studies are indicative of a broader body of evidence which shows that community strategies to engage people with CMHC in social and vocational activities can produce meaningful improvements in their mental health and well-being. Although different programmes focus on different objectives (e.g., social integration, work), they share a common emphasis on promoting an active life, personal autonomy, meaning and purpose in life, and a positive sense of self. These are all elements of the *recovery model of mental health* that has been adopted by the Australian national framework for recovery-oriented mental health services (AHMAC, 2013) and by the UK Department of Health (Department of Health, 2014). This strives to place those who suffer from various mental health conditions at the heart of their own treatment and to give them a seat at the table when it comes to the design and delivery of health services. This is because the model recognises that, like all members of the community, those who are experiencing mental health challenges need and desire sustaining relationships, meaningful occupation, and safety and respect in their lives. Community organisations offer an important means to target these goals.

What is less clear is what produces these benefits; are they a consequence of the particular activities in which people take part or of their group delivery? This is a point on which those designers of these programmes are typically silent. Nevertheless, there is a tendency for researchers to focus on the specific content of a given programme (e.g., sport, music, computer training) rather than on the group context in which it is delivered (e.g., see McGurk et al., 2005, 2010). Indeed, it is clear that, much of the time, the group context in which programmes are delivered is barely worth a mention.

We know, however, from other research in this volume (e.g., Chapter 7) that the group context in which an intervention is delivered is often a non-trivial component of its efficacy (e.g., see Gleibs, Haslam, Haslam, & Jones, 2011a; Haslam et al., 2010). It is also the case that the influence of groups can be both positive and negative. For example, support groups may be beneficial for some, but be detrimental for others (e.g., because they heighten their sense of stigma). Because it helps to bring these processes into view – and helps us to understand their impact – it is here that a social identity approach to CMHC would appear to hold particular promise. Indeed, as we will see in the next section, this approach points us to two key possibilities. First, that much of the benefit of the various family and community programmes that we have discussed arises from their capacity to build group-based social capital. Second, that when it comes to avoiding or overcoming the debilitating effects of CMHC, this group-based social capital is a particularly potent social psychological resource.

The social identity approach to CMHC

Sue Estroff (1989) described the development of schizophrenia in terms of a loss of self and of positive social roles and identity. She argued that the person's inner sense of self and public social self must overlap to an extent, and when they do not, the individual is likely to experience a "radical estrangement" or "hyperalienation" (Kovel, 1987, p. 334) of self that is a hallmark of schizophrenia. Furthermore, Claudine Herzlich and Janine Pierret (1987, p. 178) explained that by enforcing inactivity, chronic illness prevents individuals from "playing their role", marginalises them, and can provoke a feeling of loss of identity. "Who am I?" the person wonders, and, in answering this question, some may develop a stigmatised identity around their mental illness. These earlier works conceptualised identity mainly in individualised terms, but the social identity approach extends this to consider the role that social identities – such as understanding oneself to be member of a family, stigmatised minority group, or immigrant population – have to play in the development of CMHC.

Social identity protects against development of psychosis

As noted earlier, environmental factors such as social inequalities, childhood trauma and maltreatment, and negative life events in adulthood place people at an increased risk of developing CMHC. One population that exemplifies the effects of negative life events and social marginalisation is immigrants. Indeed, a meta-analysis by Elizabeth Cantor-Graae and Jean-Paul Selten (2005) observed that first-generation migrants were 2.7 times more likely to develop schizophrenia than members of the general population. And for second-generation migrants this risk was even greater: they were 4.5 times more likely to develop the condition than members of the general population.

Looking to explore these issues further, a study by Jason McIntyre, Anam Elahi and Richard Bentall (2016) focused specifically on the development of paranoia in immigrant communities. As we noted earlier, paranoia is the most common psychotic symptom (Moutoussis, et al., 2007) and is defined as undue suspiciousness about the intents and actions of others. It varies on a continuum from everyday suspiciousness to clinical paranoia that may endanger the life of the individual or others. The opposite of paranoia is trust: the expectation that others will behave in expected, generally positive, ways (Laporte, 2015, p. 22). Accordingly, because shared social identification is a basis for trust (as suggested by the connection hypothesis, H12; see Foddy, Platow, & Yamagishi, 2009; Platow, Wenzel, & Nolan, 2003), it follows that a lack or loss of social identification might be implicated in the development of paranoia.

Speaking to this point, it is apparent that the process of migration involves transitioning to an unfamiliar social, cultural, and physical environment, commonly with experiences of social disconnection and discrimination. Indeed, McIntyre and colleagues' study (2016) examined the basis for development of paranoid beliefs around exclusion and harm among people who do not feel a sense of shared identity with their neighbourhood, country, or workplace (see also McIntyre, Wickham, Barr, & Bentall, 2017). Their results showed that those who felt less connected with these social groups were more vulnerable to feelings of interpersonal threat and had lower levels of trust. Conversely, there was evidence that migrants who engaged with other members of their ingroup had a lower risk of psychosis. These findings also marry with other evidence that paranoid psychosis is more prevalent in migrant communities that are physically and psychologically set apart from the rest of society (Cantor-Graae & Selten, 2005; Veling et al., 2007) and that paranoid ideation is more common in individuals with low levels of family identification (Wakefield, Sani, Herrera, & Zeybek, 2017).

In this context, it is apparent that social identity development may be facilitated by positive contact with new groups and by maintaining cultural ties with pre-existing groups (e.g., in ways suggested by Berry, 1997). However, it is also apparent that for migrants, identification with their home culture may lead to social *disconnection* – especially when combined with perceived discrimination within the new culture – and that this will tend to have adverse consequences for mental health (e.g., in ways suggested by the social identity model of identity change, SIMIC; see Chapter 3, Figure 3.6). Consistent with this analysis, the fact that the incidence of psychotic symptoms such as paranoia is higher for second-generation migrants can be seen partly to reflect the fact that a relatively high proportion of them identify weakly with *both* their original cultural group *and* their adopted cultural group (Berry & Sabatier, 2010). Accordingly, they are particularly at risk of losing access to meaningful social identities and the psychological resources that are associated with them (McIntyre et al., 2016).

In line with this analysis, Fabian Lamster and colleagues conducted an experimental study to examine the potential association between social disconnection and paranoid beliefs among 60 healthy adults (Lamster, Nittel, Rief, Mehl, & Lincoln, 2017). This used false feedback to manipulate participants' sense of psychological isolation and found that reducing loneliness was associated with a significant reduction in paranoid beliefs, whereas the induction of loneliness tended to lead to more pronounced paranoia. Moreover, proneness to psychosis significantly moderated the impact of loneliness on paranoia. This meant that participants who were at risk of developing psychosis (measured by their reported frequency of psychotic experiences) showed a greater decrease in paranoid beliefs as a consequence of a decrease in loneliness than those who were less prone.

A similar pattern of findings was also observed in the BBC Prison Study that we discussed in Chapters 2 and 5 (Reicher & Haslam, 2006a). Recall that this involved studying healthy volunteers over a

10-day period after they had been randomly assigned to be Prisoners or Guards in a simulated prison. As we noted earlier, as the study progressed, experimental manipulations led the Prisoners to identify more strongly with each other and to resist the Guards' authority, and their insurgence contributed to a declining sense of shared identity among the Guards. In previous chapters we observed that these changes in group identification had a discernible impact on the mental health of participants. In particular, as shared identity led to marked improvement in the Prisoners' well-being, the Guards' loss of identity led them to become increasingly stressed and depressed (Haslam & Reicher, 2006; Reicher & Haslam, 2006a). At the same time, though, these changes in participants' shared identity also led the Prisoners to become more trusting of each other and the Guards to become much more paranoid.

At a quantitative level, this was seen in changes in the participants' self-reported paranoia over time (as presented in Figure 13.9). However, in qualitative terms, it was seen even more vividly in exchanges which showed the Guards to have a looming fear that the Prisoners were conspiring against them. This is exemplified by the following exchange:

TQg: They're going to lock us, lock us in somewhere.
IBg: Who's going to lock us in?
TQg: That's it, isn't it? That's what they're going to do.
IBg: Who, the guys? We've got keys.
TQg: What?
IBg: Who's going to lock us in?
TQg: That's what they'll do.
IBg: What, the others?
TQg: Yeah.
IBg: But we've got keys. [silence]
(Haslam, Reicher, Koppel, & Mirsky, 2006, p. 106)

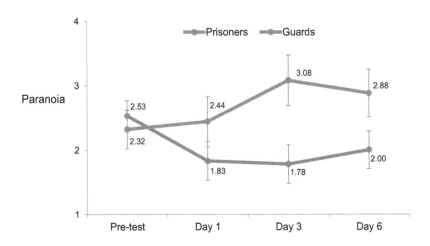

Figure 13.9 Paranoia in the BBC Prison Study

Note: At the start of the study there was no difference in the paranoia of the two groups; however, as the study progressed the Guards became significantly more paranoid than the Prisoners.

Source: Haslam, Reicher, Bentall et al., (2016)

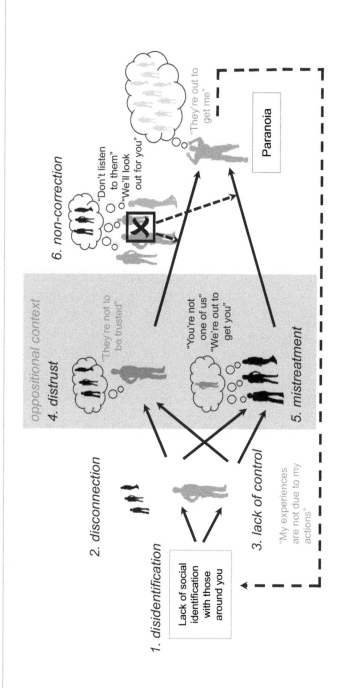

Figure 13.10 A social identity model of emergent paranoia

Note: This model suggests (1) that a lack of social identification with the people a person routinely comes into contact with leads them to have (2) a sense of social disconnection and (3) a perceived lack of control. If this occurs in a context of intergroup opposition, this in turn is a basis for (4) generalised distrust and (5) mistreatment at the hands of outgroups. Because (6) there are limited sources of ingroup support (that might provide the person with cognitive and material protection), this will tend to make them susceptible to paranoid ideation.

Source: Haslam et al. (2016)

In many ways too, the emergent dynamics in the BBC Prison Study can be seen to provide a model of how paranoia can develop over time in environments that combine social isolation with intergroup opposition (Haslam et al., 2016). As represented schematically in Figure 13.10, the starting point for this is a person's reduced sense of identification with the people by whom they are surrounded (e.g., as seen in studies of migrants; McIntyre et al., 2016). As suggested by the connection hypothesis (H12) and the agency hypotheses (H15), this lack of identification then leads to a sense of disconnection from those other people and a reduced sense that one is in control of one's own life (Greenaway et al., 2015; see also Greenaway, Haslam, & Bingley, 2017). In a context which *really is* oppositional (e.g., where migrants confront real prejudice or guards face real hostility from prisoners), these in turn are likely to feed into a sense of mistrust and to lead to the person being exposed to mistreatment from outgroup members (e.g., in the form of prejudice or bullying; Branscombe, Schmitt, & Harvey, 1999; Haslam & Reicher, 2006).

At the same time, as suggested by the support hypothesis (H14), precisely because the person is psychologically isolated, they are not in a position to benefit from ingroup help (cognitive, emotional, or material) that might protect them from (perceived) harm and also correct any misconceptions that they might have (e.g., persuading the person that things are not as bad as they imagine). In this context, then, the lack of social identity exposes a person to a range of risks which centre on perceptions of persecution that have at least some basis in social psychological reality. As we see with both Guards in BBC Prison Study and migrants around the world today, their paranoia is a cognitive concoction that is neither wholly unfounded nor entirely of their own making.

Social identity is a basis for recovery from CMHC

As well as helping us to understand the role that social processes can play in the emergence of CMHC, the social identity approach helps to explain how both formal group programmes (e.g., family-involved therapy or group CBT) and naturally occurring groups in a person's social and community environment (e.g., cultural community, family, friends, and interest groups) can play an important role in the recovery of those with CMHC. In particular, it is apparent that the formation of a new valued social identity as a member of such groups can help people transition from an illness identity (e.g., "I'm a schizophrenic") to a strength-based identity (e.g. "I'm a tenor in the choir"). This is because, as we noted in Chapter 2 (and have also observed in several other chapters), internalised membership of valued groups gives people access to a range of psychological resources, including a sense of connectedness, belonging, meaning, and purpose, that can be expected to have a positive impact on their health and well-being.

Furthermore, compared to formal mental health treatment services, naturally occurring group activities in the community are typically less focused on mental illness and therefore less likely to perpetuate a stigmatised identity. Indeed, on the contrary, joining such groups is often an expression of the individual's personal choice and autonomy and, as we noted earlier, these are valuable principles of the recovery model of mental health that are often missing from hospital and psychotherapeutic treatment options. This points to the fact that recovery (and mental health more generally) is not simply a question of (re) establishing social contact with others, but rather a consequence of people's subjective sense of belonging to social groups and of their associated perceived commonality with other ingroup members (e.g., as suggested by the identification hypothesis, H2; Sani, Herrera, Wakefield, Boroch, & Gulyas, 2012).

So what are the psychological mechanisms that underpin this transition from a mental illness–related identity (e.g., "I'm a schizophrenic") to a strength-based identity (e.g., "I'm a member of a choir")? In a qualitative study designed to explore precisely this question, Dingle and her colleagues interviewed 21 members of a Reclink choir at three different time points: as they were joining the choir and again 6 and 12 months later (Dingle, Brander, Ballantyne, & Baker, 2013). This was a heterogeneous sample, but the majority of the choir members (89%) had experienced chronic mental illness, and a smaller percentage reported having physical (28%) or intellectual (11%) disabilities.

As summarised in Figure 13.11, qualitative analysis of interview transcripts revealed three broad kinds of benefit that flowed from membership of the choir. First, there were *personal benefits* in the

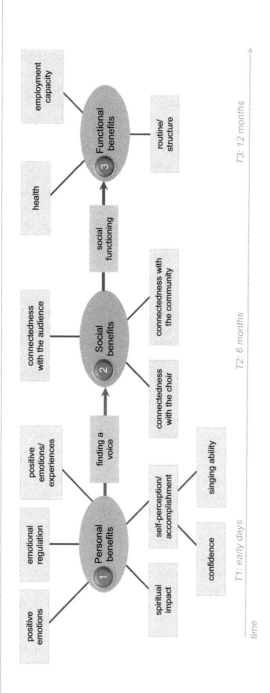

Figure 13.11 Thematic map of the benefits of choir membership for people with CMHC

Note: Participants who joined a Reclink choir identified three benefits that they derived from belonging to this group. First, it provided them with personal benefits associated with more positive emotional experiences and confidence. This in turn led to social benefits by allowing them to connect more with others both in their choir and in the wider community. This increase in social group capital then led to functional benefits in the form of improved health and better employment opportunities.

Source: Based on Dingle, Brander, Ballantyne, and Baker (2013)

form of positive emotions, emotion regulation, spiritual experience, self-understanding, and the sense of "finding a voice". Second, there were *social benefits* reflecting a sense of connectedness within the choir and with its audiences, as well as improved social functioning. And third, there were *functional benefits* in the form of better health, improved employment prospects, and a more healthy routine. Importantly too, these benefits all emerged over time, indicating that choir involvement helped participants on a personal level at first by improving their mood and their sense of achievement and esteem. This then created a platform for them to connect more with others in the choir and with audiences and others in the community. Eventually too, in ways suggested by social identity theorising, this increase in social psychological capital fed into functional changes that sustained improved social functioning and health (Dingle et al., 2013).

Dingle and colleagues built on this work in a three-phase quantitative study of 59 new recruits to a range of group arts activities organised by the charitable organisation the School of Hard Knocks (SHK; see Figure 13.12). SHK's motto is "Empowering through the Arts" and, as its website suggests, its seeks to do this through:

> Programs [that] involve students in arts and well-being activities with the country's best arts practitioners, in the highest quality rehearsal and performance venues possible, with 'performance' as a key outcome.
>
> (http://schoolofhardknocks.org.au/sohk/about/)

As the website explains:

> Students are typically referred to us by health and welfare organisations. We have strong relationships with many of these organisations who refer their clients. . . . We've developed, piloted and currently run a wide range of innovative arts programs including choral, drama,

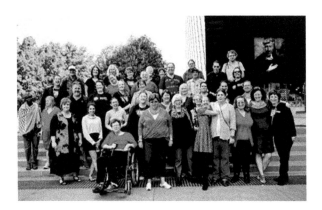

Figure 13.12 Members of the School of Hard Knocks (Queensland) creative writing group and choir

Note: The School of Hard Knocks is a charity that provides a range of arts-based programmes to disadvantaged Australians with the aim of promoting social inclusion and thereby enhancing members' health and well-being.

Source: The authors

instrumental and creative writing. We also develop and lead community choirs in under-priv-ileged areas, in association with City Councils and community and welfare organisations which enable them to engage isolated members of their communities.

In line with this philosophy, participants in the study were referred from community mental health, homeless, substance rehabilitation, and disability organisations. Three quarters had a current mental health condition, most commonly a mood disorder (45%), anxiety disorder (33%), schizophrenia (22%), or a substance use disorder (13%; Dingle, Williams, Sharman, & Jetten, 2016).

As observed in our previous research, over the period of their involvement in the SHK, partici-pants experienced significant improvement on standardised indicators of mental health (e.g., self-es-teem, life satisfaction). Importantly, though, we were also able to examine more directly the role that the development of a sense of identification with the SHK group played in this improvement. What we found was that this sense of connectedness with the group developed early on (where mean group identification was over 5 out of 7) and remained high at Time 2 (3 to 6 months later) and Time 3 (1 year later). Moreover, speaking to the importance of this for the observed health benefits, multilevel model-ling indicated that the more people identified with the SHK, the more their mental well-being improved over time (Williams, Dingle, Jetten, & Rowan, 2017). Analysis also pointed to the importance of perceived social support in this process, with a pattern of statistical interaction showing that mental well-being improved more over time for those participants who reported receiving more social support from SHK. As a corollary, though, there was no change in the mental well-being of participants with a weak sense of SHK identity and who perceived themselves to receive less social support.

As in previous studies, qualitative data from interviews with these SHK participants also provided the researchers with vivid evidence of the mechanisms through which joining an SHK group pro-gramme led to positive mental health outcomes. As indicated in Table 13.2, primary amongst these was the acquisition of a valued social identity – for example, as "choir member", "musician", or "writer".

Table 13.2 Excerpts from interviews with members of the School of Hard Knocks

Theme	*Quotation*
Social identity gain	I see myself as a participant in the choir first and foremost. At the moment I'm singing soprano but I probably identify more as an alto. – BP1207, T1
	I know a lot of people who are in various circumstances, whether it's homelessness or drug addiction or whatever, and when I sort of say, "Hey, I'm doing the choir on Friday," it provides me with a good change from that sort of thing and people often say to me, "Wow," as though they would like to be involved in something like that as well but all they've really got is their usual sort of stuff. – CH3012, T1
	Yes, I definitely am [becoming a writer]. I'm putting my name down for the next creative writing course. I've always wanted to write a children's book. – CD2601, T1
	I feel positive because I know that everybody's in the same boat. We're all in the same category as to knowing the songs and things like that. – GT0105, T2
	Being in front of people, the teamwork, talking to people and socialising. Performing gives me a goal rather than just playing music at home . . . I feel we share a common goal. – TC1109, T2

Theme	Quotation
Sense of reduced isolation through belonging and acceptance	I was living in Housing Commission which is kind of a little bit isolated and I moved into [*social housing complex*] because it's more of a community. So I've become a part of this community and I participate on several levels artistically here in the art room and also anything that comes along that I like and the [School of Hard Knocks] choir came along, I had a look at it and thought, "Yeah, this seems okay. I might be able to do some arts with these people," so I joined up to the choir. – CH3012, T1
	My confidence was really, really low. I wouldn't go near a man. I wouldn't let people touch me. I was really quite shy and it was really through that safe, supportive environment there that I started discovering again that I could actually be a part of a group and actually find a place where it was like a family I never had . . . It's usually, in the environment, it's a supportive thing. – DG1406, T1
	[S]ometimes it can be lonely when you live on your own and when you come on a Friday and you're meeting people, you're talking to people, it does uplift you more. You know what I mean? – CD2601, T1
	I appreciate the honesty, the rawness. The honesty, I think it's a unique space for that and writing is quite a solitary practice usually. Then writers, if they get together, I've never been to one, but I should imagine the Brisbane writing centre that that would be a little competitive, whereas this space there's no competitiveness and that's the way it should be, but it's very hard to find . . . Being in the space is a big deal. I get on with everybody. We all smile. It's a really warm space to come, and learn, and grow. – SW2903, T2
Making a contribution	The fact that I am gregarious, that I do try and sort of keep an eye on people's mood and behaviour and that sort of stuff so that I can quietly slip over and be of some support if somebody needs that. I see my role as [someone] that can hold a part sitting in those sopranos at the moment to try, and I'm not the only one, but it helps. – BP1207, T1
	Hey, I've done something [in creative writing group]. You don't need to ring up and tell people how good it was. You know it was good, we've all smiled at each other and laugh at the end of it, we know we've done something good. We can choose to share a bit of it to someone else and we can keep it to ourselves, and I kind of like that. – BS1110, T1
	I contribute where help is needed and I helped (another member) out at a concert . . . Just to make her not feel so anxious. She appreciated my help. – HC0502, T2
	If I know anything I could help I would help them, yeah . . . Sometimes I might chase up a chair for them or if they need to move something or whatever I can help or some knowledge I might have that they mightn't know about, things like that . . . I do because when you live on your own you realise that it's better to be helpful than not helpful. – JC0307, T2

Second, this acquired social identity was in turn associated with an enhanced sense of belonging, social connection with others, and of safety and trust within the group. And finally, third, through enactment of their new social identity, participants reported being in a position to make a positive and meaningful contribution to the group, not least by supporting *other* group members when the need arose (Dingle, Williams, Sharman, & Jetten, 2016). In this way, then, we see that although the loss of social identity can set in motion a vicious circle that leads people into psychological darkness, interventions that help them acquire or regain social identities can create a virtuous circle that brings them out into the light.

Social identification is a basis to manage mental health stigma

Although not all people with CMHC view themselves through the lens of, or ascribe to, a stigmatised identity, it is true that people with CMHC often encounter stigma and discrimination (Whitely & Campbell, 2014). This point is illustrated in research by Sokratis Dinos and colleagues (2004) which interviewed 46 individuals with mental health problems who were participating in mental health support groups, day centres, crisis centres, and hospitals (Dinos, Stevens, Serfaty, Weich, & King, 2004). Two key themes that emerged from these interviews pointed (1) to widespread stigma about mental illness and (2) to the heavy toll that this took on those at its receiving end (see also Corrigan, 2004). Amongst other things, this meant that interviewees reported a loss of social contact with others after disclosing their diagnosis, as well as frequent exposure to verbal and physical abuse.

These negative effects are in line with the group circumstance hypothesis that we discussed in Chapter 2 (in particular, H3b) and highlight the negative impact that a compromised social identity is likely to have on health and well-being. At the same time, however, there is also some evidence that when people with CMHC band together (e.g., as "us people who have a particular mental illness"), their identification with others in their ingroup provides an important basis for social support and efforts to challenge societal views about their condition (e.g., Camp, Finlay, & Lyons, 2002). Indeed, more particularly, social identity theorising would lead us to anticipate that a sense of shared identity could be a basis for group members to work together to resist stigma and reject negative ingroup stereotypes (e.g., in ways suggested by the rejection-identification model; Branscombe et al., 1999; Schmitt & Branscombe, 2002; see Chapter 4).

This possibility was explored by Jason Crabtree and colleagues (2010) in a study involving 73 participants who were members of mental illness support groups in the southwest of England (Crabtree, Haslam, Postmes, & Haslam, 2010). This revealed a complex pattern of associations between key variables that supported these counterposed social identity hypotheses, as shown in Figure 13.13. Thus, on the one hand, the researchers found that stronger identification with one's mental health group was associated with lower self-esteem (in line with H3b). On the other hand, though, this direct negative effect was also buffered by an indirect positive effect in which self-esteem was improved through the capacity for that group to provide a basis for increased social support, the rejection of negative stereotypes, and stigma resistance (in line with H7, H13, and H14).

The direct pathway that was observed in Crabtree and colleagues' study points to the fact that identification with a stigmatised group is not always positive. This was a point that we made in Chapter 9 where we saw that identification with substance-using social groups was associated with poorer outcomes following residential treatment for substance misuse (Dingle, Stark, Cruwys, & Best, 2015). In the context of CMHC, a person who embraces a social identity as "crazy" or "mentally ill" and ascribes to negative stereotypes of the mentally ill – for example, believing them to be incompetent, hopeless, and unemployable – is therefore likely to be confronted with very significant obstacles to recovery. As Crabtree and colleagues observe:

A key challenge, therefore, is to ensure that mental health support groups do more than merely confirm to those who identify with them that they are members of a problematic group that is stigmatised by others. Instead they need to ensure that they use this knowledge

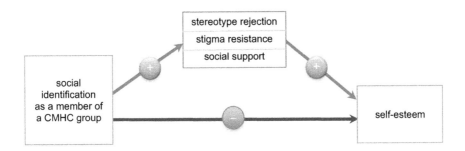

Figure 13.13 Two pathways through which social identification as a member of a CMHC group has an impact on self-esteem

Note: This figure points to a direct pathway (in blue) through which identification has a negative impact on self-esteem and an indirect pathway (in red) in which it has a positive impact as a result of being a basis for stereotype resistance, stigma rejection, and social support.

Source: Based on Crabtree et al (2010, p. 561)

as a basis for practical, political activities that not only envision social and personal change but also help to bring it about.

(Crabtree et al., 2010, p. 566)

In line with this assertion, we can see that the way in which stigmatised identities are managed is likely to have a significant bearing on the well-being of those who have them. For example, the extent to which people see their mental illness identity as permeable rather than fixed is likely to be associated with the extent to which they engage in selective disclosure and collective resistance strategies rather than those of avoidance (e.g., in ways suggested by Jones, Jetten, Haslam, & Williams, 2012; see also Chapters 4, 5, and 11). This point is confirmed in longitudinal research by Marie Ilic and colleagues which examined the use of ten identity management strategies in a sample of 367 adults with CMHC (Ilic et al., 2014). Here selective disclosure and information seeking (e.g., to and from ingroup members) emerged as adaptive identity management strategies, whereas over-compensation and withdrawal led to poorer mental health.

The agenda of working together to challenge stigmatising views of mental health is one that has been embraced through a range of public health and education campaigns that have become increasingly prominent in recent years. For example, it is seen in initiatives such as the 'R U OK Day' suicide prevention campaign, the Movember fundraiser for men's mental health, and the establishment of Mental Health Day (October 10) in more than 150 countries around the globe. These are making significant inroads in increasing public awareness and understanding of mental illness. They are also helping to correct misperceptions, counter prejudice, and remove the stigma that has historically surrounded CMHC. In this regard, it is notable that the Mental Health Australia slogan for 2016 World Mental Health Day was "Mental health begins with Me" (see Figure 13.14). This is a message that implies, correctly, that we all have a role to play in mental health – not just our own but also other people's. Indeed, because efforts to achieve a positive sense of shared social identity seem to be so important for recovery from CMHC, had we been consulted, we might have suggested that this sentiment would be captured even better by the strapline "Mental health begins with Us".

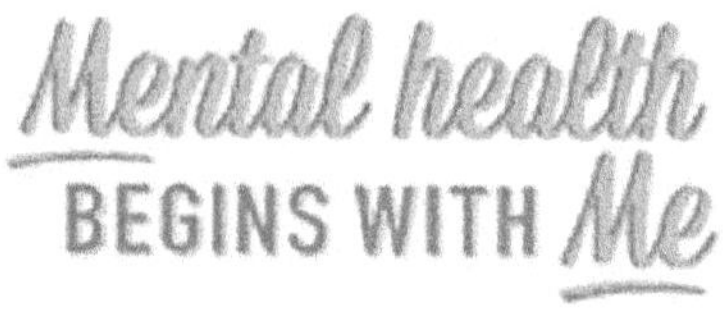

Mental health
BEGINS WITH *Me*

Figure 13.14 The Mental Health Australia slogan for the 2016 World Mental Health Day

Note: Bearing in mind the lessons of this chapter, had we been consulted, we might have suggested that this should be changed to "Mental health begins with Us".

Source: Mental Health Australia, www.mhaustralia.org

Conclusion

A growing body of research on the social identity approach to CMHC points to the fact that groups and social identities have a critical role to play in the trajectory of these conditions. More specifically, it appears that joining valued groups and thereby gaining a sense of positive social identity has the capacity to unlock resources that have profound benefits for individuals' mental health. In this, the approach offers a coherent theoretical framework that helps us better understand the proven effectiveness of community group programmes in promoting recovery from CMHC, as well as more mixed evidence for the benefits of family therapy, group psychotherapies, and supported employment programmes. In particular, what we see is that when individuals identify strongly with family (Miller, Wakefield, & Sani, 2015), mental health–related groups (Crabtree et al., 2010), and other naturally occurring groups (Dingle et al., 2013; Dingle et al., 2016), they are more likely to receive beneficial forms of social support and more likely to be able to work with others to counteract the pernicious effects of group-based discrimination.

In the clinical realm there is also preliminary evidence that an approach to treatment informed by social identity principles may be more effective in addressing the negative symptoms of CMHC (e.g., regulating negative emotions, increasing pleasure, and overcoming social isolation; see Table 13.1) than existing treatments such as medication or psychotherapies. Furthermore, compared to formal mental health treatment services, naturally occurring group activities in the community are less focused on mental illness and therefore less likely to perpetuate a stigmatised identity. Significantly too, joining such groups tends to allow for the expression of personal choice and autonomy in a manner that is entirely consistent with the recovery model of mental health (in a way that hospital and other psychotherapeutic treatments are often not). Finally, when individuals with CMHC experience depleted social networks by virtue of their condition and its treatment, it would appear that a social identity intervention such as Groups 4 Health (see Chapter 15) should have the capacity to help strengthen any pre-existing group membership while also linking people to new meaningful groups. In contrast to formal therapy groups, these naturally occurring groups are likely to endure over time and therefore would seem to hold out the promise of sustained, not just fleeting, benefit.

As things stand, however, the research that would provide conclusive evidence for this full suite of propositions remains to be conducted. Nevertheless, on the basis of the work we have reviewed in this chapter, we believe that the theoretical and empirical grounding for those propositions is very strong. Accordingly, we are optimistic not only that this much-needed research will be conducted, but also that, when it is, it will provide the necessary next step in advancing our appreciation of the potent links between social identity and CMHC.

Points for practice

A range of messages for practitioners working with people experiencing chronic mental health conditions can be drawn from the social identity approach we have outlined in this chapter.

1. *Involve people's support networks where appropriate.* Assess the nature and quality of an individual's family relationships, friendships, and broader social groups and, where suitable, include members of their support system in treatment.
2. *Encourage people with CMHC to view themselves "alongside of" the condition.* Reflective discussion about who the person was before the onset of the CMHC and who she or he is alongside of the CMHC may emphasise interests and qualities that they can explore despite the difficulties imposed by the condition.
3. *Help to link people with meaningful group activities in their community.* The School of Hard Knocks and Reclink studies that we discussed in this chapter show that participants with CMHC who stay engaged with meaningful group activities (arts based, sports, and so on) over 3- to 12-month periods improve on various measures of self-esteem, mental health, and well-being.
4. *Offer people group activities, even during inpatient treatment.* Any group that an individual with CMHC comes to identify with – including therapeutic groups, support groups, and recreational activity groups – is likely to help them feel less alone and more supported in the process of dealing with their condition. Identification with such groups will also provide access to psychological resources that they can draw upon to help in their recovery.

Resources

Further reading

As we have seen, research exploring the role that social identity and self-categorization processes play in the development and treatment of CMHC is in its infancy. Nevertheless, the following papers give a good idea of the way in which researchers are starting to explore these issues.

① Williams, E. J., Dingle, G. A., Jetten, J., & Rowan, C. (2018). *Identification with arts-based groups improves mental wellbeing in adults with chronic mental health conditions.* Manuscript under review: University of Queensland.

This longitudinal study of members of a School of Hard Knocks choir and creative writing groups found that the more people identified with the SHK group, the more their mental well-being improved over time. Likewise, those who perceived greater social support from the SHK group had greater increases in mental well-being over time. However, when participants reported having low SHK identification and low social support, there was no change in their mental well-being over time.

② Crabtree, J. W., Haslam, S. A., Postmes, T., & Haslam, C. (2010). Mental health support groups, stigma, and self-esteem: Positive and negative implications of group identification. *Journal of Social Issues, 66,* 3, 553–569.

This study of members of mental health support groups found that group identification predicted increased social support, stereotype rejection, and stigma resistance. These self-protective mechanisms in turn predicted higher levels of self-esteem – thereby buffering them from the negative implications of their stigmatised identity.

③ McIntyre, J. C., Elahi, A., Bentall, R. P. (2016). Social identity and psychosis: Explaining elevated rates of psychosis in migrant populations. *Social and Personality Psychology Compass, 10,* 619–633.

This theoretical paper proposes that cultural identities play a central role in mitigating the psychological precursors of psychosis, but that de-identification and social disconnection subsequent to migration could initiate or exacerbate psychosis across multiple generations.

Video

① Search for "Haslam paranoia" to watch a video of a talk – originally presented at the 3rd International Conference on Social Identity and Health – in which Alex Haslam outlines the social identity model of emergent paranoia and some of the evidence that supports it. www.youtube.com/watch?v=fDDclUPFH6I&feature=youtu.be   (19 minutes).

② Search for "Bentall schizophrenia" to watch a short discussion in which Richard Bentall talks about the importance of life stories in psychosis. This challenges the idea that psychosis results from problems that are "all in the brain" and instead suggests that life experiences have a very significant role to play in its development. www.youtube.com/watch?v=TRq_qBQheU0   (4 minutes).

Websites

① www.reclink.org. This is the official website of Reclink, an Australian charity that focuses on providing vulnerable adults with access to meaningful recreational activity, with the goal of improving their mental health and quality of life.

② www.schoolofhardknocks.org.au/sohk/. This is the official website of the School of Hard Knocks, an Australian charity that aims to build people's self-esteem through arts programmes in which they work towards high-quality group performances under the guidance of professional arts practitioners.

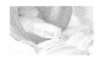

Chapter 14
Chronic physical health conditions

Chronic physical health conditions (CPHC) comprise an extremely broad category of illnesses that have become much more common over the past 100 years in Western countries. Defined by their enduring nature, the rising prevalence of such conditions is the result of a combination of factors, including more effective management of infectious diseases (previously a leading cause of death), increasing life expectancy, and lifestyle factors such as diet and exercise. For example, around 50% of Australians experience a chronic condition and 20% experience more than one, with this percentage increasing as people age (Australian Institute of Health and Welfare [AIHW], 2011). More generally, chronic conditions are the ultimate cause of death for approximately 90% of people in the developed world (AIHW, 2011).

However, what is becoming clear is that mortality rates provide an incomplete picture of the health status of a population. In addition to being the main cause of death, CPHC affect quality of life, both for the people who live with disease and for those who support them. For example, although cardiovascular disease is a leading cause of death around the world, the majority of cardiac infarctions (heart attacks) and strokes are not fatal; instead a person who has a heart attack might experience anything from return to full health after a short recovery period, through to lasting severe disability. In recognition of this, the Global Burden of Disease project (Murray et al., 2012; Vos et al., 2015) was launched by the World Health Organization in 1990 to investigate the impact of diseases on people while they are still alive. One outcome of this initiative has been the development of an index called Disability Adjusted Life Years (DALYs). This is calculated using the following three pieces of information: (1) the subjective disability caused by the illness, (2) the number of years that a person with the illness typically experiences the disability, and (3) the prevalence of the condition in the population. Because DALYs have been calculated across many countries and across many years, it provides a useful starting point for understanding what are the most disabling chronic conditions around the world. These data are summarised in Figure 14.1.

What is immediately apparent from this figure is that non-communicable diseases, which are the blue segments, account for around 75% of global disability and an even bigger proportion in industrialised Western countries. The World Health Organization uses the term *chronic condition* interchangeably with non-communicable disease (WHO, 2017b); however, some communicable diseases that have a protracted and enduring course (such as HIV) are also appropriately included in the category of chronic conditions. In this chapter, much of the evidence we draw on comes primarily from those CPHC that are the cause of the greatest burden of disease worldwide, specifically, *cardiovascular diseases* (predominantly coronary heart disease and stroke), *cancers* (particularly of the lung and liver), *musculoskeletal disorders* (chronic pain, arthritis, and chronic fatigue syndrome), *diabetes*, *sense organ disabilities* (of which hearing loss causes the largest health burden), *chronic respiratory diseases* (chronic obstructive pulmonary disease and asthma), and *neurological conditions* (epilepsy and migraine). We focus on physical disease and do not cover mental and substance use disorders here (although they can be chronic conditions) because these have already been discussed in some depth in Chapters 8, 9, and 13.

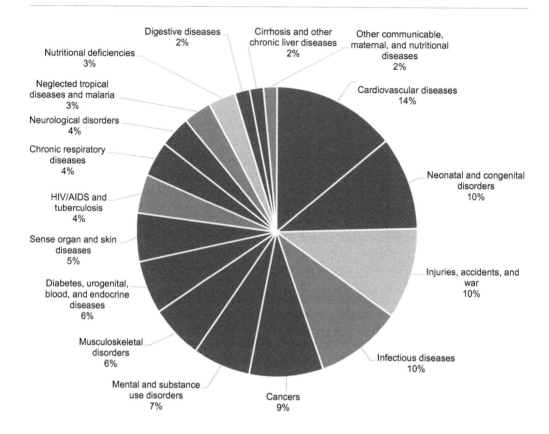

Figure 14.1 The worldwide burden of all disease

Note: Data are reported in Disability Adjusted Life Years (DALYs) as a proportion attributable to each broadly categorized disease, across all countries and age ranges for which data are available. Blue segments indicate non-communicable diseases; red segments indicate communicable diseases; green segments indicate diseases of environmental origin. The higher a country's income, the lower its burden of communicable diseases and the higher its burden of non-communicable diseases.

Source: Institute for Health Metrics and Evaluation (IHME). GBD Compare. Seattle, WA: IHME, University of Washington, 2016. Available from http://vizhub.healthdata.org/gbd-compare. (Accessed September 1, 2017)

Of course, each of these conditions could demand a chapter in its own right to fully explore issues of aetiology, course, prognosis, and treatment. These differ considerably depending on the condition. For instance, some conditions, like asthma, can have minimal impact on quality of life or life expectancy if managed well, whereas others, like lung cancer, are associated with a high likelihood of death within months of diagnosis. These differences between conditions are clearly important for their management, as already well described in a range of texts (e.g., Antman & Sabatine, 2013; Holt, Cockram, Flyvbjerg, & Goldstein, 2017; Wakley & Chambers, 2005).

But as with mental health, it is also increasingly acknowledged that – as a consequence of what can be referred to as *horizontal epidemiology* (Bailey & Williams, 2014; Cieza et al., 2015) – many also have overlapping causes, features, and risk factors. In particular, as we will see later, the social determinants of these various conditions tend to have more general rather than specific effects on health, which helps to explain why prevention and treatment strategies for various conditions often have a lot in common (AIHW, 2011). It is this commonality, underlying the social determinants, that the present chapter addresses. But before taking this perspective to explain how the social identity approach extends our understanding and management of CPHC, we first consider dominant current approaches to these conditions.

Current approaches to understanding and managing CPHC

The biomedical approach

The biomedical approach is the traditional model for managing chronic physical health conditions and underpins many modern health services, particularly tertiary care (e.g., hospital systems). In this model, intervention is warranted when a person seeks help in response to physical symptoms they experience (by contrast, see the *health promotion approach* later). Here, the initial emphasis is on *diagnosis* to determine the biological cause of these symptoms (i.e., what category of disorder in Figure 14.1 is present) and inform appropriate treatment. Diagnostic tests are diverse, but often include blood or urine samples, imaging, and/or physical examination.

Clearly diagnosis is vital to management, but it is not always straightforward. At times, it can be invasive, inconclusive, and expensive (see Figure 14.2). In some cases, too, diagnostic efforts have unintended side effects. For instance, it is recognised that x-rays – which are often used to confirm breaks and fractures to bones, pneumonia, and cancer – are best used sparingly throughout a person's life, as each exposure increases the risk of cancer (Berrington de Gonzalez & Darby, 2004). It is also the case that even accurate tests can lead to *false-positive* diagnostic errors, where the test indicates a person has a disease when they do not. For example, if an HIV test has a 98% *specificity* rate, this means that 98% of people *without* HIV will correctly receive a negative result on the test. Although this 98% accuracy rate sounds high, if large numbers of people are tested for HIV, then this 2% error rate may correspond to a significant number of healthy people being diagnosed as ill. Because of this, when a person receives a positive result, particularly for rare diseases, a number of follow-up tests are needed because, statistically, a positive result is more likely to be a *false* positive than to accurately indicate the presence of disease (Cordes & Ryan, 1995). These considerations clearly do not discredit the importance of diagnostic tests in managing CPHC. However, they should increase our awareness of how diagnostic efforts can be thwarted by the complex ways in which CPHC arise and interact, and that, in turn, can have a range of unintended consequences for patients.

The focus of the biomedical approach to CPHC is on the biological pathology that underlies symptoms of ill health. In order to relieve symptoms and the suffering associated with them, the pathological cause must be identified and, where possible, eliminated. Dealing with conditions where the underlying biological cause of illness is both easily identified and resolved is the forte of the biomedical model. Blindness caused by cataracts and pain caused by a bone fracture are both examples where this traditional model works very well and achieves excellent outcomes for most people. However, for a growing number of illnesses, the biologically based origins are not always clear or may not be plausible targets for intervention. As a result, CPHC are rarely managed by biomedical means alone. In fact, unlike infectious disease, CPHC typically have more complex and multi-pathway causes, many of which may not be biological in origin. For example, chronic back pain can be debilitating, but is rarely attributable to a clearly identifiable biological anomaly.

Because of this, patients with CPHC can sometimes find the process of diagnosis lengthy, expensive, and inconclusive. Indeed, where diagnostic testing fails to locate a biological cause for the symptoms a person is experiencing, they may be diagnosed as having *medically unexplained symptoms*. This is a catch-all diagnosis for a whole range of conditions which are described in terms of their symptoms when they have not been linked to a particular disease. Among the more common examples of medically unexplained symptoms are chronic fatigue syndrome, irritable bowel syndrome, post-concussion syndrome, and regional pain syndrome. Such conditions constitute a significant proportion of those confronted by health professionals. In fact, some estimates have suggested that around one third of symptoms reported to primary care physicians are medically unexplained (Steinbrecher, Koerber, Frieser, & Hiller, 2011).

What happens, then, when no evidence of biological pathology can be found? In this context both the physician and the person experiencing symptoms face challenges, albeit of a different nature. A medical professional with limited training in medically unexplained symptoms (Stone, 2014) might be tempted to conclude that the person is either (1) malingering (intentionally exaggerating illness; e.g., to access compensation of some kind) or (2) experiencing somatic symptoms of mental illness (e.g., where anxiety or depression manifest in terms of physical symptoms, such as fatigue or nausea; Shattock, Williamson, Caldwell, Anderson, & Peters, 2013).

In response, people who do not receive a clear diagnosis might feel alarmed at the lack of a "real" diagnosis or confused by a psychiatric label or referral if provided. They may seek the opinion of a series of health professionals – or alternative, non–evidence-based practitioners – in an effort to gain

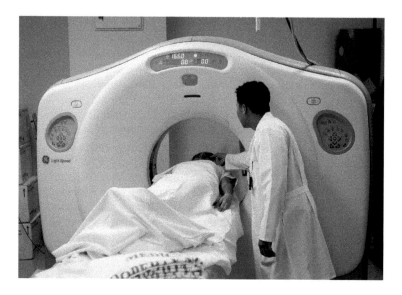

Figure 14.2 A person undergoing a full-body computerised tomography (CT) scan

Note: Diagnostic scanning, while increasingly marketed to both doctors and consumers, is also recognised as inappropriate in many cases (e.g., if a person has back pain of unknown origin). This is because there is a high chance of misidentifying abnormalities in the absence of symptoms (a false-positive result) as well as missing signs of actual disease such as cancer (a false-negative result). Additionally, such scans expose patients to a non-negligible dose of radiation (Bach et al., 2012; Black, 2000; Flynn, Smith, & Chou, 2011; Rao & Levin, 2012).

Source: Pixabay

a more conclusive diagnosis. In an attempt to demonstrate the physical reality of their symptoms, they may also become less open to suggestions that, for instance, psychological or social interventions could assist with the management of the condition (Jutel, 2010). This is unfortunate because many CPHC benefit from psychological and social interventions, and physicians who refer patients for such support are often acting on the best available evidence. Just as someone who loses their sight will benefit from psychological assistance to develop new skills to accommodate their condition, someone with chronic pain might similarly benefit from psychological interventions designed to help them better manage and tolerate their pain. However, a person's determination to 'prove' the physical reality of their chronic condition can make psychological and social approaches to intervention unattractive (see Case study 14.1).

Once CPHC are diagnosed, the biomedical approach will inform efforts to target treatment to correct the underlying biological pathology. In many cases (e.g., in treatment for diabetes, migraine, or arthritis) this cannot eliminate, or "cure", the condition as such. Here, medical intervention typically focuses on improving a person's quality of life with various management strategies – for example, through use of medication or surgical intervention to relieve symptoms. This approach can provide excellent outcomes, though it can sometimes have unintended consequences. For instance, side effects of treatment can inadvertently be worse than the symptoms they aim to relieve. A common example of this is in aggressive treatment of terminal cancer, which can extend a person's life, but can also reduce the quality of that life due to side effects such as nausea and fatigue (Brownlee et al., 2016). Another example is the use of multiple medications to manage multiple conditions, which can lead to complex pharmacological interactions and complicate symptom presentation (particularly for older people, see Chapter 7).

In recent years, a prominent and unintended consequence of the use of pharmacological symptom relief for some CPHC is the over-prescription of opiate painkillers. These very effective painkillers have been heavily marketed to primary care physicians, particularly in the United States (Van Zee, 2009), where their prescription has increased by approximately 850% (Dhalla et al., 2009). However, it is now clear that developing dependence is not an uncommon consequence of such medications. Indeed, in this same time period, researchers have found a fivefold increase in opioid use disorders (now accounting for over 2% of DALYs in the United States) and a 41% increase in overall opioid-related mortality (Dhalla et al., 2009). There has also been a marked increase in the prevalence of black market prescription opiates, as well as illegal opiates – patterns which have both been attributed to people sustaining their dependence through the most affordable means available to them (Fischer et al., 2002). Although medication undoubtedly has an important role to play in managing the symptoms of CPHC, these data remind us that biomedical approaches to treatment also come with risks and potential downsides.

The health promotion approach

Although the biomedical model is central to the management of CPHC, it is not the only approach available. In particular, it is complemented by the *health promotion* approach, and this is an approach that many health professionals would align themselves more closely with. Arising out of the disciplines of public health and epidemiology, this approach prioritises improving health and preventing the onset of chronic disease among members of the general public (Green, Tones, Cross, & Woodall, 2015). In the last 20 years, there has been growing recognition that rather than waiting for symptoms to emerge, non-communicable diseases are particularly amenable to prevention and early intervention. Typically, health promotion aims to use low-cost and minimally invasive interventions that have a broad reach within the population. The approaches used are diverse and can target any health risk factor, although they typically focus on the "big four", which have the largest influence on mortality

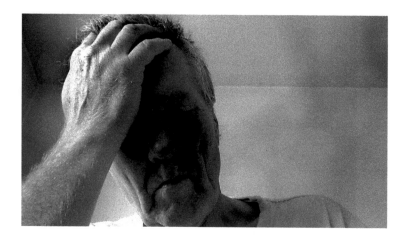

Figure 14.3 Chronic fatigue syndrome

Note: Chronic fatigue syndrome is an illness characterised by severe and disabling fatigue that lasts for at least 6 months. Like several stigmatised chronic conditions, it is only diagnosed when medical investigations fail to identify a biological cause for a person's symptoms.

Source: Pixabay

Case study 14.1 Health science as a battleground

In 2011, a large randomised controlled trial (known as PACE; White et al., 2011) was published in the journal *The Lancet*. This compared four treatments for chronic fatigue syndrome: standard medical care (SMC), adaptive pacing therapy (APT, in which patients are encouraged not to push themselves beyond their limits), cognitive behavioural therapy (CBT), and graded exercise therapy (GET; see Figure 14.3). The results indicated that both CBT and GET were superior to SMC or APT. Even though these findings seem promising from an intervention perspective, they were not greeted warmly by patient groups. In fact, the research met staunch opposition, with several high-profile support groups and online communities critiquing the methods, motives, and morals of the researchers. A petition calling for the retraction of the trial received over 10,000 signatures. Some researchers even stated that they had received death threats following their involvement in the study (Rehmeyer, 2016).

Why were these study findings so controversial? This may be easier to understand when one considers that people with chronic fatigue syndrome often report feeling discriminated against by medical professionals who imply, either explicitly or implicitly, that their condition is psychological rather than physical. For such individuals, the suggestion that they will benefit from psychological therapy may understandably be interpreted as a further claim that their symptoms are "all in the mind". Accordingly, the evidence base supporting CBT was interpreted as invalidating the physical reality of their condition. Interestingly, longer-term follow-ups of the PACE study found no difference between any of the four conditions, and treatment for chronic fatigue syndrome remains controversial (Shepherd, 2016).

and quality of life – namely, nutrition, physical activity, smoking, and alcohol use (Riekert, Ockene, & Pbert, 2013).

Examples of health promotion approaches include using healthy eating campaigns to promote the inclusion of more fruits and vegetables in children's school lunches, restrictions on where people can smoke cigarettes to prevent secondary exposure to carcinogens, and the provision of workplace facilities (e.g., secure bike storage and showers) that encourage employees to cycle to work (De Geus, De Bourdeaudhuij, Jannes, & Meeusen, 2008). Although many health promotion initiatives require changes in policy or governance, at the individual level it is often the general practitioner (GP) who bears the brunt of the load in trying to implement the health promotion approach. This is because GPs have long-term contact with their patients and are able to assess and advise not only on a person's current health concerns, but also on lifestyle risk factors (e.g., Orleans, George, Houpt, & Brodie, 1985).

The health promotion approach has been particularly important and successful in the domain of CPHC (Brownson, Haire-Joshu, & Luke, 2006). This is because many of the risk factors for CPHC are (1) *overlapping*, in that a person can reduce their risk of developing a whole range of conditions by targeting one risk factor; (2) *premorbid*, in that they are evident many years before the onset of a chronic condition; and (3) *modifiable*, in that the risk factors for CPHCs are often behaviours which can be changed (rather than purely fixed genetic vulnerabilities).

The focus on health promotion coincides with a push within the medical profession to reduce medical testing and intervention where there is emerging evidence for no demonstrable benefit (Grady & Redberg, 2010; Hudzik, Hudzik, & Polonski, 2014). Examples include recommendations to avoid the prescription of antibiotics for colds and flu viruses, imaging for lower back pain, chemotherapy in the last months of life in terminal cancer, and saline solution for cleaning cuts and grazes (Cassel et al., 2012). These initiatives offer a means of combating unnecessary medical testing and intervention (and thereby avoiding its unintended negative consequences).

One recently emerging trend in health promotion is a category of behaviour change strategies known as "nudge" policies that are largely informed by economic models of human behaviour. Popularised by Richard Thaler and Cass Sunstein, nudge policies involve light-touch interventions which aim to increase the likelihood that an average person will choose options that are better for their (or society's) health (Thaler & Sunstein, 2008). For instance, an "opt out" system for organ donation leads to a much higher percentage of people consenting to allow their organs to be transplanted after their death than an "opt in" system (Whyte et al., 2012).

An important principle of nudge interventions is that they do not involve coercion, although they may make certain behaviours more difficult, expensive, or inconvenient. This, indeed, may increase the political appeal of nudges relative to other models of health promotion that entail increased regulation. As a result, governments around the world have of late become interested in the insights that nudge approaches can bring to health policy (Ellison, 2011). However, some researchers have argued that the evidence base for nudge interventions is often patchy compared to other approaches to behaviour change, a point to which we will return in the social identity section later.

Health promotion is clearly a large and important part of the story when it comes to reducing the burden of CPHC, but the reality is that effective interventions can be difficult to devise and implement (Glasgow, Vogt, & Boles, 1999). There are several reasons for this, but probably the most important is that effective health promotion typically requires policy changes (e.g., to change laws governing organ donation) and thus need to be implemented by those with sufficient power to bring about such change. For example, although many GPs would like to focus more on early intervention and prevention in their practice, health policy and funding can be a barrier to this. In many countries, for example, people require a diagnosis in order for an appointment to be eligible for public health care funding, and publicly funded practitioners are not allotted enough time with patients to deal with anything other than their immediate health concerns (Brotons et al., 2005).

A further challenge confronted by those who are interested in health promotion is that the demands of real practice settings often mean that the implementation of evidence-based interventions is challenging and less effective than trials might suggest. This speaks to the fact that there is an important difference between *efficacy* (the performance of an intervention under ideal and controlled conditions) and *effectiveness* (the performance of an intervention in real-world health practice). Recognising this problem, Russell Glasgow and colleagues developed the RE-AIM model with a view to optimising the translation of health promotion evidence into practice (e.g., Glasgow et al., 1999; Glasgow, Lichtenstein, & Marcus, 2003). As summarised in Table 14.1, their model outlines five key principles that should guide health promotion so as to increase its public health impact. The RE-AIM framework has been very

Table 14.1 RE-AIM guidelines for developing, selecting, and evaluating programmes and policies for health promotion

RE-AIM component	Definition	Guidelines and questions to ask
Reach	Percentage and representativeness of participants	Can the programme attract a large and representative percentage of the target population? Can the programme reach those most in need and most often left out (e.g., the poor, those low in literacy and numeracy, or people with complex health issues)?
Effectiveness	Impact on key outcomes, quality of life, unanticipated outcomes, and subgroups	Does the programme produce robust effects across sub-populations? Does the programme produce minimal negative side effects and increase quality of life or broader outcomes (i.e., social capital)?
Adoption	Percentage and representativeness of settings and staff that participate	Is the programme feasible for a majority of real-world settings (given costs, expertise, time, resources, etc.)? Can it be adopted by low-resource settings and typical staff serving high-risk populations?
Implementation	Consistency and cost of delivering programme and adaptations made	Can the programme be consistently implemented across programme elements, different staff, time, etc.? Are the costs (personnel, up front, marginal, scale up, equipment) reasonable to match effectiveness?
Maintenance	Long-term changes in practice of individual and settings	Does the programme include principles to enhance long-term improvements (i.e., follow-up contact, community resources, peer support, ongoing feedback)? Can the settings sustain the programme over time without added resources and leadership?

Note: Research suggests that attending to these five components when designing an intervention will generally increase its public health impact.

Source: Gaglio and Glasgow (2011)

influential in health promotion and, in line with its goals, following these principles has been shown to increase the likelihood of interventions bringing about effective and lasting change in practice (Gaglio, Shoup, & Glasgow, 2013).

Psychological approaches

Psychological approaches to managing CPHC extend on the biomedical model to target the psychosocial factors that present with these conditions. These build on the important observation that successful prevention or management of a chronic condition often requires individual behaviour change – a key focus of psychology. Indeed, it was this insight that led to the development of the closely related subfields of health psychology and behavioural medicine, which have aimed to fill this gap in the perceived needs of people with CPHC (Davidson et al., 2003; Stanton, Revenson, & Tennen, 2006). Psychological approaches reject a dualism of physical and mental health. That is, in order for it to merit attention and treatment, the field of psychology (and particularly health psychology) does not require that a chronic condition be conceptualised in terms of either a 'real' physical disorder caused by identifiable pathological processes or in terms of a (stigmatised) mental disorder. Instead, psychological approaches emphasise that psychological factors are at work in *all* health conditions and that understanding and attending to these factors can improve peoples' health.

Psychological approaches to CPHC are diverse, but are broadly concerned with three activities: (1) identifying the psychological determinants of health behaviours which affect the risk of chronic disease such as smoking, unhealthy eating, and lack of exercise; (2) identifying which individual differences predict who will have a better or worse prognosis after being diagnosed with a chronic condition; or (3) developing and validating evidence-based psychological interventions for people with CPHC. The first of these was covered in some detail in the section on *social-cognitive models* in Chapter 10, and so in this chapter we will focus on the latter two activities.

Research on individual differences has suggested that people who cope most effectively with physical health conditions possess particular psychological traits. For instance, they are less likely to engage in catastrophising thoughts about the severity of their illness – that is, to interpret their physical symptoms as more debilitating, intense, and chronic than is warranted (Petrie, Moss-Morris, & Weinman, 1995; see Chapter 12). People who cope effectively with chronic conditions also (1) are better at regulating their behaviour (Detweiler-Bedell, Friedman, Leventhal, Miller, & Leventhal, 2008), (2) show greater optimism and conscientiousness (e.g., Cohen, Bavishi, & Rozanski, 2016) and less trait anger and hostility (Chida & Steptoe, 2009), (3) are more likely to engage in adaptive problem-solving coping (rather than emotional or avoidant coping), and (4) are found to have more positive expectations for their recovery (Scharloo et al., 1998).

Yet although it is useful to identify these features of effective coping, a potential criticism is that some of this analysis simply amounts to a redescription of effective coping rather than an explanation of it per se. However, to the extent that these psychological factors are malleable, this research is helpful in identifying appropriate targets for intervention. For instance, in one randomised controlled trial involving people with chronic lower back pain, the effectiveness of *both* physical therapy and cognitive behavioural therapy (CBT) were mediated through reduced pain catastrophising (Smeets, Vlaeyen, Kester, & Knottnerus, 2006). It is thus likely that both psychological (e.g., CBT) and non-psychological (e.g., physical therapy) interventions can be enhanced through a focus on increasing these psychological resources.

Psychological approaches have also developed evidence-based interventions for CPHC. Many psychological interventions for people experiencing CPHC include a focus on the management of comorbid depression and anxiety. This is because it is often the case that comorbid mental illness is more disabling than the chronic condition itself (Moussavi et al., 2007; Schmitz, Wang,

Malla, & Lasage, 2007). Indeed, the demands of coping with CPHC typically create psychological and social problems that exacerbate the symptoms. For instance, there is a substantial literature which suggests that comorbid anxiety increases the disability associated with conditions as diverse as arthritis, migraine, gastrointestinal disease, and respiratory disease (Sareen et al., 2006), whereas a higher incidence of depression is found in almost all physical conditions, including heart disease and diabetes (Scott et al., 2007).

Psychological intervention for comorbid mental illness is often a good way to improve quality of life and reduce the functional impairments that are associated with CPHC (Kessler, Ormel, Demler, & Strang, 2003). This is interesting because psychological interventions typically do not target physical conditions directly. Nevertheless, there is now a solid evidence base supporting the use of cognitive-behavioural therapy, mindfulness, and self-management for a number of conditions. For example, treatment guidelines for irritable bowel syndrome, chronic pain, and chronic fatigue syndrome all include psychotherapy as a component of evidence-based care (Eccleston et al., 2014; Price, Mitchell, Tidy, & Hunot, 2008; Zijdenbos, de Wit, van der Heijden, Rubin, & Quartero, 2009). It is worth noting, though, that the evidence base indicates that it is not *generalised* psychotherapy, or even generalised CBT for depression or anxiety, that is most helpful here. Rather, tailored interventions that have been validated specifically for a particular syndrome or syndromes prove to be the most effective in enhancing well-being and health (van Dessel et al., 2014).

Tailored psychological interventions for CPHC can take a number of forms. For instance, manualised forms of CBT have been developed for medically unexplained symptoms (Salkovskis et al., 2016), chronic pain (Ehde, Dillworth, & Turner, 2014), chronic fatigue syndrome (White et al., 2011), and irritable bowel syndrome (Hutton, 2005). CBT for CPHC often targets catastrophising thoughts (e.g., Thorn et al., 2007). Here research has indicated that CBT which specifically targets safety and avoidance behaviours, negative illness and symptom beliefs, and "all or nothing" behaviours are particularly effective for CPHC (Knoop, van Kessel, & Moss-Morris, 2012). Apart from targeted CBT, the other two tailored interventions for CPHC that have proved most successful to date are mindfulness for chronic pain and self-management programs, which we review next.

In the last 10 years, there has been an enormous growth in the use of mindfulness and acceptance-based psychological approaches (sometimes referred to as the 'third wave' of evidence-based psychotherapy). Chronic pain is one area where the evidence for the effectiveness of these interventions has been particularly strong. Specifically, these interventions aim to produce a shift in a person's primary appraisal of their symptoms so that rather than being seen as threatening and distressing, they are non-judgementally perceived and accepted (Day, Jensen, Ehde, & Thorn, 2014). Relatedly, an *acceptance and commitment therapy* (ACT) approach to chronic pain involves both mindfulness and an emphasis on finding ways to meet behaviour change goals that align with a person's values (Wicksell, Dahl, Magnusson, & Olsson, 2005). Although pain reduction is not the explicit goal of mindfulness and ACT interventions, people often report that by *changing their relationship with their pain* (i.e., appraising it differently, see also Chapters 5 and 12), they are no longer as distressed or impaired by it, and hence their experience is that the pain is subjectively reduced (McCracken, MacKichan, & Eccleston, 2007). Yet although the research suggesting that mindfulness and ACT can be useful for the management of chronic pain is promising (e.g., Parra-Delgado & Latorre-Postigo, 2013; Vowles, McCracken, & O'Brien, 2011), reviews of such interventions have drawn mixed conclusions, and further research is needed to establish their effectiveness (Rajguru et al., 2015).

Self-management programmes (SMPs) constitute another key way in which psychology can be harnessed to improve CPHC. These approaches have argued for a shift away from seeing people as passive recipients of health care. Instead, SMPs aim to empower individuals both to engage actively in strategies to improve their own health and to act as stakeholders in the process of making decisions about their health care (Greaves & Campbell, 2007). SMPs typically involve a combination of psychoeducation, disease and medication management strategies, as well as advice on lifestyle changes and psychological coping skills. These often take the form of structured group interventions led by a health professional. Along these lines, evidence-based manualised programmes have been developed for many conditions, such as asthma (e.g., Kotses & Harver, 1998), diabetes (e.g., Glasgow et al., 1997), and arthritis (e.g., Barlow, Turner, & Wright, 1998). SMPs are often agnostic in terms of their conceptual framework, but they are typically informed by the principles of either cognitive-behavioural theory (see Chapter 8) or self-efficacy theory (see Chapter 10). In terms of the efficacy of SMPs, research has found that although such programmes are effective in improving a person's quality of life and well-being, the benefits for their physical health status are more variable (Barlow, Wright, Sheasby, Turner, & Hainsworth, 2002).

Self-management is clearly a noble goal for those with CPHC, but there may be many obstacles that make it difficult for a person to self-manage effectively. Speaking to this point, Anthony Jerant and his colleagues conducted a study to better understand the barriers to self-management in a sample of 54 people with CPHC (most commonly multiple comorbid conditions including diabetes, arthritis, and congestive heart failure; Jerant, Friederichs-Fitzwater, & Moore, 2005). Interestingly, the most common barriers were comorbid mental health problems (particularly depression), difficulties in changing lifestyle behaviours (particularly with exercise and weight loss), and the challenges of living with the symptoms of the conditions themselves (e.g., fatigue, pain). These barriers speak to the importance of striking a balance between, on the one hand, promoting and enabling people's autonomy in managing their chronic condition and, on the other hand, avoiding policies and approaches that leave people feeling blamed and unsupported in their efforts to achieve better health outcomes. For example, whereas a sense of personal control and mastery is associated with well-being (Rodin & Langer, 1977), the perception that chronic conditions are controllable leads to an increase in stigma and blame directed at those who have these conditions (Haslam & Kvaale, 2015; Pearl & Lebowitz, 2014).

Critical perspectives on health and disability

In the approaches we have considered thus far, the health-threatening status of CPHC has very much been taken for granted. At the other end of the spectrum, however, another approach to CPHC has emphasised the contextual, subjective, and structural factors that influence health and well-being. Broadly referred to as *critical health psychology* (Hepworth, 2006), this approach aligns with sociological, feminist, and postmodern theorising and aims to highlight the way in which existing power structures (including the high status of health professionals) serve to reinforce health inequalities (St Claire, Watkins, & Billinghurst, 1996). Moreover, this is an approach to chronic conditions that emphasises social justice and often melds scientific research with social activism.

Critical approaches often adhere to tenets of social constructivism – suggesting that all of our perceptions and experiences are culturally relative, and hence that notions of health are similarly relative, with the lived experience of an individual being the most valid source of information about their reality. For this reason, critical approaches have tended to favour qualitative research methods that explore the richness of this lived experience, particularly for vulnerable population groups. Major research themes in critical health psychology have included, amongst other things, the stigma of disability (Wang, 1998) and the medicalisation of female reproductive experiences (Cahill, 2001).

In the domain of CPHC, critical health psychology has championed the view that disability arises not so much from a person's health status as from the failure of society to accommodate the needs of a particular patient group that would enable them to flourish (Oliver, 1998). One way in which society maintains or causes such disability is through what has been called *ableism*, or the tendency for structures and systems to discriminate against people whose health status is non-normative (Campbell, 2009). This might be evidenced, for example, by the requirement for a person to obtain a disability pension from a government office that is not accessible by wheelchair.

An important contribution of critical approaches has been to bring attention to assumptions about health and disability that are routinely made not only by health professionals but also by health researchers (see Figure 14.4). For instance, it is common for people to assume that a person's quality of life must *necessarily* be impaired by disability or that people will always be better off if they receive the most up-to-date medical treatment. Although these assumptions are often taken for granted, when they are put under the microscope, they often prove highly questionable.

One final contribution of critical approaches is that through their emphasis on population-led, person-oriented qualitative research, they have provided a voice – which was formerly often unheard – for people with chronic conditions. Amongst other things, this has helped to ensure that medical and health science develops in a way that meets the needs of health service users rather than just those of health care providers or scientists. Indeed, partly as a result of the lobbying of critical health researchers, all health research is increasingly expected to have input from consumer groups and a client-centred focus (Harkness, 2004).

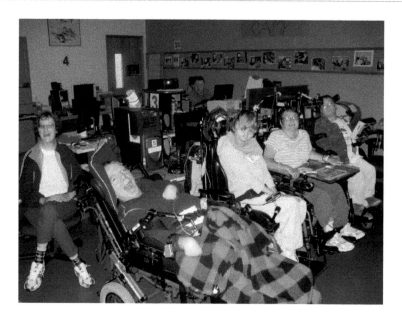

Figure 14.4 Critical health psychology: questioning assumptions and giving voice

Note: Two important contributions that critical health psychology has made to the field of CPHC are (1) to question health-related assumptions and (2) to give voice to patient groups that have traditionally been disempowered within health care systems. This picture is of a group in Seattle that was established to support and empower people who use assistive technology.

Source: Wikimedia Commons

The social identity approach to CPHC

From the earlier review, it is possible to identify at least three pervading themes of current approaches to CPHC. The first is that there is a subjective dimension to the experience of physical symptoms and disease; the second is that people with chronic conditions experience stigma; and the third is that it is necessary to adopt a social level of analysis in order to understand the interaction between a person's physical health and their social context. The social identity approach expands upon these observations in order to provide new insights into CPHC that extend upon the earlier approaches. These are unpacked in the four sections that follow and are concerned with (1) how physical symptoms are appraised, (2) how health care functions, (3) how social influence shapes the health behaviours that place a person at risk of a chronic condition, and (4) how social identity protects people against threats to physical health.

Social identities affect the way people experience, appraise, and express symptoms

Sickness and health are never givens. Instead, as we observed in Chapter 5, "there is nothing either good or bad but thinking makes it so". This means that the experience of any health condition – in terms of its symptoms, their meaning, and the degree of impairment they cause – is always subjective and psychological. More specifically, self-categorization theory argues that *all* perception – that is, the way in which people interpret the information they see, hear, feel, and so on – only occurs through the *lens* of salient self-categorizations (Turner & Oakes, 1997; Turner, Oakes, Haslam, & McGarty, 1994). To unpack this, reflect on the fact that the information available to our sensory organs at any given time is immense and at an order of magnitude greater than can be understood or usefully interpreted by our brain. Accordingly, in order to manage this vast array of data and extract meaning from it, the human mind works to *categorize* the information it receives into similar 'chunks', based on assumptions informed by our previous experience and structural features of the stimuli in question (see Figure 2.6).

To give a simple example, imagine that you are looking out over a large, empty school hall, set up ready for a performance. Rather than attending to and interpreting each complex visual stimulus individually, your mind is able to simply categorize the bulk of this information as "empty chairs", with your attention only being brought to any stimulus that does not fit this categorization. To make this example social, imagine that the hall is now full of people. In this case, your mind performs the same operation with people as it did with objects, categorizing the people in the hall as "audience". This example can be taken one step further, though, to illustrate how this categorization process is inherently self-referential. How would you perceive the audience if you were performing at a concert that day rather than simply attending a concert? What if you were a teacher at the school rather than a pupil? Clearly each of these different perspectives would affect the way you see the audience, because categorizations are always made in relation to oneself. The critical take-away point here is that all perception is *made with inherent reference to the social self.*

How, though, is this feature of human cognition relevant to CPHC? As we saw in Chapter 5 when we discussed how people's reactions to injury varied as a function of the meaning of those injuries for a salient self-definition (e.g., as a woman vs. a sports player; Levine & Reicher, 1996), *physical symptoms* (including those that may indicate underlying chronic disease) are similarly interpreted in relation to a person's self-concept. This includes social categories such as gender, ethnicity, and age, but also categories based on a person's beliefs about particular physical conditions. That is, people have existing schemas about what a particular illness looks and feels like, called an "illness representation" (Baumann, Cameron, Zimmerman, & Leventhal, 1989), and these inform their understanding of the symptoms of illness in themselves and others. Thus, as Mark Levine and Steve Reicher showed, even before a condition can be recognised as such, social identities will affect (1) whether a particular physical symptom will be noticed, (2) how serious a person thinks the symptom is, and (3) whether he or she will seek help for it.

These various points are illustrated further in qualitative interviews that Stephanie Adams and colleagues conducted with people who had been diagnosed with asthma (Adams, Pill, & Jones, 1997). They found that this population was roughly divided between "accepters", who had taken on an identity as an "asthmatic" person, and a group of "deniers/distancers", who rejected the asthmatic label and were more likely simply to think they had "a bad chest" or something similar. This latter group had a uniformly negative view of people with asthma, which may be part of the reason why they were unwilling to self-categorize in terms of this illness label.

Why, though, would someone reject a social identity that describes their symptoms? At least in part, the answer would seem to be provided by the identity restoration hypothesis (H4) that we discussed in Chapter 2, which states that *people will be motivated to restore positive identity when this is compromised by events that threaten or undermine their social identities*. Specifically, a negative evaluation of a health condition may act as a barrier to people acknowledging relevant symptoms in themselves or taking on an illness identity. This may be particularly true of conditions that are easily concealed or where the diagnosis is disputed (as is often the case with medically unexplained symptoms). Instead of taking on the illness identity, a person with a chronic condition may resist such a categorization – as did the interviewees of Stephanie Adams and her colleagues (1997) who attributed their asthma symptoms to a bad chest. Indeed, this can be interpreted as an example of individual *mobility* (see H5), in which people seek a more positive social identity by (psychologically) exiting a low-status group.

However, as we saw in Chapter 11, there are some notable downsides to individual mobility strategies of this form. In the context of CPHC, one important downside is that people who reject an illness label are less likely to believe that they require treatment for that illness and thus are less likely to adhere to a prescribed treatment regimen. For instance, in the study of people with asthma reported earlier (Adams et al., 1997), the "accepters" of the asthmatic label were more likely to be compliant with preventive medication. On the other hand, "deniers/distancers" were less likely to comply with preventative medication or to attend an asthma clinic. Perhaps as a result of this, those who denied also reported more symptoms, such as shortness of breath, that impaired their quality of life. Indeed, other research in the context of hearing loss has found that self-categorizing in terms of an illness identity can be a *necessary precondition* for even pursuing treatment in the first place (Hogan, Reynolds, Latz, & O'Brien, 2015).

As we discussed in the context of brain injury (Chapter 11), a further downside to the mobility strategy is that it means people are also less likely to receive support from (and provide support to) other people experiencing the same condition (in line with the support hypothesis, H14). Along these lines research has suggested that if people conceal stigmatised identities this can damage their health because it denies them access to the collective resources that social identity affords (Ellemers & Barreto, 2006; Quinn & Earnshaw, 2013). Speaking to this point, a study conducted by Kathleen Bogart of 106 people with multiple sclerosis found that people who identified as someone with a disability actually had lower levels of depression and anxiety (Bogart, 2015, see also Chalk, 2015).

On the other hand, there can be an upside of rejecting an illness label as self-defining, because it may enable a person to avoid the discrimination associated with membership of the group in question. Self-defining in terms of a physical condition may hold other risks too. For example, research has suggested that people who essentialise their own condition (i.e., who believe that it is something fundamental about who they are as a person) are more likely to *self-stigmatise*, holding negative attitudes about their own capacity and their likelihood of recovery (Kvaale, Haslam, & Gottdiener, 2013).

In terms of the appraisal process, too, we might predict that a strongly held illness identity will make it more likely that people will attend to certain symptoms rather than others.

In one study that explored this idea (albeit in the context of mild illness rather than CPHC), Lindsay St Claire and her colleagues examined how people experienced and appraised the physical symptoms of a cold or tinnitus (St Claire, Clift, & Dumbelton, 2008). Unsurprisingly, they found that cold sufferers reported more severe symptoms relevant to colds and tinnitus sufferers reported more severe symptoms relevant to tinnitus. What was more interesting, however, was that, in line with social identity theorising, the selective reporting of symptoms relevant to a person's condition was particularly pronounced when that person's illness identity was made salient to them. In other words, when someone thought of themselves in terms of a particular health condition (e.g., "I am a person who has tinnitus"), the symptoms relevant to that condition were particularly noticeable and apparent. In the context of CPHC, we might therefore predict that people who self-define in terms of an illness identity will be more likely to attend to and report symptoms consistent with this condition, whereas non-consistent symptoms may be ignored, minimised, or misattributed (St Claire & Clucas, 2012).

However, it is not only *illness* identities that affect the appraisal of symptoms. How a person appraises the importance and severity of a physical symptom is affected by the salience of other social identities too. As we discussed briefly in Chapter 7, this is a phenomenon that St Claire and He (2009) explored in a study on hearing loss, a chronic condition that affects as many as one in five people (Wilson et al., 1999). In this study, half of the participants were encouraged to self-categorize as older – something that the researchers achieved by highlighting 'age' in the title of the study questionnaire and asking respondents both to indicate their age and to list activities that they took part in with other older people. The remaining participants were encouraged to self-categorize as individuals (by highlighting 'the self' in the title of the study questionnaire and asking them to list activities that they engaged in personally). After this, participants were asked about their hearing. As one would expect, given that assignment to experimental conditions was random, objectively, there was no difference in the hearing performance of the groups. Nevertheless, as can be seen from Figure 14.5, the researchers found that participants who had been encouraged to self-categorize as 'older' reported many more symptoms of hearing loss. They also reported feeling that they were significantly more handicapped by them than those who self-categorized as individuals. Self-categorization as 'old' thus led participants to be more sensitive to age-related health problems and to be more concerned about their seriousness.

What, then, are the implications of these various findings for the diagnosis and treatment of CPHC? At least two points seem clear. First, it is apparent that health professionals cannot hope to understand a person's symptoms and health in a vacuum – for example, by imagining that a person's reporting of their symptoms has a straightforward correspondence to some physical reality. In particular, this is because salient social identities can help or hinder a person's sensitivity to physical health symptoms in ways that lead to these being interpreted as lying anywhere on a continuum from inconsequential to debilitating. These complex effects of *social identities* on processes of assessment, diagnosis, and treatment are ones that we are only beginning to explore and understand. Second, it is apparent that these appraisals will in turn determine whether or not people believe that they require treatment, as well as who (if anyone) they turn to in order to receive that treatment. It is to this question of how social identities affect health care choices and provision that we turn next.

The provision of effective health care services is affected by social identity processes

People who have CPHC are typically in regular and close contact with a range of health care providers. However, the nature and quality of health services, as well as a person's satisfaction with them, are all highly variable. In this regard, one important contribution of the social identity approach is to help us understand why people with CPHC do not always receive optimal care and do not always comply with a treatment regimen they are prescribed. Specifically, this is because the approach draws our attention to the importance for health care trajectories of the social identities that are salient not only for the person with CPHC but also for their health care provider.

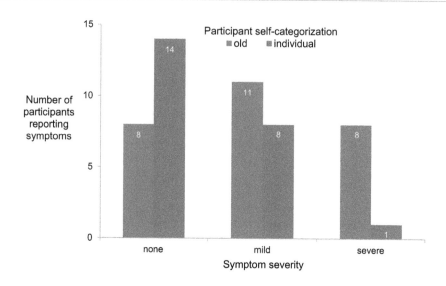

Figure 14.5 The frequency of older adults reporting symptoms of hearing loss as a function of self-categorization

Note: Pointing to the importance of self-categorization for symptom perception, when participants were led to self-categorize as old they were much more likely to report severe symptoms of hearing loss than they were when they were led to self-categorize as individuals.

Source: St Claire & He (2009)

A starting point for this discussion is the observation that, much like patients, health professionals have expectations about what people with particular chronic conditions "look like", informed by both their training and their experience. This can mean that people whose CPHC present in an unusual or counter-stereotypical way feel that they do not always receive optimal care. For example, Stuart Read and colleagues conducted qualitative interviews with people who have cerebral palsy and observed that the vast majority found the support they received for their condition to be stigmatising (Read, Morton, & Ryan, 2015). Probing further, this was because many health professionals were seen to communicate with this client group in a patronising way. However, interviewees also reported that when they did need support, they felt that they had to "enact" their cerebral palsy identity to service providers by demonstrating their high needs and similarity to other people with the condition. Indeed, interviewees reported that this strategic expression of their chronic condition was expected and necessary in order to justify their need for support.

Other research suggests that sometimes it may be the disparity between patients' and doctors' social identities that interferes with effective care. This was demonstrated in a study conducted by St Claire and Clucas (2012), which explored the way in which shared social class identity (or lack thereof) influenced the nature of the service provided by primary care physicians. What these researchers found was that doctors who were highly identified with their profession perceived their patients to be more similar to one another than those who were less highly identified. This suggests that identifying as a medical doctor (a high-status profession that traditionally aligns with the biomedical approach) can lead to reduced attention to specific patient characteristics. This echoes classic research by David Pendleton and Stephen Bochner (1980) which showed that physicians spend more time with patients

who were of upper-middle-class background (i.e., who shared their social class identity) than with those who had lower socio-economic status. They also asked more questions about their patient's health status and obtained more information in return.

This dynamic is likely to be particularly prominent for people with a CPHC, as these disproportionately affect people of lower social class (Marmot, 2005). Given that people who share social identities are more likely to trust one another (the connection hypothesis, H12) and tend to experience interactions as more supportive (the support hypothesis, H14), we would also expect that the effectiveness of health care is predicated on the capacity of a health professional to develop and sustain a sense of shared identity with their patients. Indeed, without such a shared identity, even the best planned treatment plan is likely to go awry – if for no other reason than that a patient is less likely to comply with it.

Issues of treatment adherence can also arise when health care providers do not consider the multiple identities of patients and the ways that these might facilitate or interfere with treatment. For example, people with type 1 diabetes are generally trained to self-administer their insulin, as this is required to regulate blood glucose levels and transport energy to body cells. However, a small number of people with type 1 diabetes also meet criteria for bulimia nervosa and will restrict their self-administration of insulin as a weight control strategy (often with severe adverse health consequences; Ruth-Sahd, Schneider, & Haagen, 2009). Accordingly, a health professional who attends only to a person's status as a diabetic may not uncover the real reason for a person's low adherence to treatment. In order to optimise care to such a patient, it is therefore critical for treatment providers to consider that his or her behaviour may by motivated by a different identity – that of a person with an eating disorder (Hastings, McNamara, Allan, & Marriott, 2016). This idea of identity-motivated health behaviour is one we return to in the next section.

Finally, it is instructive to reflect on the way in which a paucity of social identities can structure how people with CPHC engage with health care. People with CPHC tend to be high users of health services and are sometimes referred to by health professionals as frequent attenders. Frequent attenders illustrate well how social identities affect both (1) the way in which people make use of available health care resources and (2) the quality of care they receive. Previous research has found that frequent attenders have poor mental and physical health and typically experience at least one chronic condition which needs ongoing management (Vedsted & Christensen, 2005). Moreover, general practitioners report that frequent attenders are both the most difficult clients to manage in their caseload and a major contributor to burnout (Mathers, Jones, & Hannay, 1995). It is interesting too that alongside this, those who are characterised as frequent attenders are often the most dissatisfied with the health services they receive. What is it, then, about this group that makes them so challenging for health professionals, so dissatisfied with their doctors, and yet so persistent in presenting for care?

One answer to this question can be found in our earlier review of the research on medically unexplained symptoms. Frequent attenders are particularly likely to have chronic conditions, including a diagnosis of one of the syndromes falling under the umbrella of medically unexplained symptoms, and/ or mental health concerns (Ferrari, Galeazzi, Mackinnon, & Rigatelli, 2008; Jyväsjärvi et al., 2001). Accordingly, they are people whose health needs are unlikely to be met by a traditional biomedical approach. Furthermore, some of the reasons for frequent attendance may lie not only in their symptom profile, but also in their life circumstances. More particularly, for reasons that we explored in Chapter 3, these clients are typically socio-economically disadvantaged, lonely, and unable to access appropriate support through other means (Ellaway, Wood, & Macintyre, 1999).

With a view to exploring these patterns and their relationship to social identity in more depth, Cruwys and colleagues conducted three studies of frequent attenders (Cruwys, Wakefield, Sani, Dingle, & Jetten, 2018). These uncovered a number of interesting findings. The first was that social isolation, as indexed by the absence of social group memberships and associated identification, was a stronger and more consistent predictor of frequent attendance than mental or physical health status. Furthermore, as the results in Figure 14.6 show, an intervention to increase social group contact among a vulnerable

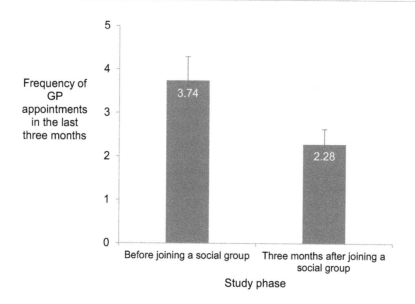

Figure 14.6 Frequency of GP appointments before and after an intervention to increase meaningful group membership

Note: Social, religious, and community organisations in many countries run recreational groups for disadvantaged people, such as free art classes, choirs, or sports teams. This study tracked 46 socially disadvantaged people with a range of chronic health problems who joined a social group (art, yoga, sewing, or indoor football). As well as a subjective increase in their mental and physical health 3 months later, the intervention resulted in participants attending an average of 1.5 fewer appointments with their general practitioner.

Source: Cruwys et al. (in press)

population (who, at the study's outset, were visiting their GP an average of more than once a month) significantly reduced the frequency of GP attendance over a 3-month period. This evidence suggests that people can be driven to seek health care not only by their physical symptoms but also by a lack of social identification. This in turn suggests that problems of health care over-utilisation cannot be fully understood – or properly addressed – without attending to the unmet social needs of patients.

Overall, then, these data suggest that social identities – both those of the patient and health care provider – interact in ways that have a critical bearing on how health care is sought, provided, and experienced. In the next section, we take a step back to examine how social identity theorising can help us understand why people engage in behaviours that place them at risk of a chronic physical condition in the first place.

Social identities can motivate both healthy behaviours and health risk behaviours

A large proportion of health promotion initiatives to prevent chronic conditions focus on education. The logic here is that people simply do not realise that behaviours such as smoking or physical inactivity are damaging their health, and if they knew the risks they would change their behaviour. Unfortunately, however, findings from these educational interventions have been somewhat disappointing (Tones, 1986), and there is little evidence that peoples' decision making is underpinned by a rational cost–benefit analysis of long-term risks to health (Slovic, Peters, Fincane, & MacGregor, 2005). One key reason for this is that health risk behaviours are often not carried out for reasons that are related to health. Driving a motorbike dangerously fast, for example, may have more to do with the fact that a person is a member of a particular bike gang than that they have been unconvinced by commercials that discourage speeding. Such observations alert us to the fact that health behaviour is often *social identity* motivated (Oyserman, Fryberg, & Yoder, 2007) rather than health motivated.

We can say that a behaviour is identity motivated when it is an enactment of the norms of a psychological salient social group (the norm enactment hypothesis, H8). Via what is called a normative influence process, people conform to the norms of the groups with which they are strongly identified. Why is normative influence such a powerful determinant of attitudes and behaviour? In line with the influence hypothesis (H9), self-categorization theory argues that this is because the social groups with which we identify provide a meaningful reference point when it comes to defining the nature of appropriate thoughts and actions (Turner, 1991). More specifically, we expect ingroup members to have a similar perspective on the world as us, and thus we draw on the beliefs and behaviours of our social groups – especially those of the individuals who are most representative of them (the prototypicality hypothesis, H10; Haslam, Reicher, & Platow, 2011) – as a guide to what we ourselves should believe and do. Accordingly, to understand and potentially modify their healthy and health risk behaviours, we should look to the norms of a person's important social groups (and those who represent them; i.e., leaders).

Speaking to this point, recent research has suggested that for every hour a person jogs, their life expectancy increases by approximately seven hours. This impressive effect is mainly because running protects against the onset of chronic disease, particularly cardiovascular disease (Lee et al., 2017). However, simply knowing that 'running is good for you' is not enough to spur most people to put on their running shoes. Instead, if we want to understand what makes a particular individual start and sustain the habit of running, it is a good idea to start by looking at how often other members of his or her social groups run and what messages they communicate about running (Madan, Lazer, & Pentland, 2010; Scarapicchia, Sabiston, Andersen, & Bengoechea, 2013; Stevens et al., 2017).

In line with this observation, as we saw in Chapters 9 and 10, there is a large body of evidence which supports the norm enactment hypothesis as an explanation for both substance use (Schofield, Pattison, Hill, & Borland, 2001) and eating behaviour (Cruwys et al., 2012; Louis, Davies, Smith, & Terry, 2007). More generally too, studies have found that membership and salience of social groups that have healthy (rather than unhealthy) norms are associated with healthier individual behaviour (e.g., Tarrant & Butler, 2011; Tarrant, Hagger, & Farrow, 2012). And in another demonstration of the importance of group-based norms for health, Juan Falomir-Pichastor and colleagues found that nurses were more likely to seek flu vaccinations – a health behaviour that has benefits for both the nurses and their patients – to the degree that they were highly identified with other nurses (Falomir-Pichastor, Toscani, & Despointes, 2009). This was because highly identified nurses tended to believe that vaccination was a professional duty, and this belief explained the relationship between their internalised professional identity and their enthusiasm for vaccination.

It is clear, too, that many of the most effective health promotion strategies make use of normative influence within their interventions. For instance, advertising campaigns in the 1980s linked Australian identity with being 'SunSmart' (i.e., using sun protection, including sunscreen; see Figure 14.7), and this ultimately led to a significant reduction in dangerous sun exposure and the incidence of skin cancer (Montague, Borland, & Sinclair, 2001; Staples et al., 2006). Indeed, the fact that national identity is likely to be both positive and important for a majority of people in the target population of a health promotion campaign, makes it a particularly viable target for such interventions. Similarly, interventions that seek to increase fruit and vegetable uptake through use of peer modelling have been found to be particularly effective among children and adults (Horne et al., 2009; Thordike, Riis, & Levy, 2016). Although some of these success stories have been claimed as evidence of the effectiveness of "nudge" policies, Frank Mols and colleagues argue that they are better understood through

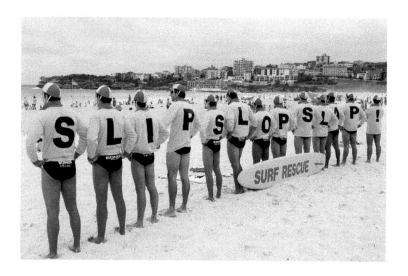

Figure 14.7 Normative influence in health promotion

Note: Effective health promotion, like the Cancer Council of Australia's "Slip, Slop, Slap!" campaign, often seeks to link
    particular behaviours to groups that are representative of targets' shared identity.

Source: Will Burgess, Reuters Pictures

a social identity lens that sees them as examples of effective normative influence (Mols, Haslam,
Jetten, & Steffens, 2015).

In sum, the norm enactment hypothesis provides an important way to understand why it is that
people often engage in health risk behaviour despite being fully aware of the health risks that these
entail. Furthermore, in this it provides clues as to how health promotion might most effectively change
such behaviour and thereby prevent or delay the onset of CPHC. Even for people with CPHC or those
who engage in risky health behaviour, understanding the key psychological processes (e.g., norms,
identities) that bring about long-term behaviour change is critical to protecting health and improving
quality of life. In drawing the chapter to a close, this is a possibility that we investigate in the next
section.

Social identities provide people with resources to manage threats to physical health

It has repeatedly been found that people who are more socially connected have better physical
health. Indeed, as we saw in Chapter 1, broadly defined social connectedness is a good predictor of
longevity and a better predictor than a range of more widely discussed factors (e.g., Holt-Lunstad,
Smith, & Layton, 2010; Holt-Lunstad, Robles, & Sbarra, 2017). Building on such research, there is
also evidence that it is not just social connectedness in general, but social identification with groups
in particular, that predicts favourable outcomes across a wide range of CPHC, including heart disease
(Haslam, O'Brien, Jetten, Vormedal, & Penna, 2005), multiple sclerosis (Wakefield, Bickley, & Sani,
2013), and cancer (Harwood & Sparks, 2003). Importantly too, social identification predicts reduced
engagement in health risk behaviours such as smoking (Schofield et al., 2001). For example, in a large
survey of adolescents, Kirsty Miller and colleagues found that the number of group identifications

young people reported was negatively associated with cigarette smoking, alcohol consumption, and the use of illicit drugs (Miller, Wakefield, & Sani, 2016).

Although this relationship between social identity and physical health has been repeatedly demonstrated (in ways that support the identification hypothesis, H2), the mechanisms here are less clear. One reason for this is that several of the mechanisms which explain how social identity protects *mental* health (e.g., psychological need satisfaction, belonging, support, control) are less plausible as mechanisms that might explain how social identity could protect physical health. Nevertheless, along lines that we discussed in previous chapters (e.g., Chapters 5, 6, and 7), there is substantial evidence that social identities provide people with more *resources* to help them cope with and effectively manage challenging life circumstances, including those associated with CPHC (consistent with H11).

In one study that speaks to this point, Juliet Wakefield and her colleagues surveyed 152 people with multiple sclerosis from around the United Kingdom who were participating in a multiple sclerosis support group (Wakefield et al, 2013). They found that identification with the support group was associated with better mental health and well-being outcomes. In another example, Lisa Nackers and her colleagues found that people with severe obesity in group-based weight loss programs lost more weight to the extent that they felt a strong connection to the group and felt there was less conflict among its members (Nackers et al., 2015).

As a result of such findings, group interventions are increasingly recognised not simply as a *cost*-effective way of delivering interventions such as self-management programmes, but as a part of what makes such interventions effective in the first place, enhancing health outcomes for those involved (see Figure 14.8). When people are asked what they find most useful about such interventions, they most often point to the sense of psychological connection to others in the group and to the social support – often very practical support, such as strategies for coping and behaviour change – that they provide (Tarrant et al., 2017). This suggests that one reason why groups improve outcomes for people with CPHC is that they promote effective coping styles. For example, people might be less likely to catastrophise symptoms to the extent that they have supportive social group networks to draw upon in managing their chronic condition. Indeed, this is apparent from studies that we reviewed in Chapter 12, which show that reassurance from an ingroup member reduces the experience of pain (Platow et al., 2007) and that the psychological salience of multiple group memberships increases performance on a challenging physical resilience task (Jones & Jetten, 2011).

There is also emergent evidence that the protective resources that social identities provide for physical health also have immunological underpinnings. Early evidence of the impact of social connectedness on the immune system came from studies on the progression of HIV (as reviewed in Chapter 4). In particular, research by Steve Cole and his colleagues found that following a diagnosis of HIV, people who are more sensitive to social rejection experience a faster deterioration of health, a reduced response to antiviral treatment, and ultimately die approximately 2 years earlier than those with HIV who are less sensitive to rejection (Cole, Kemeny, & Taylor, 1997). Although the relationship between sensitivity to rejection and social identity is unclear, this study suggests that the experience of social stress (broadly construed) is closely linked to the body's capacity to resist a threat to physical health. Interestingly, these differences are also accentuated among people who conceal their HIV-positive status (Cole, Kemeny, Taylor, & Visscher, 1996). As we discussed earlier, this points to the fact that there are advantages and disadvantages to rejecting an illness identity – with one of the disadvantages being that this removes a possible avenue to social support.

This early work led to a body of epigenetic research exploring the effect of social experiences on human biology. Here research has identified a cluster of genes, approximately 2% to 5% of the human genome, which are suppressed (or "switched off") in the context of social exclusion, loneliness, or abuse. Moreover, the fact that these genes are disproportionately implicated in disease (Cole, 2013) can help us to understand the link between social identity and physical health. In this vein, Sally Dickerson and colleagues provide a detailed description of the specific pattern of psychobiological response

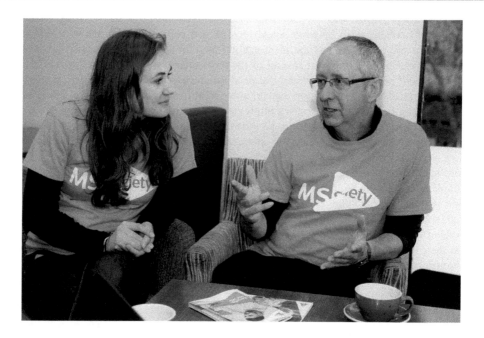

Figure 14.8 Groups as an 'active ingredient' in CPHC treatment

Note: When it comes to managing chronic physical health conditions, groups are not just an effective way of delivering information, they are an 'active ingredient' in the treatment. Indeed, it is common for people to join support groups to help them manage CPHC. This picture is of members of a support group for people with Multiple Sclerosis (MS). Evidence suggests that, providing people identify with them, such groups are an effective (not just a cost-effective) way of receiving treatment and support.

Source: The MS Society

that occurs in response to social stress (Dickerson, Grunewald, & Kemeny, 2004). This includes the expression of the stress hormone cortisol (see Chapter 5) and the regulation of proteins called cytokines, which play an important role in the immune system. Broadly speaking, this evidence suggests that social stress (particularly when such stress involves shame or a lack of control) contributes to the upregulation of the sympathetic nervous system (a component of the body's "fight or flight" system). However, as we noted in Chapter 4 (e.g., see Figure 4.3), sustained activation of the sympathetic nervous system ultimately damages physical health in a number of ways, not least by placing a greater strain on the cardiovascular system and increasing the risk of metastasising cancer and infection (for reviews, see Anisman, 2016; Chrousos, 2009; Matheson & Anisman, 2012; Uchino, 2006). Importantly, chronic stressors can lead to a dysregulation of sympathetic nervous system functioning, including a reduction in basal cortisol levels. Although low cortisol may sound like a good thing, this actually places chronically stressed people at higher risk, because they show an increased reactivity of the sympathetic nervous system in response to new stressors (McEwen, 1998, 2002; see also Chapter 6 for a discussion of the role of cortisol in trauma).

So why would it be that evolution has selected for this kind of gene expression in humans so that social suffering damages our health? How could such a system be functional? Some researchers (e.g.,

Korte, Koolhaas, Wingfield, & McEwen, 2005) have argued that the immune system is "switching" to a strategy optimised for fighting wounds and bacterial infection (which, evolutionarily speaking, would have been more likely in the context of social conflict and exclusion) and away from a strategy optimised for fighting (socially delivered) viral infections and long-term disease (the latter of which is a much more significant health threat in the modern world). For example, one type of immunological cell which is upregulated in response to social stressors are *monocytes* (Miller, Chen, & Cole, 2009). These cells are great at healing wounds, in part because they encourage the growth of new blood vessels (angiogenesis; Martin & Leibovich, 2005). However, this same process can accelerate the metastasis of cancer because cancer requires a supply of blood vessels in order to spread through the body (Carmeliet, 2005). Monocytes can also accelerate neurodegenerative disease in the brain, encourage the development of atherosclerosis, and increase the risk of asthma and pneumonia (Slavich & Cole, 2013). Stated baldly, what all this means is that social stressors like abuse, rejection, and isolation make the body much more vulnerable to chronic disease.

Although this evidence is compelling, the empirical focus in previous research has been on generalised social stress rather than on that which is linked to social identity in particular. Consistent with a social identity account, some research has found that subjective social isolation is particularly important in predicting the onset of an inflammatory epigenetic profile (Cole et al., 2007; Cole, Hawkley, Arevalo, & Cacioppo, 2011). We would go further and argue that lack or loss of social identity is the psychological core of these disparate types of social stressors (Cruwys, Haslam, Dingle, Jetten, & Haslam, 2014b; see also Chapter 5), but nevertheless this is an argument that remains to be tested empirically.

Conclusion

In the first half of this chapter we explored the range of different approaches that have previously guided efforts to understand and treat CPHC. The first of these is the biomedical approach, which seeks to diagnose and treat underlying biological pathology, or if this is not possible, to alleviate physical symptoms. The health promotion approach, on the other hand, emphasises preventative and early-intervention strategies targeted at the community more broadly with a view to increasing health-protective behaviours prior to the onset of CPHC. A third approach focuses on psychological factors, encompassing cognitive and behavioural interventions that, broadly speaking, seek to reduce unhelpful coping strategies and increase personal coping resources. In contrast, critical approaches point to the role that society plays in constructing models of health that are all too often disempowering for those with CPHC. In response, they have championed qualitative and discursive approaches to give people with CPHC a more agentic voice in health research and treatment decisions.

The second half of this chapter explored a social identity approach to CPHC, from which we can derive three important conclusions. The first is that social identities – both illness related (e.g., "asthmatic") and otherwise (e.g., gender, age) – have a central role to play in the perception of symptoms. This is seen in appraisals of their presence, form, and severity and has a major bearing on whether or not CPHC are recognised and whether or not (and how) treatment is sought. A second conclusion is that the nature and effectiveness of the health care that a person receives (and indeed whether they receive it at all) is also shaped by group memberships – those of the (potential) client, of the health care provider, and their interaction. It is therefore the case that the course and prognosis of CPHC is always partly determined by the social identities that are in play in any given health care setting. A third conclusion is that group memberships provide the underpinnings for many of the most important behaviours that have implications for our physical health – both positive and negative. For example, almost all of the behavioural risk factors identified in Figure 1.2 (e.g., smoking, exercising, taking medication, getting vaccinated) can be understood to be dictated, at least in part, by the norms of the groups to which a given person belongs and with which they identify. If our interest is in changing these behaviours, this therefore requires that we engage directly with their underpinnings in group life.

Finally, we explored the ways in which social identities function as resources to protect against health threats, both by facilitating effective coping and by reducing chronic inflammatory immune processes. However, because the science surrounding these observations is in its infancy, many of our observations here were more speculative than those in other sections. Our sense, though, is that in the years ahead this knowledge gap will close and that social identity theorising will play a pivotal role in helping to close it. At heart, this is because, as the afore-listed conclusions attest, the physical aspects of health are much more social than is commonly supposed, and a full appreciation of their social dimensions – of the form that the social identity approach affords – is necessary to engage appropriately with them in every register. Accordingly, whether our goal be analytic, diagnostic, or therapeutic, the mysteries of CPHC will prove hard to unlock without keys of this form. It is therefore by cutting social identity 'keys' more precisely that essential and much-needed forms of progress in this area are going to be made.

Points for practice

1. *Biomedical diagnosis can both affect, and be affected by, a person's perceptions of symptoms.* Self-definition in terms of an illness label (e.g., asthmatic, diabetic) can facilitate treatment seeking, treatment adherence, and access to support from fellow patients. However, such illness identities can also be stigmatising and disempowering. Health professionals should be sensitive to these disparate effects when making a diagnosis and when helping their clients to navigate these challenges.
2. *Social and psychological interventions make a valuable addition to medical treatments.* The usefulness of social and psychological interventions has been established not only for mental and psychosomatic conditions, but also for many physical conditions. Indeed, all health conditions have a psychosocial dimension, and many people can benefit from evidence-based psychosocial intervention.
3. *All stages of a person's experience of chronic physical illness are shaped by their social identities.* Amongst other things, this is because the complex interplay of internalised identities (e.g., those related to illness, gender, and class) can all have a bearing on whether symptoms are detected, how they are interpreted, the likelihood of a person seeking medical help, and the quality of help they receive.
4. *Where group interventions promote a shared sense of psychological connection among group members, then the group becomes a key ingredient of the "cure".* Group interventions are increasingly common in practice, but these are most effective where health professionals invest in building a positive sense of identification among group members. In this way, effective social identity management increases access to practical support and strategies for coping with behaviour and lifestyle change.

Resources

Further reading

The following publications provide a range of important insights into the role that social identity processes play in CPHC.

① Oyserman, D., Fryberg, S. A., & Yoder, N. (2007). Identity-based motivation and health. *Journal of Personality and Social Psychology*, *93*, 1011–1027.

This article reports findings of seven studies which show how unhealthy behaviour can be motivated by social identities.

② Mols, F., Haslam, S. A., Jetten, J., & Steffens, N. K. (2015). Why a nudge is not enough: A social identity critique of governance by stealth. *European Journal of Political Research*, *54*, 81–98.

This paper explores the social psychology of 'nudges' – interventions which have gained popularity in recent years as vehicles for health promotion.

③ Tarrant, M., Khan, S. S., Farrow, C. V., Shah, P., Daly, M., & Kos, K. (2017). Patient experiences of a bariatric group programme for managing obesity: A qualitative interview study. *British Journal of Health Psychology*, *22*, 77–93.

This paper explores the experiences of people with severe obesity in a weight loss intervention and highlights the role of group processes in facilitating positive outcomes.

Video

① Search for "identity, access and health" to watch a TEDx talk by Andrew Trotter that discusses the way in which the labels that others give us, and that we use to define ourselves, affect people's experience when accessing, or trying to access, health care – specifically in relation to HIV. www.youtube.com/watch?v=3tR3qPoROuE. This video is also relevant to the discussion of stigma in Chapter 4.   (11 minutes)

② Search for "Claire Pomeroy Social Determinants" to watch a very personal TEDx talk by Claire Pomeroy which talks about the importance of social relationships and trust for health. Amongst other things, she argues that, to be effective, health care needs to be community based and proactive rather than physician based and reactive. This video is also relevant to the discussion of social determinants of health in Chapter 3. www.youtube.com/watch?v=qykD-2AXKIU   (15 minutes)

Websites

① www.healthdata.org/gbd. This interactive website on the Global Burden of Disease has some very clever graphics which allow you to explore the burden of disease in each country and demographic group for which there are sufficient data.

Chapter 15

Unlocking the social cure: GROUPS 4 HEALTH

A key message that runs through all the chapters of this volume is that social connectedness, and group connectedness especially, is central to health behaviour and health outcomes. For example, we have shown that social groups provide people with resources to buffer the physiological effects of stress, to overcome substance misuse, to protect against depression relapse, and to cope with the consequences of injury and trauma. At the same time, groups are implicated in negative outcomes too so that, amongst other things, they can sometimes exacerbate the effects of stress and stigma and encourage problematic behaviours. Understanding these influences on good and ill health is an important first step. But bridging the gap between science and practice requires us to specify exactly how we might translate our knowledge of group and social identity processes into applied interventions. How can we furnish people with the skills to use social groups as a beneficial psychological resource in their daily lives? What would an applied social identity intervention look like? And is there any evidence that such an intervention actually works and delivers sustained benefits?

The goal of this chapter is to answer such questions by outlining a programme derived from the social identity framework that seeks to improve health by enhancing group-based social relationships. The programme, GROUPS 4 HEALTH (also referred to as G4H), aims to empower people to realise these networks and to provide them with strategies to manage these networks independently in the longer term. In this chapter we explain why G4H is needed and we summarise preliminary data that speak to its effectiveness.

Current strategies to manage social disconnection

The experience of social isolation and disconnection is common. We see it as a consequence of social disadvantage and mental health decline, but also in response to a range of common life events and transitions – encountered in the course of events such as leaving school, moving house, becoming a parent, changing jobs, and retiring. For example, this experience is portrayed by Eilis Lacey, the main character in the movie *Brooklyn*, who emigrated from Ireland to New York in the 1950s in search of a better life, but who struggled with terrible loneliness in the transition. Along these lines, Eva Wiseman (2015), writing in *The Guardian*, highlighted the unrecognised cost associated with what we tend to see as positive life changes for young people (e.g., moving cities to start a new job or to study at university). There is a downside to these changes that can exacerbate feelings of loneliness and isolation: eating alone, struggling to break into new social circles, and being forced to live with strangers. Wiseman goes on to argue that young people in Britain not only have a problem admitting they are lonely, but once they have built up the courage to confront this problem, have no-one to admit it to. Considering this wider context, it is not surprising that loneliness has been identified by some as "an epidemic in modern society" (Killeen, 1998, p. 762; see Cacioppo, Grippo, London, Goosens, & Cacioppo, 2015), and one that is a core concern for a broad array of health service providers (see also Cacioppo & Hawkley, 2009; Cacioppo & Patrick, 2008).

Nevertheless, because the risk of isolation is heightened in some populations, it is to these groups that intervention tends to be targeted. As we detailed in Chapter 7, older people are one group at elevated risk, and the evidence from this population suggests that group interventions tend generally to be more effective in treating isolation than those that are delivered one on one (e.g., Cattan & White, 1998; Cattan et al., 2005; Findlay, 2003). This point is suggested in some findings from the meta-analysis led by Christopher Masi which included studies with participants across the entire age spectrum (Masi, Chen, Hawkley, & Cacioppo, 2011). Here, among studies that utilised a non-randomised group comparison design, interventions that were group based led to significant improvements (n = 14; M effect size = $-$ .53; p < .01), but those that were individually delivered did not (n = 4; M effect size = $-$ .16; p > .3). At the same time, the analysis revealed that other interventions, targeting social skills training or the provision of opportunities for social interaction, were not particularly effective in reducing loneliness.

So what is it about group interventions that might make them especially effective in reducing loneliness in older adults? Previously, researchers have attributed this advantage to three key factors. First, groups provide a good vehicle for communication and contact with others who have similar problems and who are working towards similar goals. Second, groups provide an ideal context to develop and test relevant skills. And third, groups provide people with a supportive social environment in which to work.

Importantly, from a social identity perspective, it is not group delivery per se that is the critical mechanism through which such interventions deliver health benefits. Accordingly, it is not the case that "any group will do" – although, sadly, this is a logic that often prevails if interventions are delivered in groups merely as a strategy to save time or money. For a group to be curative, what matters is the *social identification* that people derive from internalisation of that group as part of their sense of self (e.g., see Haslam, Haslam, Jetten, Bevins, Ravenscroft, & Tonks, 2010; Haslam, Jetten, Haslam, & Knight, 2012).

Significantly, the three factors identified above are all ingredients that can help people to develop a shared sense of social identification (e.g., see Postmes, Haslam, & Swaab, 2005). The key point, then, is that group activities typically provide participants with opportunities to develop their sense of identity-based connectedness to others. Indeed, by their very nature, group interventions are often (but not always) highly conducive to the development of a sense of social identity that is shared by those facing a common threat to their well-being (e.g., "us widowers" or "us carers"). Yet the centrality of social identification to these factors has largely been ignored in the loneliness literature, and hence it has not previously been identified as a specific target for intervention.

So if group intervention is key, this still leaves the question of what form it should take in order to be maximally beneficial. This is a question on which the research literature is largely mute. Nevertheless, examination of findings from previous reviews of loneliness interventions (e.g., Cattan et al., 2005; Masi et al., 2011), as well as evidence from group-based interventions targeting other health problems that we have discussed in previous chapters (e.g., social isolation; Gleibs, Haslam, Jones, Haslam, McNeill, & Connolly, 2011b; depression; Cruwys, Dingle, Haslam, Haslam, Jetten, & Morton, 2013b; Cruwys, Dingle, Hornsey, Jetten, Oei, & Walter, 2014a; Santini, Koyanagi, Tyrovola, Haro, Donovan, Nielsen, & Kouchede, 2017; eating disorders; Cruwys et al., 2015), points to several features that appear to be shared by the most effective interventions. First, interventions seem to be more effective to the extent that they have an integrated focus on issues of social process, cognition, and behaviour – rather than looking at any one of these things in isolation. Second, interventions tend to be more effective to the extent that the groups at their heart are meaningful to their members rather than having an arbitrary or trivial basis. These two features are both therefore central to the design of GROUPS 4 HEALTH. This is grounded in social psychological theorising which seeks to explain (1) the role that social group context plays in influencing our thoughts, emotions, and behaviour (after Turner, 1982) and (2) how social connectedness and health flow from group processes that serve to build meaningful and positive social identifications (e.g., in ways suggested by *the multiple identities* and *connection hypotheses*, H11 and H12).

The social identity approach to managing social disconnection

Origins and theoretical underpinnings of GROUPS 4 HEALTH

GROUPS 4 HEALTH was developed after reviewing outcomes from various social group intervention studies that we had conducted (several of which were described in Chapter 7). These studies aimed to improve social connectedness and well-being by building meaningful social identities among vulnerable older adults. Interventions were diverse and were typically developed in response to specific questions and challenges faced by our research partners (typically, managers of care homes responsible for the care of a group of vulnerable older adults). For example, our initial group reminiscence studies were developed in part to provide a partner organisation with evidence to support their implementation of reminiscence therapy and in part to test questions that we had about the role of group process in health outcomes (Haslam et al., 2010). Likewise, we studied water clubs in light of evidence that hydration is important for older adults' health, but also to clarify whether it is the water or the club that leads to positive outcomes (Gleibs, Haslam, Haslam, & Jones, 2011a). In other care homes, men's clubs were developed to establish the benefits that meaningful group activity might have for the mental health of men in residential care (noting that men are typically a somewhat disadvantaged minority group in this context; Gleibs et al., 2011a). Similarly, our "design team" studies were developed to involve residents as groups in the process of decorating communal rooms – in recognition of the fact that space in which one does not feel 'at home' is known to contribute to poor health and reduced quality of life (Haslam et al., 2014b; Knight, Haslam, & Haslam, 2010).

As we argued in Chapter 7, a consistent finding in all of these studies was that it was not the diverse content of these interventions that delivered health benefits (e.g., the reminiscence, the water, the chosen design). Instead, the active ingredient that produced beneficial health effects in all studies was the increased sense of connectedness and belonging that resulted from engagement in meaningful group activity. In short, it was the creation and strengthening of participants' social identifications through membership in a meaningful group, club, or team that proved critical to participants' enhanced cognitive health, mental health, and well-being.

If we know that social group interventions – whatever their form – are effective, then why not just set one up and get vulnerable people to join it? There are two key reasons why such a strategy is unlikely to work in the longer term. First, and consistent with the identification hypothesis (H2), we know that *social group interventions facilitate health gain only to the extent that people identify with those groups*. Accordingly, for groups to have or retain their curative powers, they need to provide a platform for identification. Such identification may be curbed for a number of reasons. People might not be interested in the activities of the group and so have no reason to bond with it. Also, where there are changes in people's circumstances, interests, abilities, or motivations, their sense of connection with the groups they currently belong to may also undergo change. For example, a walking group that was important in supporting physical activity goals at one point in a person's life may become less important if they become frail. Similarly, a mental health support group may no longer be fit for purpose once the illness is managed (Howard, 2006, 2008).

In short, when groups no longer have purpose, function, or meaning for us, their protective capacity declines. Of course, these groups may retain their curative potential if they come to serve a different function (e.g., when a former work group continues as a friendship group), but this will not always be the case. Relying on health professionals to detect and manage these changes is far from ideal, not least because it will be very hard for them to do so in a timely fashion. The logical solution is therefore to skill up people with the knowledge and resources they need to select groups that are right for them and to manage possible changes in their social group networks themselves.

It is also important not to focus too narrowly on any one group that people may join. As we have seen in several of the preceding chapters, although one group can be an important source of support, belonging to multiple groups increases both the availability of psychological resources and the likelihood that a person can access the right resource in the situation they confront (Haslam, Holme et al., 2008; Jetten et al., 2014; 2015; Miller, Wakefield, & Sani, 2015). However, for multiple groups to be maximally effective, they must also be compatible (Iyer, Jetten, Tsivrikos, Postmes, & Haslam, 2009). Juggling multiple groups that may be at odds with one another (e.g., because they encourage contradictory health behaviours, as might be the case in gym and nightclubbing groups) can be an added source of strain and burden. On the other hand, research shows that to the extent there is perceived compatibility between groups, particularly in contexts where people experience life change, this can be protective of mental health and well-being (Iyer et al., 2009). Thus, along the lines of H11, providing they are compatible with each other, important to them, and positive, the more social identities a person has access to, *the more psychological resources they can draw upon, and the more beneficial this will be for their health.*

These observations point to the need for an intervention that puts participants at the heart of a process of connecting themselves socially with as many positive and compatible groups as possible. But even if we accept this reasoning, one can argue that it is still not clear why we need yet another intervention to tackle social disconnection. In particular, critics would say that these needs could be addressed by popular existing treatments – in particular, cognitive behavioural therapy (CBT) or interpersonal therapy (IPT).

Closer interrogation of these approaches suggests that they fall short of the prescription noted earlier. In the case of CBT, the reason for this is that it sees factors other than social disconnection as lying at the heart of psychological disorder, and accordingly it is these other (primarily cognitive) factors that it targets. Indeed, as we discussed in Chapter 8, where social disconnection is considered in CBT, it is as a secondary focus and one that is not informed by any particular theory of social relationships. In behavioural activation (often incorporated into CBT), where there is recognition of the importance of reconnecting with meaningful activities, these can involve any activities and need not be social. Although more attention is given to social factors in IPT, it focuses primarily on changes and shifts in interpersonal relationships (e.g., conflict) that affect intrapersonal well-being and, accordingly, it seeks primarily to target personal deficiencies in managing these relationships. As we also saw in Chapter 8, what this neglects is the beneficial effects of social identity–based relationships on our emotional state and health (Haslam, Cruwys, Milne, Kan, & Haslam, 2016d; Haslam et al., 2010). This, then, is the gap that GROUPS 4 HEALTH seeks to fill.

G4H is a social identity–derived intervention that seeks to improve social connectedness by building social identifications in the context of an in-vivo group experience. In targeting social disconnection, it provides a non-stigmatising context in which to manage the social issues that either cause or are responsible for exacerbating many psychological disorders (Bentall, de Sousa, Varese, Wickham, Sitko, Haarmans, & Read, 2015; Cruwys, et al., 2014a, 2014b). The intervention's design draws closely on applied social identity theorising (e.g., Haslam, 2014) and on previous studies of health and well-being informed by the *social identity model of identity change* (SIMIC, see Chapter 3; Haslam, Holme et al., 2008; Iyer, Jetten, & Tsivrikos, 2008; Jetten, Haslam, Iyer, & Haslam, 2010a).

The original focus of SIMIC was on the factors that are protective of well-being during periods of life change. As described in Chapter 3, the model highlights the importance of multiple groups and their compatibility both (1) to scaffold the development of new social identities and (2) to facilitate strengthening or reconnecting with old valued social identities to overcome any potential negative effects that life change may bring. The relevance of this model to the design of GROUPS 4 HEALTH lies in its specification of social identity processes and pathways that are broadly relevant to health (not just well-being) and to forms of social vulnerability beyond just those associated with life transitions (e.g., as set out in Chapter 3, Figure 3.6). It is on these processes and pathways, then, that the programme seeks to capitalise.

The GROUPS 4 HEALTH programme

GROUPS 4 HEALTH is composed of five modules – the 5 S's – as shown in Figure 15.1. Together, these aim to give people the knowledge and skills not only to understand the nature and importance of their social identity resources, but also to manage them effectively in the long term.

The programme is manualised, and the *GROUPS 4 HEALTH Manual* provides facilitators with a single source that (1) explains the intervention's theoretical background, rationale, and evidence base and (2) provides detailed instructions for programme delivery (Haslam, Cruwys, Haslam, Bentley, Dingle, & Jetten, 2016a; see Figure 15.2 for an outline of the program). Each module contains facilitator notes detailing the aims, content, and materials required, followed by a full description of all exercises and activities. The manual is also supplemented by a *Workbook* (Haslam, Cruwys, Haslam, Bentley, Dingle, & Jetten, 2016b), which serves as a resource for participants that they can use both during the programme and after it has ended. This is a summarised version of the facilitator's manual that identifies the main learning points and activities associated with each module and provides space (1) to make notes, (2) to complete relevant activities (both during the sessions and afterwards as homework), and (3) to document programme-related plans.

The first module of G4H, Schooling, aims to raise awareness of the benefits that social group memberships have for health. It highlights the costs of ignoring these and also notes that we can only optimise health outcomes if, rather than just relying on individualised treatments (biological and psychological), we make the most of the social group resources at our disposal. The module also emphasises the importance of empowering people to take control of their health, noting that it is possible for everyone to take steps to improve their health by working to develop, maintain, and harness group-based social resources.

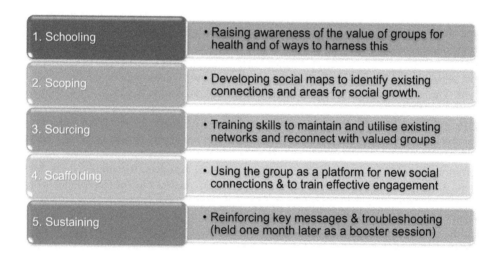

Figure 15.1 Summary of GROUPS 4 HEALTH modules – the 5 S's

Note: GROUPS 4 HEALTH is a manualised social identity–derived intervention that targets the building and maintenance of group memberships to support health and well-being. Its five modules aim to enhance knowledge of the contribution that groups make to health (Schooling), raise awareness of existing group networks (Scoping), identify networks that are important to maintain and strengthen on health grounds (Sourcing), build new social identities (Scaffolding), and review attempts to build and maintain group memberships in the context of the programme (Sustaining). Initial proof-of-concept data (Haslam et al., 2016c) show that the programme is effective in enhancing social connectedness and reducing the psychological distress associated with loneliness.

GROUPS 4 HEALTH program overview

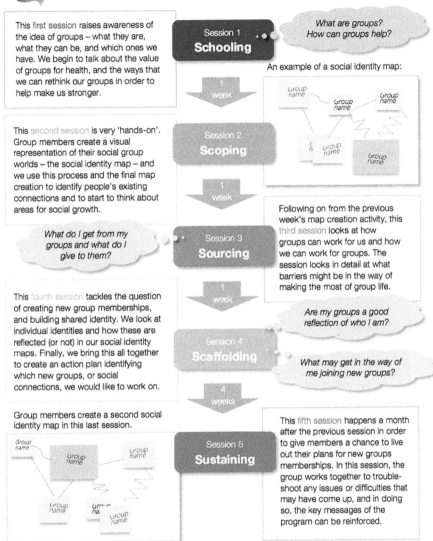

This first session raises awareness of the idea of groups – what they are, what they can be, and which ones we have. We begin to talk about the value of groups for health, and the ways that we can rethink our groups in order to help make us stronger.

Session 1
Schooling

1 week

What are groups?
How can groups help?

An example of a social identity map:

This second session is very 'hands-on'. Group members create a visual representation of their social group worlds – the social identity map – and we use this process and the final map creation to identify people's existing connections and to start to think about areas for social growth.

Session 2
Scoping

1 week

What do I get from my groups and what do I give to them?

Session 3
Sourcing

1 week

Following on from the previous week's map creation activity, this third session looks at how groups can work for us and how we can work for groups. The session looks in detail at what barriers might be in the way of making the most of group life.

This fourth session tackles the question of creating new group memberships, and building shared identity. We look at individual identities and how these are reflected (or not) in our social identity maps. Finally, we bring this all together to create an action plan identifying which new groups, or social connections, we would like to work on.

Session 4
Scaffolding

4 weeks

Are my groups a good reflection of who I am?

What may get in the way of me joining new groups?

Group members create a second social identity map in this last session.

Session 5
Sustaining

This fifth session happens a month after the previous session in order to give members a chance to live out their plans for new groups memberships. In this session, the group works together to trouble-shoot any issues or difficulties that may have come up, and in doing so, the key messages of the program can be reinforced.

Figure 15.2 An overview of the G4H programme

Note: This overview provides a brief description of the purpose and content of each of the five GROUPS 4 HEALTH modules: from psychoeducation, in Session 1, to reviewing attempts to trial plans to strengthen existing groups and join new ones, in Session 5. The programme takes place over a period of 2 months with the first four sessions taking place weekly and the final session a month later.

Source: Haslam et al. (2016a)

The aim of the second module, Scoping, is to encourage participants to think concretely about their own social group resources. This involves using *social identity mapping* (see examples in Figure 15.3) to help people construct a visual representation of their social groups that highlights existing social identities and the inter-relationships between them (Cruwys, Steffens, Haslam, Haslam, Jetten, & Dingle, 2016). Visualising one's social identities in this way provides a means for participants to gain insight into their current social functioning and a foundation on which to build as the programme progresses.

Module three, Sourcing, focuses on SIMIC's social identity continuity pathway and aims to strengthen existing valued social identities in order to sustain and make the best use of these in the longer term. With this in mind, the module helps people explore strategies to reconnect with old networks that may have been lost in the course of any upheaval or life change and to overcome barriers that may be encountered in reconnecting or managing any incompatibility between groups that might arise in the process.

The fourth module, Scaffolding, is targeted at SIMIC's social identity gain pathway. Indeed, the GROUPS 4 HEALTH programme itself contributes to this process as G4H is a new group for participants that provides them with a model of how to establish and embed new social group connections. In particular, the group provides a vehicle through which participants can trial their skills in a social group context with others who harbour similar concerns about their social connectedness. A key and tangible goal for participants here is to identify new groups that they can join and to develop a social plan of action to do so. They are then encouraged to trial these plans before returning for the final module.

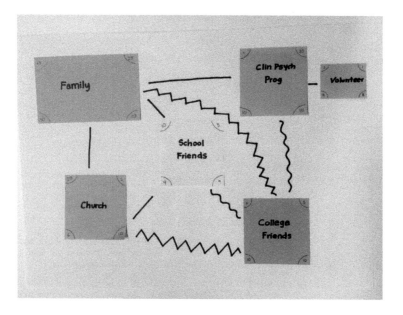

Figure 15.3 Social identity maps

Note: In these maps, the groups that participants see themselves as members of are named on the squares, and similar groups are placed closer together. The size of each square indicates the group's importance, and the lines between the squares indicate group compatibility. The map on this page was created using Post-it notes on a sheet of A3 paper (see Cruwys et al., 2016, and the Appendix for details). The map on the opposite page was made using an online mapping tool.

Source: Haslam et al. (2016a)

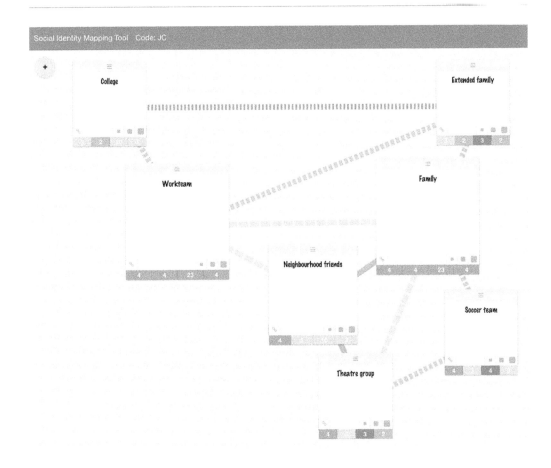

Figure 15.3 Continued

The final module, Sustaining, is held at least 1 month later, and its primary aim is to tackle any difficulties that have arisen for participants in the course of trialling their social plans. The module also engages participants in the process of reviewing their social group worlds by re-constructing their social identity maps to see how they have developed over the course of the programme. The module also invites participants to reflect on the knowledge and skills they have developed in the preceding four modules, with a view to encouraging their long-term maintenance.

Proof-of-concept evaluation

Having outlined the structure and content of G4H, an obvious next question is whether the programme achieves what it sets out to do. Does G4H improve health outcomes? Furthermore, if it has positive impact, how is this achieved? These questions were the focus on an initial proof-of-concept investigation that we conducted as a critical first stage of programme evaluation.

Proof of a programme's effectiveness lies in its capacity to achieve three things. *First*, it must be a driver of change. In the case of G4H, this means that it must lead to tangible improvements in health and well-being. *Second*, its mechanism (or mechanisms) of action must be clear and demonstrable in order that the intervention can be targeted to best effect (Walton, 2014). In line with the theory and evidence presented in previous chapters (e.g., as this relates to H2), we hypothesise that a fundamental mechanism of change in G4H is *social identification*. Specifically, we argue that G4H helps participants realise the power of their social identities (through Schooling and Scoping modules) and to develop the skills they need to make the most of their group-based relationships (through Sourcing and Scaffolding modules). Accordingly, if enhanced social identification is the means by which health improvement is achieved, then we should see not only that the programme leads to improvements in health, but also that these are the result of a strengthened sense of social identification with any combination of existing or new social groups. *Third*, the programme itself must be feasible and be seen as acceptable and relevant to both participants and facilitators (Arain, Campbell, Cooper, & Lancaster, 2010; Lancaster, Dodd, & Williamson, 2004).

These three criteria were the focus of an initial study that we conducted to assess the viability and utility of G4H (see Haslam, Cruwys, Haslam, Dingle, & Chang, 2016c). Participants were recruited via university mailing lists, campus advertising, local health centres, and practicing psychologists. The majority (90%) were undergraduate university students who were experiencing social isolation as well as affective disturbance. Although there are a range of issues associated with using student samples in psychological research (e.g., Henrich, Heine, & Norenzayan, 2010), it is also the case that this is a population that is increasingly recognised as being prone to social isolation and mental health problems (Gotlib, 1984; Iyer et al., 2009; Sarokhani et al., 2013), and we therefore deemed this to be an appropriate sample on which to test G4H. In line with this reasoning, all those who were included in the study met two key criteria. First, they reported at least mild clinical symptoms of depression and anxiety (as indexed by the DASS-21; Lovibond & Lovibond, 1995; see Appendix for details). Second, they indicated that they were either "very isolated" or "isolated" on the Hawthorne Friendship Scale (Hawthorne, 2006) or were experiencing at least moderate psychological distress as rated by the Kessler Psychological Distress Scale (the K-10; Coombs, 2005). Eighty-one participants commenced the programme, and 54 completed it, with the latter defined as (1) having filled in both T1 and T2 questionnaires and (2) having taken part in at least three of the five programme modules as well as a make-up session to complete any that had been missed.

Prior to taking part in G4H and at its completion we asked people to respond to a number of measures that indexed mental health (i.e., depression, anxiety, stress, social anxiety), social connectedness (loneliness, social adjustment), and well-being (life satisfaction, self-esteem). Social identification was also assessed using two measures. The first of these was participants' strength of identification with the G4H group, and this was included to examine identification with a new group membership common to all those who took part in the programme. The second was the strength of their identification with multiple groups, and this was intended to capture identification with the range of groups (both new and old) in participants' social networks. To establish the relevance and fidelity of G4H, we also measured programme attendance, retention, satisfaction, acceptability, and adherence.

Analysis of pre- and post-intervention data indicated that G4H led to significant improvement on all health outcomes (see Figure 15.4 and Haslam et al., 2016c, for baseline and end-of-treatment means with effect sizes). More specifically, clinical symptoms of depression declined from the moderate to mild range, and both anxiety and stress fell from the severe to moderate clinical range. In addition, there were significant positive changes in social anxiety, social functioning, self-esteem, and life satisfaction. The size of these effects ranged from small to large (see Haslam et al., 2016c). Clearly, then, the first and most important criterion for effectiveness was met: *G4H produces desired forms of health improvement*. Importantly too, follow-up data that were obtained from available participants 6 months later indicated that most of these improvements were sustained – and in fact generally *enhanced* – well after the programme had ended (see Haslam et al., 2016c).

Turning to the second effectiveness criterion, we then used hierarchical regression to explore the mechanism underlying these improvements. More particularly, we sought to establish whether health gains were associated with gains in participants' social identification, both with their G4H group and with multiple group memberships. Together, these two social identity mechanisms accounted for

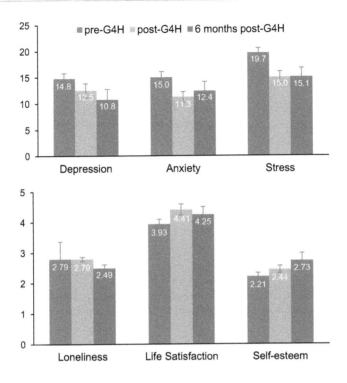

Figure 15.4 Health and well-being outcomes associated with participation in G4H

Note: The top graph shows scores on the three subscales of the DASS-21 (Lovibond & Lovibond, 1995); the bottom graph shows scores on the ULS-8 Loneliness Scale (Hays & DiMatteo, 1987), the Satisfaction with Life Scale (SWLS, Diener, Emmons, Larsen, R.J., & Griffin, 1985), and a single-item self-esteem measure ("I have high self-esteem", Robins et al., 2001; see Appendix for details of measures and interpretation of scores). Pre- and post-G4H data are provided for the 59 people who completed the programme, and the 6-month post-G4H data are from the 26 people available for follow-up.

Source: Haslam et al. (2016c)

---

significant and substantial improvement in most outcomes – notably, depression, anxiety, stress, life satisfaction, and loneliness. Thus, as the data in Table 15.1 show, the more the programme led to an increase in participants' social identification with the various groups that they belonged to, the more their mental health, well-being, and social connectedness improved. In this way, the second criterion for effectiveness was met: *The health improvements produced by G4H were associated with increases in people's sense of social identification with groups.*

The third and final criterion of programme acceptability and relevance was evaluated in three ways. First, we examined retention rates and found that around two thirds of participants who started the programme completed it. The average number of sessions attended was 3.89, with the median and mode both 5 (i.e., attendance at all sessions). Moreover, statistical analyses indicated that retention at T2 was not predicted by demographic variables (e.g., age, gender), initial symptom severity (e.g., depression, anxiety, stress, life satisfaction), or initial social isolation (e.g., number of group memberships, loneliness). Accordingly, it appears that the people who completed T2 measures were a representative subsample of those who had commenced the programme.

Table 15.1 Change in identification with G4H group and with multiple groups following participation in Groups 4 Health programme as a predictor of key outcomes

	Social identity mechanisms		G4H identification		Multiple group membership	
	R^2 change	*p*	Change in identification B	*p*	Change in identification B	*p*
Depression	.17	.003	−4.33	.008*	−2.02	.136
Anxiety	.21	<.001	−3.42	.002*	−1.94	.024*
Stress	.18	.003	−2.86	.031*	−2.32	.036*
Social anxiety	.04	.181	−0.12	.379	−0.16	.174
Life satisfaction	.26	<.001	0.13	.469	0.73	<.001*
Self-esteem	.01	.448	0.09	.422	0.07	.471
Loneliness	.17	<.001	−0.14	.030*	−0.16	.007*

Note: * denotes significant post-G4H change ($p <.05$). This table shows that increased identification with the G4H group and with multiple groups was assoicated with improvement in key outcomes (depression, anxiety, stress, life satisfaction and loneliness)

Source: Haslam et al. (2016c)

Participant satisfaction – assayed by enjoyment of the programme, interest in it, belief that it had allowed useful skills to be learned, and that these would be useful in future – provided a second indicator of programme acceptability. On all these measures the modal response (on 11-point scales with a maximum value of 10) was 7, all means were above 7, and no more than five participants provided a rating below the mid-point of the scale on any index.

To assess the experience of those who delivered the programme, G4H facilitators were also asked to rate the ease of delivery, enjoyment, and perceived value of each module (e.g., "The content of Module 2 was relevant to participants" and "I would recommend G4H to someone experiencing social isolation and mental illness"). The mean acceptability score (on a 7-point scale) was above 5 for all modules. Indeed, across the five modules, only two scores were below the mid-point of the scale. At the end of the programme all facilitators indicated that they "would recommend G4H to a person experiencing social isolation and mental illness", with all scores on this item above 5. In sum, participants and facilitators were generally engaged in and satisfied with the programme.

Finally, after each module, group facilitators were asked to anonymously report their own adherence to the manual content for that module. Here facilitators responded to a list of statements relevant to the main elements and tasks in each module (e.g., "We helped participants visualise areas for growth based on their social identity maps") rating them on 7-point scales from "not covered" to "extensively covered". To encourage honest responding, it was emphasised (1) that facilitators should use these questions as a checklist to ensure the core content had been covered (and thereby increase adherence) and (2) that the goal was to evaluate the programme, not those who had delivered it. Across 45 questions (an average of nine content components per module), none received a mean rating below the scale mid-point. In other words, it appears that the programme had generally been delivered in ways prescribed by the *Groups 4 Health Manual*. All in all then, these various indices suggest that the third criterion for effectiveness was met: *G4H was feasible and it was acceptable and relevant to both participants and facilitators.*

These early data thus give good grounds to be optimistic about G4H. Primarily this is because they suggest that the programme can improve the mental health, social connectedness, and well-being of participants. Moreover, in line with the theorising that informs this volume as a whole, it does so in part by increasing their sense of social identification with other people – that is, their sense of themselves as group members who are embedded in a network of meaningful group memberships. Importantly too, the programme is feasible to deliver and also typically proves enjoyable both for those who take part in it and for those who facilitate it.

But as with any novel intervention, there is still some way to go. Although we have been able to show that the programme produces benefits relative to a matched control group taking part in a different concurrent study (see Haslam et al., 2016c), more rigorous evaluation using randomised controlled methodology is needed. Future research also needs to address questions of programme generalisability and applicability to wider populations. Nevertheless, these initial proof-of-concept data make a good case for investing in such trials as a means of establishing whether G4H can fill the all-important gap in the intervention space that has been identified within a range of literatures (e.g., epidemiological, sociological, social psychological). A range of such trials are currently underway.

Conclusion

In showing that social identity theorising not only allows us to better understand the social determinants of health but also to take steps to harness the positive potential of meaningful social identities, GROUPS 4 HEALTH is proof of Kurt Lewin's assertion that "there is nothing so practical as a good theory" (Lewin, 1952, p. 169; see also Haslam, 2014). Indeed, as a way of wrapping up this chapter – and the book as a whole – it is useful to abstract some concrete recommendations for improving health that emerge from the previous 14 chapters, along the lines of the "top ten tips" generated by medical and social determinants research that we discussed in Chapter 3 (see Table 3.1). Here, then, these tips – which are presented in Table 15.2 – emphasise what social identity research suggests we might try to do in practice to harness the health-enhancing power of social groups.

Table 15.2 The top ten social identity tips for better health

1.	If you feel socially isolated, try to join a group.
2.	If you can, join more groups.
3.	Try to hold on to positive group memberships, especially if you are going through a challenging time.
4.	If you lose membership in an important group, seek out a new one.
5.	Invest in groups that are important to you and in groups by which you are valued.
6.	Be wary of groups that make unhealthy choices.
7.	Get support from your groups, but also give support to others in your groups.
8.	Recognise that it can sometimes be healthy to try to leave disadvantaged and stigmatised groups, whereas at other times it can also be healthy to stay.
9.	Challenge the stigma and disadvantage that produce health inequality.
10.	If you experience health problems, seek professional help – ideally from a source with which you identify.

Note: These provide an alternative to the traditional medical and alternative social determinants tips for better health first introduced in Chapter 3 (see Table 3.1). This list identifies some of the key practical points that emerge from previous chapters that are targeted in the GROUPS 4 HEALTH programme.

As with the two lists presented in Chapter 3, these tips are not always easy to put into practice. This, though, is where GROUPS 4 HEALTH comes in – drawing on what is now a rich body of social cure theorising to provide the structure and support that can help people develop meaningful group memberships and embed them into their lives.

But GROUPS 4 HEALTH is more than just a theory-informed intervention. It is also non-stigmatising and relatively cheap and easy to deliver. This is of utmost importance in a world where many existing psychological treatments serve to mark out those who receive them as in some way tainted (Conner et al., 2010; Wahl, 1999) and where one of the most basic determinants of social disconnection and poor mental health is poverty (World Health Organization, 2001; see also Chapters 3 and 8). Indeed, in this respect, GROUPS 4 HEALTH is a corrective to some of the main criticisms targeted at other health and psychological interventions: namely, that they can be unnecessarily arcane, overly psychologised, and poorly targeted. This is seen, for example, when they focus on the troubles of the relatively well educated and affluent 'worried well' rather than on those of the hard-to-treat groups that most need professional assistance (Hall & Iqbal, 2010).

However, it is unlikely that the real value of GROUPS 4 HEALTH will be established either by its efficacy (for which we claim no uniqueness) or by its mechanism (for which interest may be largely academic) – important as these things undoubtedly are. Instead, its most appealing feature is that it gives a broad range of practitioners a relatively accessible and easy-to-use platform from which to deliver social cures in the hard-to-reach places where they are most urgently needed. Tailored neither to the privileged practitioner nor to the privileged client, our ambition for G4H is thus for it to be a *democratising intervention* in which the curative power of social groups and social identities is unlocked in accessible and effective ways. However, as with the various other ambitions that we have flagged in previous chapters, this is a goal that will only be realised through collective effort. Above all else, then, this chapter – and indeed this book as a whole – should be understood as an invitation for you to contribute to that effort so that you not only read about social cures but also help to unlock them yourself.

Points for practice

Unlike the previous chapters, our discussion in this chapter has been focused almost exclusively on practical issues. The following points are probably the most important that this examination has revealed:

1. *Group interventions tend to increase participants' sense of social identification more than individual interventions.* This point makes good theoretical sense, but it is worth noting that there are not many studies in which it has been directly tested.
2. *Because and to the extent that they build participants' sense of social identification, group interventions unlock associated psychological resources.* This is a point that emerges from the range of studies – mainly conducted with older adults (see Chapter 7) – that informed the development of GROUPS 4 HEALTH.
3. *GROUPS 4 HEALTH is a group-based intervention that has been shown to reduce psychological distress associated with social disconnection, and it does this by increasing participants' sense of social identification.* The evidence that supports this point is provided by Haslam and colleagues' (2016) first proof-of-concept trial, but clearly this is a point that needs to be corroborated through more extensive and more rigorous testing. We hope that this chapter encourages readers to contribute to these efforts.

Resources

Further reading

The following resources will be useful to anyone who is looking to find out more about GROUPS 4 HEALTH – particularly if they are planning to run or take part in the programme themselves.

① Haslam, C., Cruwys, T., Haslam, S. A., Bentley, S., Dingle, G., & Jetten, J. (2016a). *GROUPS 4 HEALTH manual* (version 3.0). Social Identity and Groups Network (SIGN): University of Queensland, Australia.

This manual provides full details on how to run the GROUPS 4 HEALTH programme.

② Haslam, C., Cruwys, T., Haslam, S. A., Bentley, S., Dingle, G., & Jetten, J. (2016b). *GROUPS 4 HEALTH workbook.* (version 3.0). Social Identity and Groups Network (SIGN): University of Queensland, Australia.

This workbook is intended to be used alongside the *Manual* and provides materials (e.g., instructions, exercises, and notes) for participants in the GROUPS 4 HEALTH programme.

③ Haslam, C., Cruwys, T., Haslam, S. A., Dingle, G., & Chang, M. X.-L. (2016c). GROUPS 4 HEALTH: Evidence that a social-identity intervention that builds and strengthens social group membership improves mental health. *Journal of Affective Disorders, 194*, 188–195.

This paper provides full details of the first proof-of-concept study of the GROUPS 4 HEALTH programme.

Websites

① www.groups4health.com. This site contains information about GROUPS 4 HEALTH for both participants and researchers. In also includes details of on-going trials.

② #Groups4Health. This Twitter hashtag will direct you to a range of Tweets that flag issues related to GROUPS 4 HEALTH – including news stories, photographs, and events.

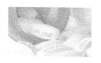

Appendix

Measures of identity, health, and well-being

This appendix presents details of a range of different measures that have been developed to assess identity, health, and well-being. It updates and extends a similar appendix to *The Social Cure* (Jetten, Haslam, & Haslam, 2012, pp. 345–367). There are two reasons why we collated these measures in that volume and why we have done so again here. First, we wanted to provide readers with a sense of how the key constructs that we have discussed in the foregoing chapters are typically assessed. Second, we were keen to provide a practical resource that readers might find useful in their own work.

As Figure A.1 indicates, the measures are organised into three sections. The first of these includes measures of identity and identification. The second section presents a range of process measures related to issues of health and well-being (e.g., assessing social isolation and social support – processes that *mediate* the relationship between social identity and health). And finally the third section includes instruments designed to assess health and well-being directly.

As in other domains, no single measure is appropriate for all settings, and it will often be necessary to adapt a measure to suit the particular health context or to address the particular issues that are being explored in a given piece of research. In most cases this process of adapting a scale will be straightforward and simply involve changing the referent in each item. However, in some cases it will be more complex, and its implications (e.g., for validity) will need to be thought through carefully. Note, too, that the measures we describe (particularly in the final two sections) are not exhaustive but rather indicative of the type of construct that it is possible to assess.

In selecting scales to include, we have tended to choose shorter general scales which are easy to administer and access (i.e., for which there is no fee for use). However, exactly which measure a practitioner or researcher chooses to administer will depend on factors such as the setting (e.g., laboratory or field), the time available for measures to be completed, the response format (e.g., multi-phase or one-shot), and the number and capacity of respondents. In particular, such things will determine whether they use longer or shorter scales and ones that are more general or ones that are more specific to a particular condition. Critically too, these choices will depend on the purposes for which data from a given measure are intended to be used (e.g., for clinical assessment vs. fine-grained analysis of psychological process).

Social identity measures

Social identification

This scale was developed by Tom Postmes and colleagues based on earlier work by Bertjan Doosje, Naomi Ellemers and Russell Spears (1995) that assessed Dutch students' identification with the category 'psychology student' (Postmes, Haslam, & Jans, 2013). The items are widely used by social and organisational psychologists (e.g., see Haslam, 2004), and the form of the scale makes it suitable as a measure of social identification with a wide range of groups. The items can easily be adapted for use in health-related settings by substituting the name of a relevant group or organisation.

Different dimensions of identification can also be assessed using other more elaborate measures (e.g., Leach, van Zomeren, Zebel, Vliek, & Spears, 2008). However, Postmes and colleagues (2013) also note that the first item of the scale ("I identify with [relevant group]") can be used as a single-item measure of social identification that is both reliable and valid. It is also highly correlated with the four-item scale ($r = .84$).

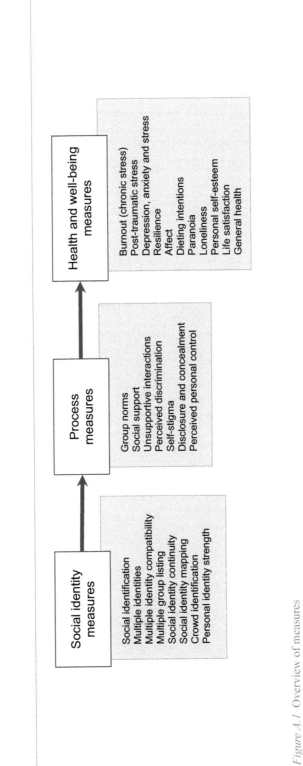

Figure A.1 Overview of measures

Social identification: Suggested items and scale

1. I identify with [members of Group X].*
2. I see myself as a [member of Group X].
3. I am pleased to be a [member of Group X].
4. I feel strong ties with [members of Group X].

Rating scale for each item: *Do not agree at all* 1 2 3 4 5 6 7 *Agree completely*

Notes: * Item used for one-item version of the scale (Postmes et al., 2013).

A 7-point Likert scale is presented here and for other scales, but researchers can adapt these as they see fit.

Social identification scale: Study comparison

Study (year published)	Sample and scale details	N	Mean (SD)	Internal reliability
Doosje, Ellemers, & Spears (1995)	First-year psychology undergraduates (Netherlands) Measuring identification with other psychology students. 4 items (1–7 Likert scale).	131	Median = 4.25	$\alpha = .83$
Gleibs, Haslam, Haslam, & Jones (2011a)	Older people living in care homes (UK). Measuring identification with care home. 4 items (1–5 Likert scale).	66	3.91 (0.96)	$\alpha = .71$
Dingle, Stark, Cruwys, & Best (2015)	Adults entering treatment in a therapeutic community. Measuring identification with that therapeutic community. 4 items (1–7 Likert scale).	132	5.16 (1.11) on entry 6.03 (1.11) on exit	$\alpha = .75$ entry $\alpha = .91$ exit

Multiple identities

This measure is used to assess the extent to which people perceive themselves as belonging to multiple social groups and is a central element of what are referred to as the Exeter Identity Transition Scales (EXITS; e.g., Haslam, Holme et al., 2008; Jetten et al., 2015). The four-item and two-item forms have been used with a range of groups (e.g., stroke survivors, Haslam, Holme et al., 2008; students entering university, Iyer, Jetten, Tsivrikos, Postmes, & Haslam, 2009; older adults residing in care, Jetten et al., 2010). It can be used to index multiple forms of group belonging at the point where people are anticipating some life change (i.e., as a Time 1 measure; Iyer et al., 2009) or retrospectively after life change has occurred (e.g., Haslam, Holme et al., 2008; where the items had the form "Before my stroke I belonged to lots of different groups"). Both scales have good internal reliability.

Multiple identities: Suggested items and scale

1. I belong to lots of different groups.*†
2. I join in the activities of lots of different groups. †
3. I am friendly with people in lots of different groups.*†
4. I have strong ties with lots of different groups.

Rating scale for each item: *Do not agree at all* 1 2 3 4 5 6 7 *Agree completely*

Note: * Items used for two-item version of the scale (Jetten et al., 2010).

　　　† Items used as basis for three-item version of the scale (Jetten et al., 2015).

Multiple identities scale: Study comparison

Study (year published)	Sample and scale details	N	Mean (SD)	Internal reliability
Haslam, Holme, Haslam, Iyer, Jetten, & Williams (2008)	Recovering stroke patients (UK). Four items (1–7 Likert scale).	53	2.94 (2.19) pre-stroke	α = .93
Iyer, Jetten, Tsivrikos, Postmes, & Haslam – Study 2 (2009)	First-year undergraduate students (UK). 4 items (1–5 Likert scale).	934	5.11 (1.69)	α = .78
Jetten, Haslam, Pugliese, Tonks, & Haslam (2010b)	Older people living in the community or residential care where they were receiving either standard or specialist dementia care (UK). 2 items (1–5 Likert scale).	17 community 15 standard care home 16 specialist dementia care	2.79 (1.37) community 1.87 (1.08) standard care home 2.72 (0.86) specialist dementia care home	r = .44
Jetten, Branscombe, Haslam et al. – Study 2 (2015)	Boys attending a private school (Australia) 3 items (1–7 Likert scale).	827	5.07 (1.42)	α = .88

Multiple identity compatibility

This measure has recently been developed to investigate the issue of identity compatibility, with a view to understanding the impact not just of group membership but also the quality of relationships between groups (for a similar measure, see also Brook, Garcia, & Fleming, 2008). This can assess compatibility between groups in the present or between those in the present and those in the past (as in Iyer et al., 2009).

Multiple identity compatibility: Suggested items and scale

1. There is harmony between being a member of my various groups.
2. On the whole, it is easy to be a member of my various groups.
3. The norms and ideals of my various groups are congruent with each other.
4. On the whole, being a member of a particular group is compatible with being a member of other groups.

Rating scale for each item: *Do not agree at all* 1 2 3 4 5 6 7 *Agree completely*

Multiple identity compatibility: Study comparison

Study (year published)	Sample and scale details	N	Mean (SD)	Internal reliability
Cruwys, Steffens, Haslam, Haslam, Jetten, & Dingle (2016)*	Community sample (Australia) 4 items (1–7 Likert scale).	186	5.18 (1.09)	α = .79

Note: * These data were collected as part of pilot testing but not reported in the published paper.

Multiple group listing

Haslam and her colleagues developed a multiple-identity scale to capture changes in group membership in the course of a life transition (Haslam, Holme et al., 2008). It first requires participants to write down the names of groups that are (or were) important to them, up to a maximum number (e.g., six). They are then asked to reflect on these groups and to indicate (1) how important this group is (or was) to them and (2) the compatibility of this group to the other groups to which they belong. This measure provides a rich source of data that can be used to examine the influence of (1) the number of group memberships, (2) the type of group memberships that respondents list, and (3) the types of group memberships that are compatible with other identities. It can also be adapted to measure other aspects of group life (e.g., the amount of support that various groups provide). The measure is intended to assess the groups that respondents belonged to *before* a life-changing event (as in the following example) and then again to assess the groups that respondents belong to currently, *after* the life-changing event. However, the measure can be used to capture multiple group membership at a single time point.

Group listings: Suggested wording and scale

This questionnaire refers to the types of groups that you [used to belong to] [and] [now belong to]. These groups could take any form – for example, they could be leisure or social groups (e.g., book group or gardening club); community groups (e.g., church group); sporting groups (e.g., rugby club); work groups (e.g., sales team); professional groups (e.g., trade union); or any others you can think of.

In the first column, list up to six groups that you belong[ed] to [before/after] [the life-changing event]. Then indicate how much you agree with the items in the next two columns.

Group memberships before [life-changing event].	How important was this group to you before [life-changing event].	How well did this group fit with your other groups before [life-changing event]?
1.	not very 1 2 3 4 5 6 7 very	not a lot 1 2 3 4 5 6 7 a great deal
2.	not at all 1 2 3 4 5 6 7 very	not a lot 1 2 3 4 5 6 7 a great deal
3.	not at all 1 2 3 4 5 6 7 very	not a lot 1 2 3 4 5 6 7 a great deal
4.	not at all 1 2 3 4 5 6 7 very	not a lot 1 2 3 4 5 6 7 a great deal
5.	not at all 1 2 3 4 5 6 7 very	not a lot 1 2 3 4 5 6 7 a great deal
6.	not at all 1 2 3 4 5 6 7 very	not a lot 1 2 3 4 5 6 7 a great deal

Multiple group listings: Study comparison

Study (year published)	Sample and scale details	N	Mean (SD)	Internal reliability
Jetten, Branscombe, Haslam et al. – Study 2 (2015)	Boys attending a private school (Australia). List up to 10 groups. *	827	2.24 (1.48) Number of groups 14.31 (7.59) Number of important groups [†]	not applicable
Cruwys, Steffens, Haslam, Haslam, Jetten, & Dingle (2016)	Members of university community (Australia). List up to 6 groups.	201	4.55 (1.79) Number of groups	not applicable

Note: * Bear in mind that the maximum number may create a frame of reference that has other implications. In particular, Young, Brown, and Hutchins (2017) note that the higher this number is, the more likely this is to make respondents feel that their social lives are deficient.

[†] Number of important groups calculated as the number of groups multiplied by their mean rated importance.

Social identity continuity

This measure was first used in research by Haslam and her colleagues to assess the degree to which stroke survivors were able to maintain their pre-stroke social group memberships (Haslam, Holme et al., 2008). The scale is another component of the Exeter Identity Transition Scales (EXITS) and typically has very good internal reliability.

Social identity continuity: Suggested items and scale

1. After [life transition] I still belong to the same groups I was a member of before [life transition].
2. After [life transition] I still join in the same group activities as before [life transition].
3. After [life transition] I am friendly with people in the same groups as I was before [life transition].
4. After [life transition] I continue to have strong ties with the same groups as before [life transition].

Rating scale for each item: *Do not agree at all* 1 2 3 4 5 6 7 *Agree completely*

Social identity continuity scale: Study comparison

Study (year published)	Sample and scale details	N	Mean (SD)	Internal reliability
Haslam, Holme, Haslam, Iyer, Jetten, & Williams (2008)	Recovering stroke patients (UK). Measuring how many pre-stroke groups people are still engaged with. 4 items (1–7 Likert scale).	53	3.94 (2.53)	α = .94
Seymour-Smith, Cruwys, Haslam, & Brodribb (2016)	Online community sample of mothers with children aged less than 12 months (US). Measuring continuity of mother's group identifications pre- and post-birth. 4 items (1–7 Likert scale).	387	4.11 (1.73)	α = .93

Social identity mapping

The nature of a person's social identity can also be established using *social identity mapping* (Cruwys et al., 2016; see also Best et al., 2014; Haslam, Best, Dingle, Mackenzie, & Beckwith, 2017). This engages participants in the process of simultaneously representing a number of key social identity constructs in a way that allows for their systematic comparison and assessment. In its basic form, mapping involves participants constructing a visual map that (1) identifies the groups to which they subjectively belong as well as their psychological importance, (2) describes theoretically relevant aspects of these group memberships (e.g., the degree to which a group membership is positive), and (3) represents the similarity and compatibility of these groups to each other. By this means, the procedure serves to create a visual representation of a person's social world that captures key features of relevant social identities and their interrelationship.

Importantly, the visual nature of the process means that, unlike standard rating scale measures, the map not only gives researchers, but also participants themselves, insight into important social identity constructs. This makes it particularly useful in therapeutic and intervention contexts where insight of this form is beneficial – as it is in addiction management (see Chapter 9, Figure 9.5; Best et al., 2014; Haslam et al., 2017) and in GROUPS 4 HEALTH (Haslam et al., 2016c; see Chapter 15). The following instructions are for the paper-and-pencil version of the mapping procedure, but an online version is also available (contact the authors for details).

This version is good to administer in face-to-face therapeutic contexts (e.g., see Jetten, Haslam, Iyer, & Haslam, 2010a), whereas an advantage of the online version is that the complex data that can be garnered from the process is collected automatically behind the scenes. Note, too, that the procedure can be customised so that the information collected in Stage 2 is adapted to the particular issues that are being addressed by the researcher or practitioner.

Stage 1: Identifying your groups

Please think about all the groups that you belong to. These groups can take any form, for example, they could be broad opinion-based or demographic groups (e.g., feminist; Australian); leisure or social groups (e.g., book group or gardening group); community groups (e.g., church group); sporting groups (e.g., rugby or tennis club); work groups (e.g., sales team); professional groups (e.g., trade union); or any others you can think of.

To start the process of social identity mapping, write down the names of each of these groups on separate Post-it notes. Remember the size of the Post-it note matters, so write down the name of each very important group on a large Post-it note, write down the names of each moderately important group on separate medium-sized Post-it notes, and write the name of each less important group on separate small Post-it notes.

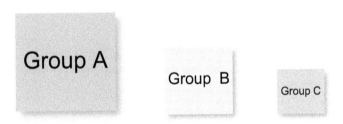

Stage 2: Thinking about your groups

1. HOW TYPICAL (OR REPRESENTATIVE) ARE YOU OF YOUR SOCIAL GROUPS?

For each group indicate how typical you are of the group and the people in it. Put this rating in the top-left corner of each Post-it note.

Use a scale from 1 to 10 where 1 indicates that you are not at all typical of the group and 10 indicates that you are very typical.

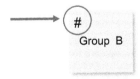

2. HOW MANY DAYS IN A MONTH DO YOU ENGAGE WITH EACH GROUP?

If it's every day, the number would be 30. If it's every week, then the number would be 4. So the range is 0–30. Write this number in the top-right corner for each group on your Post-it notes.

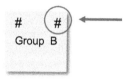

3. HOW MUCH SUPPORT DO YOU GET FROM EACH GROUP?

Now rate how much support you get from each group. Rate this on a scale from 1 (no support at all) to 10 (a very high level of support). For example, you could belong to a work-related group or a family-related group that provides you with a lot of practical support or emotional support, so the rating you might give that group would be high, for instance, an 8 or a 9. For every group, write your rating in the bottom-right corner of each Post-it note.

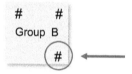

4. HOW POSITIVE DO YOU FEEL ABOUT BEING A MEMBER OF EACH GROUP?

Rate how positive you feel about being part of each group. Write your rating in the bottom-left corner of each Post-it note where 1 indicates that you are not positive at all about the group and 10 indicates that you are very positive.

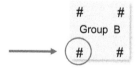

Use a scale from 1 to 10:

Stage 3: Mapping your groups in relation to each other

1. HOW DIFFERENT ARE YOUR GROUPS FROM EACH OTHER?

We know that some groups are very similar to each other because they like or do similar things, but others are very different from each other. On the sheet of A3 paper provided we would like you to show how similar and different your groups are to each other. Do this by placing your Post-it notes close together if they are similar and farther apart if they are different.

So if two groups are very similar to each other, place these close to each other, like this:

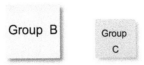

But if two groups are very different from each other (e.g., they do different things, it feels different being a part of each, they have different members), place them far from each other like this:

2. HOW EASY OR DIFFICULT IS IT TO BE A MEMBER OF YOUR GROUPS AT THE SAME TIME?

Because we typically belong to a number of groups, it can be hard at times trying to juggle them. In your social identity map, we would like you to use different lines to show how easy or hard it is to be part of different groups at the same time.

For example, if you belong to a chess club, it might be very easy to also be a member of your family but not that easy to also be a member of your rugby club.

Show the ease or difficulty of being part of multiple groups at the same time by using different types of lines.

If two groups are very easy to belong to, then join them with a straight line.

If two groups are moderately easy to belong to, join them with a wavy line

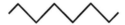

If two groups are hard to belong to, join them with a jagged line.

This is an example of what the map might look like when these lines are added:

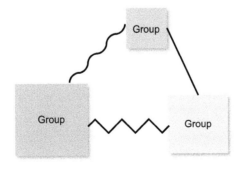

Social identity mapping: Study comparison

Study (year published)	Sample and scale details	N	Mean (SD)	Internal reliability
Cruwys, Steffens, Haslam, Haslam, Jetten, & Dingle – Study 1 (2016)	University staff and students (Australia).	201	6.52 (3.25) Number of groups 2.74 (1.53) Number of important groups* 3.41 (3.05) Number of positive groups[†] 0.51 (0.23) Group compatibility[#]	not applicable
Cruwys, Steffens et al. – Study 3 (2016)	Participants in first GROUPS 4 HEALTH trial who completed maps at T1 and T2 (Australia).	45	6.62 (1.59) T1 Number of groups 6.55 (1.60) T2 Number of groups 1.99 (0.87) T1 Number of important groups 2.44 (0.85) T2 Number of important groups 3.64 (1.70) T1 Number of positive groups 4.31 (2.02) T2 Number of positive groups 0.45 (0.19) T1 Group compatibility 0.54 (0.23) T2 Group compatibility	not applicable
Dingle, Williams, Sharman, & Jetten (2016)	Participants in School of Hard Knocks who completed maps at both T1 and T2 (Australia).	23	6.35 (2.64) T1 Number of groups 6.35 (2.37) T2 Number of groups 3.57 (2.20) T1 Number of important groups 3.30 (1.55) T2 Number of important groups 4.35 (2.53) T1 Number of positive groups 4.22 (2.10) T2 Number of positive groups	not applicable

Note: * Number of important groups is the number of large Post-it notes used in the map.

[†] Number of positive groups is the number with a positivity score of 8 or more (where maximum score is 10).

[#] Group compatibility is the proportion of groups where it was "very easy" to be a member of both groups.

Crowd identification

Crowds are not often seen as a typical social group, but seminal studies by Steve Reicher (1987) demonstrated that the same social identity and self-categorization principles that shape group behaviour also operate in large and novel crowd events (e.g., such as the Hajj; see Chapter 2). John Drury (2012) measured crowd identification retrospectively using a 2-item scale (*r* = .81) that he had previously developed with colleagues (Drury, Cocking, Reicher, Burton et al., 2009, Study 2). Working with Hani Alnabulsi, Drury then extended this to create a five-item scale (Alnabulsi & Drury, 2014). These items refer to the particular crowd context that researchers are investigating and can be adapted to make them amenable to any assessment context.

Crowd identification: Suggested items and scale

1. I felt that I was part [of this crowd].
2. I felt at one with the people around me [in the crowd].
3. I felt a sense of togetherness with others [in the crowd]. *
4. I felt unity with others [in the crowd].*
5. I felt strong ties with other people [in the crowd].

Rating scale for each item: *Disagree strongly* 1 2 3 4 5 6 7 *Agree strongly*

Note: * Items used for two-item version of the scale (Drury, Cocking, Reicher, Burton et al., 2009).

Crowd identification: Study comparison

Study (year published)	Sample and scale details	N	Mean (SD)	Internal reliability
Drury, Cocking, Reicher, Burton et al. (2009)	Participants in a simulated emergency (UK). 2 items (1–11 Likert scale).	72	6.14 (2.59)	*r* = .81

Crowd identification: Study comparison

Study (year published)	Sample and scale details	N	Mean (SD)	Internal reliability
Alnabulsi & Drury (2014)	Pilgrims attending the Hajj at Mecca (Saudi Arabia). 5 items (1–7 Likert scale).	1184	5.99 (0.91)	α = .88
Kearns, Muldoon, Msefti, & Surgenor (2017)	People who attended a suicide prevention fundraising event (responding afterwards) (Ireland). 5 items (1–7 Likert scale).	121	Total score 29.91 (7.0)	α = .97

Personal identity strength

This five-item scale was developed primarily for use with older adults to assess the extent to which people have a clear understanding of who they are (see Haslam, Jetten, Haslam, & Knight, 2012). The items were adapted from a self-clarity scale developed by Jennifer Campbell and colleagues and a personal identity strength scale devised by Gamze Baray and colleagues (Baray, Postmes, & Jetten, 2009; Campbell et al., 1996).

Personal identity strength: Suggested items and scale

Personal identity strength scale: Study comparison

1. I know what I like and what I don't like.
2. I know what my morals are.
3. I have strong beliefs.
4. I know what I want from life.
5. I am aware of the roles and responsibilities I have in my life.

Rating scale for each item: *Do not agree at all* 1 2 3 4 5 6 7 *Agree completely*

Personal identity strength: Study comparison

Study (year published)	Sample and scale details	N	Mean (SD)	Internal reliability
Jetten, Haslam, Pugliese, Tonks, & Haslam (2010b)	Older people living either in the community or in a standard care home, or in a specialist dementia care home (UK). 5 items (1–5 Likert scale).	17 community 15 standard care home 16 specialist dementia care	4.69 (0.40) community 4.13 (0.67) standard care home 4.20 (0.58) specialist dementia care home	$\alpha = .65$

Process measures

Group norms

There are a range of health contexts in which it can be useful to measure people's perceptions of group norms in order to assess both the nature of these perceived norms and their impact on behaviour. Researchers customarily differentiate between two types of norms: injunctive norms relate to perceptions of how members of a group ought to think and behave, and descriptive norms relate to perceptions of how they actually think and behave. The two measures here were developed by Cruwys and colleagues

to assess the role that changing norms play in shaping young women's eating behaviour after their participation in a group-based intervention (Cruwys, Haslam, Fox, & McMahon, 2015; see Chapter 9). As a result, in this case, the behaviours that were included in the scales all related to eating (e.g., plan to lose weight, go on a diet). However, both measures can easily be customised to assess a range of norms that are relevant to other groups and health contexts (where they might include more or fewer items).

Group norms: Suggested items and scales

Injunctive norms
1. [Members of this group] think that [behaviour A] is a good idea.
2. If I were to [behaviour B], [members of this group] would approve.
3. [Members of this group] think I should [behaviour C].
4. [Members of this group] think that [behaviour D] is a good thing.

Descriptive norms
1. How often do [members of this group] [behaviour A]?
2. How often do [members of this group] [behaviour B]?
3. How often do [members of this group] [behaviour C]?
4. How often do [members of this group] [behaviour D]?
5. How often do [members of this group] [behaviour E]?
6. How often do [members of this group] [behaviour F]?

Rating scale for injunctive norms: *Strongly disagree* 1 2 3 4 5 6 7 *Strongly Agree*

Rating scale for descriptive norms: *Never* 1 2 3 4 5 6 7 *Frequently*

Group norms scale: Study comparison

Study (year published)	*Sample and scale details*	*N*	*Mean (SD)*	*Internal reliability*
Cruwys, Haslam, Fox, & McMahon (2015)	Female students with concerns about their body, shape or weight (Australia). 4 items (1–7 Likert scale) assessed injunctive norms. 6 items (1–7 Likert scale) assessed descriptive norms.	112	Injunctive norms 4.75 (0.85) T1 2.50 (1.12) T5 (after a group intervention to prevent eating disorders) Descriptive norms 5.42 (1.10) T1 3.48 (1.63) T5 (after a group intervention to prevent eating disorders)	Injunctive norms α = .56 T1 α = .83 T5 Descriptive norms α = .92 T1 α = .96 T5

Social support

A range of different measures can be used to assess perceptions of social support. The following is a short version of a ten-item measure originally developed by Haslam, O'Brien, Jetten, Vormedal, and Penna (2005) to assess stress among patients recovering from heart surgery. The long version has good reliability, and this is not compromised if it is shortened (in versions with between three and seven items, internal reliability is generally high – with α's between .79 and .86). The measure incorporates items designed to assess the four distinct aspects of social support identified by James House: (1) emotional support (relating to an individual's sense of acceptance and self-worth), (2) companionship (affiliation and help from others), (3) instrumental support (concrete aid, material resources, financial assistance), and (4) informational support (advice to help understand and cope with one's circumstances; House, 1981). The scale can also be reworded to assess support from particular groups (e.g., "health professionals", "family") as well as a person's perceived *provision* of social support to other people (who can also be specified more clearly; e.g., "your colleagues", "other members of your family").

Received social support: Suggested items and scale

1. Do you get the emotional support you need from other people? *
2. Do you get the help you need from other people? *
3. Do you get the resources you need from other people? *
4. Do you get the advice you need from other people?

Rating scale for each item: *Not at all* 1 2 3 4 5 6 7 *Definitely*

Note: * Items used for three-item version of the scale (Haslam et al., 2005).

Provided social support: Suggested items and scale

1. Do you give other people the emotional support they need?
2. Do you give other people the help they need?
3. Do you give other people the resources they need?
4. Do you give other people the advice they need?

Rating scale for each item: *Not at all* 1 2 3 4 5 6 7 *Definitely*

Social support scales: Study comparison

Study (year published)	Sample and scale details	N	Mean (SD)	Internal reliability
Haslam, O'Brien, Jetten, Vormedal, & Penna – Study 2 (2005)	Bomb disposal officers and university bar staff (UK). Measuring received support. 3 items (1–7 Likert scale).	40	4.98	α = .81

Social support scales: Study comparison

Study (year published)	Sample and scale details	N	Mean (SD)	Internal reliability
Steffens, Jetten, Haslam, Cruwys, & Haslam (2016)	Community sample of recent retirees (Australia). Measuring both received and provided support. 4 items (1–7 Likert scale).	171	5.39 (1.38) received support 5.80 (1.06) provided support	$\alpha = .92$ received support $\alpha = .86$ provided support

Unsupportive interactions

Unsupportive interactions have been linked to reduced psychological well-being over and above the perceived unavailability of social support or the effects of stressor experiences (Ingram, Betz, Mindes, Schmitt, & Smith, 2001; Ingram, Jones, Fass, Neidig, & Song, 1999). The Unsupportive Social Interactions Inventory (USII; Ingram et al., 1999, 2001) can be used to index this construct and comprises 24 items tapping into four types of unsupportive responses: distancing, minimising, bumbling, and blaming (Ingram et al., 1999). The scale can be modified to refer to the extent to which people have unsupportive interactions with others in general, with specific sources, or with members of relevant ingroups and outgroups (e.g., "my family", "my work colleagues"; as it is by Matheson & Anisman, 2012). The measure, of which the following items are indicative, has been successfully used across diverse social and ethnic populations in North America (Cole, Matheson, & Anisman, 2007; Ingram et al., 1999; Jorden, Matheson, & Anisman, 2009).

Unsupportive interactions: Indicative items and scale

Unsupportive interactions scale: Study comparison

1. When I was talking about the issue, [members of group X] did not give me enough of their time or made me feel like I should hurry.
2. [Members of group X] didn't seem to know what to say or seemed afraid of saying/doing the "wrong" thing.
3. [Members of group X] said "I told you so" or made some similar comment to me about my situation.
4. [Members of group X] felt that I should stop worrying about the situation and just forget about it.
5. [Members of group X] refused to provide the type of help/support I was asking for.

Rating scale for each item: *Not at all* 1 2 3 4 *About every day*

Unsupportive interactions: Study comparison

Study (year published)	Sample and scale details	N	Mean (SD)	Internal reliability
Ingram, Betz, Mindes, Schmitt, & Smith (2001)	Undergraduate psychology students reporting on their most stressful life events (US). 24-item USII (0–4 Likert scale).	222	1.14 (0.70)	$\alpha = .90$

Perceived discrimination

A range of more or less sophisticated measures have been used to assess perceived discrimination as experienced by members of a range of different groups (e.g., see Branscombe, Schmitt, & Harvey, 1999; Jetten, Branscombe, Schmitt, & Spears, 2001; Schmitt, Branscombe, Kobrynowicz, & Owen, 2002). The following scale is one of the shorter measures and was developed by Teri Gartska and colleagues to assess young and older adults' perceptions of age-based discrimination (Garstka, Schmitt, Branscombe, & Hummert, 2004). The scale, however, can easily be adapted to assess perceived discrimination against other groups.

Perceived discrimination: Indicative items and scale

1. I feel like I am personally a victim of society because of my [group membership].
2. I consider myself a person who has been deprived of the opportunities that are available to others because of my [group membership].
3. [Members of my group] have been victimised by society.
4. Historically, [members of my group] have been discriminated against more than members of other groups.

Rating scale for each item: *Strongly disagree* 1 2 3 4 5 6 7 *Strongly agree*

Perceived discrimination: Study comparison

Study (year published)	Sample and scale details	N	Mean (SD)	Internal reliability
Gartska, Schmitt, Branscombe, & Hummert (2004)	Young adults (age 17 to 20). Older adults (age 64 to 91) (US). 4-items (1–7 Likert scale).	59 young adults 60 older adults	3.35 (1.07) young adults 2.49 (1.39) older adults	α = .68 young adults α = 77 older adults

Self-stigma

Self-stigma refers to a person's internalised sense that they have a stigmatised identity (in the sense of being tainted or damaged; Goffman, 1963; Corrigan, Watson, & Barr, 2006). As discussed in Chapter 4, this can arise from a number of factors, including a person's membership of a devalued group (e.g., as a person suffering from a particular mental illness; Clement et al., 2015). Self-stigma is widely recognised to be a cause of people's reluctance to seek treatment for particular health conditions, and there are a number of measures that assess this in relation to different conditions (e.g., Corrigan et al., 2006; Corrigan et al., 2012). The Self-Stigma of Seeking Help (SSOSH; Vogel, Wade, & Haake, 2006) scale was developed by David Vogel and his colleagues to assess people's reluctance to seek help from psychologists, but it can easily be adapted for other contexts (e.g., visiting a doctor).

Self-stigma of seeking help: Suggested items and scale

1. I would feel inadequate if I went to a therapist for psychological help.
2. My self-confidence would *not* be threatened if I sought professional help.[R]
3. Seeking psychological help would make me feel less intelligent.
4. My self-esteem would increase if I talked to a therapist.[R]
5. My view of myself would not change just because I made the choice to see a therapist.[R]
6. It would make me feel inferior to ask a therapist for help.
7. I would feel okay about myself if I made the choice to seek professional help.[R]
8. If I went to a therapist, I would be less satisfied with myself.
9. My self-confidence would remain the same if I sought help for a problem I could not solve.[R]
10. I would feel worse about myself if I could not solve my own problems.

Rating scale for each item: *Strongly disagree* 1 2 3 4 5 *Strongly agree*

Note: (R) = reverse scored.

Self-stigma of seeking help: Study comparison

Study (year published)	Sample and scale details	N	Mean (SD)	Internal reliability
Vogel, Wade, & Haake – Study 2 (2006)	College undergraduate students (US). 10 items (1–5 Likert scale).	470	27.2 (7.2)	α = .89
Pederson & Vogel (2007)	Male college undergraduate psychology students (US). 10 items (1–5 Likert scale).	575	29.4 (7.35)	α = .88

Disclosure and concealment

A range of measures have been developed to assess various aspects of people's willingness to conceal rather than disclose the fact that they have a particular medical condition to others (e.g., Comer, Henker, Kemeny, & Wyatt, 2000; Kahn & Hessling, 2001). This is a factor whose relevance for health and well-being was discussed in Chapter 4.

The following scale is a simple measure developed by Fernando Molero and colleagues to assess the willingness of people to tell others about their medical condition. In this case the researchers were studying HIV, but this can be adapted for other conditions.

Disclosure and concealment: Suggested items and scale

1. To what extent do you think it is best not to tell other people you have [condition]?
2. To what extent do you tell other people you have [condition]?

Rating scale for Item 1: *Best not to tell anyone* 1 2 3 4 5 *Best to tell everyone*

Rating scale for Item 2: *I do not tell anyone* 1 2 3 4 5 *I tell everyone*

Disclosure and concealment: Study comparison

Study (year published)	Sample and scale details	N	Mean (SD)	Internal reliability
Molero, Fuster, Jetten, & Moriano (2011)	People with HIV (Spain). 2 items (1–5 Likert scale).	68	3.23 (0.83)	$r = .68$

Perceived personal control

This measure was developed by Katharine Greenaway and colleagues in a series of studies that explored the impact of social identification on people's sense of control (e.g., as discussed in Chapter 2; Greenaway et al., 2015; see also Greenaway, Louis, & Hornsey, 2013). The scale has been used successfully with a wide range of populations and has good internal reliability.

Personal control: Suggested items and scale

1. I feel in control of my life.
2. I am free to live my life how I wish.
3. My experiences in life are due to my own actions.

Rating scale for each item: *Strongly disagree* 1 2 3 4 5 6 7 *Strongly agree*

Personal control: Study comparison

Study (year published)	Sample and scale details	N	Mean (SD)	Internal reliability
Greenaway, Louis, & Hornsey (2013)	Students (Australia). Priming precognition (exists, does not exist). 3 items (1–7 Likert scale).	53	5.37 (0.61) precognition exists 4.75 (1.44) precognition does not exist	$\alpha = .76$
Greenaway, Haslam, Cruwys, Branscombe, Ysseldyk, & Heldreth (2015)	Online community members (US). Priming identification (high, low, control). 3 items (1–7 Likert scale).	300	5.19 (1.10) control condition	$\alpha = .81$

Health and well-being measures

Burnout (chronic stress)

The following measure is an extension of the seven-item measure developed by Haslam and Reicher (2006) to measure stress in the BBC Prison Experiment (as discussed in Chapter 5). It has three subscales that correspond to the three core components of burnout identified by Jackson, Schwab, and Schuler (1986) and Maslach, Jackson, and Leiter (1996): (1) exhaustion, (2) lack of accomplishment, and (3) callousness (lack of concern for others). Studies in which various versions of this have been used indicate that the scale as a whole forms a reasonably reliable single measure (e.g., in a study of care workers, Gaffney & Haslam, 2002, report $\alpha = .67$ for a six-item version; see also van Dick & Haslam, 2012).

The three sub-scales also generally have satisfactory reliability, but this can be substantially improved either (1) by using the six-item scale that excludes reverse-scored items (Steffens, Haslam, Kerschreiter, Schuh, & van Dick, 2014) or (2) by rewording the reverse-scored items (e.g., I feel that I lack energy; I feel I am accomplishing nothing; I'm not concerned about the welfare of others).

Burnout: Suggested items and scale

Exhaustion
1. I feel I am working too hard. *[†]
2. I feel exhausted. [†]
3. I feel energetic [(R)]. *

Lack of accomplishment

4. I feel I am failing to achieve my goals. [†]
5. I feel frustrated. *[†]
6. I feel I am accomplishing many worthwhile things [(R)]. *

Callousness

7. I am concerned about the welfare of others [(R).] *
8. I don't really care what happens to people any more. *[†]
9. I feel I am becoming callous towards other people. *[†]

Rating scale for each item: *Not at all* 1 2 3 4 5 6 7 *Definitely*

Note: [(R)] = reverse scored.

    * Items used in seven-item scale (Haslam & Reicher, 2006).

    [†] Items used in six-item scale (i.e., excluding reverse-scored items; Steffens et al., 2014).

Burnout: Study comparison

Study (year published)	*Sample and scale details*	*N*	*Mean (SD)*	*Internal reliability*
Haslam & Reicher (2006)	British community members serving as Prisoners and Guards in the BBC Prison Experiment (UK). 6 items (1–7 Likert scale).	9 Prisoners 5 Guards	2.23 Guards Day 2 3.17 Guards Day 6 2.38 Prisoners Day 2 2.29 Prisoners Day 6	Day 2 $\alpha = .62$ Day 6 $\alpha = .59$
Steffens, Haslam, Kerschreiter, Schuh, & van Dick (2014)	Online community sample (US). 7 items (1–7 Likert scale).	699	3.08 (1.24)	$\alpha = .78$

Posttraumatic stress

The *Impact of Event Scale – Revised* (IES-R; Weiss, 2007) is commonly used to index posttraumatic stress and involves participants indicating how distressing various symptoms of PTSD have been during the past 7 days in relation to a specified traumatic event. It is a 22-item measure that assesses three dimensions of trauma symptoms: intrusiveness (I), avoidance (A), and hyperarousal (H). These dimensions can be analysed separately, but the correlations among them are often relatively high, thereby justifying use of a single summated index. The measure is frequently regarded as an index of posttraumatic stress disorder symptoms, demonstrating good specificity and sensitivity (Brewin, 2005; Sundin & Horowitz, 2002).

The total score on the measure can range from 0 to 88. There is some debate about how to interpret this, but Mark Creamer and his colleagues note that a score of 33 (a mean item score of 1.5) corresponds to the point at which PTSD symptomatology is evident (Creamer, Bell, & Failla, 2003). Nevertheless, because scores vary as a function of the nature of the traumatic event to which they relate, and because items do not map straightforwardly onto diagnostic criteria, it is imprudent to specify a generic cut-off point for PTSD diagnosis (Motlagh, 2010).

Posttraumatic stress: Suggested items and scale (I = intrusiveness, A = avoidance, H = hyperarousal)

The following is a list of difficulties people sometimes have after stressful life events. Please read each item and then indicate how distressing each difficulty has been for you *during the past 7 days* with respect to [event].

1. Any reminder brought back feelings about it. (I)
2. I had trouble staying asleep. (I)
3. Other things kept making me think about it. (I)
4. I felt irritable and angry. (H)
5. I avoided letting myself get upset when I thought about it or was reminded of it. (A)
6. I thought about it when I didn't mean to. (I)
7. I felt as if it hadn't happened or wasn't real. (A)
8. I stayed away from reminders about it. (A)
9. Pictures about it popped into my mind. (I)
10. I was jumpy and easily startled. (H)
11. I tried not to think about it. (A)
12. I was aware that I still had a lot of feelings about it, but I didn't deal with them. (A)
13. My feelings about it were kind of numb. (A)
14. I found myself acting or feeling like I was back at that time. (I)
15. I had trouble falling asleep. (H)
16. I had waves of strong feelings about it. (I)
17. I tried to remove it from my memory. (A)
18. I had trouble concentrating. (H)
19. Reminders of it caused me to have physical reactions, such as sweating, trouble breathing, nausea, or a pounding heart. (H)
20. I had dreams about it. (I)
21. I felt watchful and on guard. (H)
22. I tried not to talk about it. (A)

Rating scale for each item: 0 = not at all, 1 = a little bit, 2 = moderately, 3 = quite a bit, 4 = extremely

---

Posttraumatic stress: Study comparison

Study (year published)	Sample and scale details	N	Mean (SD)	Internal reliability
Asukai et al – Study 3 (2002)	Survivors of Kobe earthquake (Japan). 22-item IES-R.	86	Total score 41.4 (13.6) PTSD group 18.9 (16.0) non-PTSD group	α = .89 intrusion α = .84 avoidance α = .80 hyperarousal
Creamer, Bell, & Failla (2003)	Vietnam veterans admitted to hospital with PTSD; ex-service personnel (US). 22-item IES-R.	124 PTSD 159 Community	Mean subscale scores PTSD sample 2.72 (0.77) intrusion 2.30 (0.80) avoidance 2.99 (0.85) hyperarousal Community sample 1.82 (1.05) intrusion 1.75 (1.11) avoidance 1.59 (1.03) hyperarousal	α = .94 intrusion α = .87 avoidance α = .91 hyperarousal
Beck et al. (2008)	People involved in a serious motor vehicle accident (US). 22-item IES-R.	182	Mean subscale scores 1.57 (0.99) intrusion 1.44 (0.90) avoidance 1.81 (1.07) hyperarousal	α = .90 intrusion α = .86 avoidance α = .85 hyperarousal

Depression, anxiety, and stress

The *DASS-21* (a shorter version of the *DASS-42*, originally developed by Lovibond & Lovibond, 1995) is widely used to assess depression, anxiety, and stress (e.g., as discussed in Chapters 5 and 8). It contains seven items related to each of these three constructs, and scores for the items related to each construct are summed and multiplied by two to obtain an index of each. A range of studies also confirm that the instrument has very good psychometric properties and that its subscales reliably differentiate between the three constructs in a range of populations (e.g., Antony, Bieling, Cox, Enns, & Swinson, 1998; Henry & Crawford, 2005). In clinical contexts the DASS also does a good job of distinguishing between different types of clinical presentation (e.g., major depression vs. obsessive compulsive disorder; Page, Hooke, & Morrison, 2007). Here the total score can also provide a global index of a person's mental health.

Studies with representative populations – notably by Julie Henry and John Crawford – have also provided researchers with normative data that allow them to establish criteria for interpreting respondents' scores in order to classify their level of depression, anxiety, and stress as mild, moderate, severe, or extremely severe (Henry & Crawford, 2005). These are reproduced in Table A.1. Although the instrument is useful for assessing the level of an individual's disturbance relative to population norms (and hence the risk that they will encounter further difficulties), it remains the case that in therapeutic contexts, scores should be interpreted in the context of additional clinical information.

Depression, anxiety, and stress: suggested items and subscales (S = stress, A = anxiety, D = depression)

Please read each statement and circle a number 0, 1, 2, or 3 which indicates how much the statement applied to you over the past week. There are no right or wrong answers. Do not spend too much time on any statement.
1. I found it hard to wind down. (S)
2. I was aware of dryness of my mouth. (A)
3. I couldn't seem to experience any positive feeling at all. (D)
4. I experienced breathing difficulty (e.g., excessively rapid breathing, breathlessness in the absence of physical exertion). (A)
5. I found it difficult to work up the initiative to do things. (D)
6. I tended to over-react to situations. (S)
7. I experienced trembling (e.g., in the hands). (A)
8. I felt that I was using a lot of nervous energy. (S)
9. I was worried about situations in which I might panic and make a fool of myself. (A)
10. I felt that I had nothing to look forward to. (D)
11. I found myself getting agitated. (S)
12. I found it difficult to relax. (S)
13. I felt down-hearted and blue. (D)
14. I was intolerant of anything that kept me from getting on with what I was doing. (S)
15. I felt I was close to panic. (A)
16. I was unable to become enthusiastic about anything. (D)
17. I felt I wasn't worth much as a person. (D)
18. I felt that I was rather touchy. (S)
19. I was aware of the action of my heart in the absence of physical exertion (e.g., sense of heart rate increase, heart missing a beat). (A)
20. I felt scared without any good reason. (A)
21. I felt that life was meaningless. (D)

Rating scale for each item:
0 = did not apply to me at all
1 = applied to me to some degree or some of the time
2 = applied to me to a considerable degree or a good part of time
3 = applied to me most of the time

Depression, anxiety and stress: Study comparison

Study (year published)	Sample and scale details	N	Mean (SD)	Internal reliability
Brown, Chorpita, Korotitscw, & Barlow (1997)	A clinical sample presenting at two anxiety and stress clinics (US). 42 items (0–3 Likert scale).	437	10.65 (9.30) depression 10.90 (8.12) anxiety 21.10 (11.15) stress	α = .96 depression α = .89 anxiety α = .93 stress

Depression, anxiety and stress: Study comparison

Study (year published)	Sample and scale details	N	Mean (SD)	Internal reliability
Henry & Crawford (2005)	A non-clinical adult community sample (UK). 21 items (0–3 Likert scale).	1794	2.83 (3.87) depression 1.88 (2.95) anxiety 4.73 (4.22) stress	α = .96 depression α = .89 anxiety α = .90 stress
Haslam, Cruwys, Haslam, Dingle, & Chang (2016c)	Participants in first GROUPS 4 HEALTH trial before and after the intervention (Australia). 21 items (0–3 Likert scale).	56	15.70 (7.38) T1 depression 16.03 (8.39) T1 anxiety 20.28 (6.69) T1 stress 13.00 (10.37) T2 depression 11.74 (7.58) T2 anxiety 15.78 (8.83) T2 stress	α = .88 T1 depression α = .82 T1 anxiety α = .76 T1 stress

Table A.1 Criteria for interpretation of DASS-21 scores

Severity *	Depression	Anxiety	Stress
Normal	0–4	0–3	0–7
Mild	5–6	4–5	8–9
Moderate	7–10	6–7	10–12
Severe	11–13	8–9	13–16
Extremely Severe	14+	10+	17+

Note: * Labels relate to the full range of scores observed in the population at large (Henry & Crawford, 2005).

Resilience

Bruce Smith and his colleagues argue that resilience is best conceptualised as the capacity to bounce back from adversity (typically stressful or traumatic events), and they developed the six-item Brief Resilience Scale (BRS) to assess this (Smith et al., 2008). Validation studies show that the BRS is negatively correlated with perceived stress, anxiety, depression, negative affect, and physical symptoms of illness (and positively correlated with positive affect). At the same time, a large number of alternative measures have also been developed by other researchers, each of which frames resilience in a slightly different way (e.g., by asking how well respondents regulate their emotions or whether they have a positive future orientation; Oshio, Kaneko, Nagamine, & Nakaya, 2003). It is worth noting too, that in a review of 15 resilience scales, Gill Windle and her colleagues (2015) argue that none of these provides a 'gold standard' for assessment – in part due to the complexity of the phenomenon (e.g., as discussed in Chapter 6).

Resilience scale (BRS): Suggested items and scale

1. I tend to bounce back quickly after hard times.
2. I have a hard time making it through stressful events. (R)
3. It does not take me long to recover from a stressful event.
4. It is hard for me to snap back when something bad happens. (R)
5. I usually come through difficult times with little trouble.
6. I tend to take a long time to get over set-backs in my life. (R)

Rating scale for each item: *Strongly disagree* 1 2 3 4 5 *Strongly agree*

Note: (R) = reverse scored.

Resilience: Study comparison

Study (year published)	Sample and scale details	N	Mean (SD)	Internal reliability
Smith, Dalen, Wiggins, Tooley, Christopher, & Bernard (2008)	Undergraduate students; cardiac rehabilitation patients (US). 6-item BRS (1–7 Likert scale).	128 students, 112 patients	3.53 (0.69) students 3.98 (0.68) patients	α = .84 students α = .80 patients

Affect

The *Positive and Negative Affect Scale* (*PANAS*; Watson, Clark, & Tellegen, 1988) is widely used to gauge the incidence or preponderance of feelings and behaviours associated with positive affect and, independently, negative affect. The PANAS can be useful to administer as a repeated measure in order to examine changes in affect over time (e.g., following an experimental manipulation or after an intervention).

The scale consists of ten descriptors for positive affect (PA): attentive, interested, alert, excited, enthusiastic, inspired, proud, determined, strong, and active; and ten descriptors for negative affect (NA): distressed, upset-distressed, hostile, irritable-angry, scared, afraid-fearful, ashamed, guilty, nervous, and jittery. Respondents are asked to indicate the extent to which they are feeling (or have felt) each of these 20 affective states on a 5-point scale (where 1 = very slightly, 5 = extremely). Scores for the positive and negative items can then be summed to provide separate indices of PA and NA.

There is also a short-form version of the scale that includes half as many items (Thompson, 2007) – five descriptors for positive affect: attentive, alert, inspired, determined, and active; and five descriptors for negative affect: upset, hostile, afraid, ashamed, and nervous. Responses are again made on 5-point scales (although here 1=never, 5 = always). The scale has been validated in countries around the world, and its psychometric properties are similar to those of the longer scale (see Thompson, 2007).

Affect: Study comparison

Study (year published)	Sample and scale details	N	Mean (SD)	Internal reliability
Crawford & Henry (2004)	Representative sample of adults (UK). 20-item PANAS.	1003 (537 women, 466 men)	Total sample 31.31 (7.65) PA 16.00 (5.90) NA Women 30.62 (7.89) PA 16.68 (6.37) NA Men 32.06 (7.31) PA 15.20 (5.23) NA	α = .89 PA α = .85 NA
Thompson (2007)	Respondents in a range of validation studies (38 countries). 10-item PANAS-SF.	1789 (411 USA, 162 Indonesia 100 Hungary)	USA 19.73 (2.58) PA 11.27 (2.66) NA Indonesia 18.51 (2.46) PA 12.98 (2.70) NA Hungary 18.94 (2.71) PA 11.76 (2.73) NA	α = .76 PA α = .75 NA

Dieting intentions

The *Dieting Intentions Scale (DIS;* Cruwys et al., 2013) can be used to assess the likelihood that a person will engage in naturalistic (i.e., typical) dieting over the next 3 months. This is typically treated as an outcome measure rather than a process measure, because people's actual eating behaviour is notoriously difficult to observe and self-report measures of eating behaviour are very unreliable (Schoeller, 1995).

The scale has been validated with Western student and community samples, including women at risk of disordered eating. This scale is designed to be sensitive enough to detect fluctuations in a person's desire to engage in dieting behaviour, and is thus appropriate for laboratory research or interventions which aim to influence dieting intentions as an outcome. However, because naturalistic dieting typically involves both healthy and unhealthy eating behaviours, this scale is not appropriate to assess changes in dieting among clinical populations—for instance, in research that has a goal of increasing (healthy) dieting in obese patients or a goal of decreasing (unhealthy) dieting among eating-disordered patients. The seven items are averaged to create a single scale.

Dieting intentions: Suggested items and scale

1. In the next 3 months, I intend to go on a diet.
   Strongly disagree 1 2 3 4 5 6 7 *Strongly agree*
2. In the next 3 months, I intend to reduce my calorie intake.
   Strongly disagree 1 2 3 4 5 6 7 *Strongly agree*

(Continued)

Dieting intentions: Suggested items and scale

If I diet in the next 3 months, this would be. . .
3. *Harmful* 1 2 3 4 5 6 7 *Harmless*
4. *Unpleasant* 1 2 3 4 5 6 7 Pleasant
5. *Useless* 1 2 3 4 5 6 7 *Useful*
6. *Foolish* 1 2 3 4 5 6 7 *Wise*
7. *Bad* 1 2 3 4 5 6 7 *Good*

Dieting intentions: Study comparison

Study (year published)	Sample and scale details	N	Mean (SD)	Internal reliability
Cruwys, Platow, Rieger & Byrne (2013)	Study 1: Community sample of women (Australia). Study 2: Undergraduate male and female students (Australia). Study 3: Male and female students (Australia). Study 4: Community members (male and female) from English-speaking countries.	S1: 183 S2: 97 S3: 171 S4: 290	S1: 4.15 (1.43) S2: 3.90 (1.58) S3: 4.10 (1.67) S4: Men: 4.06 (1.56) Women: 4.50 (1.65)	S1: α = .91 S2: α = .93 S3: α = .94 S4: α = .92
Cruwys, Haslam, Fox, & McMahon (2015)	Women aged 15–25 years who reported body shape or weight concerns (Australia).	112	T1: 4.89 (1.19) T5 (after a group intervention to prevent eating disorders): 2.93 (1.21)	T1: α = .88 T5: α = .92

Paranoia

This three-item measure was developed by Reicher and Haslam (2006a) for screening purposes in the BBC Prison Experiment (see Chapter 5), where it had good reliability, and also in the study itself where the measure was used to assess participants' ongoing mental health (on 8 consecutive days αs ranged between .73 and .86). Other studies have used the larger 20-item scale developed by Allan Fenigstein and Peter Vanable (1992) that is also reproduced here. The two scales are highly correlated with each other ($r > .7$).

Paranoia 3-item scale: Suggested items and scale

1. Do you feel that other people can't be trusted?
2. Do you feel you are being watched and talked about by others?
3. Do you feel you might be being punished for things you haven't done?

Rating scale for each item: *Not at all* 1 2 3 4 5 6 7 *Very frequently*

Paranoia 20-item scale: Suggested items and scale

1. Someone has it in for me.
2. I sometimes feel as if I'm being followed.
3. I believe that I have often been punished without cause.
4. Some people have tried to steal my ideas and take credit for them.
5. My parents and family find more fault with me than they should.
6. No one really cares much about what happens to you.
7. I am sure I get a raw deal from life.
8. Most people will use somewhat unfair means to gain profit or advantage rather than lose it.
9. I often wonder what hidden reason another person may have for doing something nice for you.
10. It is safer to trust no-one.
11. I have often felt that strangers were looking at me critically.
12. Most people make friends because friends are likely to be useful to them.
13. Someone has been trying to influence my mind.
14. I am sure I have been talked about behind my back.
15. Most people inwardly dislike putting themselves out to help other people.
16. I tend to be on my guard with people who are somewhat more friendly than expected.
17. People have said insulting and unkind things about me.
18. People often disappoint me.
19. I am bothered by people outside, in cars, in stores, etc., watching me.
20. I have often found people jealous of my good ideas just because they had not thought of them.

Rating scale for each item: *Not at all* applicable to me 1 2 3 4 5 *Extremely applicable to me*

Paranoia: Study comparison

Study (year published)	Sample and scale details	N	Mean (SD)	Internal reliability
Freeman, Garety, Bebbington, Smith, Rollinson, Fowler, Kuipers, Ray, & Dunn (2005)	Online survey of university students (UK). Using the Fenigstein Paranoia scale (in conjunction with the Paranoia Checklist). 20 items (1–5 Likert scale).	1016	42.70 (14.30)	$\alpha > .90$
Haslam & Reicher (2006)	Community members (UK). 3 items (1–7 Likert scale).	317	2.95	$\alpha = .79$
Bentall, Rouse, Kinderman, Blackwood, Howard, Moore, Cummins, & Corcoran (2008)	Inpatient and outpatient clinics (UK). Using the Fenigstein Paranoia scale. 20 items (1–5 Likert scale).	115	30.82 (8.60) non-clinical 68.78 (13.95) diagnosed with paranoid delusions	$\alpha = .84$

Loneliness

The widely used *UCLA Loneliness Scale* was developed by Daniel Russell at the University of California, Los Angeles (Russell, 1996). The long version of the scale contains 20 items and is highly reliable (Russell, 1996, reports αs between .89 and .94 across a range of samples). However, the measure is very highly correlated (r = .91) with the shorter eight-item version reproduced here (the ULS-8; Hays & DiMatteo, 1987), and this also has high internal consistency. More recently, Mary Elizabeth Hughes and her colleagues have argued that their shorter *three-item loneliness scale* (3-ILS) is even more suitable for large surveys (Hughes, Waite, Hawkley, & Cacioppo, 2004). This has acceptable reliability and a limited number of response categories that make it very easy to administer (e.g., by telephone).

ULS-8: Suggested items and scale

1. I lack companionship.
2. There is no-one I can turn to.
3. I am an outgoing person. (R)
4. I feel left out.
5. I feel isolated from others.
6. I can find companionship when I want it. (R)
7. I am unhappy being so withdrawn.
8. People are around me but not with me.

Rating scale for each item: 1 = hardly ever, 2 = some of the time, 3 = often

Note: (R) = reverse scored.

3-ILS: Suggested items and scale

1. How often do you feel that you lack companionship?
2. How often do you feel left out?
3. How often do you feel isolated from others?

Rating scale for each item: 1 = hardly ever, 2 = some of the time, 3 = often

---

Loneliness: Study comparison

Study (year published)	*Sample and scale details*	*N*	*Mean (SD)*	*Internal reliability*
Hughes, Waite, Hawkley, & Cacioppo (2004)	Community sample (US). 3-item ILS (1–3 Likert scale).	2182	3.89 (1.34) (mean sum of all three items)	α = .72
Wu & Yao (2007)	Undergraduate students (Taiwan). 8-item ILS (1–4 Likert scale).	130	17.12 (5.92) (mean sum of all eight items)	α = .84

Personal self-esteem

Self-esteem is commonly measured using Morris Rosenberg's (1965) ten-item measure. This was originally developed on the basis of responses from over 5,000 adolescent high school students in New York. Previous studies have indicated that the scale has high reliability (αs in the range .72 to .88; Gray-Little, Williams, & Hancock, 1997). Yet although Rosenberg's scale is very popular, Robins, Hendin, and Trzesniewski (2001) argue that their single-item measure has high convergent validity with the ten-item measure and nearly identical correlations with a range of criterion measures (e.g., social desirability, psychological and physical health, academic outcomes, and demographic variables). As with other single-item measures, it also has the advantage of being a lot easier to administer.

Personal self-esteem (10 items): Suggested items and scale

1. On the whole, I am satisfied with myself.
2. At times, I think I am no good at all. [R]
3. I feel that I have a number of good qualities.
4. I am able to do things as well as most other people.
5. I feel I do not have much to be proud of. [R]
6. I certainly feel useless at times. [R]
7. I feel that I'm a person of worth, at least on an equal plane with others.
8. I wish I could have more respect for myself. [R]
9. All in all, I am inclined to feel that I am a failure. [R]
10. I take a positive attitude toward myself.

Rating scale for each item: *Strongly disagree* 0 1 2 3 4 *Strongly agree*

Note: [R] = reverse scored.

Personal self-esteem (1 item): Suggested item and scale

1. I have high self-esteem.

Rating scale for item: *Strongly disagree* 0 1 2 3 4 *Strongly agree*

Self-esteem: Study comparison

Study (year published)	Sample and scale details	N	Mean (SD)	Internal reliability
Haslam, O'Brien, Jetten, Vormedal, & Penna – Study 1 (2005)	Patients recovering from heart surgery (Norway). 10 items (1–7 Likert scale).	34	5.33	$\alpha = .64$
Greenaway, Haslam, Cruwys, Branscombe, Ysseldyk, & Heldreth – Study 4 (2015)	Online community members (US). Priming identification (high, low, control). Single item (1–7 Likert scale).	300	4.60 (1.61) control condition	not applicable
Jetten, Branscombe, Haslam et al. – Study 2 (2015)	Boys attending a private school (Australia). Single item (1–4 Likert scale).	827	3.11 (0.70)	not applicable

Life satisfaction

This can be indexed with either single-item or longer scales. Single-item measures such as the *Satisfaction with Life (SWL)* and the *Cantril Self-anchoring Striving Scale* (sometimes called the "Cantril Ladder"; Cantril, 1965; Kilpatrick & Cantril, 1960) have similar psychometric properties and predictive utility and are widely used in surveys of large populations (e.g., national censuses; Helliwell, Barrington-Leigh, Harris, & Huang, 2010; see also Diener, Lucas, Schimmack, & Helliwell, 2009). However, Ed Diener and his colleagues argue that multiple items are required to index life satisfaction as a cognitive-judgmental process, and their five-item measure, the *Satisfaction with Life Scale (SWLS)*, has proved very popular for this purpose (Diener, Emmons, Larsen, & Griffin, 1985). Yet although this may have greater statistical integrity than the single-item measure, it is obviously costlier to include in large-scale surveys.

Satisfaction with life (SWL): Suggested item and scale

All things considered, how satisfied are you with life as a whole these days?

Rating scale: *Completely dissatisfied* 0 1 2 3 4 5 6 7 8 9 10 *Completely satisfied*

Satisfaction with life scale (SWLS): Suggested items and scale

1. In most ways my life is close to ideal.
2. The conditions of my life are excellent.
3. I am satisfied with life.
4. So far I have gotten the important things I want in life.
5. If I could live my life over, I would change almost nothing.

Rating scale for each item: *Strongly disagree* 1 2 3 4 5 6 7 *Strongly agree*

Life satisfaction: Study comparison

Study (year published)	Sample and scale details	N	Mean (SD)	Internal reliability
Pavot & Diener (1993)	36 samples (e.g. college students, prison inmates, health workers) (7 countries). 5 items (1–5 Likert scale).	$14 < N < 472$	11.8 (5.6) Vietnam veterans $< M <$ 27.9 (5.7) male French Canadians (mean sum of all 3 items)	$.79 < \alpha < .89$
Haslam, Haslam, Ysseldyk, McCloskey, Pfisterer, & Brown (2014c)	Retirement village residents (Canada). 5 items (1–5 Likert scale).	40	4.50 (0.48) pre-intervention 4.60 (0.37) post-intervention	$\alpha = .80$ pre-intervention $\alpha = .77$ post-intervention

Life satisfaction: Study comparison

Study (year published)	Sample and scale details	N	Mean (SD)	Internal reliability
Chang, Jetten, Cruwys, Haslam, & Praharso (2016)	University students (China, Hong Kong, Indonesia, Malaysia, and Singapore). 5 items (1–7 Likert scale).	180 Study 1 105 Study 3	4.88 (1.17) Study 1 4.56 (1.12) Study 3	α = .87 Study 1 α = .85 Study 3

Cantril self-anchoring striving scale: Suggested item and scale

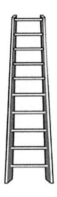

Imagine a ladder with steps numbered 0 at the bottom to 10 at the top. Suppose we say that the top of the ladder represents the best possible life for you and the bottom of the ladder represents the worst possible. If the top step is 10 and the bottom step is 0, on which step of the ladder do you feel you personally stand at the present time?

Cantril self-anchoring striving scale: Study comparison

Study (year published)	Sample and scale details	N	Mean (SD)	Internal reliability
Diener, Ng, Harter, & Arora (2010)	Respondents to Gallup World Poll (132 countries)	136,839	5.36 (2.24)	not applicable

General health

It is common – especially in large national surveys – to assess respondents' perceived health status with the following single-item measure. Aside from being easy to administer, this also has been shown to have good correspondence with objective measures of health. In particular, Karen DeSalvo and her colleagues found that there was a strong correlation between responses on this measure and assessment of a person's physical symptoms of illness ($r = .66$; DeSalvo, Fisher et al., 2006).

The measure also has good predictive utility. For example, across 22 studies, DeSalvo and colleagues found that people who had "poor" self-rated health had a mortality risk that was almost twice that of those with "excellent" self-rated health (compared to persons with "excellent" health status, the relative risk for all-cause mortality was 1.23 times greater for those whose health was "good", 1.44 times greater for those whose health was "fair", and 1.92 times greater for those whose health was "poor"; DeSalvo, Bloser, Reynolds, He, & Muntner, 2006).

General health: Suggested item and scale

How would you rate your overall physical health? ☐
Rating scale: 1 = poor, 2 = fair, 3 = good, 4 = very good, 5 = excellent

---

Points for practice

It is hard to devise hard-and-fast rules about which scales to use to assess the constructs one is interested in across a range of applied or research settings. However, the following principles are generally worth bearing in mind as you set about this task:

1. *If possible, use a validated scale (e.g., of the form included in this appendix).* There are a number of reasons why this is a sensible strategy, but the most obvious ones are (1) that it will be evident to others that the measure you are using has some provenance (and is not simply 'made up'), (2) that previous work (in particular, published validation studies) will provide you with important information about the scale's properties, and (3) that previous work will provide a benchmark against which you can interpret your own findings. All of these features will give you stronger grounds for justifying the conclusions that you want to draw from the data you obtain as a result of administering the scale in question.

2. *Use a scale that is suited to your needs.* Practitioners and researchers often have preferences for particular scales, and in some areas these preferences are widely shared (e.g., among members of particular professional groups). Nevertheless, it rarely the case that 'one size fits all', and it is important that your choice of scale is suited to the specific features and constraints of the assessment context in which you are working. For example, if you are in a field setting, it may be impractical to administer scales that have a large number of items (Postmes et al., 2013), or if you are seeking to persuade a particular group of readers of the importance of your findings, then it makes sense to employ scales that are widely used by members of that group.

3. *If necessary, be prepared to adapt scales so that they suit your needs, but ensure that you are able to justify your decision to do so.* Putting the previous two points together, it will sometimes be the case that there are no available or ideal scales that meet your assessment needs. In this case, a reasonable strategy is to tailor existing scales to make them more suitable for your purposes (e.g., to make them shorter, or to make their wording relevant to the population you are studying). If you do this, however, it is important that you are able to clearly justify the choices that you make (e.g., through reference to the decisions that others have made in previously published work).

Resources

Further reading

The following papers explore a broad range of issues that are relevant to the assessment of identity and health. They provide a good introduction to the methodological, theoretical, and practical issues that inform this process.

① Postmes, T., Haslam, S. A., & Jans, L. (2013). A single-item measure of social identification: Reliability, validity and utility. *British Journal of Social Psychology*, 52, 597–617.

This paper provides a useful discussion of the different ways in which one can measure social identification and also considers the merits of using long or short instruments to assess this and other important constructs.

② Jetten, J., Branscombe, N. R., Haslam, S. A., Haslam, C., Cruwys, T., Jones, J. M., Cui, L., Dingle, G., Liu, J., Murphy, S. C., Thai, A., Walter, Z., & Zhang, A. (2015). Having a lot of a good thing: Multiple important group memberships as a source of self-esteem. *PLoS ONE*. 10(6): e0131035.

This paper by Jetten and colleagues reports the findings of a large number of studies that examine the relationship between multiple social identities and self-esteem. As a result, it uses a range of the above measures with varied samples (e.g., children, older adults, former residents of a homeless shelter) and in a number of different settings (e.g., in Australia, Britain, China, and the United States) and gives a sense of how the measurement of relevant constructs can be tailored to the research setting.

③ Cruwys, T., Steffens, N. K., Haslam, S. A., Haslam, C., Jetten, J., & Dingle, G. A. (2016). Social Identity Mapping (SIM): A procedure for visual representation and assessment of subjective group memberships. *British Journal of Social Psychology*, 55, 613–642.

This paper introduces social identity mapping (SIM) as a method for visually representing and assessing a person's subjective network of group memberships. It reports validating data from three studies conducted with a range of samples. The studies confirm that SIM is easy to use, internally consistent, and has good convergent and discriminant validity.

References

Abbott, D. H., Keverne, E. B., Bercovitch, F. B., Shively, C. A., Mendoza, S. P., Salzman, W., . . . Sapolsky, R. M. (2003). Are subordinates always stressed? A comparative analysis of rank differences in cortisol levels among primates. *Hormones and Behavior, 43,* 67–82.

Abdou, C. M., & Fingerhut, A. W. (2014). Stereotype threat among black and white women in healthcare settings. *Culturally Diverse Ethnic Minority Psychology, 20,* 316–323.

Abrams, D., Eller, A., & Bryant, J. (2006). An age apart: The effects of intergenerational contact and stereotype threat on performance and intergroup bias. *Psychology and Aging, 21,* 691–702.

Access Economics. (2009, April). *Making choices, future dementia care: Projections, problems and preferences.* Canberra: Report for Alzheimer's Australia.

Acero, Á. R., Cano-Prous, A., Castellanos, G., Martín-Lanas, R., & Canga, A. (2017). Family identity and severe mental illness: A thematic synthesis of qualitative studies. *European Journal of Social Psychology, 47,* 611–627.

Ackerman, S. J., & Hilsenroth, M. J. (2003). A review of therapist characteristics and techniques positively impacting on the therapeutic alliance. *Clinical Psychology Review, 23,* 1–33.

Adams, S., Pill, R., & Jones, A. (1997). Medication, chronic illness and identity: The perspective of people with asthma. *Social Science and Medicine, 45,* 189–201.

Afridi, F., Li, S. X., & Ren, Y. (2015). Social identity and inequality: The impact of China's *hukou* system. *Journal of Public Economics, 123,* 17–29.

Afzal, S., Tybjærg-Hansen, A., Jensen, G. B., & Nordestgaard, B. G. (2016). Change in body mass index associated with lowest mortality in Denmark, 1976–2013. *JAMA, 315,* 1989–1996.

Agerbo, E., Mortensen, P. B., Wiuf, C., Pedersen, M. S., McGrath, J. J., Hollegaard, M. V., . . . Pedersen, C. B. (2012). Modelling the contribution of family history and variation in single nucleotide polymorphisms to risk of schizophrenia: A Danish national birth cohort-based study. *Schizophrenia Research, 134,* 246–252.

Agich, G. J. (Ed.). (1982). *Responsibility in health care.* Hingham, MA: Reidel.

Ahn, H., & Wampold, B. E. (2001). Where oh where are the specific ingredients? A meta-analysis of component studies in counseling and psychotherapy. *Journal of Counseling Psychology, 48,* 251–257.

Ajzen, I. (1991). The theory of planned behavior. *Organizational Behavior and Human Decision Processes, 50,* 179–211.

Akerlof, G. A., & Kranton, R. E. (2000). Economics and identity. *Quarterly Journal of Economics, 105,* 715–753.

Al-Anon Family Groups. (1981). *This is Al-Anon.* New York: Author.

Alexander, B. K. (2008). *The globalization of addiction: A study in the poverty of spirit.* New York: Oxford University Press.

Alexander, B. K. (2010). *Addiction: The view from Rat Park.* Retrieved from www.brucekalexander.com/articles-speeches/rat-park/148-addiction-the-view-from-rat-park

Alexander, B. K. (2017). *The dislocation theory of addiction.* Retrieved from www.brucekalexander.com/articles-speeches/dislocation-theory-addiction

Alexander, B. K., & Hadaway, P. F. (1982). Opiate addiction: The case for an adaptive orientation. *Psychological Bulletin, 92,* 367–381.

Alloy, L. B., Peterson, C., Abramson, L. Y., & Seligman, M. (1984). Attributional style and the generality of learned helplessness. *Journal of Personality and Social Psychology, 46,* 681–687.

Allsop, J., & Mulcahy, L. (1998). Maintaining professional identity: doctors' responses to complaints. *Sociology of Health and Illness, 20,* 802–824.

Alnabulsi, H., & Drury, J. (2014). Social identification moderates the effect of crowd density on safety at the Hajj. *Proceedings of the National Academy of Sciences, 111*, 9091–9096.

American Psychiatric Association. (1980). *DSM-III: Diagnostic and statistical manual of mental disorders* (3rd ed.). Washington, DC: The American Psychiatric Association.

American Psychiatric Association. (1994). *DSM-IV: Diagnostic and statistical manual of mental disorders* (4th ed.). Washington, DC: The American Psychiatric Association.

American Psychological Association. (2004). *Practice guideline for the treatment of patients with schizophrenia* (2nd ed.). APA. Retrieved from http://psychiatryonline.org/pdfaccess. ashx?ResourceID=243185&PDFSource=6

American Psychiatric Association. (2013). *Diagnostic and statistical manual of mental disorders (DSM-5).* Washington, DC: American Psychiatric Publications.

Anderson, C., Kraus, M. W., Galinsky, A. D., & Keltner, D. (2012). The local ladder effect: Social status and subjective well-being. *Psychological Science, 23*, 764–771.

Anderson, P., Beach, S. R. H., & Kaslow, N. J. (1999). Marital discord and depression: The potential of attachment theory ot guide intergrative clinical intervention. In T. Joiner & J. C. Coyne (Eds.), *The interactional nature of depression: Advances in interpersonal approaches* (pp. 271–297). Washington, DC: American Psychological Association.

Andreasen, N. C. (1987). Creativity and mental illness. *American Journal of Psychiatry, 144*, 1288–1292.

Andrews, P. W. (2015). Is serotonin an upper or a downer? The functional role of serotonin in depression and a possible mechanism of antidepressant action. *Neuroscience and Biobehavioral Reviews, 51*, 1–45.

Andrews, T. K., Rose, F. D., & Johnson, D. A. (1998). Social and behavioural effects of traumatic brain injury in children. *Brain Injury, 12*, 133–138.

Angst, J. (2012). Bipolar disorders in DSM-5: Strengths, problems and perspectives. *International Journal of Bipolar Disorders, 1*, 12.

Anguelova, M., Benkelfat, C., & Turecki, G. (2003). A systematic review of association studies investigating genes coding for serotonin receptors and the serotonin transporter: I. Affective disorders. *Molecular Psychiatry, 8*, 574–591.

Angus, J., & Reeve, P. (2006). Ageism: A threat to "aging well" in the 21st century. *Journal of Applied Gerontology, 25*, 137–152.

Anisman, H. (2016). *Health psychology*. Thousand Oaks, CA: Sage.

Ansell, N. (2011a). *Deep country*. London: Penguin.

Ansell, N. (2011b, March 11). My life as a hermit. *The Guardian*. Retrieved from www.theguardian.com/ environment/2011/mar/27/neil-ansell-my-life-as-hermit

Anson, K., & Ponsford, J. (2006). Coping and emotional adjustment following traumatic brain injury. *Journal of Head Trauma Rehabilitation, 21*, 248–259.

Antman, E. M., & Sabatine, M. S. (Eds.). (2013). *Cardiovascular therapeutics: A companion to Braunwald's heart disease* (4th ed.). Philadelphia, PA: Elsevier.

Antony, M. M., Bieling, P. J., Cox, B. J., Enns, M. W., & Swinson, R. P. (1998). Psychometric properties of the 42-item and 21-item versions of the Depression Anxiety Stress Scales in clinical groups and a community sample. *Psychological Assessment, 10*, 176–181.

Arain, M., Campbell, M. J., Cooper, C. L., & Lancaster, G. A. (2010). What is a pilot or feasibility study? A review of current practice and editorial policy. *BMC Medical Research Methodology, 10*, 67.

Aristotle. (340bc/2014). *Niomachean ethics* (C. D. C. Reeve, Trans). Indianapolis, IN: Hackett Publishing.

Armitage, C. J., & Conner, M. (2001). Efficacy of the theory of planned behaviour: A meta-analytic review. *British Journal of Social Psychology, 40*, 471–499.

Armstrong, M. J., Mottershead, T. A., Ronksley, P. E., Sigal, R. J., Campbell, T. S., & Hemmelgarn, B. R. (2011). Motivational interviewing to improve weight loss in overweight and/or obese patients: A systematic review and meta-analysis of randomized controlled trials. *Obesity Reviews, 12*, 709–723.

Armstrong-Esther, C. A., Browne, K. D., Armstrong-Esther, D. C., & Sander, L. (1996). The institutionalized elderly: Dry to the bone. *International Journal of Nursing Studies, 33*, 619–628.

Arnautovska, U., McPhedran, S., & De Leo, D. (2014). A regional approach to understanding farmer suicide rates in Queensland. *Social Psychiatry and Psychiatric Epidemiology, 49*, 593–599.

Aronson, E., & Mills, J. (1959). The effect of severity of initiation on liking for a group. *The Journal of Abnormal and Social Psychology, 59*, 177–181.

Ashforth, B. E., & Kreiner, G. E. (1999). "How can you do it?": Dirty work and the challenge of constructing a positive identity. *Academy of Management Review, 24*, 413–434.

Aspinwall, L. G., & Taylor, S. E. (1997). A stitch in time: Self-regulation and proactive coping. *Psychological Bulletin, 121*, 417–436.

Åstrosm, A. N., & Rise, J. (2001). Young adults' intention to eat healthy food: Extending the theory of planned behaviour. *Psychology and Health, 16*, 223–237.

Asukai, N., Kato, H., Kawamura, N., Kim, Y., Yamamoto, K., Kishimoto, J., . . . Nishizono-Maher, A. (2002). Reliability and validity of the Japanese-language version of the Impact of Event Scale-Revised (IES-RJ): Four studies of different traumatic events. *The Journal of Nervous and Mental Disease, 190*, 175–182.

Atkinson, Q. D., & Whitehouse, H. (2010). The cultural morphospace of ritual form: Examining modes of religiosity cross-culturally. *Evolution and Human Behavior, 32*, 50–62.

Atran, S., & Henrich, J. (2010). The evolution of religion: How cognitive by-products, adaptive learning heuristics, ritual displays, and group competition generate deep commitments to prosocial religions. *Biological Theory, 5*, 18–30.

Auerswald, C. L., & Eyre, S. L. (2002). Youth homelessness in San Francisco: A life cycle approach. *Social Science and Medicine, 54*, 1497–1512.

Australian Bureau of Statistics. (2012). *Australian health survey: Updated results, 2011–2012.* Canberra: Australian Bureau of Statistics.

Australian Centre for Posttraumatic Mental Health. (2007). *Australian guidelines for the treatment of adults with acute stress disorder and posttraumatic stress disorder.* Melbourne, Australia: Australian Centre for Posttraumatic Mental Health.

Australian Health Ministers Advisory Council. (2013). *A national framework for recovery-oriented mental health services: Policy and theory.* Australian Government Publications approval number: 10287, ISBN: 978-1-74186-012-2.

Australian Human Rights Commission. (2013). *Fact or fiction? Stereotypes of older Australians.* Sydney, Australia: 10287, ISBN: 978-1-921449-42-0.

Australian Institute of Health and Welfare. (2007). *Disability in Australia: Acquired brain injury.* Bulletin no. 55. Cat no. AUS 96. Canberra: AIHW.

Australian Institute of Health and Welfare. (2011). *Key indicators of progress for chronic disease and associated determinants: data report.* Cat. no. PHE 142. Canberra: AIHW.

Australian Institute of Health and Welfare. (2012). *Australia's health 2012.* Australia's health series No. 13. Cat. no. AUS 156. Canberra: AIHW.

Australian Institute of Health and Welfare. (2014). *Mortality inequalities in Australia 2009–2011.* AIHW, Bulletin, 124. Retrieved from www.aihw.gov.au/WorkArea/DownloadAsset.aspx?id=60129548364

Australian Institute of Health and Welfare. (2016). *Australian burden of disease study: Impact and causes of illness and death in Australia 2011.* Australian Burden of Disease Study series no. 3. BOD 4. Canberra: AIHW.

Avenanti, A., Sirigu, A., & Aglioti, S. M. (2010). Racial bias reduces empathic sensory-motor resonance with other-race pain. *Current Biology, 20*, 1018–1022.

Avina, C., & O'Donohue, W. (2002). Sexual harassment and PTSD: Is sexual harassment diagnosable trauma? *Journal of Traumatic Stress, 15*, 69–75.

Bach, P. B., Mirkin, J. N., Oliver, T. K., Azzoli, C. G., Berry, D. A., Brawley, O. W., . . . Detterbeck, F. C. (2012). Benefits and harms of CT Screening for lung cancer. *Journal of the American Medical Association, 307*, 2418–2429.

Badawy, A. A. B., Evans, C. M., & Evans, M. (1982). Production of tolerance and physical dependence in the rat by simple administration of morphine in drinking water. *British Journal of Pharmacology, 75*, 485–491.

Badawy, A. A. B., & Evans, M. (1975). The effects of ethanol on tryptophan pyrrolase activity and their comparison with those of phenobarbitone and morphine. *Advances in Experimental Medical Biology, 59*, 229–251.

Bailey, S., & Williams, R. (2014). Towards partnerships in mental healthcare. *Advances in Psychiatric Treatment*, *20*, 48–51.

Baker, A., Lee, N. K., Claire, M., Lewin, T. J., Grant, T., Pohlman, S., . . . Carr, V. J. (2005), Brief cognitive behavioural interventions for regular amphetamine users: A step in the right direction. *Addiction*, *100*, 367–378.

Baker, R. C., & Kirschenbaum, D. S. (1993). Self-monitoring may be necessary for successful weight control. *Behavior Therapy*, *24*, 377–394.

Bakouri, M., & Staerklé, C. (2015). Coping with structural disadvantage: Overcoming negative effects of perceived barriers through bonding identities. *British Journal of Social Psychology*, *54*, 648–670.

Ball, S. J., Reay, D., & David, M. (2003). Ethnic choosing: Minority ethnic students, social class, and higher education choice. *Race, Ethnicity, and Education*, *5*, 333–357.

Banas, K., Cruwys, T., De Wit, J. B. F., Johnston, M., & Haslam, S. A. (2016). When group members go against the grain: An ironic interactive effect of group identification and normative content on healthy eating. *Appetite*, *105*, 344–355.

Bandura, A. (1982). Self-efficacy mechanism in human agency. *American Psychologist*, *37*, 122–147.

Bandura, A. (1986). *Social foundations of thought and action: A social cognitive theory*. Englewood Cliffs, NJ: Prentice-Hall.

Baray, G., Postmes, T., & Jetten, J. (2009). When "I" equals "We": Exploring the relation between social and personal identity of extreme right-wing political party members. *British Journal of Social Psychology*, *48*, 625–648.

Barber, C. (2009). *Comfortably numb: How psychiatry medicated a nation*. New York, NY: Vintage Books.

Barber, S. J., & Lee, S. R. (2015). Stereotype threat lowers older adults' self-reported hearing abilities. *Gerontology*, *62*, 81–85.

Barlow, J. H., Turner, A. P., & Wright, C. C. (1998). Long-term outcomes of an Arthritis Self-Management Programme. *British Journal of Rheumatology*, *37*, 1315–1319.

Barlow, J. H., Wright, C. C., Sheasby, J., Turner, A. P., & Hainsworth, J. (2002). Self-management approaches for people with chronic conditions: A review. *Patient Education and Counseling*, *48*, 177–187.

Barnes, L. L., Mendes de Leon, C. F., Wilson, R. S., Bienias, J. L., & Evans, D. A. (2004). Social resources and cognitive decline in older African Americans and whites. *Neurology*, *63*, 2322–2326.

Barness, L. A., Opitz, J. M., & Gilbert-Barness, E. (2007). Obesity: Genetic, molecular, and environmental aspects. *American Journal of Medical Genetics Part A*, *143A*, 3016–3034.

Baron, R. S., Burgess, M. L., & Kao, C. F. (1991). Detecting and labeling prejudice: Do female perpetrators go undetected? *Personality and Social Psychology Bulletin*, *17*, 115–123.

Baron-Cohen, S. (2005). The empathizing system: A revision of the 1994 model of the mindreading system. In B. Ellis & D. Bjorklund (Eds.), *Origins of the social mind: Evolutionary psychology and child development* (pp. 468–492). New York, NY: Guildford Press.

Barreto, M. E., Ellemers, N., & Banal, S. (2006). Working under cover: performance-related self-confidence among members of contextually devalued groups who try to pass. *European Journal of Social Psychology*, *36*, 337–352.

Barreto, M. E., Ryan, M. K., & Schmitt, M. T. (2009). *The glass ceiling in the 21st century: Understanding barriers to gender equality*. Washington, D.C.: American Psychological Association.

Bartholomew, R. E., & Wessely, S. (2002). Protean nature of mass sociogenic illness: From possessed nuns to chemical and biological terrorism fears. *The British Journal of Psychiatry*, *180*, 300–306.

Başoğlu, M., Mineka, S., Paker, M., Aker, T., Livanou, M., & Gök, Ş. (1997). Psychological preparedness for trauma as a protective factor in survivors of torture. *Psychological Medicine*, *27*, 1421–1433.

Başoğlu, M., Paker, M., Özmen, E., Taşdemir, Ö., Şahin, D., Ceyhanli, A., . . . Sarimurat, N. (1996). Appraisal of self, social environment, and state authority as a possible mediator of posttraumatic stress disorder in tortured political activists. *Journal of Abnormal Psychology*, *105*, 232–236.

Bassuk, S. S., Glass, T. A., & Berkman, L. F. (1999). Social disengagement and incident cognitive decline in community-dwelling elderly persons. *Annals of Internal Medicine*, *131*, 165–173.

Bastian, B., Jetten, J., & Fasoli, F. (2011). Cleansing the soul by hurting the flesh: The guilt-reducing effect of pain. *Psychological Science*, *22*, 334–335.

Bastian, B., Jetten, J., & Ferris, L. J. (2014a). Pain as social glue shared pain increases cooperation. *Psychological Science, 25*, 2079–2085.

Bastian, B., Jetten, J., & Hornsey, M. J. (2014b). Gustatory pleasure and pain: The offset of acute physical pain enhances responsiveness to taste. *Appetite, 72*, 150–155.

Bastian, B., Jetten, J., Hornsey, M. J., & Leknes, S. (2014c). The positive consequences of pain: A biopsychosocial approach. *Personality and Social Psychology Review, 18*, 256–279.

Bastian, B., Jetten, J., & Stewart, E. (2013). Physical pain and guilty pleasures. *Social Psychological and Personality Science, 4*, 215–219.

Baumann, L. J., Cameron, L. D., Zimmerman, R. S., & Leventhal, H. (1989). Illness representations and matching labels with symptoms. *Health Psychology, 8*, 449–469.

Baxter, A. J., Scott, K. M., Ferrari, A. J., Norman, R. E., Vos, T., & Whiteford, H. A. (2014). Challenging the myth of an "epidemic" of common mental disorders: Trends in the global prevalence of anxiety and depression between 1990 and 2010. *Depression and Anxiety, 31*, 506–516.

BBC News. (2008, June 23). How care home keeps elderly healthy. *BBC News*. Retrieved from http://news.bbc.co.uk/1/hi/7466457.stm

Beadle, E. J., Ownsworth, T., Fleming, J., & Shum, D. (2016). The impact of traumatic brain injury on self-identity. A systematic review of the evidence for self concept changes. *Journal of Head Trauma Rehabilitation, 31*, 12–25.

Beals, K. P., Peplau, L. A., & Gable, S. L. (2009). Stigma management and well-being: The role of perceived social support, emotional processing, and suppression. *Personality and Social Psychology Bulletin, 35*, 867–879.

Beck, A. T. (1964). Thinking and depression II. Theory and therapy. *Archives of General Psychiatry, 10*, 561–571.

Beck, A. T. (1967). *Depression: Clinical, experimental, and theoretical aspects*. New York: Hoeber Medical Division, Harper & Row.

Beck, A. T. (1970). Cognitive therapy: Nature and relation to behavior therapy. *Behavior Therapy, 1*, 184–200.

Beck, A. T. (1979). *Cognitive therapy of depression*. New York, NY: Guilford Press.

Beck, A. T. (2005). The current state of cognitive therapy: A 40-year retrospective. *Archives of General Psychiatry, 62*, 953–959.

Beck, J. G., Grant, D. M., Read, J. P., Clapp, J. D., Coffey, S. F., Miller, L. M., & Palyo, S. A. (2008). The Impact of Event Scale-Revised: Psychometric properties in a sample of motor vehicle accident survivors. *Journal of Anxiety Disorders, 22*, 187–198.

Beck, J. S. (2011). *Cognitive behavior therapy: Basics and beyond* (2nd ed.). New York, NY: Guilford Press.

Becker, A. E. (2004). Television, disordered eating, and young women in Fiji: Negotiating body image and identity during rapid social change. *Culture, Medicine and Psychiatry, 28*, 533–559.

Becker, A. E., Burwell, R. A., Gilman, S. E., Herzog, D. B., & Hamburg, P. (2002). Eating behaviours and attitudes following prolonged exposure to television among ethnic Fijian adolescent girls. *British Journal of Psychiatry, 180*, 509–514.

Beckwith, M., Best, D., Savic, M., Haslam, C., Bathish, R., Dingle, G. A., Mackenzie, J., . . . Lubman, D. I. (2017). *Social Identity Mapping in Recovery (SIM-R): Development and application of a visual method*. Manuscript under review.

Beecher, H. K. (1946). Pain in men wounded in battle. *Annals of Surgery, 123*, 96–105.

Begeny, C. T., & Huo, Y. J. (2016). Is it always good to feel valued? The psychological benefits and costs of higher perceived status in one's ethnic minority group. *Group Processes & Intergroup Relations*. Advance online publication. doi:10.1177/1368430216656922

Bennett, D. A., Schneider, J. A., Tang, Y., Arnold, S. E., & Wilson, R. S. (2006). The effect of social networks on the relation between Alzheimer's disease pathology and level of cognitive function in old people: A longitudinal cohort study. *Lancet Neurology, 5*, 406–412.

Bennett, J. A., Perrin, N. A., Hanson, G., Bennett, D., Gaynor, W., Flaherty-Robb, M., . . . Potemka, K. (2005). Healthy aging demonstration project: Nurse coaching for behavior change in older adults. *Research in Nursing and Health, 28*, 187–197.

Bentall, R. P., De Sousa, P., Varese, F., Wickham, S., Sitko, K., Haarmans, M., & Read, J. (2015). From adversity to psychosis: Pathways and mechanisms from specific adversities to specific symptoms. *Social Psychiatry and Psychiatric Epidemiology, 49*, 1011–1022.

Bentall, R. P., Rouse, G., Kinderman, P., Blackwood, N., Howard, R., Moore, R., Cummins, S., & Corcoran, R. (2008). Paranoid delusions in schizophrenia spectrum disorders and depression. *The Journal of Nervous and Mental Disease, 196*, 375–383.

Ben-Yishay, Y. (1978). *Working approaches to remediation of cognitive deficits in brain damaged persons.* Rehabilitation Monograph. 59. New York, NY: University Medical Center.

Berchicci, M., Lucci, G., & Di Russo, F. (2013). Benefits of physical exercise on the aging brain: the role of the prefrontal cortex. *The Journals of Gerontology Series A: Biological Sciences and Medical Sciences, 68*, 1337–1341.

Berger, J., & Heath, C. (2008). Who drives divergence? Identity signaling, outgroup dissimilarity, and the abandonment of cultural tastes. *Journal of Personality and Social Psychology, 95*, 593–607.

Berger, J., & Rand, L. (2008). Shifting signals to help health: Using identity signaling to reduce risky health behaviors. *Journal of Consumer Research, 35*, 509–518.

Berkman, L. F., & Syme, S. L. (1979). Social networks, host resistance, and mortality: A nine-year follow-up study of Alameda County residents. *American Journal of Epidemiology, 109*, 186–204.

Berrington de Gonzalez, A., & Darby, S. (2004). Risk of cancer from diagnostic x-rays: Estimated for the UK and 14 other countries. *Lancet, 363*, 354–351.

Berry, J. W. (1997). Immigration, acculturation, and adaptation. *Applied Psychology: An International Review, 46*, 5–34.

Berry, J. W., & Sabatier, C. (2010). Acculturation, discrimination, and adaptation among second generation immigrant youth in Montreal and Paris. *International Journal of Intercultural Relations, 34*, 191–207.

Bertschy, K., Skorich, D. P., & Haslam, S. A. (2017). *Self-categorization and Autism: Exploring the relationship between autistic-like traits and ingroup favouritism in the minimal group paradigm.* Unpublished manuscript: University of Queensland.

Best, D. (2016). An unlikely hero? Challenging stigma through community engagement. *Drugs and Alcohol Today, 16*, 106–116.

Best, D., Beckwith, M., Haslam, C., Haslam, S. A., Jetten, J., Mawson, E., & Lubman, D. I. (2016). Overcoming alcohol and other drug addiction as a process of social identity transition: The Social Identity Model Of Recovery (SIMOR). *Addiction Research and Theory, 24*, 111–123.

Best, D., Haslam, C., Staiger, P. K., Dingle, G., Savic, M., Bathish, R., & Alexander, J. (2016). Social Networks and Recovery (SONAR): Characteristics of a longitudinal outcome study in five Therapeutic Communities in Australia. *Therapeutic Communities: The International Journal of Therapeutic Communities, 37*, 131–139.

Best, D., Lubman, D. I., Savic, M., Wilson, A., Dingle, G., Haslam, S. A., Haslam, C., & Jetten, J. (2014). Social and transitional identity: Exploring social networks and their significance in a therapeutic community setting. *Therapeutic Communities: The International Journal of Therapeutic Communities, 35*, 10–20.

Bigelow, H. J. (1850). Dr. Harlow's case of recovery from the passage of an iron bar through the head. *American Journal of the Medical Sciences, 20*, 13–22. [Facsimile provided in Macmillan, 2000].

Birmes, P., Hatton, L., Brunet, A., & Schmitt, L. (2003). Early historical literature for post-traumatic symptomatology. *Stress and Health, 19*, 17–26.

Bisogni, S., Calzolai, M., Olivini, N., Ciofi, D., Mazzoni, N., Caprilli, S., Gonzalez Lopez, J. R., & Festini, F. (2014). Cross-sectional study on differences in pain perception and behavioural distress during venipuncture between Italian and Chinese children. *Pediatric Reports, 6*, 56–60.

Bisson, J. I. (2003). Early interventions following traumatic events. *Psychiatric Annals, 33*, 37–44.

Bisson, J. I., Cosgrove, S., Lewis, C., & Roberts, N. P. (2015). Post-traumatic stress disorder. *British Medical Journal, 351*, h6161.

Bixby, W. R., Spalding, T. W., Haufler, A. J., Deeny, S. P., Mahlow, P. T., Zimmerman, J. B., & Hatfield, B. D. (2007). The unique relation of physical activity to executive function in older men and women. *Medicine and Science in Sports and Exercise, 39*, 1408–1416.

Bizumic, B., Reynolds, K. J., Turner, J. C., Bromhead, D., & Subasic, E. (2009). The role of the group in individual functioning: School identification and the psychological well-being of staff and students. *Applied Psychology, 58*, 171–192.

Bjerregaard, K., Haslam, S. A., Mewse, A., & Morton, T. A. (2015). The shared experience of caring: A study of care-workers' motivations and identifications at work. *Ageing and Society, 37*, 113–138.

Bjerregaard, K., Haslam, S. A., & Morton, T. A. (2016). How identification facilitates effective learning: The evaluation of generic versus localised professionalization training. *International Journal of Training and Development, 20*, 17–37.

Black, W. C. (2000). Overdiagnosis: An underrecognized cause of confusion and harm in cancer screening. *Journal of the National Cancer Institute, 92*, 1280–1282.

Blanchard, D. C., Spencer, R. L., Weiss, S. M., Blanchard, R. J., McEwen, B., & Sakai, R. R. (1995). Visible burrow system as a model of chronic social stress: Behavioural and neuroendocrine correlates. *Psychoneuroendocrinology, 20*, 117–134.

Blanz, M. (1999). Accessibility and fit as determinants of the salience of social categorizations. *European Journal of Social Psychology, 29*, 43–74.

Blascovich, J. (2008). Challenge, threat, and health. In J. Y. Shah & W. L. Gardner (Eds.), *Handbook of motivation science* (pp. 481–493). New York, NY: Guilford Press.

Blascovich, J., & Mendes, W. B. (2000). Challenge and threat appraisals: The role of affective cues. In J. Forgas (Ed.), *Feeling and thinking: The role of affect in social cognition* (pp. 59–82). Cambridge, UK: Cambridge University Press.

Boccia, M. L., Scanlan, J. M., Laudenslager, M. L., Berger, C. L., Hijazi, A. S., & Reite, M. L. (1997). Juvenile friends, behaviour, and immune responses to separation in bonnet marque infants. *Physiology and Behavior, 61*, 191–198.

Bogart, K. R. (2015). Disability identity predicts lower anxiety and depression in multiple sclerosis. *Rehabilitation Psychology, 60*, 105–109.

Bombardier, C., Fann, J. R., Temkin, N. R., Esselman, P. C., Barber, J., & Dikmen, S. S. (2010). Rates of major depressive disorder and clinical outcomes following traumatic brain injury. *Journal of the American Medical Association, 303*, 1938–1945.

Bombay, A., Matheson, K., & Anisman, H. (2011). The impact of stressors on second generation Indian residential school survivors. *Transcultural Psychiatry, 48*, 367–391.

Bombay, A., Matheson, K., & Anisman, H. (2014). Appraisals of discriminatory events among adult offspring of Indian residential school survivors: The influences of identity centrality and past perceptions of discrimination. *Cultural Diversity and Ethnic Minority Psychology, 20*, 75–86.

Booth-Kewley, S., & Friedman, H. S. (1987). Psychological predictors of heart disease: A quantitative review. *Psychological Bulletin, 101*, 343–362.

Bossé, R., Spiro III, A., & Kressin, N. R. (1996). The psychology of retirement. In R. T. Woods (Ed.), *Handbook of the clinical psychology of ageing* (pp. 141–157). Chichester, England: John Wiley & Sons.

Boström, G., Conradsson, M., Hörnsten, C., Rosendahl, E., Lindelöf, N., Holmberg, H., . . . Littbrand, H. (2015). Effects of a high-intensity functional exercise program on depressive symptoms among people with dementia in residential care: A randomized controlled trial. *International Journal of Geriatric Psychiatry, 31*, 868–878.

Bottrell, D. (2007). Resistance, resilience and social identities: Reframing "problem youth" and the "problem of schooling". *Journal of Youth Studies, 10*, 597–616.

Bottrell, D. (2016). Understanding "marginal" perspectives: Towards a social theory of resilience. *Qualitative Social Work, 8*, 321–339.

Bourdieu, P. (1979/1984). *Distinction: A social critique of the judgment of taste* (R. Nice, Trans.). Cambridge, MA: Harvard University Press.

Bourguignon, D., Yzerbyt, V. Y., Teixeira, C. P., & Herman, G. (2015). When does it hurt? Intergroup permeability moderates the link between discrimination and self-esteem. *European Journal of Social Psychology, 45*, 3–9.

Bowe, C. M., Lahey, L., Kegan, R., & Armstrong, E. (2003). Questioning the "big assumptions". Part II: Recognizing organizational contradictions that impede institutional change. *Medical Education, 37*, 723–733.

Bowen, S., Chawla, N., Collins, S. E., Witkiewitz, K., Hsu, S., Grow, J., . . . Marlatt, G. A. (2009). Mindfulness-Based Relapse Prevention for substance use disorders: A pilot efficacy trial. *Substance Abuse, 30*, 295–305.

Bowen, S., Witkiewitz, K., Dillworth, T. M., Chawla, N., Simpson, T. L., Ostafin, B. D., . . . Marlatt, G. A. (2006). Mindfulness meditation and substance use in an incarcerated population. *Psychology of Addictive Behaviors, 20*, 343–347.

Bradbury, C. L., Christensen, B. K., Lau, M. A., Ruttan, L. A., Arandine, A. L., & Green, R. E. (2008). The efficacy of cognitive behavior therapy in the treatment of emotional distress after acquired brain injury. *Archives of Physical Medicine and Rehabilitation, 89*, 61–68.

Brand, R. (2011). We have lost a beautiful, talented woman. *The Guardian*. Retrieved from www.theguardian.com/music/2011/jul/24/russell-brand-amy-winehouse-woman

Branscombe, N. R., & Ellemers, N. (1998). Coping with group-based discrimination: Individualistic versus group-level strategies. In J. K. Swim & C. Stangor (Eds.), *Prejudice: The target's perspective* (pp. 243–266). New York, NY: Academic Press.

Branscombe, N. R., Fernández, S., Gómez, A., & Cronin, T. (2012). Moving toward or away from a group identity: Different strategies for coping with pervasive discrimination. In J. Jetten, C. Haslam, & S. A. Haslam (Eds.), *The social cure: Identity, health and well-being* (pp. 115–131). New York, NY: Psychology Press.

Branscombe, N. R., Schmitt, M. T., & Harvey, R. D. (1999). Perceiving pervasive discrimination among African Americans: Implications for group identification and well-being. *Journal of Personality and Social Psychology, 77*, 135–149.

Branscombe, N. R., & Wann, D. L. (1994). Collective self-esteem consequences of outgroup derogation when a valued social identity is on trial. *European Journal of Social Psychology, 24*, 641–658.

Branscombe, N. R., Wann, D. L., Noel, J. G., & Coleman, J. (1993). Ingroup or outgroup extremity: Importance of the threatened identity. *Personality and Social Psychology Bulletin, 19*, 381–388.

Braveman, P. A., Cubbin, C., Egerter, S., Williams, D. R., & Pamuk, E. (2010). Socio-economic disparities in health in the United States: What the patterns tell us. *American Journal of Public Health, 100*, 186–196.

Breakwell, G. M. (1986). *Coping with threatened identities*. London: Methuen.

Bremner, J. D., Vythilingam, M., Vermetten, E., Southwick, S. M., McGlashan, T., Nazeer, A., . . . Ng, C. K. (2003). MRI and PET study of deficits in hippocampal structure and function in women with childhood sexual abuse and posttraumatic stress disorder. *American Journal of Psychiatry, 160*, 924–932.

Brett, E. A. (1993). Psychoanalytic contributions to a theory of traumatic stress. In *International handbook of traumatic stress syndromes* (pp. 61–68). New York, NY: Springer.

Brewer, M. B., & Silver, M. (1978). Ingroup bias as a function of task characteristics. *European Journal of Social Psychology, 8*, 393–400.

Brewin, C. (2005). Systematic review of screening instruments of adults at risk of PTSD. *Journal of Trauma Stress, 18*, 53–62.

Bridle, C., Riemsma, R. P., Pattenden, J., Sowden, A. J., Mather, L., Watt, I. S., & Walker, A. (2005). Systematic review of the effectiveness of health behavior interventions based on the transtheoretical model. *Psychology and Health, 20*, 283–301.

Britt, T. W., Crane, M., Hodson, S. E., & Adler, A. B. (2016). Effective and ineffective coping strategies in a low-autonomy work environment. *Journal of Occupational Health Psychology, 21*, 154–168.

Brohan, E., Elgie, R., Sartorius, N., & Thornicroft, G. (2010). Self-stigma, empowerment and perceived discrimination among people with schizophrenia in 14 European countries: the GAMIAN-Europe study. *Schizophrenia Research, 122*, 232–238.

Bromberg, P. M. (2003). Something wicked this way comes: Trauma, dissociation, and conflict: The space where psychoanalysis, cognitive science, and neuroscience overlap. *Psychoanalytic Psychology, 20*, 558–574.

Brondolo, E., Libby, D. J., Denton, E., Thompson, S., Beatty, D. L., Schwartz, J., . . . Gerin, W. (2008). Racism and ambulatory blood pressure in a community sample. *Psychosomatic Medicine, 70*, 49–56.

Brondolo, E., Libretti, M., Rivera, L., & Walsemann, K. M. (2012). Racism and social capital: The implications for social and physical well-being. *Journal of Social Issues, 68*, 358–384.

Brook, A. T., Garcia, J., & Fleming, M. A. (2008). The effects of multiple identities on psychological well-being. *Personality and Social Psychology Bulletin, 34*, 1588–1600.

Brotons, C., Björkelund, C., Bulc, M., Ciurana, R., Godycki-Cwirko, M., Jurgova, E., . . . Pullerits, L. (2005). Prevention and health promotion in clinical practice: The views of general practitioners in Europe. *Preventive Medicine, 40*, 595–601.

Brown, G. W. (1985). The discovery of expressed emotion: Induction or deduction? In J. Leff & C. Vaughn (Eds.), *Expressed emotion in families* (pp. 7–25). New York, NY: Guilford Press.

Brown, J. L., Sheffield, D., Leary, M. R., & Robinson, M. E. (2003). Social support and experimental pain. *Psychosomatic Medicine, 65*, 276–283.

Brown, L., Thurecht, L., & Nepal, B. (2012). *The cost of inaction on the social determinants of health*. University of Canberra: National Centre for Social and Economic Modelling (NATSEM).

Brown, T. A., Chorpita, B. F., Korotitsch, W., & Barlow, D. H. (1997). Psychometric properties of the depression, anxiety, stress scales (DASS) in clinical samples. *Behaviour Research Therapy, 135*, 79–89.

Brownlee, S., Chalkidoun, K., Doust, J., Elshaug, A. G., Glasziou, P., Heath, I., . . . Korenstein, D. (2016). Evidence for overuse of medical services around the world. *Lancet, 16*, 1–13.

Brownson, R. C., Haire-Joshu, D., & Luke, D. A. (2006). Shaping the context of health: A review of environmental and policy approaches in the prevention of chronic diseases. *Annual Review of Public Health, 27*, 341–370.

Brownwell, K. D., & Frieden, T. R. (2009). Ounces of prevention – the public policy case for taxes on sugared beverages. *The New England Journal of Medicine, 360*, 1805–1808.

Bruner, J. S. (1957). On perceptual readiness. *Psychological Review, 64*, 123–152.

Bryant, R. A., Nickerson, A., Creamer, M., O'Donnell, M. L., Forbes, D., Galatzer-Levy, I., . . . Silove, D. (2015). Trajectory of post-traumatic stress following traumatic injury: 6-year follow-up. *The British Journal of Psychiatry, 206*, 417–423.

Bryant, R. A., O'Donnel, M. L., Creamer, M., McFarlane, A. C., Clark, C. R., & Silove, D. (2010). The psychiatric sequelae of traumatic injury. *The American Journal of Psychiatry, 167*, 312–320.

Buckingham, S. A., & Best, D. (Eds.). (2017). *Addiction, behavioural change and social identity: The path to resilience and recovery*. London: Routledge.

Buckingham, S. A., Frings, D., & Albery, I. P. (2013). Group membership and social identity in addiction recovery. *Psychology of Addictive Behaviors, 27*, 1132–1140.

Budd, R., & Hughes, I. (2009). The Dodo Bird verdict – controversial, inevitable and important: A commentary on 30 years of meta-analyses. *Clinical Psychology and Psychotherapy, 16*, 510–522.

Bugelli, T., & Crowther, T. R. (2008). Motivational interviewing and the older population in psychiatry. *Psychiatric Bulletin, 32*, 23–25.

Burton, A. K., Tillotson, K. M., Main, C. J., & Hollis, S. (1995). Psychosocial predictors of outcome in acute and subchronic low back trouble. *SPINE, 20*, 722–728.

Burton, E., Stice, E., & Seeley, J. R. (2004). A prospective test of the stress-buffering model of depression in adolescent girls: no support once again. *Journal of Consulting and Clinical Psychology, 72*, 689–697.

Burton, P., Smit, H. J., & Lightowler, H. J. (2007). The influence of restrained and externl eating patterns on overeating. *Appetite, 49*, 191–197.

Busch-Geertsema, V., Edgar, W., O'Sullivan, E., & Pleace, N. (2010). *Homelessness and homeless policies in Europe: Lessons from research*. Brussels: FEANTSA.

Butler, A. C., Chapman, J. E., Forman, E., & Beck, A. T. (2006). The empirical status of cognitive-behavioral therapy: A review of meta-analyses. *Clinical Psychology Review, 26*, 17–31.

Butler, T. (2016). *Investigating and overcoming barriers to seeking intragroup support*. Unpublished PhD thesis. Brisbane, QLD: University of Queensland.

Cacioppo, J. T., & Cacioppo, S. (2014). Social relationships and health: The toxic effects of perceived social isolation. *Social and Personality Psychology Compass, 8*, 58–72.

Cacioppo, J. T., & Hawkley, L. C. (2009). Perceived social isolation and cognition. *Trends in Cognitive Sciences, 13*, 447–454.

Cacioppo, J. T., Hawkley, L. C., & Thisted, R. A. (2010). Perceived social isolation makes me sad: 5-year cross-lagged analyses of loneliness and depressive symptomatology in the Chicago Health, Aging, and Social Relations Study. *Psychology and Aging, 25*, 453–463.

Cacioppo, J. T., & Patrick, W. (2008). *Loneliness: Human nature and the need for social connection.* New York, NY: Norton & Company.

Cacioppo, J. T., Reis, H. T., & Zautra, A. J. (2011). Social resilience: The value of social fitness with an application to the military. *American Psychologist, 66,* 43–51.

Cacioppo, S., Grippo, A. J., London, S., Goossens, L., & Cacioppo, J. T. (2015). Loneliness: Clinical import and interventions. *Perspectives on Psychological Science, 10,* 238–249.

Cahill, H. A. (2001). Male appropriation and medicalization of childbirth: An historical analysis. *Journal of Advanced Nursing, 33,* 334–342.

Calabrese, J. R., Fatemi, S. H., Kujawa, M., & Woyshville, M. J. (1996). Predictors of response to mood stabilizers. *Journal of Clinical Psychopharmacology, 16,* 24–31.

Camp, D. L., Finlay, W. M. L., & Lyons, E. (2002). Is low self-esteem an inevitable consequence of stigma? An example from women with chronic mental health problems. *Social Science and Medicine, 55,* 823–834.

Campbell, A. (1987). Self definition by rejection: The case of gang girls. *Social Problems, 34,* 451–466.

Campbell, F. K. (2009). *Counters of ableism: The production of disability and abledness.* London: Palgrave Macmillan.

Campbell, J. D., Trapnell, P. D., Heine, S. J., Katz, I. M., Lavallee, L. F., & Lehman, D. R. (1996). Self-concept clarity: Measurement, personality correlates, and cultural boundaries. *Journal of Personality and Social Psychology, 70,* 141–156.

Canadian Psychiatric Association. (2005). Clinical practice guidelines: Treatment of schizophrenia. *The Canadian Journal of Psychiatry, 50,* 7–57.

Cantor-Graae, E., & Selten, J. P. (2005). Schizophrenia and migration: A meta-analysis and review. *American Journal of Psychiatry, 162,* 12–24.

Cantril, H. (1965). *The pattern of human concerns.* New Brunswick, NJ: Rutgers University Press.

Caplan, B., Bogner, J., Brenner, L., Beadle, E. J., Ownsworth, T., Fleming, J., & Shum, D. (2016). The impact of traumatic brain injury on self-identity: A systematic review of the evidence for self-concept changes. *Journal of Head Trauma Rehabilitation, 31,* 12–25.

Caporael, L. R., & Brewer, M. B. (1995). Hierarchical evolutionary theory: There is an alternative, and it's not creationism. *Psychological Inquiry, 6,* 31–34.

Care Quality Commission. (2011). *Dignity and nutrition inspection programme: National overview.* Newcastle upon Tyne: Care Quality Commission.

Carmeliet, P. (2005). Angiogenesis in life, disease and medicine. *Nature, 438,* 932–936.

Carroll, E., & Coetzer, R. (2011). Identity, grief, and self-awareness after traumatic brain injury. *Neuropsychological Rehabilitation, 21,* 289–305.

Carroll, L. (1916). *Alice's adventures in wonderland.* New York, NY: Samuel Gabriel Sons & Company.

Carter, H., Drury, J., Rubin, G. J., Williams, R., & Amlôt, R. (2015). Applying crowd psychology to develop recommendations for the management of mass decontamination. *Health Security, 13,* 45–53.

Cartwright, S., & Cooper, C. L. (1997). *Managing workplace stress.* Thousand Oaks, CA: Sage.

Carver, C. S. (1995). Stress and coping. In A. S. R. Manstead & M. R. C. Hewstone (Eds.), *The Blackwell encyclopedia of social psychology* (pp. 635–639). Oxford: Blackwell.

Cassel, C. K., & Guest, J. A. (2012). Choosing wisely. *The Journal of the American Medical Association, 307,* 1801–1802.

Cassin, S. E., & Von Ranson, K. M. (2005). Personality and eating disorders: A decade in review. *Clinical Psychology Review, 25,* 895–916.

Cattan, M., & White, M. (1998). Developing evidence based health promotion for older people: A systematic review and survey of health promotion interventions targeting social isolation and loneliness among older people. *Internet Journal Health Promotion, 13,* 1–9.

Cattan, M., White, M., Bond, J., & Learmouth, A. (2005). Preventing social isolation and loneliness among older people: A systematic review of health promotion interventions. *Ageing and Society, 25,* 41–67.

CDC National Center for Injury Prevention and Control. (2015). *Suicide facts at a glance 2015.* Retrieved from www.cdc.gov/violenceprevention/pdf/suicide-datasheet-a.pdf

Centre for Sport and Social Impact. (2015). *Value of a community football club.* AFL Victoria and Centre for Sport and Social Impact (LaTrobe). Retrieved from http://apo.org.au/node/53348

Chalk, H. M. (2015). Disability self-categorization in emerging adults. *Emerging Adulthood, 4*, 200–206.

Chamberlain, C., & MacKenzie, D. (2006). Homeless careers: A framework for intervention. *Australian Social Work, 59*, 198–212.

Chandler, M. J., & Lalonde, C. E. (1998). Cultural continuity as a hedge against suicide in Canada's First Nations. *Transnational Psychiatry, 35*, 191–219.

Chandler, M. J., & Lalonde, C. E. (2008). Cultural continuity as a protective factor against suicide in First Nations youth. *Horizons, 10*, 68–72.

Chandler, M. J., Lalonde, C. E., Sokol, B. W., & Hallett, D. (2003). Personal persistence, identity development, and suicide: A study of native and non-native North American adolescents. *Monographs of the Society for Research in Child Development, 68*, 1–138.

Chang, M. X-L., Jetten, J., Cruwys, T., & Haslam, C. (2017). Cultural identity and the expression of depression: A social identity perspective. *Journal of Community and Applied Social Psychology, 27*, 16–34.

Chang, M. X-L., Jetten, J., Cruwys, T., Haslam, C., & Praharso, N. (2016). The more (social group memberships) the merrier: Is this the case for Asians? *Frontiers in Psychology, 7*. doi:10.3389/fpsyg.2016.01001

Chatzisarantis, N. L. D., & Hagger, M. S. (2005). Effects of a brief intervention based on the theory of planned behavior on leisure-time physical activity participation. *Journal of Sport and Exercise Psychology, 27*, 470–487.

Chaudhury, S., Pande, V., Saini, R., & Rathee, S. P. (2005). Neuropsychiatric sequelae of head injury. *Indian Journal of Neurotrauma, 2*, 13–21.

Chida, Y., & Steptoe, A. (2009). The association of anger and hostility with future coronary heart disease: A meta-analytic review of prospective evidence. *Journal of the American College of Cardiology, 53*, 936–946.

Chrousos, G. P. (2009). Stress and disorders of the stress system. *Nature Reviews. Endocrinology, 5*, 374–381.

Cicerone, K. D., Langenbahn, D. M., Braddon, C., Malec, J. F., Kalmar, K., Fraas, M., . . . Ashman, T. (2011). Evidence-based cognitive rehabilitation: Updated review of the literature from 2003 through 2008. *Archives of Physical Medicine and Rehabilitation, 89*, 2239–2249.

Cieza, A., Anczewska, M., Ayuso-Mateos, J. L., Baker, M., Bickenbach, J., Chatterji, S., . . . PARADISE Consortium. (2015). Understanding the impact of brain disorders: towards a "horizontal epidemiology" of psychosocial difficulties and their determinants. *PLoS ONE, 10*(9), e0136271.

Cikara, M., & Van Bavel, J. J. (2014). The neuroscience of intergroup relations: An integrative review. *Perspectives in Psychological Science, 9*, 245–274.

Cikara, M., & Fiske, S. T. (2011). Bounded empathy: Neural responses to outgroup targets' (mis)fortunes. *Journal of Cognitive Neuroscience, 23*, 3791–3803.

Clare, L., Rowlands, J. M., & Quin, R. (2008). Collective strength: The impact of developing a shared social identity in early-stage dementia. *Dementia, 7*, 9–30.

Clarke, P. J., Marshall, V. W., Black, S. E., & Colantonio, A. (2002). Well-being following stroke in Canadian seniors: Findings from the Canadian study of health and aging. *Stroke, 33*, 1016–1021.

Clayton, P. J., & Darvish, H. S. (1979). Course of depressive symptoms following the stress of bereavement. In J. D. Barrett (Ed.), *Stress and Mental Disorder*, (pp. 121–136) New York: Raven Press.

Clement, S., Schauman, O., Graham, T., Maggioni, F., Evans-Lacko, S., Bezborodovs, N., . . . Thornicroft, G. (2015). What is the impact of mental health-related stigma on help-seeking? A systematic review of quantitative and qualitative studies. *Psychological Medicine, 45*, 11–27.

Clingingsmith, D., Khwaja, D., & Kremer, M. (2009). Estimating the impact of the Hajj: Religion and tolerance in Islam's global gathering. *The Quarterly Journal of Economics, 124*, 1133–1170.

Cloitre, M., Courtois, C. A., Charuvastra, A., Carapezza, R., Stolbach, B. C., & Green, B. L. (2011). Treatment of complex PTSD: Results of the ISTSS expert clinician survey on best practices. *Journal of Traumatic Stress, 24*, 615–627.

Cockell, S. J., Hewitt, P. L., Seal, B., Sherry, S., Goldner, E. M., Flett, G. L., & Remick, R. A. (2002). Trait and self-presentational dimensions of perfectionism among women with anorexia nervosa. *Cognitive Therapy and Research, 26*, 745–758.

Cocking, C., & Drury, J. (2004). Generalization of efficacy as a function of collective action and intergroup relations: Involvement in an anti-roads struggle. *Journal of Applied Social Psychology, 34*, 417–444.

Cogan, R., & Spinnato, J. A. (1988). Social support during premature labor: Effects on labor and the newborn. *Journal of Psychosomatic Obstetrics and Gynecology, 8*, 209–216.

Cohen, J. (1980). Structural consequences of psychic trauma: A new look at "Beyond the Pleasure Principle". *International Journal of Psycho-Analysis, 61*, 421–432.

Cohen, R., Bavishi, C., & Rozanski, A. (2016). Purpose in life and its relationship to all-cause mortality and cardiovascular events: A meta- analysis. *Psychosomatic Medicine, 78*, 122–133.

Cohen, S., Doyle, W. J., Turner, R., Alper, C. M., & Skoner, D. P. (2003). Sociability and susceptibility to the common cold. *Psychological Science, 14*, 389–395.

Cohen, S., & Janicki-Deverts, D. (2009). Can we improve our physical health by altering our social networks? *Perspectives on Psychological Science, 4*, 375–378.

Cohen, S., & Wills, T. A. (1985). Stress, social support and the buffering hypothesis. *Psychological Bulletin, 98*, 310–357.

Colcombe, S., & Kramer, A. F. (2003). Fitness effects on the cognitive function of older adults. *Psychological Science, 14*, 125–130.

Cole, B., Matheson, K., & Anisman, H. (2007). Academic performance and well-being: The moderating role of ethnic identity and social support. *Journal of Applied Social Psychology, 37*, 592–615.

Cole, S. W. (2013). Social regulation of human gene expression: Mechanisms and implications for public health. *American Journal of Public Health, 103*, 84–92.

Cole, S. W., Hawkley, L. C., Arevalo, J. M., & Cacioppo, J. T. (2011). Transcript origin analysis identifies antigen-presenting cells as primary targets of socially regulated gene expression in leukocytes. *Proceedings of the National Academy of Sciences, 108*, 3080–3085.

Cole, S. W., Hawkley, L. C., Arevalo, J. M., Sung, C. Y., Rose, R. M., & Cacioppo, J. T. (2007). Social regulation of gene expression in human leukocytes. *Genome Biology, 8*, R189.

Cole, S. W., Kemeny, M. E., & Taylor, S. E. (1997). Social identity and physical health: Accelerated HIV progression in rejection-sensitive gay men. *Journal of Personality and Social Psychology, 72*, 320–335.

Cole, S. W., Kemeny, M. E., Taylor, S. E., & Visscher, B. R. (1996). Elevated physical health risk among gay men who conceal their homosexual identity. *Health Psychology, 15*, 243–251.

Collicutt-McGrath, J., & Linley, P. A. (2006). Post-traumatic growth in acquired brain injury: A preliminary small scale study. *Brain Injury, 20*, 767–773.

Colville, G., & Cream, P. (2009). Post-traumatic growth in parents after a child's admission to intensive care: Maybe Nietzsche was right? *Intensive Care Medicine, 35*, 919–923.

Comer, L. K., Henker, B., Kemeny, M., & Wyatt, G. (2000). Illness disclosure and mental health among women with HIV/AIDS. *Journal of Community and Applied Social Psychology, 10*, 449–464.

Compton, M. T., & Shim, R. S. (2015). *The social determinants of mental health.* Arlington, VA: American Psychiatric Association Publishing.

Conger, J. C., Conger, A. J., Costanzo, P. R., Wright, K. L., & Matter, J. A. (1980). The effect of social cues on the eating behavior of obese and normal subjects. *Journal of Personality, 48*, 258–271.

Conner, K. O., Copeland, V. C., Grote, N. K., Koeske, G., Rosen, D., Reynolds, C. F., & Brown, C. (2010). Mental health treatment seeking among older adults with depression: The impact of stigma and race. *The American Journal of Geriatric Psychiatry, 18*, 531–543.

Connor, J. P., Young, R. M., Lawford, B. R., Saunders, J. B., Ritchie, T. L., & Noble, E. P. (2007). Heavy nicotine and alcohol use in alcohol dependence is associated with D2 dopamine receptor (DRD2) polymorphism. *Addictive Behaviors, 32*, 310–319.

Conrad, J. (1899/1999). *Lord Jim.* New York, NY: Dover Books.

Conrad, P. (1994). Wellness as virtue: Morality and the pursuit of health. *Culture, Medicine and Psychiatry, 18*, 385–401.

Conrod, P. J., Castellanos-Ryan, N., & Strang, J. (2010). Brief, personality-targeted coping skills interventions and survival as a non-drug user over a 2-year period during adolescence. *Archives of General Psychiatry, 67*, 85–93.

Coombs, T. (2005). *Australian mental health outcomes and classification network; Kessler – 10 training manual.* Sydney: NSW Institute of Psychiatry.

Cooper, C. L. (1995, February 24). Your place in the stress league. *The Sunday Times.*

Cooper, C. L., Dewe, P. J., & O'Driscoll, M. P. (2001). *Organizational stress: A review and critique of theory, research and applications.* London: Sage.

Cooper, J., Gracey, F., Malley, D., Deakins, J., & Prince, L. (2010). Integrating "doing" and "meaning" in rehabilitation: A case example. In C. Bowen, G. Yeates, & S. Palmer (Eds.), *A relational approach to rehabilitation: Thinking about relationships after brain injury* (pp. 231–256). London: Karna Books.

Cooper, L. A., Gonzales, J. J., Gallo, J. J., Rost, K. M., Meredith, L. S., Rubenstein, L. V., . . . Ford, D. E. (2003). The acceptability of treatment for depression among African-American, Hispanic, and White primary care patients. *Medical Care, 41,* 479–489.

Cooper, M. L., Russell, M., Skinner, J. B., & Windle, M. (1992). Development and validation of a three-dimensional measure of drinking motives. *Psychological Assessment, 4,* 123–132.

Cordain, L., Eaton, S. B., Sebastian, A., Mann, N., Lindeberg, S., Watkins, B. A., . . . Brand-Miller, J. (2005). Origins and evolution of the Western diet: Health implications for the 21st century. *American Journal of Clinical Nutrition, 81,* 341–354.

Cordes, R. J., & Ryan, M. E. (1995). Pitfalls in HIV testing. Application and limitations of current tests. *Postgraduate Medicine, 98,* 177–180.

Cordle, D. (2012). Protect/protest: British nuclear fiction of the 1980s. *The British Journal for the History of Science, 45,* 653–669.

Cornwell, E. Y., & Waite, L. J. (2009). Social disconnectedness, perceived isolation, and health among older adults. *Journal of Health and Social Behavior, 50,* 31–48.

Corrigan, P. W. (2004). How stigma interferes with mental health care. *American Psychologist, 59,* 614–625.

Corrigan, P. W., Lurie, B. D., Goldman, H. H., Slopen, N., Medasani, K., & Phelan, S. (2005). How adolescents perceive the stigma of mental illness and alcohol abuse. *Psychiatric Services, 56,* 544–550.

Corrigan, P. W., Michaels, P. J., Vega, E., Gause, M., Watson, A. C., & Rüsch, N. (2012). Self-stigma of mental illness scale – short form: Reliability and validity. *Psychiatry Research, 199,* 65–69.

Corrigan, P. W., Rafacz, J., & Rüsch, N. (2011). Examining a progressive model of self-stigma and its impact on people with serious mental illness. *Psychiatry Research, 189,* 339–343.

Corrigan, P. W., & Watson, A. C. (2006). The paradox of self-stigma and mental illness. *Clinical Psychology: Science and Practice, 9,* 35–53.

Corrigan, P. W., Watson, A. C., & Barr, L. (2006). The self-stigma of mental illness: Implications for self-esteem and self-efficacy. *Journal of Social and Clinical Psychology, 25,* 875–884.

Cox, B. J., Enns, M. W., Borger, S. C., & Parker, J. D. (1999). The nature of the depressive experience in analogue and clinically depressed samples. *Behaviour Research and Therapy, 37,* 15–24.

Coyne, S. M., Nelson, D. A., Robinson, S. L., & Gundersen, N. C. (2011). Is viewing ostracism on television distressing? *The Journal of Social Psychology, 151,* 213–217.

Crabtree, J. W., Haslam, S. A., Postmes, T., & Haslam, C. (2010). Mental health support groups, stigma and self-esteem: Positive and negative implications of group identification. *Journal of Social Issues, 66,* 553–569.

Crandall, C. S. (1994). Prejudice against fat people: Ideology and self-interest. *Journal of Personality and Social Psychology, 66,* 882–894.

Crandall, C. S., Eshleman, A., & O'Brien, L. (2002). Social norms and the expression and suppression of prejudice: The struggle for internalization. *Journal of Personality and Social Psychology, 82,* 359–378.

Crandall, C. S., Nierman, A., & Hebl, M. (2009). Anti-fat prejudice. In T. D. Nelson (Ed.), *Handbook of prejudice, stereotyping, and discrimination* (pp. 469–488). New York, NY: Psychology Press.

Crawford, J. R., & Henry, J. D. (2004). The Positive and Negative Affect Schedule (PANAS): Construct validity, measurement properties and normative data in a large non-clinical sample. *British Journal of Clinical Psychology, 43,* 245–265.

Creamer, M., Bell, R., & Failla, S. (2003). Psychometric properties of the Impact of Event Scale – Revised. *Behaviour Research and Therapy, 41,* 1489–1496.

Creel, S. (2001). Social dominance and stress hormones. *Trends in Ecology and Evolution, 16,* 491–497.

Crocker, J., & Luhtanen, R. (1990). Collective self-esteem and ingroup bias. *Journal of Personality and Social Psychology, 58*, 60–67.

Crocker, J., Major, B., & Steel, C. (1998). Social stigma. In D. Gilbert, S. T. Fiske, & G. Lindzey (Eds.), *Handbook of social psychology* (4th ed., pp. 504–553). Boston: McGraw-Hill.

Crombez, G., Vlaeyen, J. W. S., Heuts, P. H. T. G., & Lysens, R. (1999). Pain-related fear is more disabling than pain itself: Evidence on the role of pain-related fear in chronic back pain disability. *Pain, 80*, 329–339.

Crow, T. J. (1986). The continuum of psychosis and its implications for the structure of the gene. *British Journal of Psychiatry, 149*, 419–429.

Cruwys, T., Berry, H. L., Cassells, R., Duncan, A., O'Brien, L., Sage, B., & D'Souza, G. (2013a). *Marginalised Australians: Characteristics and predictors of exit over ten years 2001–2010*. Canberra: University of Canberra.

Cruwys, T., Bevelander, K. E., & Hermans, R. C. J. (2015). Social modeling of eating: A review of when and why social influence affects food intake and choice. *Appetite, 86*, 3–18.

Cruwys, T., Dingle, G. A., Haslam, C., Haslam, S. A., Jetten, J., & Morton, T. A. (2013b). Social group memberships protect against future depression, alleviate depression symptoms and prevent depression relapse. *Social Science and Medicine, 98*, 179–186.

Cruwys, T., Dingle, G. A., Hornsey, M. J., Jetten, J., Oei, T. P. S., & Walter, Z. C. (2014a). Social isolation schema responds to positive social experiences: Longitudinal evidence from vulnerable populations. *British Journal of Clinical Psychology, 53*, 265–280.

Cruwys, T., & Gunaseelan, S. (2016). "Depression is who I am": Mental illness identity, stigma and wellbeing. *Journal of Affective Disorders, 189*, 36–42.

Cruwys, T., Haslam, S. A., Dingle, G. A., Haslam, C., & Jetten, J., (2014). Depression and Social Identity: An integrative review. *Personality and Social Psychology Review, 18*, 215–238.

Cruwys, T., Haslam, S. A., Dingle, G. A., Jetten, J., Hornsey, M. J., Chong, E. M., & Oei, T. P. S. (2014c). Feeling connected again: Interventions that increase social identification reduce depression symptoms in community and clinical settings. *Journal of Affective Disorders, 159*, 139–146.

Cruwys, T., Haslam, S. A., Fox, N. E., & McMahon, H. (2015). "That's not what we do": Evidence that normative change is a mechanism of action in group interventions. *Behaviour Research and Therapy, 65*, 11–17.

Cruwys, T., Leverington, C. T., & Sheldon, A. M. (2016). An experimental investigation of the consequences and social functions of fat talk in friendship groups. *International Journal of Eating Disorders, 49*, 84–91.

Cruwys, T., Lizzio-Wilson, M., & Jetten, J. (2017). *Groups on my mind: Salience of group memberships reduces aggression following social rejection*. Unpublished Manuscript, University of Queensland.

Cruwys, T., & O'Kearney, R. (2008). Implications of neuroscientific evidence for the cognitive models of post-traumatic stress disorder. *Clinical Psychologist, 12*, 67–76.

Cruwys, T., Platow, M. J., Angullia, S. A., Chang, J. M., Diler, S. E., Kirchner, J. L., . . . Wadley, A. L. (2012). Modeling of food intake is moderated by salient psychological group membership. *Appetite, 58*, 754–757.

Cruwys, T., Platow, M. J., Reiger, E., & Byrne, D. G. (2013). The development and validation of the Dieting Intentions Scale. *Psychological Assessment, 25*, 264–278.

Cruwys, T., Platow, M. J., Rieger, E., Byrne, D. G., & Haslam, S. A. (2016). The social psychology of disordered eating: The Situated Identity Enactment model. *European Review of Social Psychology, 27*, 160–195.

Cruwys, T., South, E. I., Greenaway, K. H., & Haslam, S. A. (2015). Social identity reduces depression by fostering positive attributions. *Social Psychological and Personality Science, 6*, 65–74.

Cruwys, T., Steffens, N. K., Haslam, S. A., Haslam, C., Jetten, J., & Dingle, G. A. (2016). Social identity mapping: A procedure for visual representation and assessment of subjective multiple group memberships. *British Journal of Social Psychology, 55*, 613–642.

Cruwys, T., Wakefield, J. R. H., Sani, F., Dingle, G. A., & Jetten, J. (in press). A doctor a day keeps loneliness at bay? Social isolation, health status, and frequent attendance in primary care. *Annals of Behavioral Medicine*.

Cuddy, A. J., Norton, M. I., & Fiske, S. T. (2005). This old stereotype: The pervasiveness and persistence of the elderly stereotype. *Journal of Social Issues, 61*, 267–285.

Cuevas, A. G., O'Brien, K., & Saha, S. (2016). African American experiences in healthcare: "I always feel like I'm getting skipped over". *Health Psychology, 35*, 987–995.

Cuijpers, P., Geraedts, A. S., Oppen, P. Van, Andersson, G., Markowitz, J. C., & Van Straten, A. (2011). Interpersonal psychotherapy for depression: A meta-analysis. *American Journal of Psychiatry, 168*, 581–592.

Cuijpers, P., Van Straten, A., & Warmerdam, L. (2007). Behavioral activation treatments of depression: A meta-analysis. *Clinical Psychology Review, 27*, 318–326.

Cukor, D., & McGinn, L. (2006). History of child abuse and severity of adult depression: The mediating role of cognitive schema history of child abuse and severity of adult depression. *Journal of Child Sexual Abuse, 15*, 19–34.

Cusack, K., Jonas, D. E., Forneris, C. A., Wines, C., Sonis, J., Middleton, J. C., . . . Weil, A. (2016). Psychological treatments for adults with posttraumatic stress disorder: A systematic review and meta-analysis. *Clinical Psychology Review, 43*, 128–141.

Cusamano, D. L., & Thompson, J. K. (1999). Sociocultural theory: The media and society. In J. K. Thompson, L. J. Heinberg, M. Altabe, & S. Tantleff-Dunn (Eds.), *Exacting beauty: Theory, assessment, and treatment of body image disturbance* (pp. 85–124). Washington, DC: American Psychological Association.

Dai, W., Chen, L., Lai, Z., Li, Y., Wang, J., & Liu, A. (2016). The incidence of post-traumatic stress disorder among survivors after earthquakes: a systematic review and meta-analysis. *BMC Psychiatry, 16*, 188.

Danaher, K., & Branscombe, N. R. (2010). Maintaining the system with tokenism: bolstering individual mobility beliefs and identification with a discriminatory organization. *British Journal of Social Psychology, 49*, 343–362.

Dao, T. T., & LeResche, L. (2000). Gender differences in pain. *Journal of Orofacial Pain, 14*, 169–184.

Darby, A., Hay, P. J., Mond, J. M., Quirk, F., Buttner, P., & Kennedy, L. (2009). The rising prevalence of comorbid obesity and eating disorder behaviours from 1995 to 2005. *International Journal of Eating Disorders, 42*, 104–108.

Darkes, J., & Goldman, M. S. (1998). Expectancy challenge and drinking reduction: Process and structure in the alcohol expectancy network. *Experimental and Clinical Psychopharmacology, 6*, 64–76.

Dar-Nimrod, I., & Heine, S. J. (2011). Genetic essentialism: on the deceptive determinism of DNA. *Psychological Bulletin, 137*, 800–818.

Davidson, K. W., Goldstein, M., Kaplan, R. M., Kaufmann, P. G., Knatterud, G. L., Orleans, C. T., . . . Whitlock, E. P. (2003). Evidence-based behavioral medicine: What is it and how do we achieve it? *Annals of Behavioral Medicine, 26*, 161–171.

Davies, C., & Neal, M. (2000). Durkheim's altruistic and fatalistic suicide. In W. S. F. Pickering & G. Valford (Eds.), *Durkheim's suicide: A century of research and debate* (pp. 36–52). London: Routledge.

Dawe, S., & Loxton, N. J. (2004). The role of impulsivity in the development of substance use and eating disorders. *Neuroscience and Biobehavioral Reviews, 28*, 343–351.

Dax, E. C. (1961). *From asylum to community: The development of the mental hygiene service in Victoria, Australia.* Melbourne: F.W. Cheshire, for the World Federation for Mental Health.

Day, M. A. (2017). Pain and its optimal management. In J. Dorrian, E. Thorsteinsson, M. DiBenedetto, K. Lane-Krebs, M. Day, A. Hutchinson, & K. Sharman (Eds.), *Health psychology in Australia* (pp. 261–281). Cambridge: Cambridge University Press.

Day, M. A., Jensen, M. P., Ehde, D. M., & Thorn, B. E. (2014). Toward a theoretical model for mindfulness-based pain management. *The Journal of Pain, 15*, 691–703.

Dayan, E., & Bar-Hillel, M. (2011). Nudge to nobesity II: Menu positions influence food orders. *Judgement and Decision Making, 6*, 333–342.

De Geus, B., De Bourdeaudhuij, I., Jannes, C., & Meeusen, R. (2008). Psychosocial and environmental factors associated with cycling for transport among a working population. *Health Education Research, 23*, 697–708.

De Leon, G. (2000). *The therapeutic community: Theory, model and method.* New York, NY: Springer.

De Mello, M. F., Mari, J. D. J., Bacaltchuk, J., Verdeli, H., & Neugebauer, R. (2005). A systematic review of research findings on the efficacy of interpersonal therapy for depressive disorders. *European Archives of Psychiatry and Clinical Neuroscience, 255*, 75–82.

De Nooy, J. (2016). Distant (be)longings: Contemporary Australian memoirs of life in France. *Australian Journal of French Studies, 53*, 39–52.

Deacon, B. J. (2013). The biomedical model of mental disorder: A critical analysis of its validity, utility, and effects on psychotherapy research. *Clinical Psychology Review, 33*, 846–861.

Degeneffe, C. E. (2001). Family caregiving and traumatic brain injury. *Health and Social Work, 26*, 257–268.

Degenhardt, L., Mattick, R. P., & Gibson, A. (2009). Opioid dependence and management. In R. P. Mattick, R. Ali, & N. Lintzeris (Eds.), *Pharmacotherapies for the treatment of opioid dependence: Efficacy, cost-effectiveness and implementation guidelines* (pp. 1–14). Boca Raton, Florida: CRC Press.

Delahanty, D. L., Nugent, N. R., Christopher, N. C., & Walsh, M. (2005). Initial urinary epinephrine and cortisol levels predict acute PTSD symptoms in child trauma victims. *Psychoneuroendocrinology, 30*, 121–128.

Department of Health (UK). (2014). *Closing the gap: Priorities for essential change in mental health.* London: Social Care, Local Government and Care Partnership Directorate.

DePaulo, B. M., & Morris, W. L. (2006). The unrecognised stereotyping and discrimination against singles. *Current Directions in Psychological Science, 15*, 251–254.

Dermatis, H., Salke, M., Galanter, M., & Bunt, G. (2001). The role of social cohesion among residents in a therapeutic community, *Journal of Substance Abuse Treatment, 21*, 105–110.

DeSalvo, K. B., Bloser, N., Reynolds, K., He, J., & Muntner, P. (2006). Mortality prediction with a single general self-rated health question. *Journal of General Internal Medicine, 21*, 267–275.

DeSalvo, K. B., Fisher, W. P., Tran, K., Bloser, N., Merrill, W., & Peabody, J. (2006). Assessing measurement properties of two single-item general health measures. *Quality of Life Research, 15*, 191–201.

Descartes, R (1164/1972). Traité de l'homme (*Treatise of man*) T. S. Hall (trans.). Cambridge, MA: Harvard University Press.

Detweiler-Bedell, J. B., Friedman, M. A., Leventhal, H., Miller, I. W., & Leventhal, E. A. (2008). Integrating co-morbid depression and chronic physical disease management: Identifying and resolving failures in self-regulation. *Clinical Psychology Review, 28*, 1426–1446.

DeWall, C. N., Twenge, J. M., Bushman, B., Im, C., & Williams, K. (2010). A little acceptance goes a long way: Applying social impact theory to the rejection aggression link. *Social Psychological and Personality Science, 1*, 168–174.

Dhalla, I. A., Mamdani, M. M., Sivilotti, M. L. A., Kopp, A., Qureshi, O., & Juurlink, D. N. (2009). Prescribing of opioid analgesics and related mortality before and after the introduction of long-acting oxycodone. *Canadian Medical Association Journal, 181*, 891–896.

Dickens, A. P., Richards, S. H., Greaves, C. J., & Campbell, J. L. (2011). Interventions targeting social isolation in older people: A systematic review. *BMC Public Health, 11*, 647–668.

Dickerson, S. S., Gruenewald, T. L., & Kemeny, M. E. (2004). When the social self is threatened: Shame, physiology, and health. *Journal of Personality, 72*, 1191–1216.

Diener, E., & Diener, C. (1996). Most people are happy. *Psychological Science, 7*, 181–185.

Diener, E., Emmons, R. A., Larsen, R. J., & Griffin, S. (1985). The satisfaction with Life Scale. *Personality Assessment, 49*, 71–75.

Diener, E., Lucas, R., Schimmack, U., & Helliwell, J. F. (2009). *Well-Being for public policy.* New York and Oxford: Oxford University Press.

Diener, E., Ng, W., Harter, J., & Arora, R. (2010). Wealth and happiness across the world: Material prosperity predicts life evaluation, whereas psychosocial prosperity predicts positive feeling. *Journal of Personality and Social Psychology, 99*, 52–61.

Diller, L. (1976). A model for cognitive retraining in rehabilitation. *Clinical Psychologist, 29*, 13–15.

Dingle, G. A., Brander, C., Ballantyne, J., & Baker, F. A. (2013). "To be heard": The social and mental health benefits of choir singing for disadvantaged adults. *Psychology of Music, 41*, 405–421.

Dingle, G. A., Cruwys, T., & Frings, D. (2015). Social identities as pathways into and out of addiction. *Frontiers in Psychology, 6*. doi:10.3389/fpsyg.2015.01795

Dingle, G. A., Cruwys, T., Jetten, J., Johnstone, M., & Walter, Z. (2014). The benefits of participation in recreational group activities for adults at risk of homelessness. *Parity, 27*, 18–19.

Dingle, G. A., Stark, C., Cruwys, T., & Best, D. (2015) Breaking good: breaking ties with social groups may be good for recovery from substance misuse. *British Journal of Social Psychology, 54*, 236–254.

Dingle, G. A., Williams, E., Jetten, J., & Welch, J. (2017). Choir singing and creative writing enhance effective emotion regulation. *British Journal of Clinical Psychology*. Advance online publication.

Dingle, G. A., Williams, E., Sharman, L., & Jetten, J. (2016). *School of hard knocks QLD: Final evaluation report*. Brisbane: School of Psychology, The University of Queensland.

Dinos, D., Stevens, S., Serfaty, M., Weich, S., & King, M. (2004). Stigma: the feelings and experiences of 46 people with mental illness. *The British Journal of Psychiatry, 184*, 176–181.

Dionigi, R. A. (2015). Stereotypes of aging: Their effects on the health of older adults. *Journal of Geriatrics*. Article ID 954027. http://dx.doi.org/10.1155/2015/954027.

Discerning History. (2013). *Shackleton's ad: Men wanted for hazardous journey*. Retrieved from http://discerninghistory.com/2013/05/shackletons-ad-men-wanted-for-hazerdous-journey/

Dittmar, H., Halliwell, E., & Ive, S. (2006). Does Barbie make girls want to be thin? The effect of experimental exposure to images of dolls on the body image of 5- to 8-year-old girls. *Developmental Psychology, 42*, 283–292.

Dittmar, H., Halliwell, E., & Stirling, E. (2009). Understanding the impact of thin media models on women's body-focused affect: The roles of thin-ideal internalisation and weight-related self-discrepancy activation in experimental exposure effects. *Journal of Social and Clinical Psychology, 28*, 43–72.

Dixon, J., & Broom, D. H. (2007). *The seven deadly sins of obesity: How the modern world is making us fat*. Sydney: UNSW Press.

Dixon, J., Durrheim, K., Thomae, N., Tredoux, C., Kerr, P., & Quayle, M. (2015). Divide and rule, unite and resist: Contact, collective action and policy attitudes among historically disadvantaged groups. *Journal of Social Issues, 71*, 576–596.

Dohrenwend, B. P. (2006). Inventorying stressful life events as risk factors for psychopathology: Toward resolution of the problem of intracategory variability. *Psychological Bulletin, 132*, 477–495.

Doise, W., Csepeli, G., Dann, H. D., Gouge, C., Larsen, K., & Ostell, A. (1972). An experimental investigation into the formation of intergroup representations. *European Journal of Social Psychology, 2*, 202–204.

Dole, V., & Nyswander, M. (1965). A medical treatment for diacetylmorphine (heroin) addiction. *JAMA, 193*, 80–84.

Donne, J. (1624/1959). *Devotions upon emergent occasions: Together with death's duel*. Ann Arbor, PA: The University of Michigan Press.

Doosje, B., Ellemers, N., & Spears, R. (1995). Perceived intragroup variability as a function of group status and identification. *Journal of Experimental Social Psychology, 31*, 410–436.

Doosje, B., Haslam, S. A., Spears, R., Oakes, P. J., & Koomen, W. (1998). The effect of comparative context on central tendency and variability judgements and the evaluation of group characteristics. *European Journal of Social Psychology, 28*, 173–184.

Dorahy, M. J., Lewis-Fernández, R., Krüger, C., Brand, B. L., Şar, V., Ewing, J., . . . Middleton, W. (2016). The role of clinical experience, diagnosis, and theoretical orientation in the treatment of posttraumatic and dissociative disorders: A vignette and survey investigation. *Journal of Trauma & Dissociation, 18*, 206–222.

Douglas, J. M. (2012). Social linkage, self concept and well-being after severe traumatic brain injury. In J. Jetten, C. Haslam, & S. A. Haslam (Eds.), *The social cure: Identity, health and well-being* (pp. 237–254). Hove, UK: Psychology Press.

Douglas, J. M. (2013). Conceptualizing self and maintaining social connection following severe traumatic brain injury. *Brain Injury, 27*, 60–74.

Douglas, J. M., Dyson, M., & Foreman, P. (2006). Increasing leisure activity following severe brain injury: Does it make a difference? *Brain Impairment, 7*, 107–118.

Douglas, J. M., & Spellacy, F. (2000). Correlates of depression in adults with sever traumatic brain injury and their carers. *Brain Injury, 14*, 71–88.

Dovidio, J. F., Penner, L. A., Albrecht, T. L., Norton, W. E., Gaertner, S. L., & Shelton, J. N. (2008). Dispar-ities and distrust: The implications of psychological processes for understanding racial disparities in health and health care. *Social Sciences and Medical Journal, 67*, 478–486.

Doyle, D. M., & Molix, L. (2014). How does stigma spoil relationships? Evidence that perceived discrim-ination harms romantic relationship quality through impaired self-image. *Journal of Applied Social Psychology, 44*, 600–610.

Drury, J. (2012). Collective resilience in mass emergencies and disasters. In J. Jetten, C. Haslam, & S. A. Haslam (Eds.), *The social cure: Identity, health and well-being* (pp. 195–215). Hove, UK: Psychology Press.

Drury, J., Brown, R., González, R., & Miranda, D. (2016). Emergent social identity and observing social support predict social support provided by survivors in a disaster: Solidarity in the 2010 Chile earth-quake. *European Journal of Social Psychology, 46*, 209–223.

Drury, J., Cocking, C., & Reicher, S. D. (2009a). The nature of collective resilience: Survivor reactions to the 2005 London bombings. *International Journal of Mass Emergencies and Disasters, 27*, 66–95.

Drury, J., Cocking, C., & Reicher, S. D. (2009b). Everyone for themselves? A comparative study of crowd solidarity among emergency survivors. *British Journal of Social Psychology, 48*, 487–506.

Drury, J., Cocking, C., Reicher, S. D., Burton, A., Schofield, D., Hardwick, A., . . . Langston, P. (2009). Cooperation versus competition in a mass emergency evacuation: A new laboratory simulation and a new theoretical model. *Behavior Research Methods, 41*, 957–970.

Drury, J., Novelli, D., & Stott, C. (2013). Representing crowd behaviour in emergency planning guidance: "Mass panic" or collective resilience? *Resilience: International Policies, Practices and Discourses, 1*, 18–37.

Drury, J., Novelli, D., & Stott, C. (2015). Managing to avert disaster: Explaining collective resilience at an outdoor music event. *European Journal of Social Psychology, 4*, 533–547.

Drury, J., & Reicher, S. D. (2000). Collective action and psychological change: The emergence of new social identities. *British Journal of Social Psychology, 39*, 579–604.

Drury, J., & Reicher, S. D. (2005). Explaining enduring empowerment: A comparative study of collective action and psychological outcomes. *European Journal of Social Psychology, 35*, 35–58.

Drury, J., & Reicher, S. D. (2009). Collective psychological empowerment as a model of social change: Researching crowds and power. *Journal of Social Issues, 65*, 707–725.

Drury, J., & Williams, R. (2012). Children and young people who are refugees, internally displaced persons or victims or perpetrators of war, mass violence and terrorism. *Current Opinion in Psychiatry, 25*, 277–284.

Drury, J., & Winter, G. (2004). Social identity as a source of strength in mass emergencies and other crowd events. *International Journal of Mental Health, 32*, 77–93.

Dumont, M., & Provost, M. A. (1999). Resilience in adolescents: Protective role of social support, coping strategies, self-esteem, and social activities on experience of stress and depression. *Journal of Youth and Adolescence, 28*, 343–363.

Dunbar, R. I. M. (1998). The social brain hypothesis. *Brain, 9*, 178–190.

Dunbar, R. I. M. (2013). *Primate social systems*. New York, NY: Springer.

Duncan, L. E., & Keller, M. C. (2011). A critical review of the first 10 years of candidate gene-by-environ-ment interaction research in psychiatry. *American Journal of Psychiatry, 168*, 1041–1049.

Dunkel Schetter, C. (2017). Moving research on health and close relationships forward – a challenge and an obligation: Introduction to the special issue. *American Psychologist, 72*, 511–516.

Durkheim, É. (1897/1951). *Suicide* (J. A. Spaulding & G. Simpson, Trans.). New York, NY: Free Press.

Durkheim, É. (1912). *Les formes élémentaires de la vie religieuse* [The elementary forms of religious life]. Paris, France: Alcan.

Durkheim, É. (1912/1915). *The elementary forms of religious life* (J. W. Swain, Trans.). London: George Allen and Unwin.

Dutra, L., Stathopoulou, G., Basden, S. L., Leyro, T. M., Powers, M. B., & Otto, M. W. (2008). A meta-ana-lytic review of psychosocial interventions for substance use disorders. *American Journal of Psychiatry, 165*, 179–187.

Dwight-Johnson, M., Sherbourne, C. D., Liao, D., & Wells, K. B. (2000). Treatment preferences among depressed primary care patients. *Journal of General Internal Medicine, 15*, 527–534.

Dykes, J., Brunner, E. J., Martikainen, P. T., & Wardle, J. (2004). Socio-economic gradient in body size and obesity among women: The role of dietary restraint, disinhibition and hunger in the Whitehall II study. *International Journal of Obesity, 28*, 262–268.

Eberhart, N. K., Auerbach, R. P., Bigda-Peyton, J., & Abela, J. R. Z. (2011). Maladaptive schemas and depression: tests of stress generation and diathesis-stress models. *Journal of Social and Clinical Psychology, 30*, 75–104.

Eccleston, C., Palermo, T. M., Williams, A. C., Lewandowski-Holley, A., Morley, S., Fisher, E., & Law, E. (2014). Psychological therapies for the management of chronic and recurrent pain in children and adolescents. *Cochrane Database of Systematic Reviews, 5*. Retrieved from http://doi.org/10.1002/14651858. CD003968.pub4

The Economist. (2010). *Japan's population: The old and the older*. Retrieved from www.economist.com/blogs/dailychart/2010/11/japans_population

Egremont, M. (2014). *Siegfried Sassoon: A biography*. London: Picador.

Ehde, D. M., Dillworth, T. M., & Turner, J. A. (2014). Cognitive-behavioral therapy for individuals with chronic pain: Efficacy, innovations, and directions for research. *American Psychologist, 69*, 153–166.

Ehlers, A., & Clark, D. M. (2000). A cognitive model of posttraumatic stress disorder. *Behaviour Research and Therapy, 38*, 319–345.

Ehring, T., Ehlers, A., & Glucksman, E. (2008). Do cognitive models help in predicting the severity of posttraumatic stress disorder, phobia, and depression after motor vehicle accidents? A prospective longitudinal study. *Journal of Consulting and Clinical Psychology, 76*, 219–230.

Einsenstein, C. (2003). *The yoga of eating: Transcending diets and dogma to nourish the natural self*. Washington, DC: New Trends Publishing.

Eisenberg, M. E., Toumbourou, J. W., Catalano, R. F., & Hemphill, S. A. (2014). Social norms in the development of adolescent substance use: A longitudinal analysis of the International Youth Development Study. *Journal of Youth and Adolescence, 43*, 1486–1497.

Eisenberger, N. I., Lieberman, M. D., & Williams, K. D. (2003). Does rejection hurt? An FMRI study of social exclusion. *Science, 302*, 290–292.

Elkin, I., Gibbons, R. D., Shea, M. T., Sotsky, S. M., Watkins, J. T., Pilkonis, P. A., & Hedeker, D. (1995). Initial severity and differential treatment outcome in the National Institute of Mental Health Treatment of Depression Collaborative Research Program. *Journal of Consulting and Clinical Psychology, 63*, 841–847.

Ellaway, A., Wood, S., & Macintyre, S. (1999). Someone to talk to? The role of loneliness as a factor in the frequency of GP consultations. *British Journal of General Practice, 49*, 363–367.

Ellemers, N. (1993). The influence of socio-structural variables on identity enhancement strategies. *European Review of Social Psychology, 4*, 27–57.

Ellemers, N. (2001). Individual upward mobility and the perceived legitimacy of intergroup relations. In J. Jost & B. Major (Eds.), *The psychology of legitimacy: Emerging perspectives on ideology, justice, and intergroup relations* (pp. 205–222). Cambridge: Cambridge University Press.

Ellemers, N., & Barreto, M. (2006). Social identity and self-presentation at work: How attempts to hide a stigmatised identity affect emotional well-being, social inclusion and performance. *Netherlands Journal of Psychology, 62*, 51–57.

Ellemers, N., & Haslam, S. A. (2012). Social identity theory. In P. Van Lange, A. Kruglanski, & T. Higgins (Eds.), *Handbook of theories of social psychology* (pp. 379–398). London: Sage.

Ellemers, N., Kortekaas, P., & Ouwerkerk, J.W. (1999). Self-categorization, commitment to the group and group self-esteem as related but distinct aspects of social identity. *European Journal of Social Psychology, 29*, 371–389.

Ellemers, N., Van Knippenberg, A., & Wilke, H. (1990). The influence of permeability of group boundaries and stability of group status on strategies of individual mobility and social change. *British Journal of Social Psychology, 29*, 233–246.

Ellemers, N., & Van Rijswijk, W. (1997). Identity needs versus social opportunities: The use of group-level and individual-level identity management strategies. *Social Psychology Quarterly, 60,* 52–65.

Ellemers, N., Van Rijswijk, W., Bruins, J., & De Gilder, D. (1998). Group commitment as a moderator of attributional and behavioural responses to power use. *European Journal of Social Psychology, 28,* 555–573.

Ellis-Hill, C., & Horn, S. (2000). Change in identity and self-concept: A new theoretical approach to recovery following stroke. *Clinical Rehabilitation, 14,* 279–287.

Ellis-Hill, C., Payne, S., & Ward, C. (2008). Using stroke to explore the Life Thread Model: An alternative approach to understanding rehabilitation following acquired disability. *Disability and Rehabilitation, 30,* 150–159.

Ellison, N. (2011). The conservative party and the "big society". *Social Policy Review, 23,* 45–62.

Elsbach, K. D., & Kramer, R. D. (1996). Members' responses to organizational identity threats: Encountering and countering the Business Week rankings. *Administrative Science Quarterly, 41,* 442–476.

Elzinga, B. M., & Bremner, J. D. (2002). Are the neural substrates of memory the final common pathway in posttraumatic stress disorder (PTSD)? *Journal of Affective Disorders, 70,* 1–17.

Emery, C. F., & Gatz, M. (1990). Psychological and cognitive effects of an exercise program for community-residing adults. *The Gerontologist, 30,* 184–188.

Engel, G. L. (1977). The need for a new medical model: A challenge for biomedicine. *Science, 196,* 129–136.

Ensall, J. (2014, July 31). The ultimate guide to tube etiquette: 20 things you need to know to be a good commuter. *Time Out.* Retrieved November 22, 2016, from http://now-here-this.timeout.com/2014/07/31/the-ultimate-guide-to-tube-etiquette-20-things-you-need-to-know-to-be-a-good-commuter/

Epstein, L. H. (1992). The role of behavior theory in behavioral medicine. *Journal of Consulting and Clinical Psychology, 60,* 493–498.

Epstein, L. J. (2011). *George Burns: An American life.* Jefferson, NC: MacFarland and Co.

Ertel, K. A., Glymour, M. M., & Berkman, L. F. (2008). Effects of social integration on preserving memory function in a nationally representative US elderly population. *American Journal of Public Health, 98,* 1215–1220.

Estroff, S. E. (1989). Self, identity, and subjective experiences of schizophrenia: In search of the subject. *Schizophrenia Bulletin, 15,* 189–196.

Ethier, K. A., & Deaux, K. (1994). Negotiating social identity when contexts change: Maintaining identification and responding to threat. *Journal of Personality and Social Psychology, 67,* 243–251.

Etnier, J. L., & Chang, Y-K. (2009). The effect of physical activity on executive function: A brief commentary on definitions, measurement issues and the current state of the literature. *Journal of Sport and Exercise Science, 31,* 469–483.

Eyer, J., & Sterling, P. (1977). Stress-related mortality and social organization. *Review of Radical Political Economy, 9,* 1–44.

Eymard, A., & Douglas, D. (2012). Ageism among health care providers and interventions to improve their attitudes toward older adults: An integrative review. *Journal of Gerontological Nursing, 38,* 26–35.

Ezquiaga, E., Garcia, A., Pallarés, T., Bravo, M. F., & García, A. (1999). Psychosocial predictors of outcome in major depression: A prospective 12-month study. *Journal of Affective Disorders, 52,* 209–216.

Fabre, C., Chamari, K., Mucci, P., Massé-Birron, J., & Préfaut, C. (2002). Improvement of cognitive function by mental and/or individualized aerobic training in healthy elderly subjects. *International Journal of Sports Medicine, 23,* 415–421.

Fairburn, C. G., Shafran, R., & Cooper, Z. (1999). A cognitive behavioural theory of anorexia nervosa. *Behaviour Research and Therapy, 37,* 1–13.

Falloon, I. R. H., Boyd, J. L., McGill, C. W., Williamson, M., Razani, J., Moss, H. B., . . . Simpson, G. M. (1985). Family management in the prevention of morbidity of schizophrenia. Clinical outcome of a 2-year longitudinal study. *Archives of General Psychiatry, 42,* 887–896.

Falloon, I. R. H., Kydd, R. R., Coverdale, J. H., & Laidlaw, T. M. (1996). Early detection and intervention for initial episodes of schizophrenia. *Schizophrenia Bulletin, 22,* 271–282.

Falloon, I. R. H., McGill, C. W., & Boyd, J. L. (1984). *Family care of schizophrenia: a problem-solving approach to the treatment of mental illness.* New York, NY: Guilford family therapy series.

Falomir-Pichastor, J. M., Toscani, L., & Despointes, S. H. (2009). Determinants of flu vaccination among nurses: The effects of group identification and professional responsibility. *Applied Psychology: An International Review, 58,* 42–58.

Fann, J. R., Hart, T., & Schomer, K. G. (2009). Treatment for depression after traumatic brain injury: A systematic review. *Journal of Neurotrauma, 26,* 2383–2402.

Fardouly, J., Pinkus, R. T., & Vartanian, L. R. (2017). The impact of appearance comparisons made through social media, traditional media, and in person in women's everyday lives. *Body Image, 20,* 31–39. http://doi.org/10.1016/j.bodyim.2016.11.002

Farrow, C. V., Tarrant, M., & Khan, S. (2017). Using social identity to promote health: The impact of group memberships on health in the context of obesity. In S. A. Buckingham & D. Best (Eds.), *Addiction, behavioural change and social identity* (pp. 52–70). London: Routledge.

Fava, G. A., Rafanelli, C., Grandi, S., Conti, S., & Belluardo, P. (1998). Prevention of recurrent depression with cognitive behavioral therapy. *Archives of General Psychiatry, 55,* 816–820.

Fayers, P., & Machin, D. (2007). *Quality of life: The assessment, analysis and interpretation of patient-reported outcomes.* New York, NY: John Wiley & Sons.

Fenigstein, A., & Vanable, P. A. (1992). Paranoia and self-consciousness. *Journal of Personality and Social Psychology, 62,* 129–138.

Ferguson, E. (2013). Personality is of central concern to understand health: Towards a theoretical model for health psychology. *Health Psychology Review, 7*(Supp. 1), 32–70.

Fernández, S., Branscombe, N. R., Gómez, Á., & Morales, J. (2012). Influence of the social context on use of surgical-lengthening and group-empowering coping strategies among people with dwarfism. *Rehabilitation Psychology, 57,* 224–235.

Ferrari, S., Galeazzi, G. M., Mackinnon, A., & Rigatelli, M. (2008). Frequent attenders in primary care: Impact of medical, psychiatric and psychosomatic diagnoses. *Psychotherapy and Psychosomatics, 77,* 306–314.

Ferris, L. J., Jetten, J., & Bastian, B. (2017). *"It did hurt, but I enjoyed it": Pleasurable pain promotes identification by revealing the self.* Manuscript submitted for publication.

Ferris, L., Jetten, J., Molenberghs, P., Bastian, B., & Karnadewi, F. (2016). Increased pain communication following multiple group memberships salience leads to a relative reduction in pain-related brain activity. *PLoS ONE, 11*(9), e0163117.

Festinger, L. (1957). *A theory of cognitive dissonance.* Evanston, IL: Row, Peterson and Co.

Findlay, R. A. (2003). Interventions to reduce social isolation amongst older people: Where is the evidence? *Psychology and Aging, 23,* 647–658.

Finlayson, R. (2003). *We shall overcome: The history of the American Civil Rights Movement.* New York, NY: Twenty-First Century Books.

Fiore, J., Becker, J., & Coppel, D. B. (1983). Social network interactions: A buffer or a stress. *American Journal of Community Psychology, 11,* 423–439.

Fischer, B., Rehm, J., Kirst, M., Casas, M., Hall, W., Krausz, M., . . . Van Ree, J. M. (2002). Heroin-assisted treatment as a response to the public health problem of opiate dependence. *European Journal of Public Health, 12,* 228–234.

Fischler, C. (1988). Food, self and identity. *Social Science Information, 27,* 275–292.

Fitcher, M. M., & Quadflieg, N. (2007). Long-term stability of eating disorder diagnoses. *International Journal of Eating Disorders, 40,* 61–66.

Fitzpatrick, S., & Jones, A. (2005). Pursuing social justice or social cohesion? Coercion in street homelessness policies in England. *Journal of Social Policy, 34,* 389–406.

Flynn, T. W., Smith, B., & Chou, R. (2011). Appropriate use of diagnostic imaging in low back pain: a reminder that unnecessary imaging may do as much harm as good. *Journal of Orthopaedic and Sports Physical Therapy, 41,* 838–846.

Foa, E. B., Steketee, G., & Rothbaum, B. O. (1989). Behavioral/cognitive conceptualizations of post-traumatic stress disorder. *Behavior Therapy, 20,* 155–176.

Foddy, M., Platow, M. J., & Yamagishi, T. (2009). Group-based trust in strangers: The role of stereotypes and expectations. *Psychological Science, 20*, 419–422.

Folkman, S., & Moskowitz, J. T. (2004). Coping: Pitfalls and promise. *Annual Review of Psychology, 55*, 745–774.

Fonda, S. J., Wallace, R. B., & Herzog, A. R. (2001). Changes in driving patterns and worsening depressive symptoms among older adults. *Journals of Gerontology Series B: Psychological Sciences and Social Sciences, 56B*, 343–351.

Foster, M. D., & Matheson, K. (1999). Perceiving and responding to the personal/group discrimination discrepancy. *Personality and Social Psychology Bulletin, 25*, 1319–1329.

Fournier, J. C., Derubeis, R. J., Hollon, S. D., Dimidjian, S., Amsterdam, J. D., Shelton, R. C., & Fawcett, J. (2010). Antidepressant drug effects and depression severity: A patient-level meta-analysis. *Journal of the American Medical Association, 303*, 47–53.

Frable, D. E. S., Blackstone, T., & Scherbaum, C. (1990). Marginal and mindful: Deviants in social interactions. *Journal of Personality and Social Psychology, 59*, 140–149.

Frank, E., Kupfer, D. J., Thase, M. E., Mallinger, A. E., Swartz, H. A., Fagiolini, A. M., . . . Monk, T. (2005). Two-year outcomes for Interpersonal and Social Rhythm Therapy in individuals with Bipolar I disorder. *Archives of General Psychiatry, 62*, 996–1004.

Fratiglioni, L., Wang, H.-X., Ericsson, K., Maytan, M., & Winblad, B. (2000). Influence of social network on occurrence of dementia: A community-based longitudinal study. *The Lancet, 355*, 1315–1319.

Freeman, D., Garety, P. A., Bebbington, P. E, Smith, B., Rollinson, R., Fowler, D., Kuipers, E., Ray, K., & Dunn, G. (2005). Psychological investigation of the structure of paranoia in a non-clinical population. *British Journal of Psychiatry, 186*, 427–435.

French, D. P., Olander, E. K., Chisholm, A., & McSharry, J. (2014). Which behavior change techniques are most effective at increasing older adult' self-efficacy and physical behavior? A systematic review. *Annals of Behavioral Medicine, 48*, 225–234.

Freud, S. (1920/1953). Beyond the pleasure principle. In J. Strachey (Ed. and Trans.), *The standard edition of the complete psychological works of Sigmund Freud* (Vol. 18). London: Hogarth Press.

Freud, S. (1939/1953). Moses and monotheism. In J. Strachey (Ed. and Trans.), *The standard edition of the complete psychological works of Sigmund Freud* (Vol. 23). London: Hogarth Press.

Friedman, M. J. (1997). Drug treatment for PTSD. *Annals of the New York Academy of Sciences, 821*, 359–371.

Friedman, M. J., Donnelly, C. L., & Mellman, T. A. (2003). Pharmacotherapy for PTSD. *Psychiatric Annals, 33*, 57–62.

Friedman, M., & Rosenman, R. H. (1959). Association of specific overt behaviour pattern with blood and cardiovascular findings. *Journal of the American Medical Association, 169*, 1286–1296.

Friedman, M., & Rosenman, R. H. (1974). *Type A behavior and your heart*. Greenwich, CT: Fawcett.

Friel, S. (2014). Inequities in the freedom to lead a flourishing and healthy life: Issues for healthy public policy. *International Journal of Health Policy and Management, 3*, 161–163.

Frings, D., & Albery, I. P. (2015). The social identity model of cessation maintenance: Formulation and initial evidence. *Addictive Behaviors, 44*, 35–42.

Frings, D., & Albery, I. P. (2017). The social identity model of cessation maintenance. In S. A. Buckingham & D. Best (Eds.), *Addiction, behavioural change and social identity: The path to resilience and recovery* (pp. 116–136). London: Routledge.

Frings, D., Albery, I. P., & Monk, R. L. (2017). The whys and hows of psychosocial approaches to addiction. *Journal of Applied Psychology, 47*, 115–117.

Frings, D., Collins, M., Long, G., Pinto, I. R., & Albery, I. P. (2016). A test of the Social Identity Model of Cessation Maintenance: The content and role of social control. *Addictive Behaviour Reports, 3*, 77–85.

Frith, U., & Happé, F. (1994). Autism: Beyond "theory of mind". *Cognition, 50*, 115–132.

Fry, P. S., & Debats, D. L. (2009). Perfectionism and the five-factor personality traits as predictors of mortality in older adults. *Journal of Health Psychology, 14*, 513–524.

Funk, S. C. (1992). Hardiness: A review of theory and research. *Health Psychology, 11*, 335–345.

Gabriel, P. (1980). Not one of us. From the album *Peter Gabriel II*. London: Charisma records. Retrieved from www.youtube.com/watch?v=dbwQ0Wy3ljQ

Gaffney, C., & Haslam, S. A. (2002). *Burnout in care workers: The role of social identification.* Unpublished manuscript, University of Exeter.

Gaglio, B., & Glasgow, R. E. (2011). Evaluating approaches for evaluation and dissemination research. In R. Brownson, E. Proctor, & G. Colditz (Eds.), *Handbook of dissemination and implementation research* (pp. 327–358). Oxford: Oxford University Press.

Gaglio, B., Shoup, J. A., & Glasgow, R. E. (2013). The RE-AIM framework: A systematic review of use over time. *American Journal of Public Health, 103,* 38–46.

Gallagher, M., Muldoon, O. T., & Pettigrew, J. (2015). An integrative review of social and occupational factors influencing health and wellbeing. *Frontiers in Psychology, 6,* 1281. doi: 10.3389/fpsyg.2015.01281

Gallagher, S., Bennett, K. M., & Halford, J, C. G. (2006). A comparison of acute and long-term health-care personnel's attitudes towards older adults. *International Journal of Nursing Practice, 12,* 273–279.

Galletly, C., Castle, D., Dark, F., Humberstone, V., Jablensky, A., Killackey, E., . . . Tran, N. (2016). Royal Australian and New Zealand College of Psychiatrists clinical practice guidelines for the management of schizophrenia and related disorders. *Australian and New Zealand Journal of Psychiatry, 50,* 1–117.

Gangstad, B., Norman, P., & Barton, J. (2009). Cognitive processing and post-traumatic growth after stroke. *Rehabilitation Psychology, 54,* 69–75.

Garcia, D. M., Schmitt, M. T., Branscombe, N. R., & Ellemers, N. (2009). Women's reactions to ingroup members who protest discriminatory treatment: The importance of beliefs about inequality and response appropriateness. *European Journal of Social Psychology, 40,* 733–745.

García-Cabeza, I., Gómez, J., Sacristán, J. A., Edgell, E., & González de Chavez, M. (2001). Subjective response to antipsychotic treatment and compliance in schizophrenia: A naturalistic study comparing olanzapine, risperidone and haloperidol (EFESO Study). *BMC Psychiatry, 1,* 7. doi: 10.1186/1471-244x-1-7

Garske, G. G., & Thomas, K. R. (1992). Self-reported self-esteem and depression: Indexes of psychosocial adjustment following severe traumatic brain injury. *Rehabilitation Counseling Bulletin, 36,* 44–52.

Garstka, T. A., Schmitt, M. T., Branscombe, N. R., & Hummert, M. L. (2004). How young and older adults differ in their responses to perceived age discrimination. *Psychology and Aging, 19,* 326–335.

Gaspar, P. (1999). Water intake of nursing home residents. *Journal of Gerontological Nursing, 25,* 22–29.

Gee, G. C., Spencer, M., Chen, J., Yip, T., & Takeuchi, D. (2007). The association between self-reported racial discrimination and 12-month DSM-IV mental disorders among Asian Americans nationwide. *Social Science and Medicine, 64,* 1984–1996.

Geisner, I. M., Rhew, I. C., Ramirez, J. J., Lewis, M. E., Larimer, M. E., & Lee, C. M. (2017). Not all drinking events are the same: Exploring 21st birthday and typical alcohol expectancies as a risk factor for high-risk drinking and alcohol problems. *Addictive Behaviors, 70,* 97–101.

Gerard, H. B., & Matthewson, G. C. (1966). The effects of severity of initiation on liking for the group: A replication. *Journal of Experimental Social Psychology, 2,* 278–287.

Gerlach, J., & Larsen, E. B. (1999). Subjective experience and mental side-effects of antipsychotic treatment. *Acta Psychiatrica Scandinavica,* Supplement 1999, *395,* 113–117.

Ghaemi, S. N. (2009). The rise and fall of the biopsychosocial model. *The British Journal of Psychiatry, 195,* 3–4.

Ghaemi, S. N. (2011). The biopsychosocial model in psychiatry: A critique. *Existenz, 6,* 1–8.

Giamo, L. S., Schmitt, M. T., & Outten, H. R. (2012). Perceived discrimination, group identification, and life satisfaction among multiracial people: A test of the rejection-identification model. *Cultural Diversity and Ethnic Minority Psychology, 18,* 319–328.

Gil, T., Calev, A., Greenberg, D., Kugelmass, S., & Lerer, B. (1990). Cognitive functioning in post-traumatic stress disorder. *Journal of Traumatic Stress, 3,* 29–45.

Giles, H., & Reid, S. A. (2005). Ageism across the lifespan: Towards a self-categorization model of ageing. *Journal of Social Issues, 61,* 389–404.

Giles, L. C., Anstey, K. J., Walker, R. B., & Luszcz, M. A. (2012). Social networks and memory over 15 years of follow-up in a cohort of older Australians: Results from the Australian Longitudinal Study of Ageing. *Journal of Aging Research*, Article ID 856048, 1–7.

Glasgow, R. E., La Chance, P. A., Toobert, D. J., Brown, J., Hampson, S. E., & Riddle, M. C. (1997). Long term effects and costs of brief behavioural dietary intervention for patients with diabetes delivered from the medical office. *Patient Education and Counseling, 32*, 175–184.

Glasgow, R. E., Lichtenstein, E., & Marcus, A. C. (2003). Why don't we see more translation of health promotion research to practice? Rethinking the efficacy-to-effectiveness transition. *American Journal of Public Health, 93*, 1261–1267.

Glasgow, R. E., Vogt, T. M., & Boles, S. M. (1999). Evaluating the public health impact of health promotion interventions: the RE-AIM framework. *American Journal of Public Health, 89*, 1322–1327.

Glass, T. A., De Leon, C. F. M., Bassuk, S. S., & Berkman, L. F. (2006). Social engagement and depressive symptoms in late life: Longitudinal findings. *Journal of Aging and Health, 18*, 604–628.

Gleibs, I. H., Haslam, C., Haslam, S. A., & Jones, J. M. (2011a). Water clubs in residential care: Is it the water or the club that enhances health and well-being? *Psychology & Health, 26*, 1361–1377.

Gleibs, I. H., Haslam, C., Jones, J. M., Haslam, S. A., McNeill, J., & Connolly, H. (2011b). No country for old men? The role of a "Gentlemen's' Club" in promoting social engagement and psychological well-being in residential care. *Aging and Mental Health, 15*, 256–266.

Glynn, S. M. (2012). Family interventions in schizophrenia: Promise and pitfalls over 30 years. *Current Psychiatry Reports, 14*, 237–243.

Gneezy, U., List, J., & Price, M. K. (2012). *Toward an understanding of why people discriminate: Evidence from a series of natural field experiments*. NBER Working Paper No. 17855.

Goffman, E. (1963). *Stigma: Notes on the management of spoiled identity*. London, UK: Penguin books.

Goldman, L. S., Nielsen, N. H., & Champion, H. C. (1999). Awareness, diagnosis, and treatment of depression. *Journal of General Internal Medicine, 14*, 569–580.

Goldman, S. J., Herman, C. P., & Polivy, J. (1991). Is the effect of a social model on eating attenuated by hunger? *Appetite, 17*, 129–140.

Goldscheider, A. (1894). *Uber den schmerzs in physiologischer und klinischer hinsicht [A physiological and clinical view of pain]*. Berlin: Hirschwald.

Gotlib, I. H. (1984). Depression and general psychopathology in university students. *Journal of Abnormal Psychology, 93*, 19–30.

Goubert, L., Craig, K. D., Vervoort, T., Morley, S., Sullivan, M. J. L., Williams, A., . . . Crombez, G. (2005). Facing others in pain: The effects of empathy. *Pain, 118*, 286–288.

Gould, K. R., Ponsford, J. L., & Spitz, G. (2014). Association between cognitive impairments and anxiety disorders following traumatic brain injury. *Journal of Clinical and Experimental Neuropsychology, 36*, 1–14.

Gowing, L. R., Ali, R., Dunlop, A., Farrell, M., & Lintzeris, N. (2014). *National guidelines for medication-assisted treatment of opioid dependence*. Publication number 10253, Department of Health, Canberra.

Goymann, W., & Wingfield, J. C. (2004). Allostatic load, social status and stress hormones: The costs of social status matter. *Animal Behaviour, 67*, 591–602.

Gracey, F., Evans, J. J., & Malley, D. (2009). Capturing process and outcome in complex rehabilitation interventions: A Y-shaped model. *Neuropsychological Rehabilitation, 19*, 867–890.

Gracey, F., & Ownsworth, T. (2012). The experience of self in the world: The personal and social contexts of social identity change in brain injury. In J. Jetten, C. Haslam, & S. A. Haslam (Eds.), *The social cure: Identity, health and well-being* (pp. 273–295). Hove, UK: Psychology Press.

Grady, D., & Redberg, R. F. (2010). Less is more: How less health care can result in better health. *Archives of Internal Medicine, 170*, 749–750.

Gray, K., & Wegner, D. M. (2008). The sting of intentional pain. *Psychological Science, 19*, 1260–1262.

Gray-Little, B., Williams, V. S. L., & Hancock, T. D. (1997). An item response theory analysis of the Rosenberg Self-Esteem Scale. *Personality and Social Psychology Bulletin, 23*, 443–451.

Greaves, C. J., & Campbell, J. L. (2007). Supporting self-care in general practice. *British Journal of General Practice, 57*, 814–821.

Green, J., Tones, K., Cross, R., & Woodall, J. (2015). *Health promotion: Planning and strategies.* Los Angeles, CA: Sage.

Greenaway, K. H., Cruwys, T., Haslam, S. A., & Jetten, J. (2016). Social identities promote well-being because they satisfy global psychological needs. *European Journal of Social Psychology, 46*, 294–307.

Greenaway, K. H., Haslam, S. A., & Bingley, W. (2017). *Are "they" out to get me? Social disidentification, paranoia, and receptivity to conspiracy theories.* Unpublished manuscript, University of Queensland.

Greenaway, K. H., Haslam, S. A., Branscombe, N. R., Cruwys, T., Ysseldyk, R., & Heldreth, C. (2015). From "we" to "me": Group identification enhances perceived personal control with consequences for health and well-being. *Journal of Personality and Social Psychology, 109*, 53–74.

Greenaway, K. H., Louis, W. R., & Hornsey, M. J. (2013). Belief in precognition increases perceived control and loss of control increases belief in precognition. *PLoS ONE, 8*(8), e71327.

Greenaway, K. H., Wright, R., Reynolds, K. J., Willingham, J., & Haslam, S. A. (2015). Shared identity is key to effective communication. *Personality and Social Psychology Bulletin, 41*, 171–182.

Greenspan, J. D., Craft, R. M., LeResche, L., Arendt-Nielsen, L., Berkley, K. J., Fillingim, R. B., . . . Mogil, J. S. (2007). Studying sex and gender differences in pain and analgesia: A consensus report. *Pain, 132*, 26–45.

Greiwe, J. S., Cheng, B., Rubin, D. C., Yarasheski, K. E., & Semenkovich, C. F. (2001). Resistance exercise decreases skeletal muscle tumor necrosis factor α in frail elderly humans. *The Journal of the Federation of American Societies for Experimental Biology, 15*, 475–482.

Grencavage, L. M., & Norcross, J. C. (1990). Where are the commonalities among the therapeutic common factors? *Professional Psychology: Research and Practice, 21*, 372–378.

Griggs, R. A. (2015). Coverage of the Phineas Gage story in introductory psychology textbooks: Was Gage no longer Gage? *Teaching of Psychology, 42*, 195–202.

Groh, D. R., Jason, L. A., & Keys, C. B. (2008). Social network variables in alcoholics anonymous: A literature review. *Clinical Psychology Review, 28*, 430–450.

Grunze, H., Schlösser, S., Amann, B., & Walden, J. (1999). Anticonvulsant drugs in bipolar disorder. *Dialogues in Clinical Neuroscience, 1*, 24–40.

Guendelman, M. D., Cheryan, S., & Monin, B. (2011). Fitting in but getting fat: Identity threat and dietary choices among U.S. immigrant groups. *Psychological Science, 22*, 959–967.

Gujjarlamundi, H. B. (2016). Polytherapy and drug interactions in the elderly. *Journal of Midlife Health, 7*, 105–107.

Gunderson, M. (1989). Male-female wage differentials and policy responses. *Journal of Economic Literature, 27*, 46–72.

Gunthert, K. C., Cohen, L. H., & Armeli, S. (1999). The role of neuroticism in daily stress and coping. *Journal of Personality and Social Psychology, 77*, 1087–1100.

Gurin, P. (1985). Women's gender consciousness. *Public Opinion Quarterly, 49*, 143–163.

Gust, D. A., Gordon, T. P., Wilson, M. E., Ahmed-Ansari, A., Brodie, A. R., & McClure, H. M. (1991). Formation of a new social group of unfamiliar female rhesus monkeys affects the immune and pituitary adrenocortical systems. *Brain, Behavior, and Immunity, 5*, 296–307.

Güth, W., Levati, M. V., & Ploner, M. (2008). Social identity and trust: An experimental investigation. *The Journal of Socio-Economics, 37*, 1293–1308.

Gutsell, J. N., & Inzlicht, M. (2012). Intergroup differences in the sharing of emotive states: Neural evidence of an empathy gap. *Social Cognitive and Affective Neuroscience, 7*, 596–603.

Haber, M. G., Cohen, J. L., Lucas, T., & Baltes, B. B. (2007). The relationship between self-reported received and perceived social support: A meta-analytic review. *American Journal of Community Psychology, 39*, 133–144.

Hackel, L. M., Coppin, G., Wohl, M. J. A., & Van Bavel, J. J. (2015). *From groups to grits: Social identity shapes evaluations of food pleasantness.* Retrieved from http://ssrn.com/abstract=2662835

Hafer, C. L., & Olson, J. M. (1993). Beliefs in a just world, discontent and assertive actions by working women. *Personality and Social Psychology Bulletin, 19*, 30–38.

Hagger, M. S. (2009). Personality, individual differences, stress and health. *Stress and Health, 25*, 381–386.

Hajjar, E. R., Cafiero, A. C., & Hanlon, J. T. (2007). Polypharmacy in elderly patients. *The American Journal of Geriatric Pharmacotherapy, 5*, 345–351.

Halford, W. K., Price, J., Kelly, A. B., Bouma, R., & Young, R. M. (2001). Helping the female partners of men abusing alcohol: A comparison of three treatments. *Addiction, 96*, 1497–1508.

Hall, K., & Iqbal, F. (2010). *The problem with cognitive behavioural therapy*. London: Karnac books.

Hall, W., Ward, J., & Mattick, R. P. (1998). The effectiveness of methadone maintenance treatment 1: Heroin use and crime. In J. Ward, R. P. Mattick, & W. Hall (Eds.), *Methadone maintenance treatment and other opioid replacement therapies*. Amsterdam: Harwood Academic Publishers.

Handley, E. D., Rogosch, F. A., Guild, D. J., & Cicchetti, D. (2015). Neighborhood disadvantage and adolescent substance use disorder: The moderating role of maltreatment. *Child Maltreatment, 20*, 193–202.

Handley, T. E., Inder, K. J., Kelly, B. J., Attia, J. R., Lewin, T. J., Fitzgerald, M. N., & Kay-Lambkin, F. J. (2012). You've got to have friends: The predictive value of social integration and support in suicidal ideation among rural communities. *Social Psychiatry and Psychiatric Epidemiology, 47*, 1281–1290.

Harkness, J. (2004). Patient involvement: a vital principle for patient-centred health care. *World Hospitals and Health Services, 41*, 12–16.

Harlow, J. M. (1868). Recovery from the passage of an iron bar through the head. *Publications of the Massachusetts Medical Society, 2*, 327–347.

Harrison, J. A., Mullen, P. D., & Green, L. W. (1992). A meta-analysis of studies of the Health Belief Model with adults. *Health Education Research, 7*, 107–116.

Harrow, M., Goldberg, J. F., Grossman, L. S., & Meltzer, H. Y. (1990). Outcome in manic disorders: A naturalistic follow-up study. *Archives of General Psychiatry, 47*, 665–671.

Harvey, A. G. (2004). *Cognitive behavioural processes across psychological disorders: A transdiagnostic approach to research and treatment*. Oxford, UK: Oxford University Press.

Harvey, A. G., Bryant, R. A., & Tarrier, N. (2003). Cognitive behaviour therapy for post-traumatic stress disorder. *Clinical Psychology Review, 23*, 501-502.

Harvey, S. B., Hatch, S. L., Jones, M., Hull, L., Jones, N., Greenberg, N., . . . Wessely, S. (2011). Coming home: Social functioning and the mental health of UK reservists on return from deployment to Iraq or Afghanistan. *Annals of Epidemiology, 21*, 666–672.

Harwood, J., & Sparks, L. (2003). Social identity and health: An intergroup communication approach to cancer. *Health Communication, 15*, 145–159.

Haslam, C., Best, D., Dingle, G. A., Mackenzie, J., & Beckwith, M. (2017). Social Identity Mapping: Measuring social identity change in recovery from addiction. In S. Buckingham & D. Best (Eds.), *Addiction, behavioural change and social identity* (pp. 155–171). Oxford, UK: Routledge.

Haslam, C., Cruwys, T., & Haslam, S. A. (2014a). "The we's have it": Evidence for the distinctive benefits of group engagement in enhancing cognitive health in ageing. *Social Science and Medicine, 120*, 57–66.

Haslam, C., Cruwys, T., Haslam, S. A., Bentley, S. V., Dingle, G. A., & Jetten, J. (2016a). *Groups 4 Health manual* (version 3.0). Social Identity and Groups Network (SIGN). Australia: University of Queensland.

Haslam, C., Cruwys, T., Haslam, S. A., Bentley, S. V., Dingle, G. A., & Jetten, J. (2016b). *Groups 4 Health workbook*. (version 3.0). Social Identity and Groups Network (SIGN): University of Queensland, Australia.

Haslam, C., Cruwys, T., Haslam, S. A., Dingle, G. A., & Chang, M. X.-L. (2016c). Groups 4 Health: Evidence that a social-identity intervention that builds and strengthens social group membership improves mental health. *Journal of Affective Disorders, 194*, 188–195.

Haslam, C., Cruwys, T., Milne, M., Kan, C.-H., & Haslam, S. A. (2016d). Group ties protect cognitive health by promoting social identification and social support. *Journal of Aging and Health, 28*, 244–266.

Haslam, C., Dingle, G. A., Best, D., Mackenzie, J., & Beckwith, M. (2017). Social Identity Mapping: Measuring social identity change in recovery from addiction. In S. A. Buckingham & D. Best (Eds.), *Addiction, behavioural change and social identity: The path to resilience and recovery*. London: Routledge.

Haslam, C., Haslam, S. A., Jetten, J., Bevins, A., Ravenscroft, S., & Tonks, J. (2010). The social treatment: The benefits of group interventions in residential care settings. *Psychology and Aging, 25*, 157–167.

Haslam, C., Haslam, S. A., Knight, C., Gleibs, I., Ysseldyk, R., & McCloskey, L.-G. (2014). We can work it out: Group decision-making builds social identity and enhances the cognitive performance of care home residents. *British Journal of Psychology*, *105*, 17–34.

Haslam, C., Haslam, S. A., Ysseldyk, R., McCloskey, L-G., Pfisterer, K., & Brown, S. G. (2014). Social identification moderates cognitive health and well-being following story- and song-based reminiscence. *Aging and Mental Health*, *18*, 425–434.

Haslam, C., Holme, A., Haslam, S. A., Iyer, A., Jetten, J., & Williams, W. H. (2008). Maintaining group memberships: Social identity continuity predicts well-being after stroke. *Neuropsychological Rehabilitation*, *18*, 671–691.

Haslam, C. Jetten, J., & Haslam, S. A. (2012). Advancing the social cure: Implications for theory, practice and policy. In J. Jetten, C. Haslam, & S. A. Haslam (Eds.), *The social cure: Identity, health, and well-being* (pp. 319–343). Hove, UK: Psychology Press.

Haslam, C., Jetten, J., Haslam, S. A., & Knight, C. (2012). The importance of remembering and deciding together: Enhancing the health and well-being of older adults in care. In J. Jetten, C. Haslam, & S. A. Haslam (Eds.), *The social cure: Identity, health and well-being* (pp. 297–315). Hove, UK: Psychology Press.

Haslam, C., Morton, T. A., Haslam, S. A., Varnes, L., Graham, R., & Gamaz, L. (2012). "When the age is in, the wit is out": Age-related self-categorization and deficit expectations reduce performance on clinical tests used in dementia assessment. *Psychology and Aging*, *27*, 778–784.

Haslam, D. W., & James, W. P. T. (2005). Obesity. *The Lancet*, *366*, 1197–1209.

Haslam, N. (2016). Concept creep: Psychology's expanding concepts of harm and pathology. *Psychological Inquiry*, *27*, 1–17.

Haslam, N., & Kvaale, E. P. (2015). Biogenetic explanations of mental disorder: The mixed-blessings model. *Current Directions in Psychological Science*, *24*, 399–404.

Haslam, S. A. (2004). *Psychology in organizations: The social identity approach* (2nd ed.). London: Sage.

Haslam, S. A. (2014). Making good theory practical: Five lessons for an Applied Social Identity Approach to challenges of organizational, health, and clinical psychology. *British Journal of Social Psychology*, *53*, 1–20.

Haslam, S. A., Haslam, C., Jetten, J., Cruwys, T., & Dingle, G. A. (in press). The social identity approach to health. In K. Sweeny & M. Robbins (Eds.), *Wiley encyclopedia of health psychology*. Abingdon, UK: Wiley.

Haslam, S. A., Jetten, J., Haslam, C., & Knight, C. (2008). *Working with social identities to enhance neuropsychological outcomes and adjustment: The case for a social neuropsychology*. Meeting of the International Neuropsychology Society (INS), Buenos Aires, July 3–5.

Haslam, S. A., Jetten, J., O'Brien, A., & Jacobs, E. (2004). Social identity, social influence, and reactions to potentially stressful tasks: Support for the self-categorization model of stress. *Stress and Health*, *20*, 3–9.

Haslam, S. A., Jetten, J., Postmes, T., & Haslam, C. (2009). Social identity, health and well-being: An emerging agenda for applied psychology. *Applied Psychology: An International Review*, *58*, 1–23.

Haslam, S. A., Jetten, J., Reynolds, K. J., & Reicher, S. D. (2013). The dangers of isolating the individual: The need for a dynamic and socially structured model of personality. *Health Psychology Review*, *7*, 79–84.

Haslam, S. A., McMahon, C., Cruwys, T., Haslam, C., Jetten, J., & Steffens, N. K. (2018). Social cure, what social cure? The propensity to underestimate the importance of social factors for health. *Social Science and Medicine*, *198*, 14–21.

Haslam, S. A., O'Brien, A., Jetten, J., Vormedal, K., & Penna, S. (2005). Taking the strain: Social identity, social support and the experience of stress. *British Journal of Social Psychology*, *44*, 355–370.

Haslam, S. A., Oakes, P. J., Turner, J. C., & McGarty, C. (1995). Social categorization and group homogeneity: Changes in the perceived applicability of stereotype content as a function of comparative context and trait favourableness. *British Journal of Social Psychology*, *34*, 139–160.

Haslam, S. A., & Reicher, S. D. (2006). Stressing the group: Social identity and the unfolding dynamics of responses to stress. *Journal of Applied Psychology*, *91*, 1037–1052.

Haslam, S. A., & Reicher, S. D. (2012). When prisoners take over the prison: A social psychology of resistance. *Personality and Social Psychology Review, 16*, 152–179.

Haslam, S. A., Reicher, S. D., Bentall, R. P., Cruwys, T., McIntyre, J., & Haslam, C. (2016). *They're out to get me: Disidentification and the emergence of paranoia.* Paper presented at the Third International Conference on Social Identity and Health. Brisbane, June 16–19.

Haslam, S. A., Reicher, S. D., Koppel, G., & Mirsky, N. (2002). *The BBC prison experiment: The transcript.* London: British Broadcasting Company.

Haslam, S. A., Reicher, S. D., Koppel, G., & Mirsky, N. (2006). *The experiment: The transcript.* London: BBC Active and Pearson Education.

Haslam, S. A., Reicher, S. D., & Levine, R. M. (2012). When other people are heaven, when other people are hell: How social identity determines the nature and impact of social support. In J. Jetten, C. Haslam, & S. A. Haslam (Eds.), *The social cure: Identity, health and well-being* (pp. 157–174). Hove, UK: Psychology Press.

Haslam, S. A., Reicher, S. D., & Platow, M. J. (2011). *The new psychology of leadership: Identity, influence and power.* New York, NY: Psychology Press.

Haslam, S. A., Steffens, N. K., Peters, K., Boyce, R. A., Mallett, C. J., & Fransen, K. (2017). A social identity approach to leadership development: The 5R program. *Journal of Personnel Psychology, 16*, 113–124.

Haslam, S. A., & Turner, J. C. (1992). Context-dependent variation in social stereotyping 2: The relationship between frame of reference, self-categorization and accentuation. *European Journal of Social Psychology, 22*, 251–277.

Hastings, A., McNamara, N., Allan, J., & Marriott, M. (2016). The importance of social identities in the management of and recovery from "Diabulimia": A qualitative exploration. *Addictive Behaviors Reports, 4*, 78–86.

Haunschild, P. R., Moreland, R. L., & Murrell, A. J. (1994). Sources of resistance to mergers between groups. *Journal of Applied Social Psychology, 24*, 1150–1178.

Häusser, J. A., Kattenstroth, M., Van Dick, R., & Mojzisch, A. (2012). "We" are not stressed: Social identity in groups buffers neuroendocrine stress reactions. *Journal of Experimental Social Psychology, 48*, 973–977.

Havelka, M., Despot Lucanin, J., & Lucanin, D. (2009). Biopsychosocial model: The integrated approach to health and disease. *Collegial Antropologicum, 33*, 303–310.

Hawe, P., & Shiell, A. (2000). Social capital and health promotion: A review. *Social Science and Medicine, 51*, 871–885.

Hawkley, L. C., & Cacioppo, J. T. (2003). Loneliness and pathways to disease. *Brain, Behavior, and Immunity, 17*, 98–105.

Hawkley, L. C., & Cacioppo, J. T. (2010). Loneliness matters: A theoretical and empirical review of consequences and mechanisms. *Annals of Behavioral Medicine, 40*, 218–227.

Hawthorne, G. (2006). Measuring social isolation in older adults: Development and initial validation of the Friendship Scale. *Social Indicators Research, 77*, 521–548.

Hay, P. J., Mond, J. M., Buttner, P., & Darby, A. (2008). Eating disorder behaviors are increasing: findings from two sequential community surveys in South Australia. *PLoS ONE, 3*(2), e1541.

Hays, R. D., & DiMatteo, M. E. R. (1987). A short-form measure of loneliness. *Journal of Personality Assessment, 51*, 69–81.

Hedges, D. W., Allen, S., Tate, D. F., Thatcher, G. W., Miller, M. J., Rice, S. A., . . . Bigler, E. D. (2003). Reduced hippocampal volume in alcohol and substance naive Vietnam combat veterans with posttraumatic stress disorder. *Cognitive and Behavioral Neurology, 16*, 219–224.

Heilbrun, A. B., & Bloomfield, D. L. (1986). Cognitive differences between bulimic and anorexic females: Self-control deficits in bulimia. *International Journal of Eating Disorders, 5*, 209–222.

Hein, G., Silani, G., Preuschoff, K., Batson, C. D., & Singer, T. (2010). Neural responses to in-group and out-group members' suffering predict individual differences in costly helping. *Neuron, 68*, 149–160.

Heinz, W. R. W. (2009). Structure and agency in transition research. *Journal of Education and Work, 22*, 391–404.

Helliwell, J. F. (2006). Well-being, social capital and public policy. *The Economic Journal, 116*, 34–45.

Helliwell, J. F., & Barrington-Leigh, C. P. (2012). How much is social capital worth? In J. Jetten, C. Haslam, & S. A. Haslam (Eds.), *The social cure: Identity, health and well-being* (pp. 55–71). Hove, UK: Psychology Press.

Helliwell, J. F., Barrington-Leigh, C. P., Harris, A., & Huang, H. (2010). International evidence on the social context of well-being'. In D. Kahneman, E. Diener, & J. F. Helliwell (Eds.), *International differences in well-being*. Oxford: Oxford University Press.

Helliwell, J. F., Layard, R., & Sachs, J. (Eds.). (2013). *World happiness report.* New York, NY: UN Sustainable Development Solutions Network.

Henrich, J., Heine, S. J., & Norenzayan, A. (2010). Most people are not WEIRD. *Nature, 466,* 29.

Henry, J. D., & Crawford, J. R. (2005). The short-form version of the Depression Anxiety Stress Scales (DASS-21): Construct validity and normative data in a large non-clinical sample. *British Journal of Clinical Psychology, 44,* 227–239.

Hepworth, J. (2006). The emergence of critical health psychology: Can it contribute to promoting public health? *Journal of Health Psychology, 11,* 331–341.

Herington, K. J., Dingle, G. A., & Perryman, C. (2017). *Do posttraumatic symptoms influence the formation of a recovery identity in therapeutic community treatment for drug and alcohol misuse?* Presented at the UQ Centre for Health Outcomes Innovation and Clinical Education conference. Brisbane, September 8.

Herman, C. P., Koenig-Nobert, S., Peterson, J. B., & Polivy, J. (2005). Matching effects on eating: Do individual differences make a difference? *Appetite, 45,* 108–109.

Hernandez, B., Balcazar, F., Keys, C., Hidalgo, M. A., & Rosen, J. (2006). Taking it to the streets: Ethnic minorities with disabilities seek community inclusion. *Community Development, 37,* 13–25.

Herzlich, C., & Pierret, J. (1987). *Illness and self in society.* Baltimore: The Johns Hopkins University Press.

Hess, T. M., Auman, C., Colombe, S. J., & Rahhal, T. A. (2003). The impact of stereotype threat on age differences in memory performance. *Journal of Gerontology: Psychological Sciences, 58B,* 3–11.

Hess, T. M., & Hinson, J. T. (2006). Age-related variation in the influences of aging stereotypes on memory in adulthood. *Psychology and Aging, 21,* 621–625.

Hess, T. M., Hinson, J. T., & Hodges, E. A. (2009). Moderators of and mechanisms underlying stereotype threat effects on older adults' memory performance. *Experimental Aging Research, 35,* 153–177.

Hettema, J., Steele, J., & Miller, W. R. (2005). Motivational Interviewing. *Annual Review of Clinical Psychology, 1,* 91–111.

Hewa, S., & Hetherington, R. W. (1995). Specialists without spirit: Limitations of the mechanistic biomedical model. *Theoretical Medicine and Bioethics, 16,* 129–139.

Hewett, D. G., Watson, B. M., Gallois, C., Ward, M., & Leggett, B. A. (2009). Intergroup communication between hospital doctors: Implications for quality of patient care. *Social Science and Medicine, 69,* 1732–1740.

Hibbard, M. R., Uysal, S., Kepler, K., Bognay, J., & Silver, J. (1998). Axis I psychopathology in individuals with traumatic brain injury. *Journal of Head Trauma Rehabilitation, 13,* 24–39.

Hibscher, J. A., & Herman, C. P. (1977). Obesity, dieting, and the expression of obese characteristics. *Journal of Comparative and Physiological Psychology, 91,* 374–380.

Hill, A. J. (2004). Does dieting make you fat? *British Journal of Nutrition, 92,* 15–18.

Hill, J. O., & Melanson, E. L. (1999). Overview of the determinants of overweight and obesity: Current evidence and research issues. *Medicine and Science in Sports & Exercise, 31,* 515–521.

Hodgson, J., McDonald, S., Tate, R., & Gertler, P. (2005). A randomised controlled trial of a cognitive-behavioural therapy program for managing social anxiety after acquired brain injury. *Brain Impairment, 6,* 169–180.

Hoek, H. W. (2006). Incidence, prevalence and mortality of anorexia nervosa and other eating disorders. *Current Opinion in Psychiatry, 19,* 389–394.

Hogan, P. A., Reynolds, K. J., Latz, I., & O'Brien, L. (2015). Stigma and its consequences for social identity. In P. A. Hogan & R. Phillips (Eds.), *Hearing impairment and hearing disability: Towards a paradigm change in hearing services* (pp. 33–48). Dorchester, UK: Ashgate.

Hogan, T. P., Awad, A. G., & Eastwood, R. (1983). A self-report scale predictive of drug compliance in schizophrenics: Reliability and discriminative validity. *Psychological Medicine, 13,* 177–183.

Hoge, C. W., Auchterlonie, J., & Milliken, C. (2006). Mental health problems, use of mental health services, and attrition from military service after returning from deployment to Iraq or Afghanistan. *Journal of the American Medical Association, 295,* 1023–1032.

Hollies. (1969). He ain't heavy, he's my brother. From the album *Hollies sing Hollies.* London: Parlophone. Retrieved from www.youtube.com/watch?v=Jl5vi9ir49g

Hollon, S. D., Derubeis, R. J., Fawcett, J., Amsterdam, J. D., Shelton, R. C., Zajecka, J., . . . Gallop, R. (2014). Effect of cognitive therapy with antidepressant medications vs antidepressants alone on the rate of recovery in major depressive disorder: A randomized clinical trial. *JAMA Psychiatry, 71,* 1157–1164.

Holmes, T. H., & Rahe, R. H. (1967). The social readjustment rating scale. *Journal of Psychosomatic Research, 11,* 213–218.

Holt, R. I., Cockram, C., Flyvbjerg, A., & Goldstein, B. J. (Eds.). (2017). *Textbook on diabetes* (5th ed.). Chichester, UK: Wiley.

Holt-Lunstad, J., Robles, T. F., & Sbarra, D. A. (2017). Advancing social connection as a public health priority in the United States. *American Psychologist, 72,* 517–530.

Holt-Lunstad, J., Smith, T. B., & Layton, J. B. (2010). Social relationships and mortality risk: A meta-analytic review. *PLoS Medicine, 7*(7), e1000316.

Hommel, K., Madsen, M., & Kamper, A. L. (2012). The importance of early referral for the treatment of chronic kidney disease: A Danish nationwide cohort study. *BMC Nephrology, 13,* 108–116.

Honyashiki, M., Furukawa, T. A., Noma, H., Tanaka, S., Chen, P., Ichikawa, K., . . . Caldwell, D. M. (2014). Specificity of CBT for depression: a contribution from multiple treatments meta-analyses. *Cognitive Therapy and Research, 38,* 249–260.

Hopkins, N., & Reicher, S. D. (1996). The construction of social categories and processes of social change: Arguing about national identity. In G. M. Breakwell & E. Lyons (Eds.), *Changing European identities: Social psychological analyses of social change* (pp. 69–93). Oxford: Butterworth-Heinemann.

Hopkins, N., & Reicher, S. D. (2007). Social identity and health at mass gatherings. *European Journal of Social Psychology, 47,* 867–877.

Hopkins, N., Reicher, S. D., Khan, S. S., Tewari, S., Srinivasan, N., & Stevenson, C. (2016). Explaining effervescence: Investigating the relationship between shared social identity and positive experience in crowds. *Cognition and Emotion, 30,* 20–32.

Hor, K., & Taylor, M. (2010). Suicide and schizophrenia: a systematic review of rates and risk factors. *Journal of Psychopharmacology, 24*(Supplement 4), 81–90.

Horne, P. J., Hardman, C. A, Lowe, C. F., Tapper, K., Le Noury, J., Madden, P., . . . Doody, M. (2009). Increasing parental provision and children's consumption of lunchbox fruit and vegetables in Ireland: The Food Dudes intervention. *European Journal of Clinical Nutrition, 63,* 613–618.

Hornsey, M. J., & Hogg, M. A. (2000). Intergroup similarity and subgroup relations: Some implications for assimilation. *Personality and Social Psychology Bulletin, 26,* 948–958.

House, J. S. (1981). *Work stress and social support.* Reading, MA: Addison-Wesley.

Howard, J. (2006). Expecting and accepting: the temporal ambiguity of recovery identities. *Social Psychology Quarterly, 69,* 307–324.

Howard, J. (2008). Negotiating an exit: Existential, interactional, and cultural obstacles to disorder disidentification. *Social Psychology Quarterly, 71,* 177–192.

Hsieh, M., Ponsford, J. L., Wong, D. K., Schönberger, M., Taffe, J. R., & McKay, A. D. (2012). Motivational interviewing and cognitive behaviour therapy for anxiety following traumatic brain injury: A pilot randomised trial. *Neuropsychological Rehabilitation, 22,* 585–608.

Huang, Z., & Xu, K. (2006). Education of migrant workers and their children and its solutions. *Journal of Zhejiang University (Humanities and Social Sciences), 36,* 108–114.

Hudzik, B., Hudzik, M., & Polonski, L. (2014). Choosing wisely: Avoiding too much medicine. *Canadian Family Physician, 60,* 873–876.

Hughes, M. E., Waite, L. J., Hawkley, L. C., & Cacioppo, J. T. (2004). A short scale for measuring loneliness in large surveys results from two population-based studies. *Research on Aging, 26,* 655–672.

Hummert, M. L. (2011). Age stereotypes and aging. In K. W. Schaie & S. L. Willis (Eds.), *Handbook of the psychology of aging* (pp. 249–262). Amsterdam, Netherlands: Elsevier.

Hummert, M. L., Garstka, T. A., Shaner, J. L., & Strahm, S. (1994). Stereotypes of the elderly held by young, middle-aged and elderly adults. *Journal of Gerontology: Psychological Sciences, 49*, 240–249.

Hummert, M. L., Shaner, J. L., Garstka, T. A., & Henry, C. (1998). Communication with older adults: The influence of age stereotypes, context, and communicator age. *Human Communication Research, 25*, 124–151.

Hutchinson, G., Bhugra, D., Mallett, R., Burnett, R., Corridan, B., & Leff, J. (1999). Fertility and marital rates in first-onset schizophrenia. *Social Psychiatry & Psychiatric Epidemiology, 34*, 617–621.

Hutterer, J., & Liss, M. (2006). Cognitive development, memory, trauma, treatment: An integration of psychoanalytic and behavioural concepts in the light of current neuroscience research. *Journal of the American Academy of Psychoanalysis and Dynamic Psychiatry, 34*, 287–302.

Hutton, J. (2005). Cognitive behaviour therapy for irritable bowel syndrome. *European Journal of Gastro-enterology and Hepatology, 17*, 11–14.

IASP Task Force on Taxonomy. (1994). Pain terms: A current list with definitions and notes on usage. In H. Merskey & N. Bogduk (Eds.), *Classification of chronic pain* (2nd ed., pp. 207–213). Seattle: IASP Press.

Ilic, M., Reinecke, J., Bohner, G., Röttgers, H., Beblo, T., Driessen, M., Frommberger, U., & Corrigan, P. W. (2014). Managing a stigmatized identity – evidence from a longitudinal analysis about people with mental illness. *Journal of Applied Social Psychology, 44*, 464–480.

Ingram, K. M., Betz, N. E., Mindes, E. J., Schmitt, M. M., & Smith, N. G. (2001). Unsupportive responses from others concerning a stressful life event: Development of the Unsupportive Social Interactions Inventory. *Journal of Social and Clinical Psychology, 20*, 174–208.

Ingram, K. M., Jones, D. A., Fass, R. J., Neidig, J. L., & Song, Y. S. (1999). Social support and unsupportive social interactions: Their association with depression among people living with HIV. *AIDS Care, 11*, 313–329.

Inman, M. L., & Baron, R. S. (1996). Influence of prototypes on perceptions of prejudice. *Journal of Personality and Social Psychology, 70*, 727–739.

Institute for Safe Medication Practice. (2007). *Protecting U.S. citizens from inappropriate medication use: A white paper on medication safety in the U.S. and the role of community pharmacists.* Retrieved from www.ismp.org/pressroom/viewpoints/CommunityPharmacy.pdf

Iyer, A., & Jetten, J. (2011). What's left behind: Identity continuity moderates the effect of nostalgia on well-being and life choices. *Journal of Personality and Social Psychology, 101*, 94–108.

Iyer, A., Jetten, J., & Tsivrikos, D. (2008). Torn between identities: Predictors of adjustment to identity change. In F. Sani (Ed.), *Self-continuity: Individual and collective perspectives* (pp. 187–197). New York, NY: Psychology Press.

Iyer, A., Jetten, J., Tsivrikos, D., Postmes, T., & Haslam, S. A. (2009). The more (and the more compatible) the merrier: Multiple group memberships and identity compatibility as predictors of adjustment after life transitions. *British Journal of Social Psychology, 48*, 707–733.

Jackson, J. J., Hill, P. L., Payne, B. R., Roberts, S. W., & Stein-Morrow, E. A. (2012). Can an old dog learn (and want to experience) new tricks? Cognitive training increases openness to experience in older adults. *Psychology and Aging, 27*, 286–292.

Jackson, S. E., Schwab, R. L., & Schuler, R. S. (1986). Toward an understanding of the burnout phenomenon. *Journal of Applied Psychology, 71*, 630–640.

Jacobson, N. S., Dobson, K. S., Truax, P. A., Addis, M. E., Koerner, K., Gollan, J. K., . . . Prince, S. E. (1996). A component analysis of cognitive-behavioral treatment for depression. *Journal of Consulting and Clinical Psychology, 64*, 295–304.

Jasinskaja-Lahti, I., Liebkind, K., Jaakola, M., & Jaakkola Reuter, A. (2006). Perceived discrimination, social support networks, and psychological well-being among three immigrant groups. *Journal of Cross-Cultural Psychology, 37*, 293–311.

Jeffery, R. W., Rydell, S., Dunn, C. L., Harnack, L. J., Levine, A. S., Pentel, P. R., . . . Walsh, E. M. (2007). Effects of portion size on chronic energy intake. *International Journal of Behavioral Nutrition and Physical Activity, 4*, 27–32.

Jerant, A. F., Von Friederichs-Fitzwater, M. M., & Moore, M. (2005). Patients' perceived barriers to active self-management of chronic conditions. *Patient Education and Counseling, 57*, 300–307.

Jetten, J., & Branscombe, N. R. (2009). Seeking minority group memberships: Responses to discrimination when group membership is self-selected. In F. Butera & J. Levine (Eds.), *Coping with minority status: Responses to exclusion and inclusion* (pp. 155–176). New York, NY: Cambridge University Press.

Jetten, J., Branscombe, N. R., Haslam, S. A., Haslam, C., Cruwys, T., Jones, J. M., . . . Zhang, A. (2015). Having a lot of a good thing: Multiple important group memberships as a source of self-esteem. *PLoS ONE, 10*(6), e0131035.

Jetten, J., Branscombe, N. R., Iyer, A., & Asai, N. (2013). Appraising gender discrimination as legitimate or illegitimate: Antecedents and consequences. In M. K. Ryan & N. R. Branscombe (Eds.), *Handbook of gender and psychology* (pp. 306–322). London: Sage.

Jetten, J., Branscombe, N. R., Schmitt, M. T., & Spears, R. (2001). Rebels with a cause: Group identification as a response to perceived discrimination from the mainstream. *Personality and Social Psychology Bulletin, 27,* 1204–1213.

Jetten, J., Branscombe, N. R., Spears, R., & McKimmie, B. M. (2003). Predicting the paths of peripherals: The interaction of identification and future possibilities. *Personality and Social Psychology Bulletin, 29,* 130–140.

Jetten, J., Haslam, C., & Haslam S. A. (Eds.). (2012). *The social cure: Identity, health and well-being.* Hove, UK: Psychology Press.

Jetten, J., Haslam, C., Haslam, S. A., & Branscombe, N. (2009). The social cure. *Scientific American Mind, 20,* 26–33.

Jetten, J., Haslam, C., Haslam, S. A., Dingle, G. A., & Jones, J. M. (2014). How groups affect our health and well-being: The path from theory to policy. *Social Issues and Policy Review, 8,* 103–130.

Jetten, J., Haslam, C., Pugliese, C., Tonks, J., & Haslam, S. A. (2010b). Declining autobiographical memory and the loss of identity: Effects on well-being. *Journal of Clinical and Experimental Neuropsychology, 32,* 408–416.

Jetten, J., Haslam, S. A., & Barlow, F. (2013). Bringing back the system: One reason why conservatives are happier than liberals is that higher socio-economic status gives them access to more group memberships. *Social Psychological and Personality Science, 4,* 6–13.

Jetten, J., Haslam, S. A., Cruwys, T., Greenaway, K., Haslam, S. A., & Steffens, N. R. (2017). Advancing the social identity approach to health and well-being: Progressing the social cure research agenda. *European Journal of Social Psychology, 47,* 789–802.

Jetten, J., Haslam, S. A., Iyer, A., & Haslam, C. (2010a). Turning to others in times of change: Social identity and coping with stress. In S. Stürmer & M. Snyder (Eds.), *The psychology of pro-social behavior: Group processes, intergroup relations, and helping* (pp. 139–156). Oxford, UK: Blackwell.

Jetten, J., Hornsey, M. J., Spears, R., Haslam, S. A., & Cowell, E. (2010). Rule transgressions in groups: The conditional nature of newcomers' willingness to confront deviance. *European Journal of Social Psychology, 40,* 338–348.

Jetten, J., Iyer, A., Branscombe, N. R., & Zhang, A. (2013). How the disadvantaged appraise group-based exclusion: The path from legitimacy to illegitimacy. *European Review of Social Psychology, 24,* 194–224.

Jetten, J., Iyer, A., Tsivrikos, D., & Young, B. M. (2008). When is individual mobility costly? The role of economic and social identity factors. *European Journal of Social Psychology, 38,* 866–879.

Jetten, J., Iyer, A., & Zhang, A. (2017). The educational experience of low SES background students. In K. Mavor, M. Platow, & B. Bizumic (Eds.), *Self, social identity and education* (pp. 112–125). London: Routledge.

Jetten, J., O'Brien, A., & Trindall, N. (2002). Changing identity: Predicting adjustment to organizational restructure as a function of subgroup and superordinate identification. *British Journal of Social Psychology, 41,* 281–298.

Jetten, J., & Pachana, N. A. (2012). Not wanting to grow old: A social identity model of identity change (SIMIC) analysis of driving cessation among older adults. In J. Jetten, C. Haslam, & S. A. Haslam (Eds.), *The social cure: Identity, health and well-being* (pp. 97–113). Hove, UK: Psychology Press.

Jetten, J., Schmitt, M. T., Branscombe, N. R., Garza, A. A., & Mewse, A. J. (2011). Group commitment in the face of discrimination: The role of legitimacy appraisals. *European Journal of Social Psychology, 41,* 116–126.

Johnson, G., & Chamberlain, C. (2008). Homelessness and substance bbuse: Which comes first? *Australian Social Work, 61,* 342–356.

Johnson, G., & Chamberlain, C. (2011). Are the homeless mentally ill? *The Australian Journal of Social Issues, 46,* 29–48.

Johnstone, M., Jetten, J., Dingle, G. A., Parsell, C., & Walter, Z. C. (2015). Discrimination and well-being amongst the homeless: The role of multiple group membership. *Frontiers in Psychology, 6.* doi:10.3389/fpsyg.2015.00739

Johnstone, M., Jetten, J., Dingle, G. A., Parsell, C., & Walter, Z. C. (2016). Enhancing well-being of homeless individuals by building group memberships. *Journal of Community & Applied Social Psychology, 26,* 421–438.

Jones, A., Phillips, R., Parsell, C., & Dingle, G. A. (2014). *Review of systematic issues for social housing clients with complex needs.* Report to the Queensland Mental Health Commission, UQ Institute of Social Sciences Research.

Jones, E., & Wessely, S. (2005). *Shell shock to PTSD: Military psychiatry from 1900 to the Gulf War.* Hove and New York: Psychology Press.

Jones, J. M., Haslam, S. A., Jetten, J., Williams, W. H., Morris, R., & Saroyan, S. (2011). That which doesn't kill us can make us stronger (and more satisfied with life): The contribution of personal and social changes to well-being after acquired injury. *Psychology and Health, 26,* 353–369.

Jones, J. M., & Jetten, J. (2011). Recovering from strain and enduring pain: Multiple group memberships promote resilience in the face of physical challenges. *Social Psychological and Personality Science, 2,* 239–244.

Jones, J. M., Jetten, J., Haslam, S. A., & Williams, W. H. (2012). Deciding to disclose: The importance of maintaining social relationships for well-being after acquired brain injury. In J. Jetten, C. Haslam, & S. A. Haslam (Eds.), *The social cure: Identity, health, and well-being* (pp. 255–271). Hove, UK: Psychology Press.

Jones, J. M., Williams, W. H., Jetten, J., Haslam, S. A., Harris, A., & Gleibs, I. H. (2012). The role of psychological symptoms and social group memberships in the development of post-traumatic stress after traumatic injury. *British Journal of Health Psychology, 17,* 798–811.

Jones, N., Burdett, H., Wessely, S., & Greenberg, N. (2011). The subjective utility of early psychosocial interventions following combat deployment. *Occupational Medicine, 61,* 102–107.

Jones, N., Seddon, R., Fear, N. T., McAllister, P., Wessely, S., & Greenberg, N. (2012) Leadership, cohesion, morale, and the mental health of UK armed forces in Afghanistan. *Psychiatry: Interpersonal and Biological Processes, 75,* 49–59.

Jorden, S., Matheson, K., & Anisman, H. (2009). Supportive and unsupportive social interactions in relation to cultural adaptation and psychological symptoms among Somali refugees. *Journal of Cross-Cultural Psychology, 40,* 853–874.

Joseph, S. (2011). *What doesn't kill us: The new psychology of post-traumatic growth.* New York, NY: Basic Books.

Jost, J. T., & Thompson, E. P. (2000). Group-based dominance and opposition to equality as independent predictors of self-esteem, ethnocentrism, and social policy attitudes among African Americans and European Americans. *Journal of Experimental Social Psychology, 36,* 209–232.

Judd, L. (1997). The clinical course of unipolar major depressive disorders. *Archives of General Psychiatry, 54,* 989–991.

Jutel, A. (2010). Medically unexplained symptoms and the disease label. *Social Theory and Health, 8,* 229–245.

Jyväsjärvi, S., Joukamaa, M., Väisänen, E., Larivaara, P., Kivelä, S.-L., & Keinänen-Kiukaanniemi, S. (2001). Somatizing frequent attenders in primary health care. *Journal of Psychosomatic Research, 50,* 185–192.

Kahn, J. H., & Hessling, R. M. (2001). Measuring the tendency to conceal versus disclose psychological distress. *Journal of Social and Clinical Psychology, 20,* 41–65.

Kahn, R. S., Fleischhacker, W. W., Boter, H., Davidson, M., Vergouwe, Y., Keet, I. P., . . . EUFEST study group. (2008). Effectiveness of antipsychotic drugs in first episode schizophrenia and schizophreniform disorder: an open randomised clinical trial. *Lancet, 371,* 1085–1097.

Kalra, S. P., Bagnasco, M., Otukonyong, E. E., Dube, M. G., & Kalra, P. S. (2003). Rhythmic, reciprocal ghrelin and leptin signaling: new insight in the development of obesity. *Regulatory Peptides, 111*, 1–11.

Kaminer, D. (2006). Healing processes in trauma narratives: A review. *South African Journal of Psychology, 36*, 481–499.

Kang, S. K., & Chasteen, A. L. (2009). The moderating role of age-group identification and perceived threat on stereotype threat among older adults. *International Journal of Aging and Human Development, 69*, 201–220.

Kanter, R., & Caballero, B. (2012). Global gender disparities in obesity: A review. *Advances in Nutrition: An International Review Journal, 3*, 491–498.

Katona, C., & Brady, F. (in press). Complex trauma and complex responses to trauma in the asylum context. In R. Williams, S. Bailey, B. Kamaldeep, S. A. Haslam, C. Haslam, V. Kemp, & D. Maughan (Eds.), *Social scaffolding: Applying the lessons of contemporary social science to health, public mental health and healthcare*. London: Royal College of Psychiatrists.

Kavanagh, D. J. (1992). Recent developments in expressed emotion and schizophrenia. *British Journal of Psychiatry, 160*, 601–620.

Kawachi, I., & Berkman, L. F. (2000). Social cohesion, social capital, and health. In L. F. Berkman, I. Kawachi, & M. M. Glymour (Eds.), *Social epidemiology* (pp. 290–319). Oxford: Oxford University Press.

Kawachi, I., Subramanian, S. V., & Kim, D. (Eds.). (2008). *Social capital and health*. New York, NY: Springer.

Kaye, W. H., Frank, G. K., Bailer, U. F., & Henry, S. E. (2005). Neurobiology of anorexia nervosa: Clinical implications of alterations of the function of serotonin and other neuronal systems. *International Journal of Eating Disorders, 37*, 15–19.

Kearns, M., Muldoon, O. T., Msetfia, R. M., & Surgenorb, P. W. G. (2017). From darkness into light: identification with the crowd at a suicide prevention fundraiser promotes well-being amongst participants. *European Journal of Social Psychology, 47,* 878–888.

Kearon, T., Mythen, G., & Walklate, S. (2007). Making sense of emergency advice: Public perceptions of the terrorist risk. *Security Journal, 20*, 77–95.

Keinz, L. A., Schwartz, C., Trench, B., & Houlihan, D. (1995). An assessment of membership benefits in the Al-Anon program. *Alcoholism Treatment Quarterly, 12*, 31–38.

Keller, S. M., Zoellner, L. A., & Feeny, N. C. (2010). Understanding factors associated with early therapeutic alliance in PTSD treatment: Adherence, childhood sexual abuse history, and social support. *Journal of Consulting and Clinical Psychology, 78*, 974–979.

Kellezi, B., & Reicher, S. D. (2012). Social cure or social curse? The psychological impact of extreme events during the Kosovo conflict. In J. Jetten, C. Haslam, & S. A. Haslam (Eds.), *The social cure: Identity, health and well-being* (pp. 217–234). Hove, UK: Psychology Press.

Kellezi, B., Reicher, S. D., & Cassidy, C. (2009). Surviving the Kosovo conflict: A study of social identity, appraisal of extreme events, and mental well-being. *Applied Psychology: An International Review, 58*, 59–83.

Kelly, J. F., Hoeppner, B., Stout, R. L., & Pagano, M. (2012). Determining the relative importance of the mechanisms of behavior change within Alcoholic Anonymous: A multiple mediator analysis. *Addiction, 107*, 289–299.

Kelly, P. J., Deane, F. P., & Baker, A. L. (2015). Group cohesion and between session homework activities predict self-reported cognitive-behavioral skill use amongst participants of SMART recovery groups. *Journal of Substance Abuse Treatment, 51*, 53–58.

Kemp, J. J., Lickel, J. J., & Deacon, B. J. (2014). Effects of a chemical imbalance causal explanation on individuals' perceptions of their depressive symptoms. *Behaviour Research and Therapy, 56*, 47–52.

Kendler, K. S., Hettema, J. M., Butera, F., Gardner, C. O., & Prescott, C. A. (2003). Life event dimensions of loss, humiliation, entrapment, and danger in the prediction of onsets of major depression and generalized anxiety. *Archives of General Psychiatry, 60*, 789–796.

Kern, M. L., & Friedman, H. S. (2008). Do conscientious individuals live longer? A quantitative review. *Health Psychology, 27*, 505–512.

Kesey, K. (1962). *One flew over the cuckoo's nest*. New York: Penguin.

Kessler, R. C., Berglund, P., Chiu, W. T., Deitz, A. C., Hudson, J. I., Shahly, V., . . . Xavier, M. (2013). The prevalence and correlates of binge eating disorder in the World Health Organization World Mental Health Surveys. *Biological Psychiatry, 73*, 904–914.

Kessler, R. C., Ormel, J., Demler, O., & Stang, P. E. (2003). Comorbid mental disorders account for the role impairment of commonly occurring chronic physical disorders: Results from the National Comorbidity Survey. *Journal of Occupational and Environmental Medicine, 45*, 1257–1266.

Khan-Bourne, N., & Brown, R. G. (2003) Cognitive behaviour therapy for the treatment of depression in individuals with brain injury. *Neuropsychological Rehabilitation, 13*, 89–107.

Killeen, C. (1998). Loneliness: An epidemic in modern society. *Journal of Advanced Nursing, 28*, 762–770.

Kilpatrick, F. P., & Cantril, H. (1960). Self-anchoring scaling: A measure of individuals' unique reality worlds. *Journal of Individual Psychology, 16*, 158–173.

Kim, H. J., Burke, D. T., Dowds, M. M., Boone, K. A. R., & Park, G. J. (2000). Electronic memory aids for outpatient brain injury: Follow-up findings. *Brain Injury, 14*, 187–196.

Kim, H. J., Burke, D. T., Dowds, M. M., & George, J. (1999). Case study: Utility of a microcomputer as an external memory aid for a memory-impaired head injury patient during in-patient rehabilitation. *Brain Injury, 13*, 147–150.

Kim, D., Subramanian, S. V., & Kawachi, I. (2006). Bonding versus bridging social capital and their associations with self rated health: a multilevel analysis of 40 US communities. *Journal of Epidemiological Community Health, 60*, 116–122.

Kirmayer, L. J. (1999). Rhetorics of the body: medically unexplained symptoms in sociocultural perspective. In Y. Onoe, A. Janca, M. Asai, & N. Sartorious (Eds.), *Somatoform disorders: a worldwide perspective* (pp. 271–286). Japan: Springer.

Kirsch, I., Deacon, B. J., Huedo-Medina, T. B., Scoboria, A., Moore, T. J., & Johnson, B. T. (2008). Initial severity and antidepressant benefits: A meta-analysis of data submitted to the food and drug administration. *PLoS Medicine, 5*(2), e45.

Kjellgren, A., Lyden, F., & Norlander, T. (2008). Sensory isolation in flotation tanks: Altered states of consciousness and effects on well-being. *The Qualitative Report, 13*, 636–656.

Klaus, H. H., Kennell, J. H., Robertson, S. S., & Sosa, R. (1986). Effects of social support during parturition on maternal and infant morbidity. *British Medical Journal, 293*, 585–587.

Klehe, U. C., Koen, J., & Pater, I. E. (2012). Ending on the scrap heap? The experience of job loss and job search among older workers. In J. W. Hedge & W. C. Borman (Eds.), *Handbook of work and aging* (pp. 313–340). Oxford: Oxford University Press.

Klerman, G. L., Weissman, M. M., Rounsaville, B. J., & Chevron, E. S. (1984). *Interpersonal Psychotherapy of Depression*. New York, NY: Basic Books.

Klonoff, P. S., Lamb, D. G., Henderson, S. W., & Shepherd, J. (1998). Outcome assessment after milieu-based neurorehabilitation: new considerations. *Archives of Physical Medicine and Rehabilitation, 79*, 684–690.

Knight, C., Haslam, S. A., & Haslam, C. (2010). In home or at home? Evidence that collective decision making enhances older adults' social identification, well-being and use of communal space when moving to a new care facility. *Aging and Society, 30*, 1393–1418.

Knoop, H., Van Kessel, K., & Moss-Morris, R. (2012). Which cognitions and behaviours mediate the positive effect of cognitive behavioural therapy on fatigue in patients with multiple sclerosis? *Psychological Medicine, 42*, 205–213.

Kolb, L. C. (1987). A neuropsychological hypothesis explaining posttraumatic stress disorders. *American Journal of Psychiatry, 144*, 989–995.

Korte, S. M., Koolhaas, J. M., Wingfield, J. C., & McEwen, B. S. (2005). The Darwinian concept of stress: Benefits of allostasis and costs of allostatic load and the trade-offs in health and disease. *Neuroscience and Biobehavioral Reviews, 29*, 3–38.

Kotowicz, Z. (2007). The strange case of Phineas Gage. *History of the Human Sciences, 20*, 115–131.

Kotses, H., & Harver, A. (Eds.). (1998). *Self-management of asthma*. New York, NY: Marcel Dekker.

Kouchaki, M. (2011). Vicarious moral licensing: The influence of others' past moral actions on moral behavior. *Journal of Personality and Social Psychology, 101*, 702–715.

Koudenburg, N., Jetten, J., & Haslam, S. A. (2017). *The social search for self.* Unpublished manuscript, University of Groningen.

Kovacs, M., & Beck, A. T. (1978). Maladaptive cognitive structures in depression. *American Journal of Psychiatry, 135*, 525–533.

Kovel, J. (1987). Schizophrenic being and technocratic society. In D. M. Levin (Ed.), *Pathologies of the modern self: Postmodern studies on narcissism, schizophrenia, and depression* (pp. 330–348). New York, NY: New York University Press.

Kramer, A. F., Erickson, K. I., & Colcombe, S. J. (2006). Exercise, cognition, and the aging brain. *Journal of Applied Physiology, 101*, 1237–1242.

Kramer, A. F., Hahn, S., Cohen, N. J., Banich, M. B., McAuley, E., Harrison, C. R., . . . Colcombe, A. (1999). Ageing, fitness and neurocognitive function. *Nature, 400*, 418–419.

Krones, P. G., Stice, E., Batres, C., & Orjada, K. (2005). In vivo social comparison to a thin-ideal peer promotes body dissatisfaction: A randomized experiment. *International Journal of Eating Disorders, 38*, 134–142.

Kruijshaar, M. E., Barendregt, J., Vos, T., De Graaf, R., Spijker, J., & Andrews, G. (2005). Lifetime prevalence estimates of major depression: An indirect estimation method and a quantification of recall bias. *European Journal of Epidemiology, 20*, 103–111.

Kumar, R., Husain, M., Gupta, R. K., Hasan, K. M. Haris, M., Agarwal, A. K., . . . Narayana, P. A. (2009). Serial changes in the white matter diffusion tensor imaging metrics in moderate traumatic brain injury and correlation with neuro-cognitive function. *Journal of Neurotrauma, 26*, 481–495.

Kvaale, E. P., Haslam, N., & Gottdiener, W. H. (2013). The "side effects" of medicalization: a meta-analytic review of how biogenetic explanations affect stigma. *Clinical Psychology Review, 33*, 782–794.

Lalonde, R. N., & Silverman, R. A. (1994). Behavioral preference in response to social injustice: The effects of group permeability and social identity salience. *Journal of Personality and Social Psychology, 66*, 78–85.

Lambert, A. E., Watson, J. M., Stefanucci, J. K., Ward, N., Bakdash, J. Z., & Strayer, D. L. (2016). Stereotype threat impairs older adult driving. *Applied Cognitive Psychology, 30*, 22–28.

Lambert, M., Naber, D., Schacht, A., Wagner, T., Hundemer, H. P., Karow, A., . . . Schimmelmann, B. G. (2008). Rates and predictors of remission and recovery during 3 years in 392 never-treated patients with schizophrenia. *Acta Psychiatrica Scandinavica, 118*, 220–229.

Lambert, W. E., Libman, E., & Poser, E. G. (1960). The effect of increased salience of a membership group on pain tolerance. *Journal of Personality, 28*, 350–357.

Lamont, R. A., Swift, H. J., & Abrams, D. (2015). A review and meta-analysis of age-based stereotype threat: Negative stereotypes, not facts, do the damage. *Psychology and Aging, 30*, 180–193.

Lamster, F., Nittel, C., Rief, W., Mehl, S., & Lincoln, T. (2017). The impact of loneliness on paranoia: An experimental approach. *Journal of Behavior Therapy and Experimental Psychiatry, 54*, 51–57.

Lancaster, G. A., Dodd, S., & Williamson, P. R. (2004). Design and analysis of pilot studies: recommendations for good practice. *Journal of Evaluation in Clinical Practice, 10*, 307–312.

Landes, S. D., Ardelt, M., Vaillant, G. E., & Waldinger, R. J. (2014). Childhood adversity, midlife generativity, and later life well-being. *The Journals of Gerontology Series B: Psychological Sciences and Social Sciences, 69*, 942–952.

Landman, A., Cortese, D. K., & Glantz, S. (2008). Tobacco industry sociological programs to influence public beliefs about smoking. *Social Science and Medicine, 66*, 970–981.

Laney, B. B. (2009). Public health significance of neuroticism. *American Psychologist, 64*, 241–256.

Lansing, A. (2002). *Endurance: Shackleton's incredible voyage to the Antarctic.* London: Weidenfeld & Nicolson.

LaPorte, D. J. (2015). *Paranoid: Exploring suspicion from the dubious to the delusional.* Amherst, NY: Prometheus Books.

Lasky-Su, J. A., Faraone, S. V., Glatt, S. J., & Tsuang, M. T. (2005). Meta-analysis of the association between two polymorphisms in the serotonin transporter gene and affective disorders. *American Journal of Medical Genetics Part B, Neuropsychiatric Genetics, 133B*, 110–115.

Latrofa, M., Vaes, J., Pastore, M., & Cadinu, M. (2009). "United we stand, divided we fall"! The protective function of self-stereotyping for stigmatised members' psychological well-being. *Applied Psychology, 58*, 84–104.

Lazarus, A. A. (1968). Learning theory and the treatment of depression. *Behaviour Research and Therapy*, *6*, 83–89.

Lazarus, R. S. (1966). *Psychological stress and the coping process*. New York, NY: McGraw-Hill.

Lazarus, R. S. (2006). *Stress and emotion: A new synthesis*. New York, NY: Springer.

Lazarus, R. S., & Folkman, S. (1984). *Stress, appraisal and coping*. New York, NY. Springer Publishing Company.

Leach, C. W., Spears, R., Branscombe, N. R., & Doosje, B. (2003). Malicious pleasure: Schadenfreude at the suffering of another group. *Journal of Personality and Social Psychology*, *84*, 932–943.

Leach, C.W., Van Zomeren, M., Zebel, S., Vliek, M. L. W., & Spears, R. (2008). Group-level self-definition and self-investment: A hierarchical (multicomponent) model of ingroup identification. *Journal of Personality and Social Psychology*, *95*, 144–165.

Leary, M. R., Haupt, A. L., Strausser, K. S., & Chokel, J. T. (1998). Calibrating the sociometer: The relationship between interpersonal appraisals and state self esteem. *Journal of Personality and Social Psychology*, *74*, 1290–1299.

Le Bon, G. (1895). *The crowd: A study of the popular mind*. London: Ernest Benn.

Lebowitz, M. S., & Ahn, W. (2015). Emphasizing malleability in the biology of depression: Durable effects on perceived agency and prognostic pessimism. *Behaviour Research and Therapy*, *71*, 125–130.

Lee, D., Brellenthin, A. G., Thompson, P. D., Sui, X., Lee, I.-M., & Lavie, C. J. (in press). Running as a key lifestyle medicine for longevity. *Progress in Cardiovascular Diseases*. Retrieved from http://doi.org/10.1016/j.pcad.2017.03.005

Leknes, S., Brooks, J. C. W., Wiech, K., & Tracey, I. (2008). Pain relief as an opponent process: A psychophysical investigation. *European Medical Journal*, *28*, 794–801.

Lenz, A. S., Henesy, R., & Callender, K. (2016). Effectiveness of seeking safety for co-occurring posttraumatic stress disorder and substance use. *Journal of Counseling and Development*, *94*, 51–61.

Leo, R. J., & Narendran, R. (1999). Anticonvulsant use in the treatment of bipolar disorder: A primer for primary care physicians. *Primary Care Companion to the Journal of Clinical Psychiatry*, *1*, 74–84.

Lerner, M. J., & Miller, D.T. (1978). Just world research and the attribution process: Looking back and ahead. *Psychological Bulletin*, *85*, 1030–1051.

Levin, H. S., McCauley, S. R., Josic, C. P., Boake, C., Brown, S. A., Goodman, H. S., . . . Brundage, S. I. (2005). Predicting depression following mild traumatic brain injury. *Archives of General Psychiatry*, *62*, 523–528.

Levine, M., & Murnen, S. K. (2009). "Everybody knows that mass media are/are not (pick one) a cause of eating disorders": A critical review of evidence for a causal link between media, negative body image, and disordered eating in females. *Journal of Social and Clinical Psychology*, *28*, 9–42.

Levine, R. M. (1999). Identity and illness: The effects of identity salience and frame of reference on evaluation of illness and injury. *British Journal of Health Psychology*, *4*, 63–80.

Levine, R. M., Prosser, A., Evans, D., & Reicher, S. D. (2005). Identity and emergency intervention: How social group membership and inclusiveness of group boundaries shapes helping behaviour. *Personality and Social Psychology Bulletin*, *31*, 443–453.

Levine, R. M., & Reicher, S. D. (1996). Making sense of symptoms: Self-categorization and the meaning of illness and injury. *British Journal of Social Psychology*, *35*, 245–256.

Levine, R. M., & Thompson, K. (2004). Identity, place and bystander intervention: Social categories and helping after natural disasters. *Journal of Social Psychology*, *144*, 229–245.

Levy, B. R., Slade, M. D., Kunkel, S. R., & Kasl, S. V. (2002). Longevity increased by positive self-perceptions of aging. *Journal of Personality and Social Psychology*, *83*, 261–270.

Lewin, K. (1935). Psycho-sociological problems of a minority group. *Journal of Personality*, *3*, 175–187.

Lewin, K. (1948). *Field theory in social science*. New York, NY: Harper and Row.

Lewin, K. (1952). *Field theory in social science: Selected theoretical papers*. London: Tavistock.

Lewinsohn, P. M. (1975). Engagement in pleasant activities and depression level. *Journal of Abnormal Psychology*, *84*, 729–731.

Lewis, S., Thomas, S. L., Blood, R. W., Castle, D., Hyde, J., & Komesaroff, P. A. (2011). "I'm searching for solutions": Why are obese individuals turning to the Internet for help and support with "being fat"? *Health Expectations, 14*, 339–350.

Lezak, M. D., Howiesen, D. B., Bigler, E. D., & Tranel, D. (2012). *Neuropsychological Assessment* (5th ed.). New York, NY: Oxford University Press.

Li, H. K., & Dingle, G. A. (2012). Using the Drinking Expectancy Questionnaire (revised scoring method) in clinical practice. *Addictive Behaviours, 37*, 198–204.

Lichtenstein, P., Yip, B. H., Björk, C., Pawitan, Y., Cannon, T. D., Sullivan, P. F., & Hultman, C. M. (2009). Common genetic determinants of schizophrenia and bipolar disorder in Swedish families: a population-based study. *Lancet, 373*, 234–239.

Lifton, R. J. (1988). Understanding the traumatized self. In J. P. Wilson, Z. Harel, & B. Kahana (Eds.), *Human adaptation to extreme stress* (pp. 7–31). New York, NY: Springer.

Link, B. G., Struening, E. L., Neese-Todd, S., Asmussen, S., & Phelan, J. C. (2001). Stigma as a barrier to recovery: The consequences of stigma for the self-esteem of people with mental illnesses. *Psychiatric services, 52*, 1621–1626.

Linley, P. A., & Joseph, S. (2004). Positive change following trauma and adversity: A review. *Journal of Traumatic Stress, 17*, 11–21.

Linville, P. W. (1985). Self-complexity and affective extremity: Don't put all of your eggs in one cognitive basket. *Social Cognition, 3*, 94–120.

Linville, P. W. (1987). Self-complexity as a cognitive buffer against stress-related illness and depression. *Journal of Personality and Social Psychology, 52*, 663–676.

Lipworth, L., Abelin, T., & Conelly, R. R. (1970). Socio-economic factors in the prognosis of cancer patients. *Journal of Chronic Disability, 23*, 105–116.

Litz, B. T., Gray, M. J., Bryant, R. A., & Adler, A. B. (2002). Early intervention for trauma: Current status and future directions. *Clinical Psychology: Science and Practice, 9*, 112–134.

Loftus, E. F., & Pickrell, J. E. (1995). The formation of false memories. *Psychiatric Annals, 25*, 720–725.

Longmore, R. J., & Worrell, M. (2007). Do we need to challenge thoughts in cognitive behavior therapy? *Clinical Psychology Review, 27*, 173–187.

López-Cevallos, D. F., Harvey, S. M., & Warren, J. T. (2014). Medical mistrust, perceived discrimination, and satisfaction with health care among young-adult rural Latinos. *The Journal of Rural Health, 30*, 344–351.

López-Muñoz, F., Alamo, C., Cuenca, E., Shen, W. W., Clervoy, P., & Rubio, G. (2005). History of the discovery and clinical introduction of chlorpromazine. *Annals of Clinical Psychiatry, 17*, 113–135.

Loughnan, S., Bastian, B., & Haslam, N. (2014). The psychology of eating animals. *Current Directions in Psychological Science, 23*, 104–108.

Loughran, T. (2012). Shell shock, trauma, and the First World War: The making of a diagnosis and its histories. *Journal of the History of Medicine and Allied Sciences, 67*, 94–119.

Louis, W. R., Davies, S., Smith, J. R., & Terry, D. (2007). Pizza and pop and the student identity: The role of referent group norms in healthy and unhealthy eating. *The Journal of Social Psychology, 147*, 57–74.

Lovibond, S. H., & Lovibond, P. F. (1995). *Manual for the Depression Anxiety Stress Scales* (2nd ed.). Sydney: Psychology Foundation.

Lowe, M. R., & Kral, T. V. E. (2006). Stress-induced eating in restrained eaters may not be caused by stress or restraint. *Appetite, 46*, 16–21.

Lowe, M. R., & Timko, C. A. (2004). Dieting: really harmful, merely ineffective or actually helpful? *British Journal of Nutrition, 92*, 19–22.

Lowe, R. D., & Muldoon, O. T. (2014). Shared national identification in Northern Ireland: An application of psychological models of group inclusion post conflict. *Group Processes & Intergroup Relations, 17*, 602–616.

Loxton, N. J., Bunker, R. J., Dingle, G. A., & Wong, V. (2015). Drinking not thinking: A prospective study of personality traits and drinking motives on alcohol consumption across first year university. *Personality and Individual Differences, 79*, 134–139.

Luborsky, L., Rosenthal, R., Diguer, L., Andrusyna, T. P., Berman, J. S., Levitt, J. T., . . . Krause, E. D. (2002). The dodo bird verdict is alive and well – mostly. *Clinical Psychology: Science and Practice, 9,* 2–12.

Luce, B. R., Mauskopf, J., Sloan, F. A., Ostermann, J., & Paramore, L. C. (2006). The return on investment in health care: From 1980 to 2000. *Value in Health, 9,* 146–156.

Luhtanen, R., & Crocker, J. (1991). Self-esteem and intergroup comparison: Toward a theory of collective self-esteem. In J. Suls & T. A. Wills (Eds.), *Social comparison: Contemporary theory and research* (pp. 211–234). Hillsdale, NJ: Lawrence Erlbaum.

Lundahl, B. W., Kunz, C., Brownell, C., Tollefson, D., & Burke, B. L. (2010). A meta-analysis of motivational interviewing: Twenty-five years of empirical studies. *Research on Social Work Practice, 20,* 137–160.

Lynch, P., & Stagoll, B. (2002). Promoting equality: Homelessness and discrimination. *Deakin Law Review, 7,* 295–321.

MacDonald, G., & Leary, M. R. (2005). Why does social exclusion hurt? The relationship between social and physical pain. *Psychological Bulletin, 131,* 202–223.

Macmillan, M. (2000). *An odd kind of fame: Stories of Phineas Gage.* Cambridge, MA: MIT Press.

Macmillan, M. (2008). Phineas Gage: Unravelling the myth. *The Psychologist, 21,* 828–832.

Macmillan, M., & Lena, M. L. (2010). Rehabilitating Phineas Gage. *Neuropsychological Rehabilitation, 20,* 641–658.

Madan, A., Lazer, D., & Pentland, A. S. (2010). Social sensing: Obesity, unhealthy eating and exercise in face-to-face networks. *Wireless Health,* 104. Retrieved from http://dspace.mit.edu/openaccess-disseminate/1721.1/65376

Magerøy, N. (2009). *Health among Navy personnel. A cross-sectional study in the Royal Norwegian Navy.* Retrieved from http://bora.uib.no/handle/1956/3678?show=full

Magnus, A., Haby, M. M., Carter, R., & Swinburn, B. (2009). The cost-effectiveness of removing television advertising of high-fat and/or high-sugar food and beverages to Australian children. *International Journal of Obesity, 33,* 1094–1102.

Major, B., Gramzow, R. H., McCoy, S. K., Levin, S., Schmader, T., & Sidanius, J. (2002a). Perceiving personal discrimination: The role of group status and legitimizing ideology. *Journal of Personality and Social Psychology, 82,* 269–282.

Major, B., & O'Brien, L. T. (2005). The social psychology of stigma. *Annual Review of Psychology, 56,* 393–421.

Major, B., Quinton, W. J., & McCoy, S. K. (2002b). Antecedents and consequences of attributions to discrimination: Theoretical and empirical advances. In M. P. Zanna (Ed.), *Advances in experimental social psychology* (Vol. 34, pp. 251–300). San Diego, CA: Academic Press.

Major, B., & Schmader, T. (2001). Legitimacy and the construal of social disadvantage. In J. Jost & B. Major (Eds.), *The psychology of legitimacy: Emerging perspectives on ideology, power, and intergroup relations* (pp. 176–204). New York, NY: Cambridge University Press.

Major, B., & Testa, M. (1989). Social comparisons processes and judgments of entitlement and satisfaction. *Journal of Experimental Social Psychology, 25,* 101–120.

Makino, M., Tsuboi, K., & Dennerstein, L. (2004). Prevalence of eating disorders: A comparison of Western and Non-Western countries. *Medscape General Medicine, 6,* 49.

Malec, J. F. (2001). Impact of comprehensive day treatment on societal participation for persons with acquired brain injury. *Archives of Physical Medicine and Rehabilitation, 82,* 885–895.

Malivert, M., Fatséas, M., Denis, C., Langlois, E., & Auriacombe, M. (2012). Effectiveness of therapeutic communities: A systematic review. *European Addiction Research, 18,* 1–11.

Manogue, K. R., Leshner, A. I., & Candland, D. K. (1975). Dominance status and adrenocortical reactivity to stress in squirrel monkeys, *Primates, 16,* 457–463.

Marchiori, D., Waroquier, L., & Klein, O. (2012). "Split them!" smaller item sizes of cookies lead to a decrease in energy intake in children. *Journal of Nutrition Education and Behavior, 44,* 251–255.

Markle-Reid, M., & Browne, G. (2003). Conceptualisations of frailty in relation to older adults. *Journal of Advanced Nursing, 44,* 58–68.

Marlatt, A., & Gordon, J. (1985). *Relapse prevention: Maintenance strategies in the treatment of addictive behaviors*. New York, NY: Guilford Press.

Marmot, M. (2004). *Status syndrome: How our social standing affects your health and life expectancy*. London, UK: Bloomsburry Publishing.

Marmot, M. (2005). Social determinants of health inequalities. *Lancet, 365*, 1099–1104.

Marmot, M. (2015). *The health gap: The challenge of an unequal world*. London, UK: Bloomsbury.

Marmot, M., & Wilkinson, R. (Eds.). (2005). *Social determinants of health*. Oxford: Oxford University Press.

Martin, D. J., Garske, J. P., & Davis, M. K. (2000). Relation of the therapeutic alliance with outcome and other variables: A meta-analytic review. *Journal of Consulting and Clinical Psychology, 68*, 438–450.

Martin, P. (2016). *The sickening mind: Brain, behaviour, immunity and disease* (2nd ed.). London: Harper Collins.

Martin, P., & Leibovich, S. J. (2005). Inflammatory cells during wound repair: The good, the bad and the ugly. *Trends in Cell Biology, 15*, 599–607.

Martiny, S. E., & Rubin, M. (2016). Towards a clearer understanding of social identity theory's self-esteem hypothesis. In S. McKeown, R. Haji, & N. Ferguson (Eds.), *Understanding peace and conflict through social identity theory: Contemporary global perspectives* (pp. 19–32). New York, NY: Springer.

Masi, C. M., Chen, H-Y., Hawkley, L. C., & Cacioppo, J. T. (2011). A meta-analysis of interventions to reduce loneliness. *Personality and Social Psychology Review, 15*, 219–266.

Maslach, C., & Jackson, S. E. (1981). The measurement of experienced burnout. *Journal of Occupational Behavior, 2*, 99–113.

Maslach, C., Jackson, S. E., & Leiter, M. P. (1996). *Maslach Burnout Inventory manual* (3rd ed.). Palo Alto, CA: Consulting Psychologists Press.

Maslach, C., & Leiter, M. P. (1997). *The truth about burnout*. San Francisco, CA: Josey-Bass.

Master, S. L., Eisenberger, N. I., Taylor, S. E., Naliboff, B. D., Shirinyan, D., & Lieberman, M. D. (2009). A picture's worth: Partner photographs reduce experimentally induced pain. *Psychological Science, 20*, 1316–1318.

Mathers, N., Jones, N., & Hannay, D. (1995). Heartsink patients: A study of their general practitioners. *The British Journal of General Practice: The Journal of the Royal College of General Practitioners, 45*, 293–296.

Matheson, C., Robertson, H. D., Elliott, A. M., Iversen, L., & Murchie, P. (2016). Resilience of primary healthcare professionals working in challenging environments: A focus group study. *British Journal of General Practice, 66*, 507–515.

Matheson, K., & Anisman, H. (2012). Biological and psychosocial responses to discrimination. In J. Jetten, C. Haslam, & S. A. Haslam (Eds.), *The social cure: Identity, health and well-being* (pp. 133–153). Hove, UK: Psychology Press.

Matheson, K., Jorden, S., & Anisman, H. (2008). Relations between trauma experiences and psychological, physical and neuroendocrine functioning among Somali refugees: Mediating role of coping with acculturation stressors. *Journal of Immigrant and Minority Health, 10*, 291–304.

Matheson, K., McQuaid, R. J., & Anisman, H. (2016). Group identity, discrimination, and well-being: Confluence of psychosocial and neurobiological factors. *Current Opinion in Psychology, 11*, 35–39.

Matthews, K. A. (1988). Coronary heart disease and Type A behaviors: Update on, and alternative to, the Booth-Kewley and Friedman (1987) quantitative review. *Psychological Bulletin, 104*, 373–380.

Mattick, R. P., Breen, C., & Gibson, A. (2009). The place of buprenorphine in the management of opioid dependence. In R. P. Mattick, R. Ali, & N. Lintzeris (Eds.), *Pharmacotherapies for the treatment of opioid dependence: Efficacy, cost-effectiveness and implementation guidelines* (pp. 1–14). Boca Raton, Florida: CRC Press.

Mawson, E., Best, D., Beckwith, M., Dingle, G. A., & Lubman, D. I. (2015). Social identity, social networks and recovery capital in emerging adulthood: A pilot study. *Substance Abuse Treatment, Prevention, and Policy, 10*, 45.

McAllister, T. W. (2008). Neurobehavioral sequelae of traumatic brain injury: Evaluation and Management. *World Psychiatry, 7*, 3–10.

McAuley, E., Kramer, A. F., & Colcombe, S. J. (2004). Cardiovascular fitness and neurocognitive function in older adults: A brief review. *Brain, Behavior, and Immunity 18*, 214–220.

McCracken, L. M., MacKichan, F., & Eccleston, C. (2007). Contextual cognitive-behavioral therapy for severely disabled chronic pain sufferers: Effectiveness and clinically significant change. *European Journal of Pain, 11*, 314–322.

McEwen, B. S. (1998). Stress, adaptation, and disease: Allostasis and allostatic load. *Annals of the New York Academy of Sciences, 840*, 33–44.

McEwen, B. S. (2002). Sex, stress and the hippocampus: Allostasis, allostatic load and the aging process. *Neurobiology of Aging, 23*, 921–939.

McFall, M. E., Murburg, M. M., Ko, G. N., & Veith, R. C. (1990). Autonomic responses to stress in Vietnam combat veterans with posttraumatic stress disorder. *Biological Psychiatry, 27*, 1165–1175.

McGrath, J. J., Mortensen, P. B., Visscher, P. M., & Wray, N. R. (2013). Where GWAS and epidemiology meet: Opportunities for the simultaneous study of genetic and environmental risk factors in schizophrenia. *Schizophrenia Bulletin, 39*, 955–959.

McGurk, S. R., Mueser, K. T., & Pascaris, A. (2005). Cognitive training and supported employment for persons with severe mental illness: One-year results from a randomized controlled trial. *Schizophrenia Bulletin, 31*, 898–909.

McGurk, S. R., Schiano, D., Mueser, K. T., & Wolfe, R. (2010). Implementation of the thinking skills for work program in a psychosocial clubhouse. *Psychiatric Rehabilitation Journal, 33*, 190–199.

McIntyre, J., Elahi, A., & Bentall, R. P. (2016). Social identity and psychosis: Explaining elevated rates of psychosis in migrant populations. *Social and Personality Psychology Compass, 10*, 619–633.

McIntyre, J., Wickham, S., Barr, B., & Bentall, R. P. (2017). Social identity and psychosis: Associations and psychological mechanisms. *Schizophrenia Bulletin*. Advance online publication. doi:10.1093/schbul/sbx110

McKetin, R., Kothe, A., Baker, A., Lee, N. K., Ross, J., & Lubman, D. (2017). Predicting abstinence from methamphetamine use after residential rehabilitation: Findings from the Methamphetamine Treatment Evaluation Study. *Drug and Alcohol Review, 37*, 70–78.

McLaren, N. (1998). A critical review of the biopsychosocial model. *Australian and New Zealand Journal of Psychiatry, 32*, 86–92.

McLaren, S., & Challis, C. (2009). Resilience among men farmers: The protective roles of social support and sense of belonging in the depression-suicidal ideation relation. *Death Studies, 33*, 262–276.

McLeod, J. D., Hallett, T., & Lively, K. J. (2015). Beyond three faces: Toward an integrated social psychology of inequality. *Advances in Group Processes, 25*, 1–29.

McNally, R. J. (2003). Progress and controversy in the study of posttraumatic stress disorder. *Annual Review of Psychology, 54*, 229–252.

McNally, R. J., Lasko, N. B., Macklin, M. L., & Pitman, R. K. (1995). Autobiographical memory disturbance in combat-related posttraumatic stress disorder. *Behaviour Research and Therapy, 33*, 619–630.

McNamara, N., Stevenson, C., & Muldoon, O. T. (2013). Community identity as resource and context: A mixed method investigation of coping and collective action in a disadvantaged community. *European Journal of Social Psychology, 43*, 393–403.

McNeal, E. T., & Cimbolic, P. (1986). Antidepressants and biochemical theories of depression. *Psychological Bulletin, 99*, 361–374.

McNeil, J. K., LeBlanc, E. M., & Joyner, M. (1991. The effect of exercise on depressive symptoms in moderately depressed elderly. *Psychology and Aging, 6*, 487–488.

McPhedran, S., & De Leo, D. (2013a). Miseries suffered, unvoiced, unknown? Communication of suicidal intent by men in "Rural" Queensland, Australia. *Suicide and Life-Threatening Behavior, 43*, 589–597.

McPhedran, S., & De Leo, D. (2013b). Risk factors for suicide among rural men: Are farmers more socially isolated? *International Journal of Sociology and Social Policy, 33*, 762–772.

McPherson, J. (2012). Does narrative exposure therapy reduce PTSD in survivors of mass violence? *Research on Social Work Practice, 22*, 29–42.

McQuaid, R. J., McInnis, O. A., Matheson, K., & Anisman, H. (2015). Distress of ostracism: Oxytocin receptor gene polymorphism confers sensitivity to social exclusion. *Social Cognitive and Affective Neuroscience, 10*, 1153–1159.

McQuilken, M., Zahniser, J. H., Novak, J., Starks, R. D., Olmos, A., & Bond, G. R. (2003). The Work Project Survey: Consumer perspectives on work. *Journal of Vocational Rehabilitation, 18*, 59–68.

Meier, P. S., Barrowclough, C., & Donmall, M. C. (2005). The role of the therapeutic alliance in the treatment of substance misuse: A critical review of the literature. *Addiction, 100*, 304–316.

Melzack, R., & Wall, P. D. (1965). Pain mechanism: A new theory. *Science, 150*, 971–979.

Mendoza-Denton, R., Downey, G., Purdie, V. J., Davis, A., & Pietrzak, J. (2002). Sensitivity to status-based rejection: Implications for African American students' college experience. *Journal of Personality and Social Psychology, 83*, 896–918.

Menzies, D. (2011). The case for a worldwide ban on smoking in public places. *Current Opinion in Pulmonary Medicine, 17*, 116–122.

Merckelbach, H., Jelicic, M., & Jonker, C. (2012). Planting a misdiagnosis of Alzheimer's disease in a person's mind. *Acta Neuropsychiatrica, 24*, 60–62.

Messer, S. B., & Wampold, B. E. (2002). Let's face facts: Common factors are more potent than specific therapy ingredients. *Clinical Psychology: Science and Practice, 9*, 21–25.

Mezuk, B., & Rebok, G. W. (2008). Social integration and social support among older adults following driving cessation. *Journals of Gerontology Series B: Psychological Sciences and Social Sciences, 63B*, 298–303.

Migone, P. (1994, April). The problem of real trauma and the future of psychoanalysis. *International Forum of Psychoanalysis, 3*, 89–96.

Miklowitz, D. J. (2008). *Bipolar disorder: A family-focused approach* (2nd ed.). New York, NY: Guilford Press.

Miklowitz, D. J., O'Brien, M. P., Schlosser, D. A., Addington, J., Candan, K. A., Marshall, C., . . . Cannonet, T. D. (2014). Family-Focused Treatment for adolescents and young adults at high risk for psychosis: Results of a randomized trial. *Journal of the American Academy of Child and Adolescent Psychiatry, 53*, 848–858.

Miklowitz, D. J., Otto, M. W., Frank, E., Reilly-Harrington, N. A., Wisniewski, S. R., Kogan, J. N., . . . Araga, M. (2007). Psychosocial treatments for bipolar depression: A 1-year randomized trial from the Systematic Treatment Enhancement Program. *Archives of General Psychiatry, 64*, 419–426.

Miller, G., Chen, E., & Cole, S. W. (2009). Health psychology: Developing biologically plausible models linking the social world and physical health. *Annual Review of Psychology, 60*, 501–524.

Miller, K., Wakefield, J. R. H., & Sani, F. (2015). Identification with social groups is associated with mental health in adolescents: evidence from a Scottish community sample. *Psychiatry Research, 228*, 340–346.

Miller, K., Wakefield, J. R. H., & Sani, F. (2016). Greater number of group identifications is associated with healthier behaviour in adolescents. *British Journal of Developmental Psychology, 34*, 291–305.

Miller, P. M. (Ed.). (2013). *Interventions for addiction: Comprehensive addictive behaviors and Disorders* (Vol. 3). San Diego, CA: Academic Press.

Miller, T. Q., Smith, T. W., Turner, C. W., Guijarro, M. L., & Hallet, J. A. (1996). A meta-analytic review of research on hostility and physical health. *Psychological Bulletin, 119*, 332–348.

Miller, W. R., & Rollnick, S. (1991). *Motivational interviewing: Preparing people to change addictive behavior*. New York, NY: Guilford Press.

Miller, W. R., & Rollnick, S. (2002). *Motivation interviewing: Preparing people for change* (2nd ed.). New York, NY: Guilford Press.

Milton, K. (1999). Nutritional characteristics of wild primate foods: Do the diets of our closest living relatives have lessons for us?. *Nutrition, 15*, 488–498.

Milton, K. (2000). Hunter-gatherer diets: A different perspective. *American Journal of Clinical Nutrition, 71*, 665–667.

Miyamoto, S., Duncan, G. E., Marx, C. E., & Lieberman, J. A. (2005). Treatments for schizophrenia: a critical review of pharmacology and mechanisms of action of antipsychotic drugs. *Molecular Psychiatry, 10*, 79–104.

Molero, F., Fuster, M. J., Jetten, J., & Moriano, J. A. (2011). Living with HIV/AIDS: A psychosocial perspective on coping with prejudice and discrimination. *Journal of Applied Social Psychology, 41*, 609–626.

Mols, F., Haslam, S. A., Steffens, N., & Jetten, J. (2015). Why a Nudge is not enough: A social identity critique of governance by stealth. *European Journal of Political Research, 54*, 81–98.

Monroe, S. M., Rohde, P., Seeley, J. R., & Lewinsohn, P. M. (1999). Life events and depression in adolescence: Relationship loss as a prospective risk factor for first onset of major depressive disorder, *Journal of Abnormal Psychology, 108*, 606–614.

Montague, M., Borland, R., & Sinclair, C. (2001). Slip! Slop! Slap! and SunSmart, 1980–2000: Skin cancer control and 20 years of population-based campaigning. *Health Education and Behavior, 28*, 290–305.

Montalan, B., Lelard, T., Godefroy, O., & Mouras, H. (2012). Behavioral investigation of the influence of social categorization on empathy for pain: A minimal group paradigm study. *Frontiers in Psychology, 3*, 389. doi:10.3389/fpsyg.2012.00389

Moore, S. E., Scott, J. G., Ferrari, A. J., Mills, R., Dunne, M. P., Erskine, H. E., . . . Norman, R. E. (2015). Burden attributable to child maltreatment in Australia. *Child Abuse and Neglect, 48*, 208–220.

Moorer, A. (2014). *It's gonna feel good (when it stops hurting). From the album* Crows. Salem, MA: Rykodisk. Retrieved from www.youtube.com/watch?v=pxycEwz87JI&list=PLcJBUAv6rM 6Pito5eOtQ8donWdUnRFIoR&index=73

Moos, R. H. (2008). Active ingredients of substance use focused self help groups. *Addiction, 103*, 387–396.

Morgan, V. A., Waterreus, A., Jablensky, A., Mackinnon, A., McGrath, J. J., Carr, V., . . . Saw, S. (2011). *People Living with Psychotic Illness 2010*. Canberra: Australian Government. Retrieved from www. health.gov.au/internet/main/publishing.nsf/Content/717137A2F9B9FCC2CA257BF0001C118F/$File/psych10.pdf

Morris, D. B. (1991). *The culture of pain*. Berkeley, CA: University of California Press.

Morris, D. J. (2015). *The evil hours: A biography of post-traumatic stress disorder*. Boston, MA: Houghton Mifflin Harcourt.

Morris, W. L., Sinclair, S., & DePaulo, B. M. (2007). No shelter for singles: The perceived legitimacy of marital status discrimination. *Group Processes & Intergroup Relations, 10*, 457–470.

Mosely, L. G., & Arntz, A. (2007). The context of a noxious stimulus affects the pain it evokes. *Pain, 133*, 64–71.

Moses, H., Matheson, D. H., Cairns-Smith, S., George, B. P., Palisch, C., & Dorsey, E. R. (2015). The anatomy of medical research: US and international comparisons. *JAMA, 313*, 174–189.

Motion, A. (2009, November 7). An equal voice. *The Guardian*. Retrieved November 21, 2016, from www. guardian.co.uk/books/2009/nov/07/andrew-motion-remembrance-day-poem

Motlagh, H. (2010). Impact of Event Scale-Revised. *Journal of Physiotherapy, 56*, 203.

Motowidlo, S. J., Packard, J. S., & Manning, M. R. (1986). Occupational stress: Its causes and consequences for job performance. *Journal of Applied Psychology, 71*, 618–629.

Moussavi, S., Chatterji, S., Verdes, E., Tandon, A., Patel, V., & Ustun, B. (2007). Depression, chronic diseases, and decrements in health: Results from the World Health Surveys. *Lancet, 370*, 851–858.

Moutoussis, M., Williams, J., Dayan, P., & Bentall, R. P. (2007). Persecutory delusions and the conditioned avoidance paradigm: Towards an integration of the psychology and biology of paranoia. *Cognitive Neuropsychiatry, 12*, 495–510.

Mowrer, O. H. (1960). *Learning theory and behavior*. New York, NY: Wiley.

Mrazek, P. J., & Haggerty, R. J. (1994). *Reducing risks for mental disorders: Frontiers for preventive intervention research*. Washington, DC: National Academies Press.

Muenchberger, H., Kendall, E., & Neal, R. (2008). Identity transition following brain injury: A dynamic process of contraction, expansion and tentative balance. *Brain Injury, 22*, 979–992.

Mueser, K. T., Glynn, S. M., Cather, C., Xie, H., Zarate, R., Fox Smith, L., . . . Feldman, J. (2013). A randomized controlled trial of family intervention for co-occurring substance use and severe psychiatric disorders. *Schizophrenia Bulletin, 39*, 658–672.

Mukherjee, S. (2010). *The emperor of all maladies: A biography of cancer*. New York, NY: Simon and Schuster.

Muldoon, O. T. (2013). Understanding the impact of political violence in childhood: A theoretical review using a social identity approach. *Clinical Psychology Review, 33*, 929–939.

Muldoon, O. T., Acharya, K., Jay, S., Adhikari, K., Pettigrew, J., & Lowe, R. D. (2017). Community identity and collective efficacy: A social cure for traumatic stress in post-earthquake Nepal. *European Journal of Social Psychology, 47*, 904–915.

Muldoon, O. T., & Downes, C. (2007). Social identification and post-traumatic stress symptoms in post-conflict Northern Ireland. *The British Journal of Psychiatry, 191*, 146–149.

Muldoon, O. T., & Lowe, R. D. (2012). Social identity, groups, and post-traumatic stress disorder. *Political Psychology, 33*, 259–273.

Muldoon, O. T., Schmid, K., & Downes, C. (2009). Political violence and psychological well-being: The role of social identity. *Applied Psychology, 58*, 129–145.

Mullen, B., Brown, R., & Smith, C. (1992). Ingroup bias as a function of salience, relevance, and status: An integration. *European Journal of Social Psychology, 22*, 103–122.

Münsterberg, H. (1913). *Psychology and industrial efficiency*. Boston: Houghton Mifflin.

Murphy, K. M., & Topel, R. H. (Eds.). (2010). *Measuring the gains from medical research: An economic approach*. Chicago, IL: University of Chicago Press.

Murray, C. J. L., Vos, T., Lozano, R., Naghavi, M., Flaxman, A. D., Michaud, C., . . . Lopez, A. D. (2012). Disability-adjusted life years (DALYs) for 291 diseases and injuries in 21 regions, 1990–2010: A systematic analysis for the Global Burden of Disease Study 2010. *The Lancet, 380*, 2197–2223.

Myers, J. K., Lindenthal, J. J., & Pepper, M. P. (1971). Life events and psychiatric impairment. *The Journal of Nervous and Mental Disease, 152*, 149–157.

Myrtek, M. (2001). Meta-analyses of prospective studies on coronary heart disease, type A personality, and hostility. *International Journal of Cardiology, 79*, 245–251.

Nackers, L. M., Dubyak, P. J., Lu, X., Anton, S. D., Dutton, G. R., & Perri, M. G. (2015). Group dynamics are associated with weight loss in the behavioral treatment of obesity. *Obesity, 23*, 1563–1569.

Nadler, A. (2010). Interpersonal and intergroup helping relations as power relations: Implications for real-world helping. In S. Stürmer & M. Snyder (Eds.), *The psychology of pro-social behavior: Group processes, intergroup relations, and helping* (pp. 269–287). Oxford: Blackwell.

Nadort, M., Arntz, A., Smit, J. H., Giesen-Bloo, J., Eikelenboom, M., Spinhoven, P., . . . Van Dyck, R. (2009). Implementation of outpatient schema therapy for borderline personality disorder with versus without crisis support by the therapist outside office hours: A randomized trial. *Behaviour Research and Therapy, 47*, 961–973.

Najavits, L. M. (2002). *Seeking Safety: A treatment manual for PTSD and substance abuse*. New York, NY: Guilford Press.

Nakagawa, Y., & Shaw, R. (2004). Social capital: A missing link to disaster recovery. *International Journal of Mass Emergencies and Disasters, 22*, 5–34.

Nalder, E., Fleming, J., Cornwell, P., Foster, M., Ownsworth, T., Shields, C., & Haines, T. (2012) Recording sentinel events in the life course of individuals with acquired brain injury: A preliminary study. *Brain Injury, 26*, 1381–1396.

Nasser, M., Katzman, M. A., & Gordon, R. A. (2001). *Eating disorders and cultures in transition*. East Sussex: Psychology Press.

National Institute for Health and Clinical Excellence. (2014). *Psychosis and schizophrenia in adults: Prevention and management*. London: National Institute for Health and Clinical Excellence.

National Treatment Agency for Substance Misuse. (2006). *Models of care for treatment of adult drug misusers: Update 2006*. London, UK: Department of Health.

Neumark-Sztainer, D. (2003). Obesity and eating disorder prevention: An integrated approach? *Adolescent Medicine, 14*, 159–173.

Neuvonen, E., Rusanen, M., Solomon, A., Ngandu, T., Laatikainen, T., Soininen, H., Kivipelto, M., & Tolppanen, A-M. (2014). Late-life cynical distrust, risk of incident dementia, and mortality in a population-based cohort. *Neurology, 82*, 2205–2212.

Newheiser, A. K., & Barreto, M. (2014). Hidden costs of hiding stigma: Ironic interpersonal consequences of concealing a stigmatised identity in social interactions. *Journal of Experimental Social Psychology, 52*, 58–70.

Nietzsche, F. (1888). *Twilight of the idols* (R. J. Hollingdale, Trans., 1977). Harmondsworth: Penguin.

Nock, M. K. (2010). Why do people hurt themselves? New Insights into the nature and function of self-injury. *Current Directions in Psychological Science, 18*, 78–83.

Norris, F. H., & Kaniasty, K. (1996). Received and perceived social support in times of stress: A test of the social support deterioration deterrence model. *Journal of Personality and Social Psychology, 71*, 498–511.

Norton, K. I., Olds, T. S., Olive, S., & Dank, S. (1996). Ken and Barbie at life size. *Sex Roles, 34*, 287–294.

Notter, M. L., MacTavish, K. A., & Shamah, D. (2008), Pathways toward resilience among women in rural trailer parks. *Family Relations, 57*, 613–624.

Novelli, D., Drury, J., Reicher, S. D., & Stott, C. (2013). Crowdedness mediates the effect of social identification on positive emotion in a crowd: A survey of two crowd events. *PLoS ONE, 8*(11), e78983.

Nuechterlein, K. H., & Dawson, M. E. (1984). A heuristic vulnerability/stress model of schizophrenic episodes. *Schizophrenia Bulletin, 10*, 300–312.

Oakes, P. J. (1987). The salience of social categories. In J. C. Turner, M. A. Hogg, P. J. Oakes, S. D. Reicher, & M. S. Wetherell (Eds.), *Rediscovering the social group: A self-categorization theory* (pp. 117–141). Oxford: Blackwell.

Oakes, P. J., Haslam, S. A., & Turner, J. C. (1994). *Stereotyping and social reality*. Oxford: Blackwell.

Oakes, P. J., Turner, J. C., & Haslam, S. A. (1991). Perceiving people as group members: The role of fit in the salience of social categorizations. *British Journal of Social Psychology, 30*, 125–144.

O'Brien, A., Haslam, S. A., Jetten, J., Humphrey, L., O'Sullivan, L., Postmes, T., Eggins, R. A., & Reynolds, K. J. (2004). Cynicism and disengagement among devalued employee groups: The need to ASPIRe. *Career Development International, 9*, 28–44.

Oddy, M., Coughlan, T., Tyerman, A., & Jenkins, D. (1985). Social adjustment after closed head injury: a further follow-up seven years after injury. *Journal of Neurology, Neurosurgery and Psychiatry, 48*, 564–568.

Oei, T. P. S., McAlinden, N. M., & Cruwys, T. (2014). Exploring mechanisms of change: The relationships between cognitions, symptoms, and quality of life over the course of group cognitive-behaviour therapy. *Journal of Affective Disorders, 168C*, 72–77.

O'Farrell, T. J., & Clements, K. (2012). Review of outcome research on marital and family therapy in treatment for alcoholism. *Journal of Marital and Family Therapy, 38*, 122–144.

O'Farrell, T. J., & Fals-Stewart, W. (2006). *Behavioural couples therapy for alcoholism and drug abuse*. New York, NY: Guilford Press.

Ogden, J. (2003). Some problems with social cognition models: A pragmatic and conceptual analysis. *Health Psychology, 22*, 424–428.

Oh, H., Chung, M. H., & Labianca, G. (2004). Group social capital and group effectiveness: The role of informal socializing ties. *Academy of Management Journal, 47*, 860–875.

Oliver, M. (1998). Theories of disability in health practice and research. *British Medical Journal, 317*, 1446–1449.

Orbell, S., Lidierth, P., Henderson, C. J., Geeraert, N., Uller, C., Uskul, A. K., & Kyriakaki, M. (2009). Social-cognitive beliefs, alcohol, and tobacco use: A prospective community study of change following a ban on smoking in public places. *Health Psychology, 28*, 753–761.

Orleans, C. T., George, L. K., Houpt, J. L., & Brodie, K. H. (1985). Health promotion in primary care: A survey of U.S. family practitioners. *Preventive Medicine, 14*, 636–647.

Orsillo, S. M., Heimberg, R. G., Juster, H. R., & Garrett, J. (1996). Social phobia and PTSD in Vietnam veterans. *Journal of Traumatic Stress, 9*, 235–252.

Oshio, A., Kaneko, H., Nagamine, S., & Nakaya, M. (2003). Construct validity of the adolescent resilience scale. *Psychological reports, 93*, 1217–1222.

Otten, S., Mummendey, A., & Blanz, M. (1996). Intergroup discrimination in positive and negative outcome allocations: Impact of stimulus valence, relative group status, and relative group size. *Personality and Social Psychology Bulletin, 22*, 568–581.

Outten, H. R., Schmitt, M. T., Garcia, D. M., & Branscombe, N. R. (2009). Coping options: Missing links between minority group identification and psychological well-being. *Applied Psychology, 58*, 146–170.

Owen, M., Sellwood, W., Kan, S., Murray, J., & Sarsam, M. (2015). Group CBT for psychosis: A longitudinal, controlled trial with inpatients. *Behavior Research and Therapy, 65,* 76–85.

Ownsworth, T. (2014). *Self-identity after brain injury.* London: Psychology Press.

Ownsworth, T., Fleming, J., Haines, T., Cornwell, P., Kendall, M., Nalder, E., & Gordon, C. (2011). Development of depressive symptoms during early community reintegration after traumatic brain injury. *Journal of the International Neuropsychological Society, 17,* 112–119.

Ownsworth, T., & Haslam, C. (2016). Impact of rehabilitation on self-concept following traumatic brain injury: An exploratory systematic review of intervention and methodology. *Neuropsychological Rehabilitation, 26,* 1–35.

Oyserman, D., Fryberg, S. A., & Yoder, N. (2007). Identity-based motivation and health. *Journal of Personality and Social Psychology, 93,* 1011–1027.

Page, A. C., Hooke, G. R., & Morrison, D. L. (2007). Psychometric properties of the Depression Anxiety Stress Scales (DASS) in depressed clinical samples. *British Journal of Clinical Psychology, 46,* 283–297.

Palinkas, L. A., & Suedfeld, P. (2008). Psychological effects of polar expeditions. *The Lancet, 371,* 153–163.

Palomares, N. A. (2004). Gender schematicity, gender identity salience, and gender-linked language use. *Human Communication Research, 30,* 556–588.

Pandey, K., Stevenson, C., Shankar, S., Hopkins, N., & Reicher, S. D. (2014). Cold comfort at the Magh Mela: Social identity processes and physical hardship. *British Journal of Social Psychology, 53,* 675–690.

Papinczak, Z. E., Connor, J. P., Feeney, G. F. X., Young, R. M., & Gullo, M. J. (2017). Treatment seeking in cannabis dependence: The role of social cognition. *Drug and Alcohol Dependence, 170,* 142–146.

Paradies, Y., Ben, J., Denson, N., Elias, A., Priest, N., Pieterse, A., . . . Gee, G. (2015). Racism as a determinant of health: A systematic review and meta-analysis. *PLoS ONE, 10*(9), e0138511.

Paradies, Y., Truong, M., & Priest, N. (2014). A systematic review of the extent and measurement of healthcare provider racism. *Journal of General Internal Medicine 29,* 364–387.

Parra-Delgado, M., & Latorre-Postigo, J. M. (2013). Effectiveness of mindfulness-based cognitive therapy in the treatment of fibromyalgia: A randomized trial. *Cognitive Therapy and Research, 37,* 1015–1026.

Parsell, C. (2011). Homeless identities: Enacted and ascribed. *British Journal of Sociology, 62,* 442–461.

Pascoe, E. A., & Smart Richman, L. (2009). Perceived discrimination and health: A meta-analytic review. *Psychological Bulletin, 135,* 531–554.

Patai, E. Z., Gadian, D. G., Cooper, J. M., Dzieciol, A. M., Mishkin, M., & Vargha-Khadem, F. (2015). Extent of hippocampal atrophy predicts degree of deficit in recall. *Proceedings of the National Academy of Sciences, 112,* 12830–12833.

Pavot, W., & Diener, E. (1993). Review of the satisfaction with life scale. *Psychological Assessment, 5,* 164–172.

Paxton, S. J., Eisenberg, M. E., & Neumark-Sztainer, D. (2006). Prospective predictors of body dissatisfaction in adolescent girls and boys: A five-year longitudinal study. *Developmental Psychology, 42,* 888–899.

Paykel, E. S. (1994). Life events, social support and depression. *Acta Psychiatrica Scandinavica. Supplementum, 377,* 50–58.

Pearl, R. L., & Lebowitz, M. S. (2014). Beyond personal responsibility: effects of causal attributions for overweight and obesity on weight-related beliefs, stigma, and policy support. *Psychology and Health, 29,* 1176–1191.

Pedersen, B. K., & Hoffman-Goetz, L. (2000). Exercise and the immune system: Regulation, integration, and adaptation. *Physiological reviews, 80,* 1055–1081.

Pederson, E. L., & Vogel, D. L. (2007). Men's gender role conflict and their willingness to seek counseling: A mediation model. *Journal of Counseling Psychology, 54,* 373–384.

Pelletier, L. G., & Dion, S. C. (2007). An examination of general and specific motivational mechanisms for the elations between body dissatisfaction and eating disorders. *Journal of Social and Clinical Psychology, 26,* 303–333.

Pendleton, D. A., & Bochner, S. (1980). Communication of medical information in general practice consultations as a function of patients' social class. *Social Science & Medicine, 14,* 669–673.

Pennebaker, J. W. (1993). Putting stress into words: Health, linguistic, and therapeutic implications. *Behaviour Research and Therapy, 31*, 539–548.

Pennebaker, J. W., & Keough, K. A. (1999). Revealing, organizing, and reorganizing the self in response to stress and emotion. In R. J. Contrada & R. D. Ashmore (Eds.), *Self, social identity, and physical health: Interdisciplinary explorations* (pp. 101–121). New York, NY: Oxford University Press.

Perälä, J., Suvisaari, J., Saarni, S. I., Kuoppasalmi, K., Isometsä, E., Pirkola, S., . . . Lönnqvist, J. (2007). Lifetime prevalence of psychotic and bipolar I disorders in a general population. *Archives of General Psychiatry, 64*, 19–28.

Perreault, S., & Bourhis, R. Y. (1999). Ethnocentrism, social identification, and discrimination. *Personality and Social Psychology Bulletin, 25*, 92–103.

Perry, Y., Henry, J. D., Sethi, N., & Grisham, J. R. (2011). The pain persists: How social exclusion affects individuals with schizophrenia. *British Journal of Clinical Psychology, 50*, 339–349.

Perryman, C., & Dingle, G. A. (2015). A systematic review of the methodologies used in research related to adult drug and alcohol rehabilitation in therapeutic communities published 2000–2013. *Therapeutic Communities: The International Journal of Therapeutic Communities, 36*, 193–208.

Perryman, C., Dingle, G. A., & Clark, D. (2016). Changes in posttraumatic stress disorders symptoms during and after therapeutic community drug and alcohol treatment. *Therapeutic Communities: The International Journal of Therapeutic Communities, 37*, 170–183.

Petrie, K., Moss-Morris, R., & Weinman, J. (1995). The impact of catastrophic beliefs on functioning in chronic fatigue syndrome. *Journal of Psychosomatic Research, 39*, 31–37.

Pharoah, F., Mari, J., Rathbone, J., & Wong, W. (2010). Family intervention for schizophrenia. *Cochrane Database Systematic Review, 12*.

Phelan, J., Link, B. G., Moore, R. E., & Stueve, A. (1997). The stigma of Homelessness: The impact of the label "homeless" on attitudes toward poor persons. *Social Psychology Quarterly, 60*, 323–337.

Pietromonaco, P. R., & Collins, N. L. (2017). Interpersonal mechanisms linking close relationships to health. *American Psychologist, 72*, 531–542.

Piette, J. D., Heisler, M., & Wagner, T. H. (2004). Cost-related medication underuse among chronically III adults: The treatments people forgo, how often, and who is at risk. *American Journal of Public Health, 94*, 1782–1787.

Pilkington, P. D., Reavley, N. J., & Jorm, A. F. (2013). The Australian public's beliefs about the causes of depression: Associated factors and changes over 16 years. *Journal of Affective Disorders, 150*, 356–362.

Pinel, E. C. (1999). Stigma consciousness: The psychological legacy of social stereotypes. *Journal of Personality and Social Psychology, 76*, 114–128.

Pinker, S. (2015). *The village effect: Why face-to-face contact matters*. New York, NY: Random House.

Pinquart, M., Duberstein, P. R., & Lyness, J. M. (2007). Effects of psychotherapy and other behavioral interventions on clinically depressed older adults: A meta-analysis. *Aging and Mental Health, 11*, 645–657.

Pinquart, M., & Schindler, I. (2007). Changes of life satisfaction in the transition to retirement: A latent-class approach. *Psychology and Aging, 22*, 442–455.

Plagemann, A., Harder, T., Brunn, M., Harder, A., Roepke, K., Wittrock-Staar, M., . . . Dudenhausen, J. W. (2009). Hypothalamic proopiomelanocortin promoter methylation becomes altered by early overfeeding: an epigenetic model of obesity and the metabolic syndrome. *The Journal of Physiology, 587*, 4963–4976.

Platow, M. J., Haslam, S. A., Foddy, M., & Grace, D. M. (2003). Leadership as the outcome of self-categorization processes. In D. van Knippenberg & M. A. Hogg (Eds.), *Leadership and power: Identity processes in groups and organizations* (pp. 34–47). London: Sage.

Platow, M. J., & Hunter, J. A. (2017). Intergroup relations and conflict: Revisiting Sherif's Boys' camp studies. In J. R. Smith & S. A. Haslam (Eds.), *Social psychology: Revisiting the classic studies* (2nd ed., pp. 146–163). London: Sage.

Platow, M. J., Hunter, J. A., Branscombe, N. R., & Grace, D. M. (2014). Social creativity in Olympic medal counts: Observing the expression of ethnocentric fairness. *Social Justice Research, 27*, 283–304.

Platow, M. J., Voudouris, N. J., Gilford, N., Jamieson, R., Najdovski, L., Papaleo, N., . . . Terry, L. (2007). In-group reassurance in a pain setting produces lower levels of physiological arousal: Direct support for a self-categorization analysis of social influence. *European Journal of Social Psychology, 37*, 649–660.

Platow, M. J., Wenzel, M., & Nolan, M. (2003). The importance of social identity and self-categorization processes for creating and responding to fairness. In S. A. Haslam, D. v. Knippenberg, M. J. Platow., & N. Ellemers (Eds.). *Social identity at work: Developing theory for organizational practice* (pp. 261–276). New York: Psychology Press.

Playford, E. D., Siegert, R., Levack, W., & Freeman, J. (2009). Areas of consensus and controversy about goal setting in rehabilitation: a conference report. *Clinical Rehabilitation, 23*, 334–344.

Polivy, J., & Herman, C. P. (1985). Dieting and binging: A causal analysis. *Amercian Psychologist, 40*, 193–201.

Ponsford, J., Lee, N. K., Wong, D. K., McKay, A. D., Haines, K., Always, Y., . . . O'Donnell, M. L. (2016). Efficacy of motivational interviewing and cognitive behavioural therapy for anxiety and depression symptoms following traumatic brain injury. *Psychological Medicine, 46*, 1079–1090.

Postmes, T. (2003). A social identity approach to communication in organizations. In S. A. Haslam, D. van Knippenberg, M. J. Platow, & N. Ellemers (Eds.), *Social identity at work: Developing theory for organizational practice* (pp. 81–97). Philadelphia, PA: Psychology Press.

Postmes, T., & Branscombe, N. R. (2002). Influence of long-term racial environmental composition on subjective well-being in African Americans. *Journal of Personality and Social Psychology, 83*, 735–751.

Postmes, T., Branscombe, N. R., Spears, R., & Young, H. (1999). Comparative processes in personal and group judgments: Resolving the discrepancy. *Journal of Personality and Social Psychology, 76*, 320–338.

Postmes, T., Haslam, S. A., & Jans, L. (2013). A single-item measure of social identification: Reliability, validity and utility. *British Journal of Social Psychology, 52*, 597–617.

Postmes, T., Haslam, S. A., & Swaab, R. (2005). Social influence in small groups: An interactive model of identity formation. *European Review of Social Psychology, 16*, 1–42.

Postmes, T., & Jetten, J. (2006). *Individuality and the group: Advances in social identity*. London: Sage.

Powers, M. B., Vedel, E., & Emmelkamp, P. M. G. (2008). Behavioral couples therapy (BCT) for alcohol and drug use disorders: A meta-analysis. *Clinical Psychology Review, 28*, 952–962.

Prabha, S. C., Kommu, J. V. S., & Rudhran, V. (2012). Schizophrenia in women and children: A selective review of literature from developing countries. *International Review of Psychiatry, 24*, 467–482.

Praharso, N. F., Tear, M. J., & Cruwys, T. (2017). Stressful life transitions and wellbeing: A comparison of the stress buffering hypothesis and the social identity model of identity change. *Psychiatry Research, 247*, 265–275.

Prendergast, M., Podus, D., Finney, J., Greenwell, L., & Roll, J. (2006). Contingency management for treatment of substance use disorders: A meta-analysis. *Addiction, 101*, 1546–1560.

Presnell, K., Stice, E., & Tristan, J. (2008). Experimental investigation of the effects of naturalistic dieting on bulimic symptoms: Moderating effects of depressive symptoms. *Appetite, 50*, 91–101.

Price, J., Cole, V., & Goodwin, G. M. (2009). Emotional side-effects of selective serotonin reuptake inhibitors: Qualitative study. *The British Journal of Psychiatry, 195*, 211–217.

Price, J. R., Mitchell, E., Tidy, E., & Hunot, V. (2008). Cognitive behaviour therapy for chronic fatigue syndrome in adults. *Cochrane Database of Systematic Reviews, 3*. Retrieved from http://doi.org/10.1002/14651858.CD001027.pub2

Prigatano, G. P. (1986). Personality and psychosocial consequences of brain injury. In G. P. Prigatano, D. J. Fordyce, H. K. Zeiner, J. R. Roueche, M. Pepping, & B. C. Wood (Eds.), *Neuropsychological rehabilitation after brain injury* (pp. 29–50). Baltimore: The John Hopkins University Press.

Prigatano, G. P., & Pliskin, N. (2002). *Clinical neuropsychology and cost-outcome research: An introduction*. Hove, UK: Psychology Press.

Prochaska, J. O., & DiClemente, C. C. (1982). Transtheoretical therapy: Toward a more integrative model of change. *Psychotherapy: Theory, Research & Practice, 19*, 276–288.

Prochaska, J. O., & Velicer, W. F. (1997). The transtheoretical change model of health behavior. *American Journal of Health Promotion, 12*, 38–48.

Procidano, M. E. (1992). The nature of perceived social support: Findings of meta-analytic studies. In C. D. Spielberger & J. N. Butcher (Eds.), *Advances in personality assessment*. Hillsdale, NJ: Erlbaum.

Project MATCH Research Group. (1998). Matching patients with alcohol disorders to treatments: Clinical implications from Project MATCH. *Journal of Mental Health, 7*, 589–602.

Puhl, R. M., & Brownell, K. D. (2001). Bias, discrimination, and obesity. *Obesity, 9*, 788–805.

Puhl, R. M., & Heuer, C. A. (2010). Obesity stigma: Important considerations for public health. *American Journal of Public Health, 100*, 1019–1028.

Putnam, R. D. (1993). *Making democracy work: Civic traditions in modern Italy*. Princeton, NJ: Princeton University Press.

Putnam, R. D. (2000). *Bowling alone: The collapse and revival of American community*. New York, NY: Simon & Schuster.

Putnam, R. D., & Feldstein, L. (2004). *Better together: Restoring the American community*. New York, NY: Simon & Schuster.

Qi, L., & Cho, Y. A. (2008). Gene-environment interaction and obesity. *Nutrition Reviews, 66*, 684–694.

Queensland Mental Health Commission. (2015). *Everybody needs a home – changing Queensland's social housing policy for people with complex needs*. Retrieved from www.qmhc.qld.gov.au/work/research/social-housing/

Quinn, D. M., & Earnshaw, V. A. (2013). Concealable stigmatized identities and psychological wellbeing. *Social and Personality Psychology Compass, 7*, 40–51.

Raghubir, P., & Krishna, A. (1999). Vital dimensions in volume perception: Can the eye fool the stomach? *Journal of Marketing Research, 36*, 313–326.

Ragland, D. R., Satariano, W. A., & MacLeod, K. A. (2005). Driving cessation and increased depressive symptoms. *Journal of Gerontology: Medical Sciences, 60A*, 399–403.

Rahhal, T. A., Hasher, L., & Colombe, S. J. (2001). Instructional manipulations and age differences in memory: Now you see them, now you don't. *Psychology and Aging, 16*, 697–706.

Rajguru, P., Kolber, M. J., Garcia, A. N., Smith, M. T., Patel, C. K., & Hanney, W. J. (2015). Use of mindfulness meditation in the management of chronic pain: a systematic review of randomized controlled trials. *American Journal of Lifestyle Medicine, 9*, 176–184.

Ramachandrappa, S., & Farooqi, I. S. (2011). Genetic approaches to understanding human obesity. *Journal of Clinical Investigation, 121*, 2080–2086.

Ramanathapillai, R. (2006). The politicizing of trauma: A case study of Sri Lanka. *Peace and Conflict: Journal of Peace Psychology, 12*, 1–18.

Rankin, L. E., Jost, J. T., & Wakslak, C. J. (2009). System justification and the meaning of life: Are the existential benefits of ideology distributed unequally across racial groups? *Social Justice Research, 22*, 312–333.

Rao, V. M., & Levin, D. C. (2012). The overuse of diagnostic imaging and the choosing wisely initiative. *Annals of Internal Medicine, 157*, 574–577.

Raphael, D. (2000). Health inequities in the United States: Prospects and solutions. *Journal of Public Health Policy, 21*, 394–427.

Rauch, S., Shin, L. M., & Phelps, E. (2006). Neurocircuitry models of posttraumatic stress disorder and extinction: Human neuroimaging research – past, present, and future. *Biological Psychiatry, 60*, 376–382.

Ravindran, L. N., & Stein, M. B. (2009). Pharmacotherapy of PTSD: Premises, principles, and priorities. *Brain Research, 1293*, 24–39.

Ravndal, E., & Vaglum, P. (1994). Self-reported depression as a predictor of dropout in a hierarchical Therapeutic Community. *Journal of Substance Abuse Treatment, 11*, 471–479.

Rea, M. M., Tompson, M. C., Miklowitz, D. J., Goldstein, M. J., Hwang, S., & Mintz, J. (2003). Family-focused treatment versus individual treatment for bipolar disorder: Results of a randomized clinical trial. *Journal of Consulting and Clinical Psychology, 71*, 482–492.

Read, S. A., Morton, T. A., & Ryan, M. K. (2015). Negotiating identity: A qualitative analysis of stigma and support seeking for individuals with cerebral palsy. *Disability and Rehabilitation, 37*, 1162–1169.

Reaves, S., Bush Hitchon, J., Park, S.-Y., & Woong Yun, G. (2004). If looks could kill: Digital manipulation of fashion models. *Journal of Mass Media Ethics, 19*, 56–71.

Redersdorff, S., Martinot, D., & Branscombe, N. R. (2004). The impact of thinking about group-based disadvantages or advantages on women's well-being: An experimental test of the rejection-identification model. *Current Psychology of Cognition, 22*, 203–222.

Redlich, C. A., Sparer, J., & Cullen, M. R. (1997). Sick-building syndrome. *The Lancet, 349*, 1013–1016.

Reed, A. (2012). *Clean*. New York, NY: Simon & Schuster.

Rees, S., Steel, Z., Creamer, M., Teesson, M., Bryant, R., McFarlane, A. C., . . . Silove, D. (2014). Onset of common mental disorders and suicidal behavior following women's first exposure to gender based violence: a retrospective, population-based study. *BMC Psychiatry, 14*, 1–8.

Rehmeyer, J. (2016, September 21). Bad science misled millions with chronic fatigue syndrome. Here's how we fought back. *STATNews*. Retrieved from www.statnews.com/2016/09/21/chronic-fatigue-syndrome-pace-trial/

Reicher, S. D. (1987). Crowd behaviour as social action. In J. C. Turner, M. A. Hogg, P. J. Oakes, S. D. Reicher, & M. S. Wetherell (Eds.), *Rediscovering the social group: A self-categorization theory* (pp. 171–202). Oxford: Blackwell.

Reicher, S. D., & Haslam, S. A. (2006a). Rethinking the psychology of tyranny: The BBC Prison Study. *British Journal of Social Psychology, 45*, 1–40.

Reicher, S. D., & Haslam, S. A. (2006b). Tyranny revisited: Groups, psychological well-being and the health of societies. *The Psychologist, 19*, 146–150.

Reicher, S. D., & Haslam, S. A. (2010). Beyond help: A social psychology of collective solidarity and social cohesion. In S. Stürmer & M. Snyder (Eds.), *The psychology of pro-social behavior: Group processes, intergroup relations, and helping* (pp. 289–309). Oxford, UK: Blackwell.

Reicher, S. D., & Haslam, S. A. (2012). Change we can believe in: The role of social identity, cognitive alternatives and leadership in group mobilization and social transformation. In B. Wagoner, E. Jensen, & J. Oldmeadow (Eds.), *Culture and social change: Transforming society through the power of ideas* (pp. 53–73). London: Routledge.

Reicher, S. D., Haslam, S. A., & Hopkins, N. (2005). Social identity and the dynamics of leadership: Leaders and followers as collaborative agents in the transformation of social reality. *The Leadership Quarterly, 16*, 547–568.

Reininghaus, U., Priebe, S., & Bentall, R. P. (2013). Testing the psychopathology of psychosis: Evidence for a general psychosis dimension. *Schizophrenia Bulletin, 39*, 884–895.

Resick, P. A., Monson, C. M., & Rizvi, S. L. (2014). Posttraumatic stress disorder. In D. H. Barlow, (Ed.), *Clinical handbook of psychological disorders: A step-by-step treatment manual* (4th ed., pp. 65–122). New York, NY: Guilford Press.

Resick, P. A., & Schnicke, M. K. (1992). Cognitive processing therapy for sexual assault victims. *Journal of Consulting and Clinical Psychology, 60*, 748–756.

Reynolds, K. J., & Branscombe, N. R. (Eds.). (2015). *Psychology of change: Life contexts, experience and identities*. New York, NY: Psychology Press.

Reynolds, K. J., Turner, J. C., Branscombe, N. R., Mavor, K. I., Bizumic, B., & Subašić, E. (2010). Interactionism in personality and social psychology: An integrated approach to understanding the mind and behaviour. *European Journal of Personality, 24*, 458–482.

Ricciardelli, L. A., & McCabe, M. P. (2002). Psychometric evaluation of the Body Change Inventory: An assessment instrument for adolescent boys and girls. *Eating Behaviors, 3*, 45–59.

Richmond Fellowship QLD. (2015). *Annual Report 2015: The future in focus, today*. Retrieved from www.rfq.com.au/wp-content/uploads/2015/11/RFQ_AnnualReport15_WEB.pdf

Riecansky, I., Paul, N., Kölble, S., Stieger, S., & Lamm, C. (2015). Beta oscillations reveal ethnicity ingroup bias in sensorimotor resonance to pain of others. *Social Cognitive and Affective Neuroscience, 10*, 893–901.

Riekert, K. A., Ockene, J. K., & Pbert, L. (2013). *The handbook of health behavior change* (4th ed.). New York, NY: Springer.

Robins, R. W., Hendin, H. M., & Trzesniewski, K. H. (2001). Measuring global self-esteem: Construct validation of a single-item measure and the Rosenberg Self-Esteem Scale. *Personality and Social Psychology Bulletin, 27*, 151–161.

Roccas, S. (2003). The effects of status on identification with multiple groups. *European Journal of Social Psychology, 33*, 351–366.

Rodin, J., & Langer, E. J. (1977). Long-term effects of a control-relevant intervention with the institutionalized aged. *Journal of Personality and Social Psychology, 35*, 897–902.

Rolling Stones. (1966). *Mother's little helper. From the album* Aftermath. London: Decca records. Retrieved from www.youtube.com/watch?v=tfGYSHy1jQs

Rollman, G. B. (1998). Culture and pain. In S. S. Kazarian & D. R. Evans (Eds.), *Cultural clinical psychology: Theory, research, and practice* (pp. 267–286). New York, NY: Oxford University Press.

Room, R. (2005). Stigma, social inequality and alcohol and drug use. *Drug Alcohol Review, 24*, 143–155.

Rosch, E. (1978). Principles of categorization. In E. Rosch & B. B. Lloyd (Eds.), *Cognition and categorization* (pp. 27–48). Hillsdale, NJ: Erlbaum.

Rose, S. C., Bisson, J. I., Churchill, R., & Wessely, S. (2002). Psychological debriefing for preventing post-traumatic stress disorder (PTSD). *The Cochrane Library, 2*.

Rosenberg, M. (1965). *Society and the adolescent self-image*. Princeton, NJ: Princeton University Press.

Rosenman, R., Friedman, M., Straus, R., Wurm, M., Kositchek, R., Hahn, W., & Werthessen, N. (1964). A predictive study of coronary heart disease. *Journal of the American Medical Association, 189*, 15–22.

Rosenstock, I. M. (1990). The health belief model: Explaining health behavior through expectancies. In K. Glanz, F. M. Lewis, & B. K. Rimer (Eds.), *Health behavior and health education: Theory, research, and practice* (pp. 39–62). San Francisco, CA: Jossey-Bass.

Rosenstock, I. M., Strecher, V. J., & Becker, M. H. (1994). The health belief model and HIV risk behavior change. In R. J. DiClemente & J. L. Peterson (Eds.), *Preventing AIDS: Theories and methods of behavioral interventions* (pp. 5–24). New York, NY: Plenum.

Rosenthal, B., & Marx, R. D. (1979). Modeling influences on the eating behavior of successful and unsuccessful dieters and untreated normal weight individuals. *Addictive Behaviors, 4*, 215–221.

Rothbard, J. C., & Shaver, P. R. (1994). Continuity of attachment across the life span. In M. B. Sperling & H. B. William (Ed.), *Attachment in adults: Clinical and developmental perspectives* (pp. 31–71). New York, NY: Guilford Press.

Rothbaum, B. O., & Davis, M. (2003). Applying learning principles to the treatment of Post-Trauma reactions. *Annals of the New York Academy of Sciences, 1008*, 112–121.

Rowland, B., Evans-Whipp, T., Hemphill, S. A., Leung, R., Livingston, M., & Toumbourou, J. T. (2016). The density of alcohol outlets and adolescent alcohol consumption: An Australian longitudinal analysis. *Health and Place, 37*, 43–49.

Rozin, P. (1996). Towards a psychology of food and eating: from motivation to module to model to marker, morality, meaning, and metaphor. *Current Directions in Psychological Science, 5*, 18–24.

Rubak, S., Sandbaek, A., Lauritzen, T., & Christensen, B. (2005). Motivational interviewing: A systematic review and meta-analysis. *British Journal of General Practice, 55*, 305–312.

Rubin, M. (2012). Social class differences in social integration among students in higher education: A meta-analysis and recommendations for future research. *Journal of Diversity in Higher Education, 5*, 22–38.

Rubin, M., & Hewstone, M. (1998). Social identity theory's self-esteem hypothesis: A review and some suggestions for clarification. *Personality and Social Psychology Review, 2*, 40–62.

Rubin, M., & Wright, C. L. (2017). Time and money explain social class differences in students' social integration at university. *Studies in Higher Education, 42*, 315–330.

Rüsch, N., Angermeyer, M. C., & Corrigan, P. W. (2005). Mental illness stigma: Concepts, consequences, and initiatives to reduce stigma. *European Psychiatry, 20*, 529–539.

Rüsch, N., Zlati, A., Black, G., & Thornicroft, G. (2014). Does the stigma of mental illness contribute to suicidality? *The British Journal of Psychiatry, 205*, 257–259.

Russell, D. W. (1996). UCLA Loneliness Scale (Version 3): Reliability, validity, and factor structure. *Journal of Personality Assessment, 66*, 20–40.

Ruth-Sahd, L. A., Schneider, M., & Haagen, B. (2009). Diabulimia: What it is and how to recognize it in critical care. *Dimensions of Critical Care Nursing, 28*, 147–153.

Ryan, M. K., & Haslam, S. A. (2007). The glass cliff: Exploring the dynamics surrounding the appointment of women to precarious leadership positions. *Academy of Management Review, 32*, 549–572.

Ryn, M. V., & Burke, J. (2000). The effect of patient race and socio-economic status on physicians' perceptions of patients. *Social Science and Medicine, 50*, 813–828.

Sachdev, I., & Bourhis, R. Y. (1987). Status differentials and intergroup behaviour. *European Journal of Social Psychology, 17*, 277–293.

Sachser, N., & Prove, E. (1986). Social status and plasma-testosterone-titers in male guinea pigs. *Ethology, 71*, 103–114.

Sacks, O. (2015). *On the move: A life*. London: Picador.

Saeri, A. K., Cruwys, T., Barlow, F. K., Stronge, S., & Sibley, C. G. (2017). Social connectedness improves public mental health: Investigating bidirectional relationships in the New Zealand attitudes and values survey. *Australian & New Zealand Journal of Psychiatry*. Advance on-line publication. doi: 10.1177/0004867417723990

Saguy, A. C., & Gruys, K. (2010). Morality and health: news media constructions of overweight and eating disorders. *Social Problems, 57*, 231–250.

Salas, C. E., Casassus, M., Rowlands, L., Pimm, S., & Flanagan, D. A. J. (2016). "Relating through sameness": A qualitative study of friendship and social isolation after traumatic brain injury. *Neuropsychological Rehabilitation*. Advance on-line publication. doi:10.1080/09602011.2016.1247730

Salazar, A. M., Warden, D. L., Schwab, K., Spector, J., Braverman, S., Walter, J., . . . Ellenbogen, R. G. (2000). Cognitive rehabilitation for traumatic brain injury: A randomized trial. Defense and Veteran's Head Injury Program (DVHIP) study group. *Journal of the American Medical Association, 283*, 3075–3081.

Salkovskis, P. M., Gregory, J. D., Sedgwick-Taylor, A., White, J., Opher, S., & Ólafsdóttir, S. (2016). Extending cognitive-behavioural theory and therapy to medically unexplained symptoms and long-term physical conditions: A hybrid transdiagnostic/problem specific approach. *Behaviour Change, 33*, 1–21.

Salomons, T. V., Johnstone, T., Backonja, M-M., & Davidson, R. J. (2004). Perceived controllability modulates the neural response to pain. *The Journal of Neuroscience, 24*, 7199–7203.

Sander, A. M., Roebuck, T. M., Sturchen, M. A., Sherer, M., & High, W. M. (2001). Long-term maintenance of gains obtained in post-acute rehabilitation by persons with traumatic brain injury. *Journal of Head Trauma Rehabilitation, 16*, 356–373.

SANE Australia. (2010). Social inclusion and mental illness. *SANE Research Bulletin, 12*. Retrieved from www.sane.org/images/PDFs/1007_info_rb12.pdf and the ISSN is 1832–8385

Sani, F. (2008). *Self continuity: Individual and collective perspectives*. New York, NY: Psychology Press.

Sani, F. (2012). Group identification, social relationships, and health. In J. Jetten, C. Haslam, & S. A. Haslam (Eds.), *The social cure: Identity, health and well-being* (pp. 21–37). Hove, UK: Psychology Press.

Sani, F., Bowe, M., & Herrera, M. (2008). Perceived collective continuity and social well-being: Exploring the connections. *European Journal of Social Psychology, 38*, 365–374.

Sani, F., Herrera, M., Wakefield, J. R. H., Boroch, O., & Gulyas, C. (2012). Comparing social contact and group identification as predictors of mental health. *British Journal of Social Psychology, 51*, 781–790.

Sani, F., Madhok, V., Norbury, M., Dugard, P., & Wakefield, J. R. H. (2015). Greater number of group identifications is associated with healthier behaviour: Evidence from a Scottish community sample. *British Journal of Health Psychology, 20*, 466–481.

Sani, F., Magrin, M. E., Scrignaro, M., & McCollum, R. (2010). Ingroup identification mediates the effects of subjective ingroup status on mental health. *British Journal of Social Psychology, 49*, 883–893.

Santini, Z. I., Koyanagi, A., Tyrovola, S., Haro, J. M., Donovan, R. J., Nielsen, L., & Kouchede, V. (2017). The protective properties of Act-Belong-Commit indicators against incident depression, anxiety, and cognitive impairment among older Irish adults: Findings from a prospective community-based study. *Experimental Gerontology, 91*, 79–87.

Sapolsky, R. M. (2004). Social status and health in humans and other animals. *Annual Review of Anthropology, 33*, 393–418.

Sapolsky, R. M. (2017). *Behave: The biology of humans at our best and worst*. New York, NY: Random House.

Sareen, J., Jacobi, F., Cox, B. J., Belik, S.-L., Clara, I., & Stein, M. B. (2006). Disability and poor quality of life associated with comorbid anxiety disorders and physical conditions. *Archives of Internal Medicine, 166*, 2109–2116.

Saris, W. H. M., Blair, S. N., Van Baak, M. A., Eaton, S. B., Davies, P. S. W., Di Pietro, L., . . . Wyatt, H. (2003). How much physical activity is enough to prevent unhealthy weight gain? Outcome of the IASO 1st Stock Conference and consensus statement. *Obesity Reviews, 4*, 101–114.

Sarokhani, D., Delpisheh, A., Veisani, Y., Sarokhani, M. T., Manesh, R. E., & Sayehmiri, K. (2013). Prevalence of depression among university students: A systematic review and meta-analysis study. *Depression Research and Treatment*, Article ID 373857. doi:10.1155/2013/373857

Sassoon, S. (1983). *The war poems*. London: Faber.

Saunders, P. (2008). Measuring wellbeing using non-monetary indicators: Deprivation and social exclusion. *Family Matters, 78*, 8–17.

Sawada, N., Uchida, H., Suzuki, T., Watanabe, K., Kikuchi, T., Handa, T., & Kashima, H. (2009). Persistence and compliance to antidepressant treatment in patients with depression: A chart review. *BMC Psychiatry, 9*, 38. doi: 10.1186/1471-244X-9-38

Saxena, S., Thornicroft, G., Knapp, M., & Whiteford, H. (2007). Resources for mental health: Scarcity, inequity, and inefficiency. *The Lancet, 370*, 878–889.

Scarapicchia, T. M. F., Sabiston, C. M., Andersen, R. E., & Bengoechea, E. G. (2013). The motivational effects of social contagion on exercise participation in young female adults. *Journal of Sport and Exercise Psychology, 35*, 563–575.

Schaafsma, J. (2013). Through the lens of justice: Just world beliefs mediate relationships between perceived discrimination and subjective well-being. *International Journal of Intercultural Relations, 37*, 450–458.

Scharloo, M., Kaptein, A. A., Weinman, J., Hazes, J. M., Willems, L. N. A., Bergman, W., & Rooijmans, H. G. M. (1998). Illness perceptions, coping and functioning in patients with rheumatoid arthritis, chronic obstructive pulmonary disease and psoriasis. *Journal of Psychosomatic Research, 44*, 573–585.

Scheepers, D. T., & Ellemers, N. (2005). When the pressure is up: The assessment of social identity threat in low and high status groups. *Journal of Experimental Social Psychology, 41*, 192–200.

Scheepers, D. T., Ellemers, N., & Sintemaartensdijk, N. (2009). Suffering from the possibility of status loss: Physiological responses to social identity threat in high status groups. *European Journal of Social Psychology, 39*, 1075–1092.

Schlaff, C. (1993). From dependency to self-advocacy: Redefining disability. *American Journal of Occupational Therapy, 47*, 943–948.

Schirmer, J., Mylek, M., Peel, D., & Yabsley, B. (2015). *People and communities: The 2014 regional well-being survey*. Canberra: The University of Canberra.

Schmid, K., & Muldoon, O. T. (2015). Perceived threat, social identification, and psychological well-being: The effects of political conflict exposure. *Political Psychology, 36*, 75–92.

Schmid, K., Muldoon, O. T., & Lowe, R. D. (2017). *Effects of perceived threat and social identification on psychological wellbeing: A longitudinal analysis of the threat-identification model*. Unpublished manuscript, University of Limerick.

Schmitt, M. T., & Branscombe, N. R. (2002). The meaning and consequences of perceived discrimination in disadvantaged and privileged social groups. *European Review of Social Psychology, 12*, 167–199.

Schmitt, M. T., Branscombe, N. R., & Postmes, T. (2003). Women's emotional responses to the pervasiveness of gender discrimination. *European Journal of Social Psychology, 33*, 297–312.

Schmitt, M. T., Branscombe, N. R., Postmes, T., & Garcia, A. (2014). The consequences of perceived discrimination for psychological well-being: A meta-analytic review. *Psychological Bulletin, 140*, 921–948.

Schmitt, M. T., Davies, K., Hung, M., & Wright, S. C. (2010). Identity moderates the effects of Christmas displays on mood, self-esteem, and inclusion. *Journal of Experimental Social Psychology, 46*, 1017–1022.

Schmitt, M. T., Spears, R., & Branscombe, N. R. (2003). Constructing a minority group identity out of shared rejection. *European Journal of Social Psychology, 33*, 1–12.

Schmitz, N., Wang, J., Malla, A., & Lesage, A. (2007). Joint effect of depression and chronic conditions on disability: Results from a population-based study. *Psychosomatic Medicine, 69*, 332–338.

Schofield, P. E., Pattison, P. E., Hill, D. J., & Borland, R. (2001). The influence of group identification on the adoption of peer group smoking norms. *Psychology and Health, 16*, 1–16.

Scholliers, P. (2001). *Food, drink and identity: Cooking, eating and drinking in Europe since the Middle Ages*. Oxford: Berg Publishers.

Schwarzer, R., & Leppin, A. (1991). Social support and health: A theoretical and empirical overview. *Journal of Social and Personal Relationships, 8*, 99–127.

Scott, K. M., Bruffaerts, R., Tsang, A., Ormel, J., Alonso, J., Angermeyer, M. C., . . . Von Korff, M. (2007). Depression-anxiety relationships with CPHC: Results from the World Mental Health surveys. *Journal of Affective Disorders, 103*, 113–120.

Scott, J. A. N., Teasdale, J. D., Paykel, E. S., Johnson, A. L., Hayhurst, H., Moore, R., . . . Garland, A. (2012). Effects of cognitive therapy on psychological symptoms and social functioning in residual depression. *British Journal of Psychiatry, 177*, 440–446.

Seeman, T. E., Miller-Martinz, D. M., Merkin, S. S., Lachman, M. E., Tun, P. T., & Karlamangla, A. S. (2011). Histories of social engagement and adult cognition: Midlife in the U.S. Study. *The Journals of Gerontology Series B: Psychological Sciences and Social Sciences, 66B*, 41–52.

Seifert, R. (1996). The second front: The logic of sexual violence in wars. *Women's Studies International Forum, 19*, 35–43.

Seifert, T. (2005). Anthropomorphic characteristics of centerfold models: Trends towards slender figures over time. *International Journal of Eating Disorders, 37*, 271–274.

Seligman, M. (1975). *Helplessness: On depression, development, and death*. San Francisco: W.H. Freeman.

Sellers, R. M., & Shelton, J. N. (2003). The role of racial identity in perceived racial discrimination. *Journal of Personality and Social Psychology, 84*, 1079–1092.

Seltzer, M. (1997). Wound culture: Trauma in the pathological public sphere. *October, 80*, 3–26.

Selye, H. M. D. (1946). The general adaptation syndrome and dissonances of adaptation. *The Journal of Clinical Endocrinology, 6*, 118–135.

Selye, H. M. D. (1956). *The stress of life*. New York, NY: McGraw-Hill.

Semmer, N., & Meier, L. L. (2003). Individual differences, work stress and health. In M. J. Schabracq, J. A. M. Winnubst, & C. Cooper (Eds.), *Handbook of work and health psychology*, (2nd ed., pp. 83–120). Chichester, UK: Wiley.

Sempértegui, G. A., Karreman, A., Arntz, A., & Bekker, M. H. J. (2013). Schema therapy for borderline personality disorder: A comprehensive review of its empirical foundations, effectiveness and implementation possibilities. *Clinical Psychology Review, 33*, 426–447.

Sentell, T. L., & Halpin, H. A. (2006). Importance of adult literacy in understanding health disparities. *Journal of General Internal Medicine, 21*, 862–866.

Serdarevic, M., & Lemke, S. (2013). Motivational interviewing with the older adult. *International Journal of Mental Health Promotion, 15*, 240–249.

Seymour-Smith, M., Cruwys, T., Haslam, S. A., & Brodribb, W. (2017). Loss of group memberships predicts depression in postpartum mothers. *Social Psychiatry and Psychiatric Epidemiology, 52*, 201–210.

Shackleton, E. H. (1920). *South: The story of Shackleton's last expedition, 1914–1917*. London: Macmillan.

Shah, R., & Waller, G. (2000). Parental style and vulnerability to depression: The role of core beliefs. *The Journal of Nervous and Mental Disease, 188*, 19–25.

Shankar, S., Stevenson, C., Pandey, K., Tewari, S., Hopkins, N., & Reicher, S. D. (2013). A calming cacophony: Social identity can shape the experience of loud noise. *Journal of Environmental Psychology, 36*, 87–95.

Shapiro, K. J. (1998). *Animal models of human psychology*. Seattle, WA: Hogrefe & Huber.

Shattock, L., Williamson, H., Caldwell, K., Anderson, K., & Peters, S. (2013). "They've just got symptoms without science': Medical trainees' acquisition of negative attitudes towards patients with medically unexplained symptoms. *Patient Education and Counseling, 91*, 249–254.

Shea, M. E., & Pritchard, M. E. (2007). Is self-esteem the primary predictor of disordered eating? *Personality and Individual Differences, 42*, 1527–1537.

Shearer, J., & Gowing, L. R. (2004). Pharmacotherapies for problematic psychostimulant use: A review of current research. *Drug and Alcohol Review, 23*, 203–211.

Sheikh, J. I., Woodward, S. H., & Leskin, G. A. (2003). Sleep in post-traumatic stress disorder and panic: Convergence and divergence. *Depression and Anxiety, 18*, 187–197.

Shepherd, B. (2002). *A war of nerves: Soldiers and psychiatrists 1914–1994*. London: Random House.

Shepherd, C. (2016). Patient reaction to the PACE trial. *The Lancet Psychiatry, 3,* 7–8.

Sherif, M. (1956). Experiments in group conflict. *Scientific American, 195,* 54–58.

Sherif, M. (1966). *Group conflict and co-operation: Their social psychology*. London: Routledge and Kegan Paul.

Sherman, R. A., Sherman, C. J., & Parker, L. (1984). Chronic phantom and stump pain among American veterans: Results of a survey. *Pain, 18,* 83–95.

Shin, L. M., Rauch, S. L., & Pitman, R. K. (2006). Amygdala, medial prefrontal cortex, and hippocampal function in PTSD. *Annals of the New York Academy of Sciences, 1071,* 67–79.

Shipley, B. A., Weiss, A., Der, G., Taylor, M. D., & Deary, I. J. (2007). Neuroticism, extroversion, and mortality in the UK Health and Lifestyles survey: A 21 year prospective cohort study. *Psychosomatic Medicine, 69,* 923–931.

Shorter, E. (1997). *A history of psychiatry: From the era of the asylum to the age of prozac*. New York, NY: Wiley.

Sidanius, J., & Pratto, F. (1999). *Social dominance: An intergroup theory of social hierarchy and oppression*. New York, NY: Cambridge University press.

Siegler, I. C., Elias, M. F., & Bosworth, H. B. (2012). Aging and health. In A. Baum, T. A. Revenson, & J. Singer (Eds.), *Handbook of health psychology* (2nd ed., pp. 617–633). New York, NY: Guilford Press.

Siegrist, J., & Marmot, M. (2006). *Social inequalities in health: New evidence and policy implications*. Oxford, UK: Oxford University Press.

Silva, J., Ownsworth, T., Shields, C., & Fleming, J. (2011). Enhanced appreciation of life following acquired brain injury: Posttraumatic growth at 6 months post-discharge. *Brain Impairment, 12,* 93–104.

Simon, B., & Klandermans, B. (2001). Politicized collective identity: A social psychological analysis. *American Psychologist, 56,* 319–331.

Singh, M. K., & Gotlib, I. H. (2014). The neuroscience of depression: Implications for assessment and intervention. *Behaviour Research and Therapy, 62,* 60–73.

Singh-Manoux, A., Marmot, M., & Adler, N. E. (2005). Does subjective social status predict health and change in health status better than objective status? *Psychosomatic Medicine, 67,* 855–861.

Sklar, L. S., & Anisman, H. (1981). Stress and cancer. *Psychological Bulletin, 89,* 369–406.

Skorich, D. P., Gash, T. B., Stalker, K. L., Zheng, L., & Haslam, S. A. (2017). Exploring the cognitive foundations of the shared attention mechanism: Evidence for a relationship between self-categorization and shared attention across the Autism Spectrum. *Journal of Autism and Developmental Disorders, 47,* 1341–1353.

Skorich, D. P., May, A. R., Talipski, L. A., Hall, M. H., Dolstra, A. J., Gash, T. B., & Gunningham, B. H. (2016). Is social categorization the missing link between weak central coherence and mental state inference abilities in autism? Preliminary evidence from a general population sample. *Journal of Autism and Developmental Disorders, 46,* 862–881.

Slavich, G. M., & Cole, S. W. (2013). The emerging field of human social genomics. *Clinical Psychological Science, 1,* 331–348.

Sledge, W. H., Boydstun, J. A., & Rahe, A. J. (1980). Self-concept changes related to war captivity. *Archives of General Psychiatry, 37,* 430–443.

Sloan, D. M., Bovin, M. J., & Schnurr, P. P. (2012). Review of group treatment for PTSD. *Journal of Rehabilitation Research and Development, 49,* 689–701.

Slovic, P., Peters, E., Finucane, M. L., & MacGregor, D. G. (2005). Affect, risk, and decision making. *Health Psychology, 24,* 835–840.

Smeets, R. J. E. M., Vlaeyen, J. W. S., Kester, A. D. M., & Knottnerus, J. A. (2006). Reduction of pain catastrophizing mediates the outcome of both physical and cognitive-behavioral treatment in chronic low back pain. *Journal of Pain, 7,* 261–271.

Smink, F. R. E., Van Hoeken, D., & Hoek, H. W. (2012). Epidemiology of eating disorders: Incidence, prevalence and mortality rates. *Current Psychiatry Reports, 14,* 406–414.

Smith, B. W., Dalen, J., Wiggins, K., Tooley, E., Christopher, P., & Bernard, J. (2008). The brief resilience scale: Assessing the ability to bounce back. *International Journal of Behavioral Medicine, 15,* 194–200.

Smith, D. E., Heckemeyer, C. M., Kratt, P. P., & Mason, D. A. (1997). Motivational interviewing to improve adherence to a behavioral weight-control program for older obese women with NIDDM. *Diabetes Care, 20*, 52–54.

Smith, D. H., Meaney, D. F., & Shull, W. H. (2003). Diffuse axonal injury in head trauma. *Journal of Head Trauma Rehabilitation, 18*, 307–316.

Smith, H. J., Tyler, T. R., & Huo, Y. J. (2003). Interpersonal treatment, social identity and organizational behavior. In S. A. Haslam, D. van Knippenberg, M. J. Platow, & N. Ellemers (Eds.), *Social identity at work: Developing theory for organizational practice* (pp. 155–171). Philadelphia, PA: Psychology Press.

Smith, J. R., Louis, W. R., & Tarrant, M. (2016). University students' social identity and health behaviours in K. I. Mavor, M. J. Platow, & B. Bizumic (Eds.), *The Self, Social Identity, and Education* (pp. 159–175). London: Psychology Press.

Smith, L. G. E., & Postmes, T. (2011). Shaping stereotypical behaviour through the discussion of social stereotypes. *British Journal of Social Psychology, 50*, 74–98.

Smith, M. E. (2005). Bilateral hippocampal volume reduction in adults with post-traumatic stress disorder: A meta-analysis of structural MRI studies. *Hippocampus, 15*, 798–807.

Smith, T. W., & Spiro, A. (2002). Personality, health and aging: Prolegomenon for the next generation. *Journal of Personality Research, 36*, 363–394.

Sniehotta, F. (2009). An experimental test of the Theory of Planned Behavior. *Applied Psychology: Health and Well-Being, 1*, 257–270.

Sniehotta, F., Presseau, J., & Araújo-Soares, V. (2014). Time to retire the theory of planned behaviour. *Health Psychology Review, 8*, 1–7.

Snow, D. A., & Anderson, L. (1993). *Down on their luck: A study of homeless street people.* Berkeley, CA: University of California Press.

Soderhamn, O., Lindencrona, C., & Gustavsson, S. M. (2001). Attitudes towards older adults among nursing students and registered nurses in Sweden. *Nurse Education Today, 21*, 225–229.

Sofsky, W. (1993). *The order of terror: The concentration camp.* Princeton, NJ: Princeton University Press.

Solnit, R. (2009). *A paradise built in hell: The extraordinary communities that arise in disaster.* New York, NY: Viking.

Spahlholz, J., Bear, N., Köning, H. H., Riedel-Heller, S. G., & Luck-Sikorski, C. L. (2016). Obesity and discrimination: A systematic review and meta-analysis of observational studies. *Obesity Reviews, 17*, 43–55.

Spears, R. (2010). Group rationale, collective sense: Beyond intergroup bias. *British Journal of Social Psychology, 49*, 1–20.

Spears, R., & Leach, C. W. (2004). Intergroup schadenfreude: Conditions and consequences. In L. Z. Tiedens & C. W. Leach (Eds.), *The social life of emotions* (pp. 336–355). New York, NY: Cambridge University Press.

St Claire, L., Clift, A., & Dumbelton, L. (2008). How do I know what I feel? Evidence for the role of self-categorization in symptom perceptions. *European Journal of Social Psychology, 38*, 173–186.

St Claire, L., & Clucas, C. (2012). In sickness and in health: Influences of social categorizations on health-related outcomes. In J. Jetten, C. Haslam, & S. A. Haslam (Eds.), *The social cure: Identity, health, and well-being* (pp. 75–95). Hove, UK: Psychology Press.

St Claire, L., & He, Y. (2009). How do I know if I need a hearing aid? Further support for the self-categorization approach to symptom perception. *Applied Psychology: An International Review, 58*, 24–41.

St Claire, L., Watkins, C. J., & Billinghurst, B. (1996). Differences in meanings of health: An exploratory study of general practitioners and their patients. *Family Practice, 13*, 511–516.

Stacy, R., Brittain, K., & Kerr, S. (2002). Singing for health: An exploration of the issues. *Health Education, 102*, 156–162.

Stam, R. (2007). PTSD and stress desensitisation: A tale of brain and body. *Neuroscience and Biobehavioral Reviews, 31*, 530–557.

Stanton, A. L., Revenson, T. A., & Tennen, H. (2006). Health psychology: Psychological adjustment to chronic disease. *Annual Review of Psychology, 58*, 565–592.

Staples, M. P., Elwood, M., Burton, R. C., Williams, J. L., Marks, R., & Giles, G. G. (2006). Non-melanoma skin cancer in Australia: The 2002 national survey and trends since 1985. *Medical Journal of Australia, 184,* 6–10.

Starchina, Y., Parfenov, V., Chazova, I., Sinitsyn, V., Pustovitova, T., Kolos, I., & Ustyuzhanin, D. (2007). Cognitive function and the emotional state of stroke patients on antihypertensive therapy. *Neuroscience and Behavioral Physiology, 37,* 13–17.

Steele, C. M., & Aronson, J. (1995). Stereotype threat and the intellectual test performance of African Americans. *Journal of Personality and Social Psychology, 69,* 797–811.

Steele, C. M., Spencer, S. J., & Aronson, J. (2002). Contending with group image: The psychology of stereotype and social identity threat. In M. P. Zanna (Ed.), *Advances in experimental social psychology* (pp. 379–440). New York, NY: Academic Press.

Steffen, P. R., McNeilly, M., Anderson, N., & Sherwood, A. (2003). Effects of perceived racism and anger inhibition on ambulatory blood pressure in African Americans. *Psychosomatic Medicine, 65,* 746–750.

Steffens, N. K., Cruwys, T., Haslam, C., Jetten, J., & Haslam, S. A. (2016). Social group memberships in retirement are associated with reduced risk of premature death: Evidence from a longitudinal cohort study. *BMJ Open, 6,* e010164. doi: 10.1136/bmjopen-2015-010164

Steffens, N. K., Haslam, S. A., Kerschreiter, R., Schuh, S. C., & Van Dick, R. (2014). Leaders enhance group members' work engagement and reduce their burnout by crafting social identity. *Zeitschrift für Personalforschung (German Journal of Research in Human Resource Management), 28,* 183–204.

Steffens, N. K., Haslam, S. A., Reicher, S. D., Platow, M. J., Fransen, K., Yang, J., . . . Boen, F. (2014). Leadership as social identity management: Introducing the Identity Leadership Inventory (ILI) to assess and validate a four-dimensional model. *Leadership Quarterly, 25,* 1001–1024.

Steffens, N. K., Haslam, S. A., Schuh, S. C., Jetten, J., & Van Dick, R. (2016). A meta-analytic review of social identification and health in organizational contexts. *Personality and Social Psychology Review, 21,* 303–335.

Steinbrecher, N., Koerber, S., Frieser, D., & Hiller, W. (2011). The prevalence of medically unexplained symptoms in primary care. *Psychosomatics, 52,* 263–271.

Steptoe, A., Shankar, A., Demakakos, P., & Wardle, J. (2013). Social isolation, loneliness, and all-cause mortality in older men and women. *Proceedings of the National Academy of Sciences, 110,* 5797–5801.

Stevens, M., Rees, T., Coffee, P., Steffens, N. K., Haslam, S. A., & Polman, R. (2017). A social identity approach to understanding and promoting physical activity. *Sports Medicine.* Advance online publication, *47,* 1911–1918.

Stewart, J. J., Giles, J., Paterson, J. E., & Butler, S. J. (2005). Knowledge and attitudes towards older people: New Zealand students entering health professional degrees. *Physical and Occupational Therapy in Geriatrics, 23,* 25–36.

Stewart, N. A. J., & Lonsdale, A. J. (2016). It's better together: The psychological benefits of singing in a choir. *Psychology of Music, 44,* 1240–1254.

Stewart, T. L., Latu, I. M., Branscombe, N. R., & Denney, H. T. (2010). Yes we can! Prejudice reduction through seeing (inequality) and believing (in social change). *Psychological Science, 21,* 1557–1562.

Stice, E., & Agras, W. S. (1998). Predicting onset and cessation of bulimic behaviors during adolescence: A longitudinal grouping analysis. *Behavior Therapy, 29,* 257–276.

Stice, E., Cameron, R., Killen, J., Hayward, C., & Taylor, C. B. (1999). Naturalistic weight-reduction efforts prospectively predict growth in relative weight and onset of obesity among female adolescents. *Journal of Consulting and Clinical Psychology, 67,* 967–974.

Stice, E., Marti, C. N., & Rohde, P. (2013). Prevalence, incidence, impairment, and course of the proposed DSM-5 eating disorder diagnoses in an 8-year prospective community study of young women. *Journal of Abnormal Psychology, 122,* 445–457.

Stone, L. (2014). Blame, shame and hopelessness: Medically unexplained symptoms and the "heartsink" experience. *Australian Family Physician, 43,* 191–195.

Stout, R. L., Kelly, J. F., Magill, M., & Pagano, M. E. (2012). Association between social influences and drinking outcomes across three years. *Journal of Studies on Alcohol and Drugs, 73,* 489–499.

Stuber, J., Meyer, I., & Link, B. G. (2008). Stigma, prejudice, discrimination and health. *Social Science and Medicine, 67*, 351–357.

Styron, T., & Janoff-Bulman, R. (1997). Childhood attachment and abuse: Long-term effects on adult attachment, depression, and conflict resolution. *Child Abuse and Neglect, 21*, 1015–1023.

Suedfeld, P. (1997). The social psychology of "Invictus": Conceptual and methodological approaches to indomitability'. In C. McGarty & S. A. Haslam (Eds.), *The message of social psychology: Perspectives on mind in society* (pp. 328–341). Oxford: Blackwell.

Suedfeld, P., & Bow, R. A. (1999). Health and therapeutic applications of chamber and flotation restricted environmental stimulation therapy (REST). *Psychology and Health, 14*, 545–566.

Sullivan, M. J., Rodgers, W. M., & Kirsch, I. (2001). Catastrophizing, depression and expectancies for pain and emotional distress. *Pain, 91*, 147–154.

Sullivan, M. J., Tripp, D. A., & Santor, D. (2000). Gender differences in pain and pain behavior: The role of catastrophizing. *Cognitive Therapy and Research, 24*, 121–134.

Suls, J. M., Luger, T., & Martin, R. (2010). The biopsychosocial model and the use of theory in health psychology. In J. M. Suls, K. W. Davidson, & R. M. Kaplan (Eds.), *Handbook of health psychology and behavioural medicine* (pp. 15–27). New York, NY: Guilford Press.

Sundin, E. C., & Horowitz, M. J. (2002). Impact of Event Scale: Psychometric properties. *British Journal of Psychiatry, 180*, 205–209.

Sundin, J., Jones, N., Greenberg, N., Rona, R. J., Hotopf, M., Wessely, S., & Fear, N. T. (2010). Mental health among commando, airborne and other UK infantry personnel. *Occupational Medicine, 60*, 552–529.

Swift, H. J., Abrams, D., & Marques, S. (2013). Threat or boost? Social comparison affects older people's performance differently depending on task domain. *Journals of Gerontology B: Psychological Sciences and Social Sciences, 68*, 23–30.

Swim, J. K., Mallett, R., Russo-Devosa, Y., & Stangor, C. (2005). Judgments of sexism: A comparison of the subtlety of sexism measures and sources of variability in judgments of sexism. *Psychology of Women Quarterly, 29*, 406–411.

Swinburn, B., Egger, G., & Raza, F. (1999). Dissecting obesogenic environments: The development and application of a framework for identifying and prioritizing environmental interventions for obesity. *Public Health Nutrition, 7*, 123–146.

Syme, S. L., & Berkman, L. F. (1976). Social class, susceptibility and sickness. *American Journal of Epidemiology, 104*, 1–8.

Szreter, S., & Woolcock, M. (2004). Health by association? Social capital, social theory, and the political economy of public health. *International Journal of Epidemiology, 33*, 650–667.

Tabuteau-Harrison, S., Haslam, C., & Mewse, A. (2016). Adjusting to living with multiple sclerosis: The role of social groups. *Neuropsychological Rehabilitation, 26, 36–59.*

Tajfel, H. (1972). La catégorisation sociale (English Trans.). In S. Moscovici (Ed.), *Introduction à la psychologie sociale* (Vol. 1, pp. 272–302). Paris: Larousse.

Tajfel, H. (Ed.). (1978). *Differentiation between social groups: Studies in the social psychology of intergroup relations*. London: Academic Press.

Tajfel, H., Flament, C., Billig, M. G., & Bundy, R. F. (1971). Social categorization and intergroup behaviour. *European Journal of Social Psychology, 1*, 149–177.

Tajfel, H., & Turner, J. C. (1979). An integrative theory of intergroup conflict. In W. G. Austin & S. Worchel (Eds.), *The social psychology of intergroup relations* (pp. 33–47). Monterey, CA: Brooks/Cole.

Tajfel, H., & Turner, J. C. (1986). The social identity theory of intergroup behaviour. In S. Worchel & W. G. Austin (Eds.), *Psychology of intergroup relations* (pp. 7–24). Chicago, IL: Nelson-Hall.

Tangney, J. P., Baumeister, R. F., & Boone, A. L. (2004). High self-control predicts good adjustment, less pathology, better grades, and interpersonal success. *Journal of Personality, 72*, 271–324.

Tarrant, M., & Butler, K. (2011). Effects of self-categorization on orientation towards health. *British Journal of Social Psychology, 50*, 121–139.

Tarrant, M., Hagger, M., & Farrow, C. V. (2012). Promoting positive orientation towards health through social identity. In J. Jetten, C. Haslam, & S. A. Haslam (Eds.), *The social cure: Identity, health, and well-being* (pp. 39–54). Hove, UK: Psychology Press.

Tarrant, M., Khan, S. S., Farrow, C. V., Shah, P., Daly, M., & Kos, K. (2017). Patient experiences of a bariatric group programme for managing obesity: A qualitative interview study. *British Journal of Health Psychology, 22*, 77–93.

Tate, R. L., Harris, R. D., Cameron, I. D., Myles, B. M., Winstanley, J. B., Hodgkinson, A. E., . . . Harradine, P. G. (2006). Recovery of impairments after severe traumatic brain injury: Findings from a prospective, multicenter study. *Brain Impairment, 7*, 1–15.

Taylor, L. F., & Tovin, M. M. (2000). Student physical therapists' attitudes toward working with elderly patients. *Physical and Occupational Therapy in Geriatrics, 18*, 21–37.

Taylor, S. E. (2007). Social support. In H. S. Friedman & R. C. Silver (Eds.), *Foundations of Health Psychology* (pp. 145–171). New York, NY: Oxford University Press.

Tedeschi, R. G., & Calhoun, L. G. (2004). Post-traumatic growth: Conceptual foundations and empirical evidence. *Psychological Inquiry, 15*, 1–18.

Teesson, M., Ross, J., Darke, S., Lynskey, M., Ali, R., Ritter, A., & Cooke, R. (2006). One year outcomes for heroin dependence: Findings from the Australian Treatment Outcome Study (ATOS). *Drug and Alcohol Dependence, 83*, 174–180.

Temerlin, M. K., & Temerlin, J. W. (1982). Psychotherapy cults: An iatrogenic perversion. *Psychotherapy: Theory, Research and Practice, 19*, 131–141.

Temkin, N. R., Corrigan, J. D., Dikmen, S. S., & Marchamer, J. (2009). Social functioning after traumatic brain injury. *Journal of Head Trauma Rehabilitation, 24*, 460–467.

Teng, F., & Chen, Z. (2012). Does social support reduce distress caused by ostracism? It depends on the level of one's self-esteem. *Journal of Experimental Social Psychology, 48*, 1192–1195.

Tennant, C. (2002). Life events, stress and depression: A review of recent findings. *Australian and New Zealand Journal of Psychiatry, 36*, 173–182.

Terry, D., & O'Brien, A. (2001). Status, legitimacy and ingroup bias in the context of an organizational merger. *Group Processes and Intergroup Relations, 4*, 271–289.

Tewari, S., Khan, S., Hopkins, N., Srinivasan, N., & Reicher, S. D. (2012). Participation in mass gatherings can benefit well-being: Longitudinal and control data from a North Indian Hindu pilgrimage event. *PloS ONE, 7*(10), e47291.

Thaler, R. H., & Sunstein, C. R. (2008). *Nudge: Improving decisions about health, wealth, and happiness.* US: Yale University Press.

Thoburn, J., & O'Connell, C. (2016). *Psychological support for trauma victims.* Workshop delivered at the International Conference of Psychology, Dubai, October, 22.

Thoits, P. (2013). Dimensions of life events that influence psychological distress: An evaluation and synthesis of the literature. In H. B. Kaplan (Ed.), *Psychosocial stress: Trends in theory and research* (pp. 33–106). New York, NY: Academic Press.

Thoits, P. A. (1983). Multiple identities and psychological well-being: A reformulation and test of the social isolation hypothesis. *American Sociological Review, 48*, 174–187.

Thomas, K. C., Ellis, A. R., Konrad, T. R., Holzer, C. E., & Morrissey, J. P. (2009). County-level estimates of mental health professional shortage in the United States. *Psychiatric Services, 60*, 1323–1328.

Thompson, E. R. (2007). Development and validation of an internationally reliable short-form of the positive and negative affect schedule (PANAS). *Journal of Cross-cultural Psychology, 38*, 227–242.

Thompson, J. K., & Stice, E. (2001). Thin-ideal internalization: Mounting evidence for a new risk factor for body-image disturbance and eating pathology. *Current Directions in Psychological Science, 10*, 181–183.

Thompson, J. K., Van den Berg, P., Roehrig, M., Guarda, A. S., & Heinberg, L. J. (2004). The sociocultural attitudes towards appearance scale-3 (SATAQ-3): Development and validation. *The International Journal of Eating Disorders, 35*, 293–304.

Thorn, B. E., Pence, L. B., Ward, L. C., Kilgo, G., Clements, K. L., Cross, T. H., . . . Tsui, P. W. (2007). A randomized clinical trial of targeted cognitive behavioral treatment to reduce catastrophizing in chronic headache sufferers. *The Journal of Pain, 8*, 938–949.

Thorndike, A. N., Riis, J., & Levy, D. E. (2016). Social norms and financial incentives to promote employees' healthy food choices: A randomized controlled trial. *Preventive Medicine, 86*, 12–18.

Tiggemann, M., & Zaccardo, M. (2015). "Exercise to be fit, not skinny": The effect of fitspiration imagery on women's body image. *Body Image, 15*, 61–67.

Todis, B., Sohlberg, M. M., Hood, D., & Fickas, S. (2005). Making electronic mail accessible: Perspectives of people with acquired cognitive impairments, caregivers, and professionals. *Brain Injury, 19*, 389–401.

Tomaka, J., Blascovich, J., Kelsey, R. M., & Leitten, C. L. (1993). Subjective, physiological, and behavioral effects of threat and challenge appraisal. *Journal of Personality and Social Psychology, 65*, 248–260.

Tomaka, J., Thompson, S., & Palacios, R. (2006). The relation of social isolation, loneliness, and social support to disease outcomes among the elderly. *Journal of Aging and Health, 18*, 359–384.

Tomita, H., Ohbayashi, M., Nakahara, K., Hasegawa, I., & Miyashita, Y. (1999). Top-down signal from prefrontal cortex in executive control of memory retrieval. *Nature, 401*, 699–703.

Tones, B. K. (1986). Health education and the ideology of health promotion: a review of alternative approaches. *Health Education Research, 1*, 3–12.

Trace, S. E., Baker, J. H., Peñas-Lledó, E., & Bulik, C. M. (2013). The genetics of eating disorders. *Annual Review of Clinical Psychology, 9*, 589–620.

Tracie, M., Elkin, I., Imber, S. D., Sotsky, S. M., Watkins, J. T., Collins, F., . . . Parloff, M. B. (1992). Course of depressive symptoms over follow-up: Findings from the National Institute of Mental Health Treatment of Depression Collaborative Research Program. *Archives of General Psychiatry, 49*, 782–787.

Tsang, H. W., & Chen, E. Y. (2007). Perceptions on remission and recovery in schizophrenia. *Psychopathology, 40*, 469.

Tsang, H. W., Leung, A. Y., Chung, R. C. K., Bell, M., & Cheung, W. (2010). Review on vocational predictors – A systematic review of predictors of vocational outcomes among individuals with schizophrenia: An update since 1998. *Australia and NZ Journal of Psychiatry, 44*, 495–504.

Tucker, J. L., & Kelley, V. A. (2000). The influence of patient sociodemographic characteristics on patient satisfaction. *Military Medicine, 165*, 72–76.

Turner, B. S., & Wainwright, S. P. (2003). Corps de ballet: The case of the injured ballet dancer. *Sociology of Health and Illness, 25*, 269–288.

Turner, J. C. (1975). Social comparison and social identity: Some prospects for intergroup behaviour. *European Journal of Social Psychology, 5*, 5–34.

Turner, J. C. (1982). Towards a redefinition of the social group. In H. Tajfel (Ed.), *Social Identity and Intergroup Relations* (pp. 15–40). Cambridge: Cambridge University Press.

Turner, J. C. (1985). Social categorization and the self-concept: A social cognitive theory of group behaviour. In E. J. Lawler (Ed.), *Advances in group processes* (Vol. 2, pp. 77–122). Greenwich, CT: JAI Press.

Turner, J. C. (1991). *Social influence*. Milton Keynes: Open University Press.

Turner, J. C. (2005). Explaining the nature of power: A three-process theory. *European Journal of Social Psychology, 35*, 1–22.

Turner, J. C., Hogg, M. A., Oakes, P. J., Reicher, S. D., & Wetherell, M. S. (1987). *Rediscovering the social group: A self-categorization theory.* Oxford, UK: Blackwell.

Turner, J. C., & Oakes, P. J. (1986). The significance of the social identity concept for social psychology with reference to individualism, interactionism, and social influence. *British Journal of Social Psychology, 25*, 237–252.

Turner, J. C., & Oakes, P. J. (1997). The socially structured mind. In C. McGarty & S. A. Haslam (Eds.), *The message of social psychology* (pp. 355–373). Oxford: Blackwell.

Turner, J. C., Oakes, P. J., Haslam, S. A., & McGarty, C. (1994). Self and collective: Cognition and social context. *Personality and Social Psychology Bulletin, 20*, 454–463.

Turner, R. J., & Lloyd, D. A. (1995). Lifetime traumas and mental health: The significance of cumulative adversity. *Journal of Health and Social Behavior, 36*, 360–376.

Tuval-Mashiach, R., Freedman, S., Bargai, N., Boker, R., Hadar, H., & Shalev, A. Y. (2004). Coping with trauma: Narrative and cognitive perspectives. *Psychiatry, 67*, 280–293.

Twamley, E. W., & Davis, M. C. (1999). The sociocultural model of eating disturbance in young women: The effects of personal attributes and family environment. *Journal of Social and Clinical Psychology, 18*, 467–489.

Twenge, J. M., Baumeister, R. F., Tice, D. M., & Stucke, T. S. (2001). If you can't join them, beat them: Effects of social exclusion on aggressive behaviour. *Journal of Personality and Social Psychology, 81,* 1058–1069.

Twenge, J. M., & Campbell, W. K. (2001). Age and birth cohort differences in self-esteem: A cross-temporal meta-analysis. *Personality and Social Psychology Review, 5,* 321–344.

Twomey, S. (2010, January). Phineas Gage: Neuroscience's most famous patient. *Smithsonian.* Retrieved from www.smithsonianmag.com/history/phineas-gage-neurosciences-most-famous-patient-11390067/

Tyerman, A. (1987). *Self concept and psychological change in the rehabilitation of the severely head injured person.* Unpublished Doctoral Thesis, University of London.

Tyerman, A., & Humphrey, M. (1984). Changes in self-concept following severe head injury. *International Journal of Rehabilitation Research, 7,* 11–23.

Tyrka, A. R., Waldron, I., Graber, J. A., & Brooks-Gunn, J. (2002). Prospective predictors of the onset of anorexic and bulimic syndromes. *International Journal of Eating Disorders, 32,* 282–290.

Uchino, B. N. (2006). Social support and health: A review of physiological processes potentially underlying links to disease outcomes. *Journal of Behavioral Medicine, 29,* 377–387.

Ulijaszek, S. J. (2002). Human eating behaviour in an evolutionary ecological context. *Proceedings of the Nutrition Society, 61,* 517–526.

Ulijaszek, S. J., & Lofink, H. (2006). Obesity in biocultural perspective. *Annual Review of Anthropology, 35,* 337–360.

Ulman, R. B., & Brothers, D. (2013). *The shattered self: A psychoanalytic study of trauma.* London: Routledge.

Underwood, P. W. (2000). Social support: The promise and reality. In B. H. Rice (Ed.), *Handbook of stress, coping and health* (pp. 367–391). Newbury Park, CA: Sage.

United Nations. (2013). *World population ageing 2013.* New York, NY: United Nations Publications (Department of Economic and Social Affairs Population Division).

Unruh, A. M. (1996). Gender variations in clinical pain experience. *Pain, 65,* 123–167.

Vaananen, A., Koskinen, A., Joensuu, M., Kivimak, M., Vahtera, J., Kouvonen, A., & Jappinen, P. (2008). Lack of predictability at work and risk of acute myocardial infarction: An 18-year prospective study of industrial employees. *American Journal of Public Health, 98,* 2264–2271.

Vaillant, G. E. (2002). *Aging well: Surprising guideposts to a happier life from the landmark Harvard study of adult development.* Boston: Little, Brown and Company.

Vaillant, G. E. (2012). *Triumphs of experience.* Cambridge, MA: Harvard University Press.

Van den Berg, P., & Neumark-Sztainer, D. (2007). Fat 'n happy 5 years later: Is it bad for overweight girls to like their bodies? *The Journal of Adolescent Health : Official Publication of the Society for Adolescent Medicine, 41,* 415–417.

Van den Berg, P., Neumark-Sztainer, D., Hannan, P. J., & Haines, J. (2007). Is dieting advice from magazines helpful or harmful? Five-year associations with weight-control behaviors and psychological outcomes in adolescents. *Pediatrics, 119,* 30–36.

Van Dessel, N., Den Boeft, M., Van der Wouden, J. C., Kleinstäuber, M., Leone, S. S., . . . Van Marwijk, H. (2014). Non-pharmacological interventions for somatoform disorders and medically unexplained physical symptoms (MUPS) in adults. *Cochrane Database of Systematic Reviews, 11.* Retrieved from http://doi.org/10.1002/14651858.CD011142.pub2

Van Dick, R., & Haslam, S. A. (2012). Stress and well-being in the workplace: Support for key propositions from the social identity approach. In J. Jetten, C. Haslam, & S. A. Haslam (Eds.), *The social cure: Identity, health, and well-being* (pp. 175–194). Hove, UK: Psychology Press.

Van Horn, J., Irimia, A., Torgerson, C., Chambers, M., Kikinis, R., & Toga, A. (2012). Mapping connectivity damage in the case of Phineas Gage. *PLoS ONE, 7*(5), e37454.

Van Praag, H., Shubert, T., Zhao, C., & Gage, F. H. (2005). Exercise enhances learning and hippocampal neurogenesis in aged mice. *Journal of Neuroscience, 25,* 8680–8685.

Van Stralen, M. M., Vries, H. D., Mudde, A. N., Bolman, C., & Lechner, L. (2009). Determinants of initiation and maintenance of physical activity among older adults: A literature review. *Health Psychology Review, 3,* 147–207.

Van Tulder, M., Malmivaara, A., & Koes, B. (2007). Repetitive strain injury. *The Lancet, 369,* 1815–1822.

Van Zee, A. (2009). The promotion and marketing of OxyContin: Commercial triumph, public health tragedy. *American Journal of Public Health, 99,* 221–227.

Vartanian, L. R. (2009). When the body defines the self: Self-concept clarity, internalization, and body image. *Journal of Social and Clinical Psychology, 28,* 94–126.

Vartanian, L. R., & Novak, S. A. (2011). Internalized societal attitudes moderate the impact of weight stigma on avoidance of exercise. *Obesity, 19,* 757–762.

Vase, L., Skyt, I., & Hall, K. T. (2016). Placebo, nocebo, and neuropathic pain. *Pain, 157,* 98–105.

Vasterling, J. J., Brailey, K., Constans, J. I., & Sutker, P. B. (1998). Attention and memory dysfunction in posttraumatic stress disorder. *Neuropsychology, 12,* 125–133.

Veale, D. (2008). Behavioural activation for depression. *Advances in Psychiatric Treatment, 14,* 29–36.

Vedsted, P., & Christensen, M. B. (2005). Frequent attenders in general practice care: A literature review with special reference to methodological considerations. *Public Health, 119,* 118–137.

Veling, W., Selten, J. P., Susser, E., Laan, W., Mackenbach, J. P., & Hoek, H. W. (2007). Discrimination and the incidence of psychotic disorders among ethnic minorities in the Netherlands. *International Journal of Epidemiology, 36,* 761–768.

Vezzali, L., Cadamuro, A., Versari, A., Giovannini, D., & Trifiletti, E. (2015). Feeling like a group after a natural disaster: Common ingroup identity and relations with outgroup victims among majority and minority young children. *British Journal of Social Psychology, 54,* 519–538.

Vezzali, L., Drury, J., Cadamuro, A., & Versari, A. (2015). Sharing distress increases helping and contact intentions via one-group representation and inclusion of the other in the self: Children's prosocial behaviour after an earthquake. *Group Processes and Intergroup Relations, 19,* 314–327.

Victor, C., Scambler, S., Bond, J., & Bowling, A. (2000). Being alone in later life: Loneliness, social isolation and living alone. *Reviews in Clinical Gerontology, 10,* 407–417.

Vitousek, K., & Manke, F. (1994). Personality variables and disorders in anorexia nervosa and bulimia nervosa. *Journal of Abnormal Psychology, 103,* 137–147.

Von Dawans, B., Kirschbaum, C., & Heinrichs, M. (2011). The Trier Social Stress Test for Groups (TSST-G): A new research tool for controlled simultaneous social stress exposure in a group format. *Psychoneuroendocrinology, 36,* 514–522.

Von Frey, M. (1894). Beitrage zur physiologie des schmerzsinns [Contributions to the physiology of pain]. *Akademie der Wissenschaften zu Leipzig [Proceedings of the Saxony Academy of Sciences at Leipzig], 46,* 185–196.

Vos, T., Barber, R. M., Bell, B., Bertozzi-Villa, A., Biryukov, S., Bolliger, I., . . . Murray, C. J. L. (2015). Global, regional, and national incidence, prevalence, and years lived with disability for 301 acute and chronic diseases and injuries in 188 countries, 1990–2013: A systematic analysis for the Global Burden of Disease Study 2013. *The Lancet, 386,* 743–800.

Voss, M. W., Prakash, R. S., Erickson, K. I., Bassak, C., Chaddock, L., Kim, J. S., . . . Kramer, A. F. (2010). Plasticity of brain networks in a randomized intervention trial of exercise training in older adults. *Frontiers in Aging Neuroscience, 2,* 32. doi:10.3389/fnagi.2010.00032

Vowles, K. E., McCracken, L. M., & O'Brien, J. Z. (2011). Acceptance and values-based action in chronic pain: A three-year follow-up analysis of treatment effectiveness and process. *Behaviour Research and Therapy, 49,* 748–755.

Vredenburg, K., Flett, G. L., & Krames, L. (1993). Analogue versus clinical depression: A critical reappraisal. *Psychological Bulletin, 113,* 327–344.

Wade, T. D., Wilksch, S. M., Paxton, S. J., Byrne, S. M., & Austin, S. B. (2015). How perfectionism and ineffectiveness influence growth of eating disorder risk in young adolescent girls. *Behaviour Research and Therapy, 66,* 56–63.

Wahl, O. F. (1999). Mental health consumers' experience of stigma. *Schizophrenia Bulletin, 25,* 467–478.

Wahler, E. A., & Otis, M. D. (2014). Social stress, economic hardship, and psychological distress as predictors of sustained abstinence from substance use after treatment. *Substance Use and Misuse, 49,* 1820–1832.

Wakefield, J. R. H., Bickley, S., & Sani, F. (2013). The effects of identification with a support group on the mental health of people with multiple sclerosis. *Journal of Psychosomatic Research, 74,* 420–426.

Wakefield, J. R. H., Sani, F., Herrera, M., & Zeybek, A. (2017). On the association between greater family identification and lower family ideation among non-clinical individuals: Evidence from Cypriot and Spanish students. *Journal of Social and Clinical Psychology*, *36*, 396–418.

Wakley, G., & Chambers, R. (Eds.). (2005). *Chronic disease management in primary care: Quality and outcomes*. New York, NY: Taylor and Francis.

Waldron, B., Casserly, L. M., & O'Sullivan, C. (2013). Cognitive behavioural therapy for depression and anxiety in adults with acquired brain injury. What works for whom? *Neuropsychological Rehabilitation*, *23*, 64–101.

Walsh, R. S., Fortune, D. G., Gallagher, S., & Muldoon, O. T. (2014). Acquired brain injury: Combining social psychological and neuropsychological perspectives. *Health Psychology Review*, *8*, 458–472.

Walter, Z. C., Jetten, J., Dingle, G. A., Parsell, C., & Johnstone, M. (2015a). Two pathways through adversity: Predicting well-being and housing outcomes among homeless service users. *British Journal of Social Psychology*, *55*, 357–374.

Walter, Z. C., Jetten, J., Parsell, C., & Dingle, G. A. (2015b). The impact of self-categorizing as "homeless" on well-being and service use. *Analyses of Social Issues and Public Policy*, *15*, 333–356.

Walton, G. M. (2014). The new science of wise psychological interventions. *Current Directions in Psychological Science*, *23*, 73–82.

Walton, G. M., & Cohen, G. L. (2003). Stereotype lift. *Journal of Experimental Social Psychology*, *39*, 456–467.

Wang, C. C. (1998). Portraying stigmatized conditions: Disabling images in public health. *Journal of Health Communication*, *3*, 149–159.

Wang, C. E. A., Halvorsen, M., Eisemann, M., & Waterloo, K. (2010). Stability of dysfunctional attitudes and early maladaptive schemas: A 9-year follow-up study of clinically depressed subjects. *Journal of Behavior Therapy and Experimental Psychiatry*, *41*, 389–396.

Wang, M. (2007). Profiling retirees in the retirement transition and adjustment process: Examining the longitudinal change patterns of retirees' psychological well-being. *Journal of Applied Psychology*, *92*, 455–474.

Wann, D. L., & Branscombe, N. R. (1990). Die hard and fair-weather fans: Effects of identification on BIRGing and CORFing tendencies. *Journal of Sport and Social Issues*, *14*, 103–117.

Wansink, B., & Van Ittersum, K. (2012). Fast food restaurant lighting and music can reduce calorie intake and increase satisfaction. *Psychological Reports*, *111*, 228–232.

Ward, R. A. (1984). The marginality and salience of being old: When is age relevant? *The Gerontologist*, *24*, 227–232.

Warner, R., Hornsey, M. J., & Jetten, J. (2007). Why minority group members resent impostors. *European Journal of Social Psychology*. *37*, 1–18.

Watson, D., Clark, L. A., & Tellegen, A. (1988). Development and validation of brief measures of positive and negative affect: the PANAS scales. *Journal of Personality and Social Psychology*, *54*, 1063–1070.

Wearden, A. J., Tarrier, N., Barrowclough, C., Zastowny, T. R., & Rahill, A. A. (2000). A review of expressed emotion research in health care. *Clinical Psychology Review*, *20*, 633–666.

Webb, H., Jones, B. J., McNeill, K., Lim, L., Frain, A. J., O'Brien, K. J., . . . Cruwys, T. (2017). Smoke signals: The decline of brand identity predicts reduced smoking behaviour following the introduction of plain packaging. *Addictive Behaviors Reports*, *5*, 49–55.

Wegge, J., Van Dick, R., Fisher, G. K., Wecking, C., & Moltzen, K. (2006). Work motivation, organisational identification, and well-being in call centre work. *Work & Stress*, *20*, 60–83.

Weiner, B. (1985). An attributional theory of achievement motivation and emotion. *Journal of Personality and Social Psychology*, *92*, 548–573.

Weiss, A., & Costa, P. T. Jr. (2005). Domain and facet personality predictors of all-cause mortality among Medicare patients aged 65 to 100. *Psychosomatic Medicine*, *67*, 724–733.

Weiss, J. (1970). Somatic effects of predictable and unpredictable shock. *Psychosomatic Medicine*, *32*, 397–414.

Weiss D. S. (2007) The Impact of Event Scale: Revised. In Wilson J. P., Tang C. S. (Eds) *Cross-cultural assessment of psychological trauma and PTSD*. International and Cultural Psychology Series. Boston, MA: Springer.

Weissman, M. M. (2006). A brief history of interpersonal psychotherapy. *Psychiatric Annals, 36*, 553–557.

Wells, Y., Foreman, P., Gething, L., & Petralia, W. (2004). Nurses' attitudes toward aging and older adults: Examining attitudes and practices among health services providers in Australia. *Journal of Gerontological Nursing, 30*, 5–13.

West, L. A., Cole, S., Goodkind, D., & He, W. (2014). *65+ in the United States: 2010*. P23–P212. US Census Bureau. Washington, DC: US Government Printing Office.

West, R. (2005). Time for a change: Putting the Transtheoretical (Stages of Change) Model to rest. *Addiction, 100*, 1036–1039.

Westgate, E. C., Wormington, S. V., Oleson, K. C., & Lindgren, K. P. (2017). Productive procrastination: Academic procrastination style predicts academic and alcohol outcomes. *Journal of Applied Social Psychology, 47*, 124–135.

Wexler, D., Mendelson, J., Leiderman, P. H., & Solomon, P. (1958). Sensory deprivation: A technique for studying psychiatric aspects of stress. *AMA Archives of Neurology and Psychiatry, 79*, 225–233.

White, K. M., Smith, J. R., Terry, D. J., Greenslade, J. H., & McKimmie, B. M. (2009). Social influence in the theory of planned behaviour: The role of descriptive, injunctive, and in-group norms. *British Journal of Social Psychology, 48*, 135–158.

White, P. D., Goldsmith, K., Johnson, A. L., Potts, L., Walwyn, R., Decesare, J. C., . . . Sharpe, M. (2011). Comparison of adaptive pacing therapy, cognitive behaviour therapy, graded exercise therapy, and specialist medical care for chronic fatigue syndrome (PACE): A randomised trial. *The Lancet, 377*, 823–836.

Whiteley, P. F. (1999). The origins of social capital. In J. W. van Deth, M. Maraffi, K. Newton, & P. F. Whiteley (Eds.), *Social capital and European democracy* (pp. 25–44). Abingdon, UK: Routledge.

Whitely, R., & Campbell, R. D. (2014). Stigma, agency and recovery amongst people with severe mental illness. *Social Science and Medicine, 107*, 1–18.

Whiteside, U., Chen, E., Neighbors, C., Hunter, D., Lo, T., & Larimer, M. (2007). Difficulties regulating emotions: Do binge eaters have fewer strategies to modulate and tolerate negative affect? *Eating Behaviors, 8*, 162–169.

Whyte, K. P., Selinger, E., Caplan, A. L., & Sadowski, J. (2012). Nudge, nudge or shove, shove – the right way for nudges to increase the supply of donated cadaver organs. *The American Journal of Bioethics, 12*, 32–39.

Wicklund, R. A. (1990). Zero-variable theories in the analysis of social phenomena. *European Journal of Personality, 4*, 37–55.

Wicksell, R. K., Dahl, J., Magnusson, B., & Olsson, G. L. (2005). Using acceptance and commitment therapy in the rehabilitation of an adolescent female with chronic pain: a case example. *Cognitive and Behavioral Practice, 12*, 415–423.

Wilcox, K., Vallen, B., Block, L., & Fitzsimons, G. J. (2009). Vicarious goal fulfillment: When the mere presence of a healthy option leads to an ironically indulgent decision. *Journal of Consumer Research, 36*, 380–393.

Wilgus, J, & Wilgus, B. (2009). Face to face with Phineas Gage. *Journal of the History of Neuroscience: Basic and Clinical Perspectives, 18*, 340–345.

Wilkinson, R., & Pickett, K. (2009). *The spirit level: Why more equal societies almost always do better*. London, UK: Allen Lane.

Williams, D. R. (2005). The health of U.S. racial and ethnic populations. *The Journals of Gerontology Series B: Psychological Sciences and Social Sciences, 60*, 53–62.

Williams, D. R., & Mohammed, S. A. (2009). Discrimination and racial disparities in health: Evidence and needed research. *Journal of Behavioral Medicine, 32*, 20–47.

Williams, E., Dingle, G. A., Jetten, J., & Rowan, C. (2017). *Identification with arts-based groups improves mental wellbeing in adults with chronic mental health conditions*. Manuscript under review.

Williams, K. D., Cheung, C. K. T., & Choi, W. (2000). Cyberostracism: Effects of being ignored over the Internet. *Journal of Personality and Social Psychology, 79*, 748–762.

Williams, K. D., & Jarvis, B. (2006). Cyberball: A program for use in research on interpersonal ostracism and acceptance. *Behavior Research Methods, 38*, 174–180.

Williams, R., & Drury, J. (2009). Psychosocial resilience and its influence on managing mass emergencies and disasters. *Psychiatry, 8*, 293–296.

Williams, R., & Drury, J. (2011). Personal and collective psychosocial resilience: Implications for children, young people and their families involved in war and disasters. In D. T. Cook & J. Wall (Eds.), *Children and armed conflict* (pp. 57–75). London, UK: Palgrave Macmillan.

Williams, W. H., Evans, J. J., & Fleminger, S. (2003). Neurorehabilitation and cognitive-behaviour therapy of anxiety disorders after brain injury: An overview and a case illustration of obsessive-compulsive disorder. *Neuropsychological Rehabilitation, 13*, 133–148.

Williams, W. H., Mewse, A. J., Tonks, J., Mills, S., Burgess, C. N., & Cordan, G. (2010). Traumatic brain injury in a prison population: Prevalence and risk for re-offending. *Brain Injury, 24*, 1184–1188.

Willinge, A., Touyz, S., & Charles, M. (2006). How do body-dissatisfied and body-satisfied males and females judge the size of thin female celebrities? *International Journal of Eating Disorders, 39*, 576–582.

Wilson, B. A. (2002). Towards a comprehensive model of cognitive rehabilitation. *Neuropsychological Rehabilitation 12*, 97–110.

Wilson, B. A. (2008). Neuropsychological rehabilitation. *Annual Review of Clinical Psychology, 4*, 141–162.

Wilson, B. A., Gracey, F., Evans, J. J., & Bateman, A. (2009). *Neuropsychological rehabilitation: Theory, models, therapy and outcomes.* Cambridge, UK: Cambridge University Press.

Wilson, B. A., Winegardner, J., & Ashworth, F. (2014). *Life after brain injury: Survivors' stories.* Hove, East Sussex: Psychology Press.

Wilson, G. (2000). *Understanding old age: Critical and global perspectives.* London: Sage.

Wilson, J. P., Friedman, M. J., & Lindy, J. D. (Eds.). (2012). *Treating psychological trauma and PTSD.* New York, NY: Guilford Press.

Wimo, A., & Prince, M. (2010). *World Alzheimer Report 2010: The global economic impact of dementia.* London: Alzheimer's Disease International.

Windle, G., Bennett, K. M., & Noyes, J. (2011). A methodological review of resilience measurement scales. *Health and quality of life outcomes, 9*, 8.

Windsor, T. D., Anstey, K. J., Butterworth, P., Lusczc, M. A., & Andrews, G. (2007). The role of perceived control in explaining depressive symptoms associated with driving cessation in a longitudinal study. *Gerontologist, 46*, 215–223.

Winehouse, A. (2006). *Rehab. From the album* Back to black. London: Island records. Retrieved from www.youtube.com/watch?v=KUmZp8pR1uc

Wiseman, C. V., Gray, J. J., Mosimann, J. E., & Ahrens, A. H. (1992). Cultural expectations of thinness in women: An update. *International Journal of Eating Disorders, 11*, 85–89.

Wiseman, E. (2015, November 15). You don't have to be old to be lonely. *The Guardian.* Retrieved from www.theguardian.com/lifeandstyle/2015/nov/15/you-dont-have-to-be-old-to-be-lonely

Witkiewitz, K., & Bowen, S. (2010). Depression, craving, and substance use following a randomized trial of Mindfulness-Based Relapse Prevention. *Journal of Consulting and Clinical Psychology, 78*, 362–374.

Witkiewitz, K., & Marlatt, G. A. (2004). Relapse prevention for alcohol and drug problems: That was Zen, this is Tao. *American Psychologist, 59*, 224–235.

Wolfe, C. D. A., Crichton, C. L., Heuschmann, P. U., McKevitt, C. J., Toschke, A. M., Grieve, A. P., & Rudd, A. G. (2011). Estimates of outcomes up to ten years after stroke: Analysis from the prospective South London Stroke Register. *PLoS Medicine, 8*(5), e1001033.

Wolff, B. B. (1985). Ethnocultural factors influencing pain and illness behavior. *The Clinical Journal of Pain, 1*, 23–30.

Woods, A., Willison, K., Kington, C., & Gavin, A. (2008). Palliative care for people with severe persistent mental illness: A review of the literature. *The Canadian Journal of Psychiatry/La Revue Canadienne de Psychiatrie, 53*, 725–736.

Woods, B., Spector, A., Jones, C., Orrell, M., & Davies, S. (2005). Reminiscence therapy for dementia. *Cochrane Database of Systematic Reviews, 2*. Article No.: CD001120

Woods, R. T., Bruce, E., Edwards, R. T., Elvish, R., Hoare, Z., Hounsome, B., . . . Russell, I. T. (2012). REM-CARE: Reminiscence groups for people with dementia and their family caregivers – Effectiveness and cost-effectiveness pragmatic multicenter randomized trial. *Health Technology Assessment, 16*, 1–116.

Work Group on Substance Use Disorders, Kleber, H. D., Weiss, R. D., Anton, R. F., Rounsaville, B. J., George, T. P., . . . Regier, D. (2006). Treatment of patients with substance use disorders, Second Edition. *American Journal of Psychiatry, 163,* 5–82.

World Bank. (2012). *Women, business and the law 2012: Removing barriers to economic inclusion.* Retrieved from http://wbl.worldbank.org/~/media/FPDKM/WBL/Documents/Reports/2012/Women-Business-and-the-Law-2012.pdf

World Health Organization. (2001a). *International classification of functioning, disability and health.* Geneva, Switzerland: WHO.

World Health Organization. (2001b). *The world health report 2001: Mental health: New understanding, new hope.* New York, NY: World Health Organization.

World Health Organization. (2008). *The global burden of disease 2004.* Geneva, Switzerland: WHO.

World Health Organisation. (2017a). *Global Health Observatory (GHO) datat: Overweight and obesity.* Retrieved from www.who.int/gho/ncd/risk_factors/overweight/en/

World Health Organization. (2017b). *Non-communicable diseases fact sheet.* Retrieved from www.who.int/mediacentre/factsheets/fs355/en/, June 2017

World Health Organization, & United Nations Children's Fund. (1978). *Primary health care: A joint report.* Geneva: WHO.

Wray, N. R., Pergadia, M. L., Blackwood, D. H. R., Penninx, B. W. J. H., Gordon, S. D., Nyholt, D. R., . . . Sullivan, P. F. (2012). Genome-wide association study of major depressive disorder: New results, meta-analysis, and lessons learned. *Molecular Psychiatry, 17,* 36–48.

Wright, C. J., Zeeman, H., & Biezaitis, V. (2016). Holistic practice in traumatic brain injury rehabilitation: Perspectives of health practitioners. *PLoS One, 11*(6), e0156826.

Wright, S. C., Taylor, D. M., & Moghaddam, F. M. (1990). Responding to membership in a disadvantaged group: From acceptance to collective protest. *Journal of Personality and Social Psychology, 58,* 994–1003.

Wu, C-H., & Yao, G. (2007). Psychometric analysis of the short form UCLA Loneliness Scale (ULS-8) in Taiwanese undergraduate students. *Personality and Individual Differences, 44,* 1762–1771.

Wuthnow, R. (1994). *Sharing the journey: Support groups and America's new quest for community.* New York, NY: Simon and Schuster.

Wykes, T., Steel, C., Everitt, B., & Tarrier, N. (2008). Cognitive behavior therapy for schizophrenia: Effect sizes, clinical models, and methodological rigor. *Schizophrenia Bulletin, 34,* 523–537.

Xu, X., Zuo, Z., Wang, W., & Han, S. (2009). Do you feel my pain? Racial group membership modulates empathic neural responses. *The Journal of Neuroscience, 29,* 8525–8529.

Xygalatas, D., Mitkidis, P., Fischer, R., Reddish, P., Skewes, J., Geertz, A. W., Roepstorff, A., & Bulbulia, J. (2013). Extreme rituals promote prosociality. *Psychological Science, 24,* 1602–1605.

Yates, P. J. (2003). Psychological adjustment, social enablement and community integration following acquired brain injury. *Neuropsychological Rehabilitation, 13,* 291–306.

Yehuda, R., & McFarlane, A. C. (1995). Conflict between current knowledge about posttraumatic stress disorder and its original conceptual basis. *American Journal of Psychiatry, 152,* 1705–1713.

Yeomans, M. R., Leitch, M., & Mobini, S. (2008). Impulsivity is associated with the disinhibition but not restraint factor from the Three Factor Eating Questionnaire. *Appetite, 50,* 469–476.

Yildiz, A. A., & Verkuyten, M. (2011). Inclusive victimhood: Social identity and the politicization of collective trauma among Turkey's Alevis in Western Europe. *Peace and Conflict: Journal of Peace Psychology, 17,* 243–269.

Ylvisaker, M., & Feeney, T. (2000). Reconstruction of identity after brain injury. *Brain Impairment, 1,* 12–28.

Ylvisaker, M., McPherson, K., Kayes, N., & Pellett, E. (2008). Metaphoric identity mapping: Facilitating goal setting and engagement in rehabilitation after traumatic brain injury. *Neuropsychological Rehabilitation, 18,* 713–741.

Young, J. E., Klosko, J. S., & Weishaar, M. (2003). *Schema therapy: A practitioner's guide.* New York, NY: Guilford Press.

Young, S. G., Brown, C. M., & Hutchins, B. (2017). Ease-of-retrieval provides meta-cognitive information about social affiliation. *Social Cognition, 35,* 54-65.

Zadro, L., Williams, K. D., & Richardson, R. (2004). How low can you go? Ostracism by a computer is sufficient to lower self-reported levels of belonging, control, self esteem, and meaningful existence. *Journal of Experimental Social Psychology, 40*, 560–567.

Zhang, A., Jetten, J., Iyer, A., & Cui, L. (2013). "It will not always be this way": Cognitive alternatives improve self-esteem in contexts of segregation. *Social Psychological and Personality Science, 4*, 159–166.

Zhou, X., & Gao, D. G. (2008). Social support and money as pain management mechanisms. *Psychological Inquiry, 19*, 127–144.

Zijdenbos, I. L., De Wit, N. J., Van der Heijden, G. J., Rubin, G., & Quartero, A. O. (2009). Psychological treatments for the management of irritable bowel syndrome. *Cochrane Database of Systematic Reviews*, 1. Retrieved from http://doi.org/10.1002/14651858.CD006442.pub2

Zink, T., Regan, S., Jacobson, C. J., & Pabst, S. (2003). Cohort, period, and aging effects: A qualitative study of older women's reasons for remaining in abusive relationships. *Violence against Women, 9*, 1429–1441.

Zywiak, W. H., Neighbors, C. J., Martin, R. A., Johnson, J. E., Eaton, C. A., & Rohsenow, D. J. (2009). The important people drug and alcohol interview: Psychometric properties, predictive validity, and implications for treatment. *Journal of Substance Abuse Treatment, 36*, 321–330.

Zywiak, W. H., Stout, R. L., Longabaugh, R., Dyck, I., Connors, G. J., & Maisto, S. A. (2006). Relapse-onset factors in Project MATCH: The Relapse Questionnaire. *Journal of Substance Abuse Treatment, 31*, 341–345.

 Author index

Abbott, D. H. 40, 49
Abdou, C. M. 80
Abela, J. R. Z. 161
Abelin, T. 56
Abrams, D. 142, 144
Abramson, L. Y. 168
Access Economics 131
Acero, Á. R. 289
Ackerman, S. J. 97
Adams, S. 320
Addington, J. 290
Addis, M. E. 161
Adhikari, K. 121, 126
Adler, A. B. 93, 115
Adler, N. E. 46
Afridi, F. 78
Afzal, S. 222
Agarwal, A. K. 230
Agerbo, E. 284
Agich, G. J. 44
Aglioti, S. M. 268
Agras, W. S. 214
Ahmed-Ansari, A. 40
Ahn, H. 161
Ahn, W. 158
Ahrens, A. H. 211
Ajzen, I. 7, 207
Aker, T. 127
Akerlof, G. A. 56
Alamo, C. 285
Al-Anon Family Groups 184
Albery, I. P. 183, 189, 195, 196
Albrecht, T. L. 80
Alexander, B. K. 176, 188
Alexander, J. 19, 26, 185, 187, 189, 197
Ali, R. 122, 179
Allan, J. 323, 372
Alloy, L. B. 168
Allsop, J. 141
Alnabulsi, H. 27, 118, 357
Alonso, J. 316
Alper, C. M. 162
Always, Y. 232
Amann, B. 286
American Psychiatric Association 107, 157, 206

American Psychological Association 288
Amlôt, R. 127
Amsterdam, J. D. 157–159
Anczewska, M. 308
Andersen, R. E. 325
Anderson, C. 46
Anderson, K. 310
Anderson, L. 59
Anderson, N. 68
Anderson, P. 161
Andreasen, N. C. 170
Andrews, G. 148
Andrews, P. W. 158
Andrews, T. K. 244
Andrusyna, T. P. 170
Angermeyer, M. C. 281
Angst, J. 280
Anguelova, M. 159
Angullia, S. A. 325
Angus, J. 65
Anisman, H. 11, 66, 68, 86, 108, 116, 254, 257, 258, 273, 328, 361
Ansell, N. 16
Anson, K. 244
Anstey, K. J. 131, 148
Antman, E. M. 308
Anton, R. F. 179
Anton, S. D. 327
Antony, M. M. 367
Araga, M. 288, 289
Arain, M. 340
Arandine, A. L. 232
Araújo-Soares, V. 209
Ardelt, M. 131
Arendt-Nielsen, L. 259
Arevalo, J. M. 329
Aristotle 254
Armeli, S. 87
Armitage, C. J. 209
Armstrong, E. (2003) 3
Armstrong, M. J. (2011) 209
Armstrong-Esther, C. A. (1996) 152
Armstrong-Esther, D. C. (1996) 152
Arnautovska, U. 12
Arnold, S. E. 138

Arntz, A. 168, 254
Aronson, E. 265
Aronson, J. 142
Arora, R. 377
Asai, N. 146
Ashforth, B. E. 230, 245
Ashman, T. 236
Ashworth, F. 230, 236
Asmussen, S. 244
Aspinwall, L. G. 91
Åstrosm, A. N. 219
Asukai, N. 367
Atkinson, Q. D. 261
Atran, S. 265
Attia, J. R. 162
Auchterlonie, J. 112
Auerbach, R. P. 161
Auerswald, C. L. 59
Auman, C. 142
Auriacombe, M. 185
Austin, S. B. 206
Australian Bureau of Statistics 204
Australian Health Ministers Advisory Council 293
Australian Human Rights Commission 140
Australian Institute of Health and Welfare 37, 133, 203, 229, 307
Avenanti, A. 268
Avina, C. 108
Awad, A. G. 286
Ayuso-Mateos, J. L. 308
Azzoli, C. G. 310

Bacaltchuk, J. 163
Bach, P. B. 310
Backonja, M-M. 258
Badawy, A. A. B. 175
Bagnasco, M. 206
Bailer, U. F. 206
Bailey, S. 308
Bakdash, J. Z. 142
Baker, A. L. 187
Baker, A. 181
Baker, F. A. 17, 206, 297, 298
Baker, J. H. 17, 206, 297, 298
Baker, M. 187
Baker, R. C. 206
Bakouri, M. 52, 53, 56
Balcazar, F. 20
Ball, S. J. 44, 56
Ballantyne, J. 17, 297, 298
Baltes, B. B. 91
Banal, S. 74, 169, 320

Banas, K. 222
Bandura, A. 7, 56, 87
Banich, M. B. 20, 134, 136, 148, 150
Baray, G. 358
Barber, C. 158
Barber, J. 230
Barber, R. M. 142
Barber, S. J. 142
Barendregt, J. 157
Bargai, N. 112
Bar-Hillel, M. 218
Barlow, D. H. 368
Barlow, F. 27, 57
Barlow, J. H. 317
Barnes, L. L. 138
Barness, L. A. 215
Baron, R. S. 75
Baron-Cohen, S. 247
Barr, L. 68, 294, 362
Barreto, M. E. 65, 74, 169, 320
Barreto, M. 74, 169, 320
Barrington-Leigh, C. P. 44, 376
Barrowclough, C. 188, 283
Bartholomew, R. E. 92
Barton, J. 246
Basden, S. L. 181, 182
Başoğlu, M. 127
Bassak, C. 134
Bassuk, S. S. 131, 138, 162
Bastian, B. 126, 220, 260–263, 267, 271, 276
Bateman, A. 235
Bathish, R. 191, 192, 352
Batres, C. 213
Batson, C. D. 268
Baumann, L. J. 319
Baumeister, R. F. 206, 273
Bavishi, C. 315
Baxter, A. J. 157
BBC News 152, 153
Beach, S. R. H. 161
Beadle, E. J. 233
Beals, K. P. 71
Bear, N. 65
Beatty, D. L. 67, 68
Bebbington, P. E, 273
Beblo, T. 303
Beck, A. T. 5, 160, 161, 162, 231, 232
Beck, J. G. (2008) 367
Becker, A. E. 213
Becker, J. 162
Becker, M. H. 208
Beckwith, M. 191, 192, 352

Beecher, H. K. 256
Begeny, C. T. 46
Bekker, M. H. J. 168
Belik, S.-L. 316
Bell, B. 158, 307
Bell, M. 292
Bell, R. 366, 367
Belluardo, P. 158
Ben, J. 82
Bengoechea, E. G. 325
Benkelfat, C. 159
Bennett, D. A. 138, 140
Bennett, D. 136
Bennett, J. A. 136
Bennett, K. M. 138, 140
Bentall, R. P. 278, 280, 294, 295, 335, 373
Bentley, S. V. 336
Ben-Yishay, Y. 235
Berchicci, M. 134, 148, 150
Bercovitch, F. B. 134, 148, 150
Berger, C. L. 40
Berger, J. 219
Berglund, P. 204, 316
Bergman, W. 315
Berkley, K. J. 259
Berkman, L. F. 8, 27, 36, 37, 60, 131, 137, 162
Berman, J. S. 170
Bernard, J. 370
Berrington de Gonzalez, A. 309
Bertschy, K. 247
Berry, D. A. 310
Berry, H. L. 26, 36, 55, 164
Berry, J. W. 49, 294
Bertozzi-Villa, A. 158, 307
Best, D. 17, 55, 169, 187, 189, 192, 199, 302, 352
Betz, N. E. 361
Bevelander, K. E. 221
Bevins, A. 333
Bezborodovs, N. 362
Bhugra, D. 281
Bickenbach, J. 308
Bickley, S. 244, 326
Bieling, P. J. 367
Bienias, J. L. 138
Biezaitis, V. 235
Bigda-Peyton, J. 161
Bigelow, H. J. 249
Bigler, E. D. 230
Billig, M. G. 14
Billinghurst, B. 317
Bingley, W. 297
Birmes, P. 107

Biryukov, S. 158, 307
Bisogni, S. 259
Bisson, J. I. 108, 109, 115
Bixby, W. R. 134
Bizumic, B. 29
Bjerregaard, K. 27, 131
Björk, C. 283, 314
Björkelund, C. 313
Black, G. 169
Black, S. E. 239
Black, W. C. 310
Blackstone, T. 71
Blackwood, N. 373
Blackwood, D. H. R. 159
Blair, S. N. 211, 215
Blanchard, D. C. 39
Blanchard, R. J. 39
Blanz, M. 25, 46, 166
Blascovich, J. 41, 90
Block, L. 222
Blood, R. W. 224
Bloomfield, D. L. 206
Bloser, N. 378
Boake, C. 30, 95, 231
Boccia, M. L. 40
Bochner, S. 80, 322
Boen, F. 27, 222, 365
Bogart, K. R. 320
Bognay, J. 230
Bogner, J. 234
Bohner, G. 303
Boker, R. 112
Boles, S. M. 313
Bolliger, I. 158, 307
Bolman, C. 136
Bombardier, C. 136
Bombay, A. 116
Bond, G. R. 137
Bond, J. 138
Boone, A. L. 206
Boone, K. A. R. 236
Booth-Kewley, S. 135
Borger, S. C. 165
Borland, R. 325
Boroch, O. 18, 163, 275, 297
Bossé, R. 146
Boström, G. 134
Bosworth, H. B. 133
Boter, H. 286
Bottrell, D. 120
Bouma, R. 184
Bourdieu, P. 44, 56

Bourguignon, D. 70
Bourhis, R. Y. 46, 77
Bovin, M. J. 127
Bow, R. A. 92
Bowe, C. M. 3
Bowe, M. 54
Bowen, S. 182
Bowling, A. 137
Boyce, R. A. 2
Boyd, J. L. 289
Boydstun, J. A. 98
Bradbury, C. L. 232
Braddon, C. 236
Brady, F. 127
Brailey, K. 114
Brand, B. L. 115
Brand, R. 189, 190
Brander, C. 17, 297
Brand-Miller, J. 211
Branscombe, N. R. 19, 20, 48, 49, 52, 53, 57, 66,
    71–77, 80, 99, 146, 190, 209, 223, 268, 297,
    302, 349, 351, 362, 364, 375
Braveman, P. A. 36
Braverman, S. 236
Bravo, M. F. 162
Brawley, O. W. 310
Breakwell, G. M. 53
Breen, C. 178
Brellenthin, A. G. 325
Bremner, J. D. 110
Brenner, L. 234
Brett, E. A. 111, 112
Brewer, M. B. 5, 14
Brewin, C. 366
Bridle, C. 209
Britt, T. W. 93
Brittain, K. 17
Brodie, A. R. 40
Brodie, K. H. 313
Brodribb, W. 55, 352
Brohan, E. 281
Bromberg, P. M. 112
Bromhead, D. 29
Brondolo, E. 67, 68
Brook, A. T. 349
Brooks, J. C. W. 261
Brooks-Gunn, J. 206
Broom, D. H. 211, 215
Brothers, D. 111
Brotons, C. 313
Brown, C. 351
Brown, G. W. 283

Brown, J. L. 232, 263
Brown, J. 368
Brown, L. 42
Brown, R. G. 232, 263
Brown, R. 46, 125
Brown, S. A. 231
Brown, S. G. 376
Brown, T. A. 368
Browne, G. 141
Browne, K. D. 152
Brownell, C. 181
Brownell, K. D. 210
Brownlee, S. 311
Brownson, R. C. 313
Brownwell, K. D. 225
Bruce, E. 152
Bruffaerts, R. 316
Bruins, J. 30
Brundage, S. I. 231
Bruner, J. S. 23
Brunet, A. 107
Brunn, M. 214
Brunner, E. J. 215
Bryant, J. 142
Bryant, R. A. 108
Bryant, R. 162
Buckingham, S. A. 191, 197, 201–202
Budd, R. 170
Bugelli, T. 136
Bulbulia, J. 265
Bulc, M. 313
Bulik, C. M. 206
Bundy, R. F. 14
Bunker, R. J. 135
Bunt, G. 186
Burdett, H. 244, 246
Burgess, C. N. 75
Burgess, M. L. 55
Burke, B. L. 181
Burke, D. T. 236
Burke, J. 80
Burnett, R. 281
Burton, A. K. 258
Burton, A. 357
Burton, E. 162
Burton, P. 214
Burton, R. C. 325
Burwell, R. A. 213
Busch-Geertsema, V. 47
Bush Hitchon, J. 213
Bushman, B. 273
Butera, F. 162

Butler, A. C. 161
Butler, K. 325
Butler, S. J. 140
Butler, T. 97
Butterworth, P. 148
Buttner, P. 204
Byrne, D. G. 203, 225
Byrne, S. M. 206

Caballero, B. 204
Cacioppo, J. T. 97, 125–126, 129, 137, 162–163, 329, 332–333, 374
Cacioppo, S. 162
Cadamuro, A. 125
Cadinu, M. 73
Cafiero, A. C. 133
Cahill, H. A. 317
Cairns-Smith, S. 3
Calabrese, J. R. 286
Caldwell, D. M. 161
Caldwell, K. 310
Calev, A. 114
Calhoun, L. G. 108
Callender, K. 115
Calzolai, M. 259
Cameron, I. D. 230
Cameron, L. D. 319
Cameron, R. 223
Camp, D. L. 302
Campbell, A. 20
Campbell, F. K. 318
Campbell, J. D. 358
Campbell, J. L. 138
Campbell, M. J. 340
Campbell, R. D. 302
Campbell, T. S. 209
Campbell, W. K. 207
Canadian Psychiatric Association. 288
Candan, K. A. 290
Candland, D. K. 39
Canga, A. 289
Cannonet, T. D. 290
Cano-Prous, A. 289
Cantril, H. 376
Caplan, A. L. 313
Caplan, B. 234
Caporael, L. R. 5
Caprilli, S. 259
Carapezza, R. 115
Care Quality Commission 141
Carmeliet, P. 329
Carr, V. J. 181

Carr, V. 281
Carroll, E. 232
Carroll, L. 170
Carter, H. 127
Carter, R. 225
Cartwright, S. 89
Carver, C. S. 90
Casas, M. 311
Casassus, M. 231
Cassel, C. K. 313
Cassells, R. 371
Casserly, L. M. 232
Cassidy, C. 122
Cassin, S. E. 206
Castellanos, G. 289
Castellanos-Ryan, N. 135
Catalano, R. F. 188
Cather, C. 289
Cattan, M. 138, 333
CDC National Center for Injury Prevention and Control 288
Centre for Sport and Social Impact 1–2
Ceyhanli, A. 127
Chaddock, L. 134
Chalk, H. M. 320
Chalkidoun, K. 311
Challis, C. 12, 31
Chamari, K. 134
Chamberlain, C. 47
Chambers, M. 228
Chambers, R. 308
Champion, H. C. 157
Chandler, M. J. 59–60
Chang, J. M. 325
Chang, M. X-L. 24, 377
Chang, Y-K. 134
Chapman, J. E. 161
Charles, M. 213
Charuvastra, A. 115
Chasteen, A. L. 142
Chatterji, S. 308, 315
Chatzisarantis, N. L. D. 209
Chaudhury, S. 230
Chawla, N. 182
Chazova, I. 239
Chen, E. Y. 292
Chen, E. 207, 329
Chen, H-Y. 333
Chen, J. 68
Chen, L. 108
Chen, P. 161
Chen, Z. 275

Cheng, B. 134
Cheryan, S. 219, 225
Cheung, C. K. T. 283
Cheung, W. 292
Chevron, E. S. 163, 288
Chida, Y. 315
Chisholm, A. 136
Chiu, W. T. 204
Cho, Y. A. 214
Choi, W. 283
Chokel, J. T. 273
Chong, E. M. 335
Chorpita, B. F. 368
Chou, R. 310
Christensen, B. K. 232
Christensen, B. 209
Christensen, M. B. 323
Christopher, N. C. 110
Christopher, P. 370
Chrousos, G. P. 328
Chung, M. H. 44
Chung, R. C. K. 292
Churchill, R. 115
Cicchetti, D. 176
Cicerone, K. D. 236
Cieza, A. 308
Cikara, M. 268
Cimbolic, P. 158
Ciofi, D. 259
Ciurana, R. 313
Claire, M. 181
Clapp, J. D. 367
Clara, I. 316
Clark, C. R. 230
Clark, D. M. 123
Clark, D. 186
Clarke, P. J. 239
Clayton, P. J. 88
Clement, S. 362
Clements, K. L. 316
Clements, K. 184
Clervoy, P. 285
Clift, A. 321
Clingingsmith, D. 267
Cloitre, M. 115
Clucas, C. 80, 321–322
Cockell, S. J. 206
Cocking, C. xix 30, 117, 123, 357
Cockram, C. 308
Coetzer, R. 232
Coffee, P. 325
Coffey, S. F. 367

Cogan, R. 263
Cohen, G. L. 144
Cohen, J. L. 91
Cohen, J. 112
Cohen, L. H. 87
Cohen, N. J. 134
Cohen, R. 315
Cohen, S. 44, 162
Colantonio, A. 239
Colcombe, A. 134
Colcombe, S. J. 136
Colcombe, S. 134
Cole, B. 361
Cole, S. W. 327, 329
Cole, S. 137
Cole, V. 159
Coleman, J. 48
Collicutt-McGrath, J. 245
Collins, F. 158
Collins, M. 197
Collins, N. L. 263
Collins, S. E. 182
Colombe, S. J. 142
Colville, G. 108
Comer, L. K. 363
Compton, M. T. 36
Conelly, R. R. 56
Conger, A. J. 221
Conger, J. C. 221
Conner, K. O. 344
Conner, M. 209
Connolly, H. 333
Connor, J. P. 178, 182
Connors, G. J. 188
Conrad, J. 200
Conrad, P. 222
Conradsson, M. 134
Conrod, P. J. 135
Constans, J. I. 114
Conti, S. 158
Cooke, R. 185
Coombs, T. 340
Cooper, C. L. 89, 102, 340
Cooper, J. M. 110
Cooper, J. 233
Cooper, L. A. 25
Cooper, M. L. 181
Cooper, Z. 206
Copeland, V. C. 344
Coppel, D. B. 162
Coppin, G. 220
Corcoran, R. 373

Cordain, L. 211
Cordan, G. 55
Cordes, R. J. 309
Cordle, D. 95
Cornwell, E. Y. 137
Cornwell, P. 231
Corridan, B. 230
Corrigan, J. D. 231
Corrigan, P. W. 68, 169, 189, 281, 302, 362
Cortese, D. K. 87
Cosgrove, S. 108–109
Costa, P. T. Jr. 135
Costanzo, P. R. 221
Coughlan, T. 231
Courtois, C. A. 115
Coverdale, J. H. 283
Cowell, E. 72
Cox, B. J. 165, 316, 367
Coyne, S. M. 273
Crabtree, J. W. 19, 30, 146, 169, 302–305
Craft, R. M. 259
Craig, K. D. 263
Crandall, C. S. 65, 209
Crane, M. 93
Crawford, J. R. 367–369, 371
Cream, P. 108
Creamer, M. 366–367
Creel, S. 39
Crichton, C. L. 230
Crocker, J. 46, 67
Crombez, G. 258
Cronin, T. 19, 77
Cross, R. 311
Cross, T. H. 316
Crow, T. J. 280
Crowther, T. R. 136
Cruwys, T. 6, 17, 19, 24, 26–27, 34, 36, 55–56,
    110, 116, 148, 150, 154, 161–165, 167–171,
    173, 191–194, 199, 201, 203, 215, 216–217,
    219–222, 225, 238, 240, 273–274, 281, 291,
    302, 323–325, 329, 333, 335–336, 338, 340,
    345, 348, 350–352, 356, 358–359, 361, 364,
    369, 371–372, 375, 377
Csepeli, G. 97
Cubbin, C. 36
Cuddy, A. J. 139
Cuenca, E. 285
Cuevas, A. G. 80
Cui, L. 58, 78, 379
Cuijpers, P. 161
Cukor, D. 161
Cullen, M. R. 92

Cummins, S. 373
Cusack, K. 114
Cusamano, D. L. 211

D'Souza, G. 371
Dahl, J. 316
Dai, W. 108
Dalen, J. 370
Daly, M. 331
Danaher, K. 223
Dank, S. 213
Dann, H. D. 97
Dao, T. T. 259
Darby, A. 204
Darby, S. 309
Dark, F. 288
Darke, S. 185
Darkes, J. 182
Dar-Nimrod, I. 169, 207
Darvish, H. S. 88
David, M. 44
Davidson, K. W. 315
Davidson, M. 286
Davidson, R. J. 258
Davies, C. 35n1
Davies, K. 220
Davies, P. S. W. 215
Davies, S. 151
Davis, A. 69
Davis, M. C. 214
Davis, M. K. 25
Davis, M. 115
Dawe, S. 206
Dawson, M. E. 283
Dax, E. C. 290
Day, M. A. 252, 316
Dayan, E. 218
Dayan, P. 278
De Bourdeaudhuij, I. 313
De Geus, B. 313
De Gilder, D. 30
De Graaf, R. 157
De Leo, D. 12, 31
De Leon, C. F. M. 162
De Leon, G. 185, 200
De Mello, M. F. 163
De Nooy, J. 48
De Sousa, P. 335
De Wit, J. B. F. 222
De Wit, N. J. 316
Deacon, B. J. 5, 158, 160, 173
Deakins, J. 233

Deane, F. P. 187
Deary, I. J. 135
Deaux, K. 19, 53, 57
Debats, D. L. 135
Decesare, J. C. 316
Deeny, S. P. 134
Degeneffe, C. E. 231
Degenhardt, L. 178–179
Deitz, A. C. 204
Delahanty, D. L. 110
Delpisheh, A. 340
Demakakos, P. 137
Demler, O. 316
Den Boeft, M. 316
Denis, C. 185
Dennerstein, L. 213
Denney, H. T. 146
Denson, N. 82
Denton, E. 68
Department of Health (UK) 293
DePaulo, B. M. 65, 75
Der, G. 135
Dermatis, H. 186
Derubeis, R. J. 158–159
DeSalvo, K. B. 378
Despointes, S. H. 325
Despot Lucanin, J. 3
Detterbeck, F. C. 310
Detweiler-Bedell, J. B. 315
DeWall, C. N. 273
Dewe, P. J. 102
Dhalla, I. A. 311
Di Pietro, L. 215
Di Russo, F. 134
Dickens, A. P. 138
Dickerson, S. S. 327–328
DiClemente, C. C. 208
Diener, C. 48
Diener, E. 341, 376, 377
Diguer, L. 170
Dikmen, S. S. 230–231
Diler, S. E. 325
Diller, L. 235
Dillworth, T. M. 182, 316
Dimidjian, S. 159
Dingle, G. A. 17, 19, 26–27, 44, 47, 49, 55, 70,
    116, 123, 135, 154, 165, 168–170, 173, 181,
    185–186, 191–194, 199, 201, 240, 281, 283,
    291, 297–300, 302, 304–305, 323, 329, 333,
    336, 338, 340, 345, 348, 350–352, 356,
    369, 379
Dinos, D. 302

Dion, S. C. 214
Dionigi, R. A. 144
Discerning History 262
Dittmar, H. 213–214
Dixon, J. 76, 211, 215
Dobson, K. S. 161
Dodd, S. 340
Dohrenwend, B. P. 89
Doise, W. 28, 97
Dole, V. 178
Dolstra, A. J. 248
Donmall, M. C. 188
Donne, J. 17
Donnelly, C. L. 111
Donovan, R. J. 170, 333
Doody, M. 325
Doosje, B. 166, 268, 346, 348
Dorahy, M. J. 115
Dorsey, E. R. 3
Douglas, D. 401
Douglas, J. M. 140, 232, 237–238, 240, 246, 248
Doust, J. 311
Dovidio, J. F. 80
Dowds, M. M. 236
Downes, C. 121
Downey, G. 69
Doyle, D. M. 67
Doyle, W. J. 162
Driessen, M. 303
Drury, J. 26–28, 30, 45, 76, 108, 117–120,
    123–127, 129, 357
Dube, M. G. 206
Duberstein, P. R. 136
Dubyak, P. J. 327
Dudenhausen, J. W. 214
Dugard, P. 165, 173, 190
Dumbelton, L. 321
Dumont, M. 87
Dunbar, R. I. M. 17
Duncan, A. 371
Duncan, G. E. 284
Duncan, L. E. 283
Dunkel Schetter, C. 263
Dunlop, A. 179
Dunn, C. L. 218
Dunn, G. 373
Dunne, M. P. 162
Durkheim, É. 29, 35, 265, 270
Durrheim, K. 34
Dutra, L. 181–182
Dutton, G. R. 327
Dwight-Johnson, M. 158

Dyck, I. 182
Dykes, J. 215
Dyson, M. 237
Dzieciol, A. M. 110

Earnshaw, V. A. 169, 320
Eastwood, R. 283
Eaton, C. A. 188
Eaton, S. B. 211, 215
Eberhart, N. K. 161
Eccleston, C. 316
Edgar, W. 47
Edgell, E. 286
Edwards, R. T. 152
Egerter, S. 36
Egger, G. 211
Eggins, R. A. 27
Egremont, M. 104, 128
Ehde, D. M. 316
Ehlers, A. 5, 113–114, 123
Ehring, T. 114
Eikelenboom, M. 168
Einsenstein, C. 220
Eisemann, M. 168
Eisenberg, M. E. 188, 206
Eisenberger, N. I. 254
Elahi, A. 294, 306
Elgie, R. 281
Elias, A. 82
Elias, M. F. 133
Elkin, I. 158, 163
Ellaway, A. 323
Ellemers, N. 19, 21, 30, 41, 48, 52, 74, 76–77, 169, 245, 320, 346, 348
Ellenbogen, R. G. 236
Eller, A. 142
Elliott, A. M. 125
Ellis, A. R. 157
Ellis-Hill, C. 232, 234–235
Ellison, N. 313
Elsbach, K. D. 20
Elshaug, A. G. 311
Elvish, R. 152
Elwood, M. 325
Elzinga, B. M. 110
Emery, C. F. 134
Emmelkamp, P. M. G. 184
Emmons, R. A. 341, 376
Engel, G. L. 4–5, 158
Enns, M. W. 165, 367
Ensall, J. 124
Epstein, L. H. 5

Epstein, L. J. 145
Erickson, K. I. 134
Ericsson, K. 138
Erskine, H. E. 162
Ertel, K. A. 131, 137–138
Eshleman, A. 65
Esselman, P. C. 230
Estroff, S. E. 293
Ethier, K. A. 19, 53, 57
Etnier, J. L. 134
EUFEST study group 286
Evans, C. M. 175
Evans, D. A. 138
Evans, D. 30, 95, 103
Evans, J. J. 231, 233–235
Evans, M. 175
Evans-Lacko, S. 362
Evans-Whipp, T. 175
Everitt, B. 287
Ewing, J. 115
Eyer, J. 86
Eymard, A. 140
Eyre, S. L. 59
Ezquiaga, E. 162

Fabre, C. 134
Fagiolini, A. M. 288
Failla, S. 366–367
Fairburn, C. G. 206
Falloon, I. R. H. 283, 289
Falomir-Pichastor, J. M. 325
Fals-Stewart, W. 184
Fann, J. R. 230, 232
Faraone, S. V. 159
Farooqi, I. S. 204
Farrell, M. 179
Farrow, C. V. 7, 25, 65, 325
Fasoli, F. 261
Fass, R. J. 361
Fatemi, S. H. 286
Fatséas, M. 185
Fava, G. A. 158
Fawcett, J. 158–159
Fayers, P. 161
Fear, N. T. 112
Feeney, G. F. X. 182
Feeney, T. 234
Feeny, N. C. 115
Feldman, J. 289
Feldstein, L. 8
Fenigstein, A. 372
Ferguson, E. 135

Fernández, S. 19–20, 77
Ferrari, A. J. 157, 162
Ferrari, S. 323
Ferris, L. J. 126, 260, 266–267, 271
Festinger, L. 265
Festini, F. 259
Fickas, S. 231
Fillingim, R. B. 259
Findlay, R. A. 333
Fingerhut, A. W. 80
Finlay, W. M. L. 302
Finlayson, R. 78
Finney, J. 181
Finucane, M. L. 325
Fiore, J. 162
Fischer, B. 311
Fischer, R. 260
Fischler, C. 224
Fisher, E. 316
Fisher, G. K. 29
Fisher, W. P. 377
Fiske, S. T. 139
Fitcher, M. M. 207
Fitzgerald, M. N. 176
Fitzpatrick, S. 59
Fitzsimons, G. J. 222
Flaherty-Robb, M. 136
Flament, C. 14
Flanagan, D. A. J. 231
Flaxman, A. D. 307
Fleischhacker, W. W. 286
Fleming, J. 233, 245
Fleming, M. A. 231, 349
Fleminger, S. 231
Flett, G. L. 165
Flyvbjerg, A. 308
Flynn, T. W. 310
Foa, E. B. 113
Foddy, M. 28, 294
Folkman, S. 90, 92, 94, 123
Fonda, S. J. 148
Forbes, D. 108
Ford, D. E. 25
Foreman, P. 140, 237
Forman, E. 161
Forneris, C. A. 114
Fortune, D. G. 232
Foster, M. D. (1999) 75
Foster, M. (2012) 231
Fournier, J. C. 159
Fowler, D. 373
Fox Smith, L. 289
Fox, N. E. 6, 172, 221, 359, 372

Fraas, M. 236
Frable, D. E. S. 71
Frain, A. J. 189
Frank, E. 288
Frank, G. K. 206, 288
Fransen, K. 4, 17, 24, 27, 55, 191, 247, 297
Fratiglioni, L. 138
Freedman, S. 112
Freeman, D. 373
Freeman, J. 234
French, D. P. 136, 285
Freud, S. 111, 112
Frieden, T. R. 225
Friedman, H. S. 135
Friedman, M. A. 135, 315
Friedman, M. J. 111
Friedman, M. 86, 135
Friel, S. 36, 57, 60
Frieser, D. 310
Frings, D. 19, 116, 183, 189, 193–197
Frith, U. 247
Frommberger, U. 303
Fry, P. S. 135
Fryberg. S. A. 25, 219, 325
Funk, S. C. 87
Furukawa, T. A. 161
Fuster, M. J. 73, 364

Gable, S. L. 71
Gabriel, P. 267
Gadian, D. G. 110
Gaertner, S. L. 80
Gaffney, C. 365
Gage, F. H. 134
Gaglio, B. 314, 315
Galanter, M. 186
Galatzer-Levy, I. 108
Galeazzi, G. M. 323
Galinsky, A. D. 46
Gallagher, M. 26
Gallagher, S. 140, 232
Galletly, C. 288
Gallo, J. J. 25
Gallois, C. 28
Gallop, R. 157, 158
Gamaz, L. 10, 12, 26, 30, 44, 142, 273, 303, 333, 346, 358
Gangstad, B. 246
Gao, D. G. 263
Garcia, A. N. 316
Garcia, A. 66, 162
Garcia, D. M. 52, 76
Garcia, J. 349

García-Cabeza, I. 286
Gardner, C. O. 162
Garety, P. A. 373
Garland, A. 161
Garrett, J. 114
Garske, G. G. 244
Garske, J. P. 25
Garstka, T. A. 65, 73, 77, 141, 362
Garza, A. A. 77, 190
Gash, T. B. 247
Gaspar, P. 152
Gatz, M. 134
Gause, M. 362
Gavin, A. 278
Gaynor, W. 136
Gee, G. C. 68
Gee, G. 66, 67, 70
Geeraert, N. 190
Geertz, A.W. 260, 265
Geisner, I. M. 182
George, B. P. 3
George, J. 236
George, L. K. 283, 313
George, T. P. 179
Gerard, H. B. 265
Gerin, W. 68
Gerlach, J. 285
Gertler, P. 232
Gething, L. 140
Ghaemi, S. N. 5
Giamo, L. S. 73
Gibbons, R. D. 163
Gibson, A. 178
Giesen-Bloo, J. 168
Gil, T. 114
Gilbert-Barness, E. 215
Giles, G. G. 325
Giles, H. 140, 144
Giles, J. 140, 144
Giles, L. C. (2012) 131
Gilford, N. 94, 270, 271, 327
Gilman, S. E. 213
Giovannini, D. 125
Glantz, S. 87
Glasgow, R. E. 313–315, 317
Glass, T. A. 131, 162
Glasziou, P. 311
Glatt, S. J. 159
Gleibs, I. H. 7, 29, 97, 152, 153, 172, 293, 333, 334, 348
Gleibs, I. 97, 153
Glucksman, E. 114
Glymour, M. M. 131

Glynn, S. M. 289
Gneezy, U. 69
Godefroy, O. 267
Godycki-Cwirko, M. 313
Goffman, E. 63, 64, 232, 362
Gök, Ş. 127
Goldberg, J. F. 286
Goldman, H. H. 189, 281
Goldman, L. S. 157
Goldman, M. S., 182
Goldman, S. J. (1991) 221
Goldner, E. M. 206
Goldscheider, A. 255
Goldsmith, K. 311, 316
Goldstein, B. J. 308
Goldstein, M. J. 290
Goldstein, M. 315
Gollan, J. K. 161
Gómez, Á. 19, 77
Gómez, J. 286
Gonzales, J. J. 25
González de Chavez, M. 286
Gonzalez Lopez, J. R. 259
González, R. 125
Goodkind, D. 137
Goodman, H. S. 30, 95, 231
Goodwin, G. M. 159
Goossens, L. 162
Gordon, C. 230, 245
Gordon, J. 182
Gordon, R. A. 213
Gordon, S. D. 159
Gordon, T. P. 40
Gotlib, I. H. 158, 340
Gottdiener, W. H. 320
Goubert, L. 263
Gouge, C. 28
Gould, K. R. 230
Gowing, L. R. 179
Goymann, W. 40
Graber, J. A. 206
Grace, D. M. 20, 28
Gracey, F. 233–235, 240, 248
Grady, D. 313
Graham, T. 362
Gramzow, R. H. 67
Grandi, S. 158
Grant, D. M. 367
Grant, T. 181
Gray, J. J. 211
Gray, K. 258
Gray, M. J. 115
Gray-Little, B. 375

Greaves, C. J. 138, 317
Green, B. L. 115
Green, J. 311
Green, L. W. 209
Green, R. E. 232
Greenaway, K. H. 26, 28, 31, 45, 56, 165–167, 297, 364, 375
Greenberg, D. 114
Greenberg, N. 55, 112, 244, 249, 303
Greenslade, J. H. 219
Greenspan, J. D. 259
Greenwell, L. 181
Gregory, J. D. 316
Greiwe, J. S. 134
Grencavage, L. M. 161
Grieve, A. P. 230
Griffin, S. 341, 376
Griggs, R. A. 277, 249
Grippo, A. J. 162, 332
Grisham, J. R. 283
Groh, D. R. 186
Grossman, L. S. 286
Grote, N. K. 344
Grow, J. 182
Gruenewald, T. L. 327, 328
Grunze, H. 286
Gruys, K. 222
Guarda, A. S. 214
Guendelman, M. D. 219
Guest, J. A. 313
Guijarro, M. L. 135
Guild, D. J. 176
Gujjarlamundi, H. B. 133
Gullo, M. J. 182
Gulyas, C. 18, 163, 275, 297
Gunaseelan, S. 169
Gundersen, N. C. 273
Gunderson, M. 65
Gunningham, B. H. 247
Gunthert, K. C. 87
Gupta, R. K. 230
Gurin, P. 75
Gust, D. A. 40
Gustavsson, S. M. 140
Güth, W. 28
Gutsell, J. N. 268

Haagen, B. 323
Haarmans, M. 335
Haber, M. G. 91
Haby, M. M. 225
Hackel, L. M. 220

Hadar, H. 112
Hadaway, P. F. 176
Hafer, C. L. 75
Hagger, M. S. 5, 209
Hagger, M. 25
Haggerty, R. J. 172
Hahn, S. 134
Hahn, W. 102
Haines, J. 213
Haines, K. 232
Haines, T. 230
Hainsworth, J. 317
Haire-Joshu, D. 313
Hajjar, E. R. 133
Halford, J, C. G. 140
Halford, W. K. 184
Hall, K. T. 258
Hall, K. 344
Hall, M. H. 248
Hall, W. 311
Hallet, J. A. 135
Hallett, D. 60
Hallett, T. 9
Halliwell, E. 213
Halpin, H. A. 67
Halvorsen, M. 168
Hamburg, P. 213
Hampson, S. E. 317
Han, S. 268
Hancock, T. D. 375
Handa, T. 157
Handley, E. D. 176
Handley, T. E. 162
Hanlon, J. T. 133
Hannan, P. J. 213
Hannay, D. 323
Hanney, W. J. 316
Hanson, G. 136
Happé, F. 247
Harder, A. 214
Harder, T. 214
Hardman, C. A, 325
Hardwick, A. 357
Haris, M. 230
Harkness, J. 318
Harlow, J. M. 227
Harnack, L. J. 211, 218
Haro, J. M. 333
Harradine, P. G. 230
Harris, A. 376
Harris, R. D. 230
Harrison, C. R. 150

Harrison, J. A. 209
Harrow, M. 286
Hart, T. 232
Harter, J. 377
Harver, A. 317
Harvey, A. G. 5, 114
Harvey, R. D. 82
Harvey, S. B. 112
Harvey, S. M. 80
Harwood, J. 326
Hasan, K. M. 230
Hasegawa, I. 110
Hasher, L. 142
Haslam, C. 2, 4, 7, 10, 17, 19, 24, 26–31, 34, 44,
    46, 53, 55, 56, 72, 78, 80, 94, 96–97, 99, 103,
    108, 126, 129, 131, 142, 144, 146, 148, 150,
    152–155, 158, 163, 165–166, 169, 172–173,
    191, 218, 220–221, 233, 235–240, 244–245,
    247–248, 250, 273, 293, 295–297, 302–303,
    305, 317, 325–326, 329, 333–336, 338, 340,
    343, 345–346, 348–353, 356, 358–361, 365,
    369, 372, 375–376, 379
Haslam, D. W. 215
Haslam, N. 158, 317, 320
Haslam, S. A. 2, 4, 7, 10, 17–19, 23–31, 34,
    44, 46, 49, 51, 53–57, 65, 72, 78, 80, 84,
    92–94, 96–97, 99, 101, 103, 108, 126, 129,
    131, 135, 139, 142, 144, 146, 148, 150,
    152–155, 158, 163, 165–167, 169–170,
    172–173, 191, 215, 220–222, 225, 233,
    235–240, 244–245, 247–248, 250, 273,
    293–297, 302–303, 305, 317, 319–320,
    325–326, 329, 331, 333–336, 338, 340, 343,
    345–346, 348–353, 356, 358–361, 365, 369,
    372–373, 375–376, 379
Hastings, A. 323
Hatch, S. L. 112
Hatfield, B. D. 134
Hatton, L. 107
Haufler, A. J. 134
Haunschild, P. R. 53
Haupt, A. L. 273
Häusser, J. A. 94
Havelka, M. 3, 5
Hawe, P. 43–44
Hawkley, L. C. 137, 162–163, 329, 332–333, 374
Hawthorne, G. 340
Hay, P. J. 204
Hayhurst, H. 316
Hayward, C. 223
Hazes, J. M. 315
He, J. 378

He, W. 137
He, Y. 322
Heath, C. 219
Heath, I. 311
Hebl, M. 209
Heckemeyer, C. M. 136
Hedeker, D. 163
Hedges, D. W. 110
Heilbrun, A. B. 206
Heimberg, R. G. 114
Hein, G. 268
Heinberg, L. J. 214
Heine, S. J. 169, 207, 340, 358
Heinrichs, M. 94
Heinz, W. R. W. 56
Heisler, M. 133
Heldreth, C. 364, 375
Helliwell, J. F. 31, 44, 376
Hemmelgarn, B. R. 209
Hemphill, S. A. 175, 188
Henderson, C. J. 190
Henderson, S. W. 236
Hendin, H. M. 375
Henesy, R. 115
Henker, B. 363
Henrich, J. 265, 340
Henry, C. 141
Henry, J. D. 283, 371
Henry, S. E. 206
Hepworth, J. 317
Herington, K. 122–123, 186
Herman, C. P. 215, 221, 222
Herman, G. 70
Hermans, R. C. J. 221, 225
Hernandez, B. 20
Herrera, M. 18, 54, 163, 275, 294, 297
Herzlich, C, 293
Herzog, A. R. 148
Herzog, D. B. 213
Hess, T. M. 142, 145–146
Hessling, R. M. 363
Hetherington, R. W. 5
Hettema, J. M. 162
Hettema, J. 179
Heuer, C. A. 210
Heuschmann, P. U. 230
Heuts, P. H. T. G. 258
Hewa, S. 5
Hewett, D. G. 28
Hewitt, P. L. 206
Hewstone, M. 47
Hibbard, M. R. 230

Hibscher, J. A. 215
Hidalgo, M. A. 20
High, W. M. 236
Hijazi, A. S. 40
Hill, A. J.213
Hill, D. J. 325–326
Hill, J. O. 206
Hill, P. L. 135
Hiller, W. 310
Hilsenroth, M. J. 97
Hinson, J. T. 142, 145
Hoare, Z. 152
Hodges, E. A. 145
Hodgkinson, A. E. 230
Hodgson, J. 232
Hodson, S. E. 93
Hoek, H. W. 204, 211, 294
Hoeppner, B. 186
Hoffman-Goetz, L. 134
Hogan, P. A. 320
Hogan, T. P. 286
Hoge, C. W. 112
Hogg, M. A. 15, 49
Hollegaard, M. V. 284
Hollies 30
Hollis, S. 258
Hollon, S. D. 157–159
Holmberg, H. 134
Holme, A. 26, 44, 53, 55, 126, 154, 235–237,
    239–240, 335, 348–352
Holmes, T. H. 87–89
Holt, R. I. 308
Holt-Lunstad, J. 2–3, 326
Holzer, C. E. 157
Hommel, K. 80
Honyashiki, M. 161
Hood, D. 231
Hooke, G. R. 367
Hopkins, N. 12, 25, 29, 31, 53, 260, 268–269, 272
Hor, K. 288
Horn, S. 232
Horne, P. J. 325
Hornsey, M. J. 48–49, 72, 260–261, 276, 333, 364
Hörnsten, C. 134
Hotopf, M. 366
Houlihan, D. 184
Hounsome, B. 152
Houpt, J. L. 313
House, J. S. 91
Howard, J. 334
Howard, R. 278
Howiesen, D. B. 230

Hsieh, M. 232
Hsu, S. 182
Huang, H. 376
Huang, Z. 58
Hudson, J. I. 204
Hudzik, B. 313
Hudzik, M. 313
Huedo-Medina, T. B. 159
Hughes, I. 170
Hughes, M. E. 374
Hull, L. 112
Hultman, C. M. 283
Humberstone, V. 288
Hummert, M. L. 65, 73, 77, 139, 141, 362
Humphrey, L. 27
Humphrey, M. 233
Hundemer, H. P. 286
Hung, M. 220
Hunot, V. 316
Hunter, D. 207
Hunter, J. A. 20–21
Huo, Y. J. 46
Husain, M. 230
Hutchinson, G. 281
Hutterer, J. 110
Hutton, J. 316
Hwang, S. 289–290
Hyde, J. 224

IASP Task Force on Taxonomy 252
Ichikawa, K. 161
Ilic, M. 303
Im, C. 273
Imber, S. D. 158
Inder, K. J. 176
Ingram, K. M. 361
Inman, M. L. 75
Institute for Safe Medication Practice 133
Inzlicht, M. 268
Iqbal, F. 344
Irimia, A. 228
Isometsä, E. 278
Ive, S. 213
Iversen, L. 125
Iyer, A. 26, 44, 54–58, 61, 74, 78, 82, 94, 146, 237,
    273–274, 335, 340, 348–349, 352–353

Jaakkola Reuter, A. 73
Jaakola, M. 73
Jablensky, A. 281, 288
Jackson, J. J. 135
Jackson, S. E. 86, 99

Jacobi, F. 316
Jacobs, E. 94, 270
Jacobson, C. J. 20
Jacobson, N. S. 161
James, W. P. T. 215
Jamieson, R. 276
Janicki-Deverts, D. 44
Jannes, C. 313
Janoff-Bulman, R. 161
Jans, L. 346, 379
Jappinen, P. 43
Jarvis, B. 283
Jasinskaja-Lahti, I. 73
Jason, L. A. 186
Jay, S. 126
Jeffery, R. W. 211, 218
Jelicic, M. 144
Jenkins, D. 231
Jensen, G. B. 222
Jensen, M. P. 316
Jerant, A. F. 317
Jetten, J. 4, 10–11, 17, 24, 26–27, 31, 34, 44,
    46–49, 53–58, 61, 70–75, 77–78, 82, 84, 94,
    96, 103, 126, 129, 135, 146, 148, 154–155,
    165, 169–170, 173, 190, 215, 218, 235–237,
    244, 246, 248, 250, 260–261, 267, 270–271,
    273–274, 276, 281, 283, 300, 302–303, 305,
    323, 326–327, 329, 331, 333, 335–336, 338,
    345–346, 348–353, 356, 358, 359–362, 364,
    375, 377, 379
Joensuu, M. 43
Johnson, A. L. 161, 316
Johnson, B. T. 159
Johnson, D. A. 244
Johnson, G. 47
Johnson, J. E. 188
Johnston, M. 222
Johnstone, T. 258
Jonas, D. E. 114
Jones, A. 13
Jones, B. J. 189
Jones, C. 151
Jones, D. A. 361
Jones, E. 108, 112
Jones, J. M. 26, 270–271, 273–274
Jones, M. 112
Jones, N. 112
Jonker, C. 144
Jorden, S. 108, 361
Jorm, A. F. 158
Joseph, S. 108, 123, 245
Josic, C. P. 231

Jost, J. T. 69–70
Joukamaa, M. 323
Joyner, M. 134
Judd, L. 158
Jurgova, E. 313
Juster, H. R. 114
Jutel, A.. 311
Juurlink, D. N. 311
Jyväsjärvi, S. 323

Kahn, J. H. 363
Kahn, R. S. 286
Kalmar, K. 236
Kalra, P. S. 206
Kalra, S. P. 206
Kaminer, D. 112
Kamper, A. L. 80
Kan, C.-H. 335
Kan, S. 287
Kaneko, H. 369
Kang, S. K. 142
Kaniasty, K. 91, 97
Kanter, R. 204
Kao, C. F. 75
Kaplan, R. M. 315
Kaptein, A. A. 315
Karlamangla, A. S. 131
Karnadewi, F. 271
Karow, A. 286
Karreman, A. 168
Kashima, H. 159
Kasl, S. V. 144
Kaslow, N. J. 161
Kato, H. 367
Katona, C. 127
Kattenstroth, M. 94
Katz, I. M. 358
Katzman, M. A. 213
Kaufmann, P. G. 315
Kavanagh, D. J. 283–284
Kawachi, I. 8, 44
Kawamura, N. 367
Kaye, W. H. 206
Kayes, N. 234
Kay-Lambkin, F. J. 176
Kearns, M. 357
Kearon, T. 95
Keet, I. P. 286
Kegan, R. 3
Keinänen-Kiukaanniemi, S. 323
Keinz, L. A. 184
Keller, M. C. 115

Keller, S. M. 283
Kelley, V. A. 25
Kellezi, B. 121–122
Kelly, A. B. 184
Kelly, B. J. 162
Kelly, J. F. 186–187
Kelly, P. J. 187
Kelsey, R. M. 90
Keltner, D. 46
Kemeny, M. E. 71, 327–328
Kemeny, M. 69, 363
Kemp, J. J. 158
Kendall, E. 227
Kendall, M. 230
Kendler, K. S. 162
Kennedy, L. 204
Kennell, J. H. 263
Keough, K. A. 115
Kepler, K. 230
Kern, M. L. 135
Kerr, P. 76
Kerr, S. 17
Kerschreiter, R. 365
Kesey, K. 169
Kessler, R. C. 204, 316, 340
Kester, A. D. M. 315
Keverne, E. B. 49
Keys, C. B. 186
Keys, C. 20
Khan, S. S. 331
Khan, S. 7, 12
Khan-Bourne, N. 232
Khwaja, D. 267
Kikinis, R. 228
Kikuchi, T. 157
Kilgo, G. 316
Killackey, E. 288
Killeen, C. 332
Killen, J. 223
Kilpatrick, F. P. 376
Kim, D. 44
Kim, H. J. 236
Kim, J. S. 134
Kim, Y. 367
Kinderman, P. 373
King, M. 304
Kington, C. 278
Kirchner, J. L. 325
Kirmayer, L. J. 92
Kirsch, I. 159, 258
Kirschbaum, C. 94
Kirschenbaum, D. S. 206

Kirst, M. 311
Kishimoto, J. 367
Kivelä, S.-L. 323
Kivimak, M. 43
Kivipelto, M. 135
Kjellgren, A. 92
Klandermans, B. 75
Klaus, H. H. 263
Kleber, H. D. 179
Klehe, U. C. 146
Klein, O. 211
Kleinstäuber, M. 316
Klerman, G. L. 163, 288
Klonoff, P. S. 236
Klosko, J. S. 168
Knapp, M. 157
Knatterud, G. L. 315
Knight, C. 27, 29, 155, 236, 333–334, 358
Knoop, H. 316
Knottnerus, J. A. 315
Ko, G. N. 110
Koen, J. 146
Koenig-Nobert, S. 221
Koerber, S. 310
Koerner, K. 161
Koes, B. 92
Koeske, G. 344
Kogan, J. N. 288–289
Kolb, L. C. 109
Kolber, M. J. 316
Kölble, S. 268
Kolos, I. 239
Koolhaas, J. M. 329
Komesaroff, P. A. 224
Kommu, J. V. S. 281
Köning, H. H. 65
Konrad, T. R. 157
Koomen, W. 166
Kopp, A. 311
Koppel, G. 101, 295
Korenstein, D. 311
Korotitsch, W. 368
Korte, S. M. 329
Kortekaas, P. 77
Kos, K. 331
Kositchek, R. 102
Koskinen, A. 43
Kothe, A. 185
Kotowicz, Z. 249
Kotses, H. 317
Kouchaki, M. 222
Kouchede, V. 170, 333

Koudenburg, N. 16–17
Kouvonen, A. 43
Kovacs, M. 162
Kovel, J. 293
Koyanagi, A. 170, 333
Kral, T. V. E. 214
Kramer, A. F. 134, 136, 148
Kramer, R. D. 20
Krames, L. 165
Kranton, R. E. 56
Kratt, P. P. 136
Kraus, M. W. 46
Krause, E. D. 170
Krausz, M. 311
Kreiner, G. E.245
Kremer, M. 267
Kressin, N. R. 146
Krishna, A. 218
Krones, P. G. 213
Krüger, C. 115
Kruijshaar, M. E. 157
Kugelmass, S. 114
Kuipers, E. 373
Kujawa, M. 286
Kumar, R. 230
Kunkel, S. R. 144
Kunz, C. 181
Kuoppasalmi, K. 278
Kupfer, D. J. 288
Kvaale, E. P. 158, 317, 320
Kydd, R. R. 283
Kyriakaki, M. 190

La Chance, P. A. 317
Laan, W. 294
Laatikainen, T. 135
Labianca, G. 44
Lachman, M. E. 131
Lahey, L. 3
Lai, Z. 108
Laidlaw, T. M. 283
Lalonde, C. E. 59–60
Lalonde, R. N. 48
Lamb, D. G. 236
Lambert, A. E. (2016) 142
Lambert, M. (2008) 286
Lambert, W. E. (1960) 269
Lamm, C. 268
Lamont, R. A. 144
Lamster, F. 294
Lancaster, G. A. 340
Landes, S. D. 131

Landman, A. 87
Laney, B. B. 135
Langenbahn, D. M. 236
Langer, E. J. 317
Langlois, E. 185
Langston, P. 26, 45
Lansing, A. 262
LaPorte, D. J. 294
Larimer, M. E. 182
Larimer, M. 207
Larivaara, P. 323
Larsen, E. B. 285
Larsen, K. 28, 97
Larsen, R. J. 341, 376
Lasko, N. B. 114
Lasky-Su, J. A. 159
Latorre-Postigo, J. M. 316
Latrofa, M. 73
Latu, I. M. 146
Latz, I. 320
Lau, M. A. 232
Laudenslager, M. L. 40
Lauritzen, T. 209
Lavallee, L. F. 20, 138, 207, 302, 317, 340, 358
Lavie, C. J. 325
Law, E. 316
Lawford, B. R. 178, 182
Layard, R. 31
Layton, J. B. 2, 326
Lazarus, A. A. 160
Lazarus, R. S. 90, 123, 258
Lazer, D. 325
Le Bon, G. 120
Le Noury, J. 325
Leach, C. W. 268, 346
Learmouth, A. 138
Leary, M. R. 254, 263, 273
LeBlanc, E. M. 134
Lebowitz, M. S. 317
Lechner, L. 136
Lee, C. M. 182
Lee, D. 325
Lee, I.-M. 325
Lee, N. K. 181, 185, 187, 232
Lee, S. R. 142
Leff, J. 281
Leggett, B. A. 28
Lehman, D. R. 358
Leibovich, S. J. 329
Leiderman, P. H. 92
Leitch, M. 206
Leiter, M. P. 101, 364

Leitten, C. L. 90
Leknes, S. 261
Lelard, T. 267
Lemke, S. 136
Lena, M. L. 227, 249
Lenz, A. S. 115
Leo, R. J. 286
Leone, S. S. 316
Leppin, A. 91, 97
Lerer, B. 114
LeResche, L. 259
Lerner, M.J. 69
Lesage, A. 315
Leshner, A. I. 39
Leskin, G. A. 110
Leung, A. Y. 292
Leung, R. 175
Levack, W. 234
Levati, M. V. 28
Leventhal, E. A. 315
Leventhal, H. 315
Leverington, C. T. 221
Levin, D. C. 310
Levin, H. S. 231
Levin, S. 67, 70
Levine, A. S. 211, 218
Levine, M. 213
Levine, R. M. 30, 80, 93, 95, 97, 141, 166, 319
Levitt, J. T. 170
Levy, B. R. 144
Levy, D. E. 325
Lewandowski-Holley, A. 316
Lewin, K. 54, 270, 343
Lewin, T. J. 181, 162
Lewinsohn, P. M. 160, 162
Lewis, C. 108, 109
Lewis, M. E. 182
Lewis, S. 224
Lewis-Fernández, R. 115
Leyro, T. M. 181, 182
Lezak, M. D. 230
Li, H. K. 181
Li, S. X. 78
Li, Y. 108
Liao, D. 158
Libby, D. J. 68
Libman, E. 269
Libretti, M. 67
Lichtenstein, E. 283
Lichtenstein, P. 314
Lickel, J. J. 158
Lidierth, P. 190
Lieberman, J. A. 284

Lieberman, M. D. 254, 263
Liebkind, K. 73
Lifton, R. J. 112, 114, 256
Lightowler, H. J. 214
Lim, L. 189
Lincoln, T. 294
Lindeberg, S. 211
Lindelöf, N. 134
Lindencrona, C. 140
Lindenthal, J. J. 88
Lindgren, K. P. 184
Lindy, J. D. 111
Link, B. G. 66, 189, 244
Linley, P. A. 108, 123, 245
Lintzeris, N. 179
Linville, P. W. 55
Lipworth, L. 56
Liss, M. 110
List, J. 69
Littbrand, H. 387
Litz, B. T. 115
Liu, A. 108
Livanou, M. 127
Lively, K. J. 9
Livingston, M. 175
Lizzio-Wilson, M. 273
Lloyd, D. A. 108
Lo, T. 207
Lofink, H. 211
Loftus, E. F. 144
London, S. 42, 104, 162, 332
Long, G. 196–197
Longabaugh, R. 182, 188
Longmore, R. J. 161
Lönnqvist, J. 278
Lonsdale, A. J. 17
Lopez, A. D. 307
López-Cevallos, D. F. 80
López-Muñoz, F. 285
Loughnan, S. 220
Loughran, T. 108
Louis, W. R. 364
Lovibond, P. F. 340, 341, 367
Lovibond, S. H. 340, 341, 367
Lowe, C. F. 325
Lowe, M. R. 213, 214, 223
Lowe, R. D. 108, 121
Loxton, N. J. 135, 206
Lozano, R. 307
Lu, X. 327
Lubman, D. I. 19, 27, 185, 187, 189, 191, 192, 197, 352
Luborsky, L. 170

Lucanin, D. 3, 5
Lucas, R. 376
Lucas, T. 91
Lucci, G. 134
Luce, B. R. 1
Luck-Sikorski, C. L. 65
Luger, T. 5
Luhtanen, R. 46
Luke, D. A. 313
Lundahl, B. W. 181
Lurie, B. D. 279
Lusczc, M. A. 148
Lyden, F. 92
Lynch, P. 66
Lyness, J. M. 136
Lynskey, M. 185
Lyons, E. 302
Lysens, R. 258

McAlinden, N. M. 161
McAllister, P. 55, 169, 244, 249, 303
McAllister, T. W. 229
McAuley, E. 136
McCabe, M. P. 204
McCauley, S. R. 231
McCloskey, L.-G. 376
McClure, H. M. 40
McCollum, R. 46
McCoy, S. K. 67
McCracken, L. M. 316
McDonald, S. 232
MacDonald, G. 254
McEwen, B. S. 328–329
McFall, M. E. 110
McFarlane, A. C. 108
Machin, D. 161
McGarty, C. 18, 23, 139, 247, 319
McGill, C. W. 289
McGinn, L. 161
McGlashan, T. 110
McGrath, J. J. 245, 283
MacGregor, D. G. 325
McGurk, S. R. 292–293
McInnis, O. A. 273
McIntyre, J. 294, 297
Macintyre, S. 323
McKay, A. D. 232
Mackenbach, J. P. 294
MacKenzie, D. 191
Mackenzie, J. 191, 352
McKetin, R. 185
McKevitt, C. J. 230
MacKichan, F. 316

Mackinnon, A. 323
McKimmie, B. M. 72, 219
McLaren, N. 5
McLaren, S. 12, 31
McLeod, J. D. 9
MacLeod, K. A. 148
Macklin, M. L. 114
McMahon, C. 2–3
McMahon, H. 6, 172, 221, 359, 372
Macmillan, M. 227, 249
McNally, R. J. 108, 114
McNamara, N. 51, 52, 73, 323
McNeal, E. T. 158
McNeil, J. K. 134
McNeill, J. 333
McNeill, K. 189
McNeilly, M. 68
McPhedran, S. 12, 31
McPherson, J. 112
McPherson, K. 232–234
McQuaid, R. J. 66, 273
McQuilken, M. 292
McSharry, J. 136
MacTavish, K. A. 56
Madan, A. 325
Madden, P. 325
Madhok, V. 165, 190
Madsen, M. 80
Magerøy, N. 112
Maggioni, F. 184, 208, 362
Magill, M. 187
Magnus, A. 225
Magnusson, B. 316
Magrin, M. E. 46
Mahlow, P. T. 134
Main, C. J. 258
Maisto, S. A. 182
Major, B. 64, 67, 68, 70, 75
Makino, M. 213
Malec, J. F. 236
Malivert, M. 185
Malla, A. 316
Mallett, C. J. 353
Mallett, R. 75, 281
Malley, D. 233–234
Mallinger, A. E. 288
Malmivaara, A. 92
Mamdani, M. M. 311
Manesh, R. E. 340
Manke, F. 206–207
Mann, N. 211
Manning, M. R. 86
Manogue, K. R. 39

Marchamer, J. 231
Marchiori, D. 211
Marcus, A. C. 314
Mari, J. D. J. 163
Mari, J. 289
Markle-Reid, M. 141
Marks, R. 325
Marlatt, A. 182
Marlatt, G. A. 182
Marmot, M. 8, 36, 42–43, 46, 58, 60–62, 172, 323
Marques, S. 144
Marriott, M. 323
Marshall, C. 290
Marshall, V. W. 239
Marti, C. N. 204
Martikainen, P. T. 215
Martin, D. J. 25
Martin, P. 43, 329
Martin, R. A. 188
Martin, R. 5
Martín-Lanas, R. 289
Martinot, D. 73
Martiny, S. E. 47
Marx, C. E. 284
Marx, R. D. 221
Masi, C. M. 137, 333
Maslach, C. 86, 99, 101, 364
Mason, D. A. 136
Massé-Birron, J. 134
Master, S. L. 263
Mather, L. 209
Mathers, N. 323
Matheson, C. 125
Matheson, D. H. 3
Matheson, K. 66, 68, 75, 108, 116, 278, 328, 361
Matter, J. A. 221
Matthews, K. A. 135
Matthewson, G. C. 265
Mattick, R. P. 178
Mauskopf, J. 1
Mavor, K. I. 7
Mawson, E. 191
May, A. R. 247
Maytan, M. 138
Mazzoni, N. 259
Meaney, D. F. 230
Medasani, K. 189, 281
Meeusen, R. 313
Mehl, S. 294
Meier, L. L. 87
Meier, P. S. 188
Melanson, E. L. 206, 215

Mellman, T. A. 111
Meltzer, H. Y. 286
Melzack, R. 254, 257
Mendelson, J. 92
Mendes de Leon, C. F. 138
Mendes, W. B. 41
Mendoza, S. P. 40, 49
Mendoza-Denton, R. 69
Menzies, D. 190
Merckelbach, H. 144
Meredith, L. S. 25
Merkin, S. S. 131
Merrill, W. 377–378
Messer, S. B. 161, 170
Mewse, A. J. 55, 190
Mewse, A. 27, 131, 244
Meyer, I. 189
Mezuk, B. 148
Michaels, P. J. 362
Michaud, C. 307
Middleton, J. C. 114
Middleton, W. 115
Miklowitz, D. J. 288–290
Miller, D. T. 69
Miller, G. 329
Miller, I. W. 315
Miller, K. 304, 327, 335
Miller, L. M. 367
Miller, M. J. 110
Miller, T. Q. 135
Miller, W. R. 136, 179
Miller-Martinz, D. M. 131
Milliken, C. 112
Mills, J. 265
Mills, R. 162
Mills, S. 55
Milne, M. 335
Milton, K. 211
Mindes, E. J. 361
Mineka, S. 127
Mintz, J. 289–290
Miranda, D. 125
Mirkin, J. N. 310
Mirsky, N. 101, 295
Mishkin, M. 110
Mitchell, E. 316
Mitkidis, P. 260, 265
Miyamoto, S. 284
Miyashita, Y. 110
Mobini, S. 206
Moghaddam, F. M. 48
Mogil, J. S. 259

Mohammed, S. A. 68, 71
Mojzisch, A. 94
Molenberghs, P. 271
Molero, F. 73, 364
Molix, L. 67
Mols, F. 218, 325–326, 331
Moltzen, K. 29
Mond, J. M. 204
Monin, B. 219, 225
Monk, R. L. 183
Monk, T. 288
Monroe, S. M. 162
Monson, C. M. 107
Montague, M. 325
Montalan, B. 267
Moore, M. 317
Moore, R. 161, 373
Moore, S. E. 162
Moore, T. J. 159
Moorer, A. 261
Moos, R. H. 186
Morales, J. 19
Moreland, R. L. 53
Morgan, V. A. 281
Moriano, J. A. 73, 364
Morley, S. 316
Morris, D. B. 261
Morris, D. J. 107
Morris, R. 316
Morris, W. L. 65, 75
Morrison, D. L. 367
Morrissey, J. P. 157
Mortensen, P. B. 283
Morton, T. A. 27, 131, 322, 333
Moses, H. 3
Mosimann, J. E. 211
Moskowitz, J. T. 92
Moss, H. B. 289
Moss-Morris, R. 315, 316
Motion, A. 108
Motlagh, H. 366
Motowidlo, S. J. 86
Mottershead, T. A. 209
Mouras, H. 267
Moussavi, S. 315
Moutoussis, M. 278, 294
Mowrer, O. H. 113
Mrazek, P. J. 172
Msetfia, R. M. 357
Mucci, P. 134
Mudde, A. N. 136
Muenchberger, H. 227, 243

Mueser, K. T. 289
Mukherjee, S. xviii
Mulcahy, L.141
Muldoon, O. T. 26, 51, 73, 108, 121, 126, 232
Mullen, B. 46, 209
Mullen, P. D. 46, 209
Mummendey, A. 46
Münsterberg, H. 89
Muntner, P. 378
Murakami, H. 269
Murburg, M. M. 110
Murchie, P. 125
Murnen, S. K. 213
Murphy, K. M. 3
Murray, C. J. L. 287, 307
Murray, J. 287
Murrell, A. J. 53
Myers, J. K. 88
Myles, B. M. 230
Myrtek, M. 87
Mythen, G. 95

Naber, D. 286
Nackers, L. M. 327
Nadler, A. 97
Nadort, M. 168
Nagamine, S. 369
Naghavi, M. 307
Najavits, L. M. 115
Najdovski, L. 94, 270, 271, 327
Nakagawa, Y. 126
Nakahara, K. 110
Nakaya, M. 369
Nalder, E. 231
Naliboff, B. D. 263
Narayana, P. A. 230
Narendran, R. 286
Nasser, M. 213
National Institute for Health and Clinical
    Excellence 288
National Treatment Agency for Substance Misuse
    179
Nazeer, A. 110
Neal, M. 35
Neal, R. 227
Neese-Todd, S. 244
Neidig, J. L. 361
Neighbors, C. J. 188
Neighbors, C. 207
Nelson, D. A. 273
Nepal, B. 42
Neugebauer, R. 163

Neumark-Sztainer, D. 205, 206, 210, 213
Neuvonen, E. 135
Newheiser, A. K. 74
Ng, C. K. 110
Ng, W. 377
Ngandu, T. 135
Nickerson, A. 108
Nielsen, L. 170, 333
Nielsen, N. H. 157
Nierman, A. 209
Nietzsche, F. 68
Nishizono-Maher, A. 367
Nittel, C. 294
Noble, E. P. 178
Nock, M. K. 261
Noel, J. G. 48
Noma, H. 161
Norbury, M. 165, 190
Norcross, J. C. 161
Nordestgaard, B. G. 222
Norenzayan, A. 340
Norlander, T. 92
Norman, P. 246
Norman, R. E. 157, 162
Norris, F. H. 91, 97
Norton, K. I. 213
Norton, M. I. 139
Norton, W. E. 80
Notter, M. L. 59
Novak, J. 292
Novak, S. A. 210
Novelli, D. 117–120
Nuechterlein, K. H. 283
Nugent, N. R. 110
Nyholt, D. R. 159
Nyswander, M. 178

O'Brien, A. 27, 53, 54, 64, 68, 84, 94, 98, 270, 326, 360, 375
O'Brien, J. Z. 316
O'Brien, K. J. 189
O'Brien, K. 80
O'Brien, L. T. 54, 64, 68, 84, 326, 360, 375
O'Brien, L. 53, 65, 320
O' Brien, M. P. 290
O'Connell, C. 114
O'Donnel, M. L. 108
O'Donohue, W. 108
O'Farrell, T. J. 184
O'Kearney, R. 110
O'Sullivan, C. 232
O'Sullivan, E. 47

O'Sullivan, L. 27, 94, 270
Oakes, P. J. 4, 15, 18, 23, 46, 76, 139, 141, 166, 168, 172, 196, 215, 216, 217, 247, 319
Ockene, J. K. 313
Oddy, M. 231
O'Driscoll, M. P. 102
Oei, T. P. S. 161, 333
Ogden, J. 209
Oh, H. 44
Ohbayashi, M. 110
Ólafsdóttir, S. 316
Olander, E. K. 136
Olds, T. S. 213
Oleson, K. C. 184
Olive, S. 213
Oliver, M. 317
Oliver, T. K. 310
Olivini, N. 259
Olmos, A. 292
Olson, J. M. 75
Olsson, G. L. 316
Opher, S. 316
Opitz, J. M. 215
Orbell, S. 190
Orjada, K. 213
Orleans, C. T. 313
Ormel, J. 316
Orrell, M. 151
Orsillo, S. M. 114
Oshio, A. 369
Ostafin, B. D. 182
Ostell, A. 28, 97
Ostermann, J. 1
Otis, M. D. 176
Otten, S. 46
Otto, M. W. 181, 182
Otukonyong, E. E. 206
Outten, H. R. 52, 73
Ouwerkerk, J.W. 77
Owen, M. 287
Ownsworth, T. 227–231, 233, 240, 245, 248
Oyserman, D. 25, 219, 325
Özmen, E. 127

Pabst, S. 20
Pachana, N. A. 55, 148
Packard, J. S. 86
Pagano, M. E. 187
Pagano, M. 186
Page, A. C. 367
Paker, M. 127
Palacios, R. 137

Palermo, T. M. 316
Palinkas, L. A. 86
Palisch, C. 3
Pallarés, T. 162
Palomares, N. A. 25
Palyo, S. A. 367
Pamuk, E. 36
Pande, V. 230
Pandey, K. 268–269, 272
Papaleo, N. 276
Papinczak, Z. E. 182
Paradies, Y. 66–67, 82
PARADISE Consortium 308
Paramore, L. C. 1
Parfenov, V. 239
Park, G. J. 213
Park, S.-Y. 236
Parker, J. D. 165
Parker, L. 255
Parloff, M. B. 158
Parra-Delgado, M. 316
Parsell, C. 44, 47, 49, 70, 169, 281
Pascaris, A. 292
Pascoe, E. A. 66–67
Pastore, M. 73
Patai, E. Z. 110
Patel, C. K. 315
Patel, V. 315
Pater, I. E.
Paterson, J. E. 140
Patrick, W. 257, 332
Pattenden, J. 209
Pattison, P. E. 325
Paul, N. 268
Pavot, W. 376
Pawitan, Y. 283
Paxton, S. J. 206, 210
Paykel, E. S. 162
Payne, B. R. 135
Payne, S. 234
Pbert, L. 313
Peabody, J. 377–378
Pearl, R. L. 317
Pedersen, B. K. 134
Pedersen, C. B. 284
Pedersen, M. S. 284
Pederson, E. L. 363
Pelletier, L. G. 214
Pellett, E. 232–234
Peñas-Lledó, E. 206
Pence, L. B. 316
Pendleton, D. A. 80

Penna, S. 54, 326
Pennebaker, J. W. 115, 122
Penner, L. A. 80
Penninx, B. W. J. H. 159
Pentel, P. R. 218
Pentland, A. S. 325
Peplau, L. A. 71
Pepper, M. P. 88
Perälä, J. 278
Pergadia, M. L. 159
Perreault, S. 77
Perri, M. G. 327
Perrin, N. A. 136
Perry, Y. 283
Perryman, C. 123, 185–186
Peters, E. 325
Peters, K. 4
Peters, S. 310
Peterson, C. 168
Peterson, J. B. 221
Petralia, W. 140
Petrie, K. 315
Pettigrew, J. 26, 126
Pfisterer, K. 376
Pharoah, F. 289
Phelan, J. C. 244
Phelan, S. 189
Phelps, E. 110
Phillips, R. 281
Pickett, K. 36, 38, 62
Pickrell, J. E. 144
Pierret, J. 293
Pieterse, A. 82
Pietromonaco, P. R. 263
Pietrzak, J. 69
Piette, J. D. 133
Pilkington, P. D. 158
Pilkonis, P. A. 163
Pill, R. 320
Pimm, S. 231
Pinel, E. C. 69
Pinker, S. 12, 31
Pinquart, M. 136, 146
Pinto, I. R. 196–197
Pirkola, S. 278
Pitman, R. K. 110, 114
Plagemann, A. 214
Platow, M. J. 20–21, 25, 28, 94, 203, 222, 225, 270–271, 276, 294, 325, 327
Playford, E. D. 234
Pleace, N. 47
Pliskin, N. 236

Ploner, M. 28
Podus, D. 181
Pohlman, S. 181
Polivy, J. 221, 222
Polman, R. 325
Polonski, L. 313
Ponsford, J. L. 230
Ponsford, J. 232, 244
Poser, E. G. 269
Postmes, T. 19, 26, 31, 34, 44, 49, 55, 57, 66, 72,
    75–76, 97, 146, 169, 235, 237, 246, 273, 302,
    305, 333, 335, 346, 348–349, 358, 379
Potemka, K. 136
Potts, L. 311, 316
Powers, M. B. 181–182, 184
Prabha, S. C. 281
Praharso, N. F. 162, 377
Prakash, R. S. 134
Pratto, F. 69–70
Préfaut, C. 134
Prendergast, M. 181
Prescott, C. A. 162
Presnell, K. 223
Presseau, J. 209
Preuschoff, K. 268
Price, J. R. 316
Price, J. 159, 184
Price, M. K. 69
Priebe, S. 280
Priest, N. 67, 82
Prigatano, G. P. 235–236
Prince, L. 233
Prince, M. 131
Prince, S. E. 161
Pritchard, M. E. 206
Prochaska, J. O. 207–208
Procidano, M. E. 91
Project MATCH Research Group 186
Prosser, A. 30, 95
Prove, E. 39
Provost, M. A. 87
Pugliese, C. 31, 55, 248
Puhl, R. M. 210
Pullerits, L. 313
Purdie, V. J. 69
Pustovitova, T. 239
Putnam, R. D. 7–8, 27, 36, 43, 58

Qi, L. 214
Quadflieg, N. 207
Quartero, A. O. 316
Quayle, M. 76

Queensland Mental Health Commission 281
Quin, R. 30, 240
Quinn, D. M. 169, 320
Quinton, W. J. 67
Quirk, F. 204
Qureshi, O. 311

Rafacz, J. 281
Rafanelli, C. 158
Raghubir, P. 218
Ragland, D. R. 148
Rahe, A. J. 98
Rahe, R. H. 88–89
Rahhal, T. A. 142
Rahill, A. A. 283
Rajguru, P. 316
Ramachandrappa, S. 204
Ramanathapillai, R. 122
Ramirez, J. J. 182
Rand, L. 219
Rankin, L. E. 69–70
Rao, V. M. 310
Raphael, D. 45
Rathbone, J. 289
Rathee, S. P. 230
Rauch, S. L. 110
Rauch, S. 110, 123
Ravenscroft, S. 333
Ravindran, L. N. 111
Ravndal, E. 186
Ray, K. 86, 373
Raza, F. 211
Razani, J. 289
Rea, M. M. 289–290
Read, J. P. 367
Read, J. 335
Read, S. A. 322
Reaves, S. 213
Reavley, N. J. 158
Reay, D. 44
Rebok, G. W. 148
Redberg, R. F. 313
Reddish, P. 260, 263
Redersdorff, S. 73
Redlich, C. A. 92
Reed, A. 191
Rees, S. 162
Rees, T. 325
Reeve, P. 65
Regan, S. 20
Regier, D. 179
Rehm, J. 311

Rehmeyer, J. 311
Reicher, S. D. 12, 15, 25, 29–30, 45–46, 49–51,
   53, 76, 78, 80, 93, 95, 97, 99–101, 103,
   117–118, 120–123, 129, 135, 141, 166, 215,
   222, 260, 268, 294–295, 297, 319, 325, 357,
   364–365, 372–373
Reid, S. A. 144
Reiger, E. 371
Reilly-Harrington, N. A. 288–289
Reinecke, J. 303
Reininghaus, U. 280
Reis, H. T. 97, 126
Reite, M. L. 40
Remick, R. A. 206
Ren, Y. 78
Resick, P. A. 107–108, 112–114, 117, 127
Revenson, T. A. 315
Reynolds, C. F. 344
Reynolds, K. J. 29, 320, 364
Reynolds, K. 378
Rhew, I. C. 182
Ricciardelli, L. A. 204
Rice, S. A. 110
Richards, S. H. 138
Richardson, R. 273
Richmond Fellowship QLD 291
Riddle, M. C. 317
Riecansky, I. 268
Riedel-Heller, S. G. 65
Rief, W. 294
Rieger, E. 203, 225
Riekert, K. A. 313
Riemsma, R. P. 209
Rigatelli, M. 323
Riis, J. 325
Rise, J. 219
Ritchie, T. L. 178
Ritter, A. 185
Rivera, L. 67
Rizvi, S. L. 107
Roberts, N. P. 108–109
Roberts, S. W. 135
Robertson, H. D. 125
Robertson, S. S. 263
Robins, R. W. 341, 375
Robinson, M. E. 263
Robinson, S. L. 273
Robles, T. F. 2, 326
Roccas, S. 47–48, 52
Rodgers, W. M. 258
Rodin, J. 317
Roebuck, T. M. 236

Roehrig, M. 214
Roepke, K. 214
Roepstorff, A. 260, 265
Rogosch, F. A. 176
Rohde, P. 162, 204
Rohsenow, D. J. 188
Roll, J. 186
Rolling Stones 154
Rollinson, R. 373
Rollman, G. B. 258
Rollnick, S. 136, 179
Rona, R. J. 112
Ronksley, P. E. 209
Rooijmans, H. G. M. 315
Room, R. 189
Rosch, E. 24
Rose, F. D. 244
Rose, R. M. 329
Rose, S. C. 115
Rosen, D. 344
Rosen, J. 20
Rosenberg, M. 375
Rosendahl, E. 134
Rosenman, R. H. 86
Rosenman, R. 102
Rosenstock, I. M. 207–208
Rosenthal, B. 221
Rosenthal, R. 170
Ross, J. 185–186
Rost, K. M. 25
Rothbard, J. C. 161
Rothbaum, B. O. 113, 115
Röttgers, H. 303
Rounsaville, B. J. 163, 288
Rouse, G. 373
Rowan, C. 300, 305
Rowland, B. 175
Rowlands, J. M. 30, 240
Rowlands, L. 231
Rozanski, A. 315
Rozin, P. 222
Rubak, S. 209
Rubenstein, L. V. 25
Rubin, D. C. 134
Rubin, G. J. 127
Rubin, G. 316
Rubin, M. 47, 57–58
Rubio, G. 285
Rudd, A. G. 230
Rudhran, V. 281
Rusanen, M. 135
Rüsch, N. 169, 281

Russell, D. W. 373–374
Russell, I. T. 152
Russell, M. 181
Russo-Devosa, Y. 75
Ruth-Sahd, L. A. 323
Ruttan, L. A. 232
Ryan, M. E. 309
Ryan, M. K. 65, 322
Rydell, S. 211, 218
Ryn, M. V. 80

Saarni, S. I. 278
Sabatier, C. 294
Sabatine, M. S. 308
Sabiston, C. M. 325
Sachdev, I. 46
Sachs, J. 31
Sachser, N. 39
Sacks, O. 278–279, 290
Sacristán, J. A. 286
Sadowski, J. 313
Saeri, A. K. 27
Sage, B. 36
Saguy, A. C. 222
Saha, S. 80
Şahin, D. 127
Saini, R. 230
Sakai, R. R. 39
Salas, C. E. 231
Salazar, A. M. 236
Salke, M. 186
Salkovskis, P. M. 316
Salomons, T. V. 258
Salzman, W. 40, 49
Sandbaek, A. 209
Sander, A. M. 236
Sander, L. 152
SANE Australia 281
Sani, F. 18, 27, 46, 54–55, 61–62, 163, 165,
    173, 190, 237, 244, 275, 294, 297, 304, 323,
    326–327, 335
Santini, Z. I. 170, 333
Santor, D. 259
Sapolsky, R. M. 11, 36, 39, 43
Şar, V. 115
Sareen, J. 316
Sarimurat, N. 127
Saris, W. H. M. 211, 215
Sarokhani, D. 340
Sarokhani, M. T. 340
Saroyan, S. 244–246
Sarsam, M. 287

Sartorius, N. 281
Sassoon, S. 104–105, 109, 126–128
Satariano, W. A. 148
Saunders, J. B. 178
Saunders, P. 36
Savic, M. 19, 27, 185, 191–192, 197–198,
    352–353
Saw, S. 281
Sawada, N. 157
Saxena, S. 157
Sayehmiri, K. 340
Sbarra, D. A. 2, 326
Scambler, S. 137
Scanlan, J. M. 40
Scarapicchia, T. M. F. 325
Schaafsma, J. 69
Schacht, A. 286
Scharloo, M. 315
Schauman, O. 362
Scheepers, D. T. 41, 52
Scherbaum, C. 71
Schiano, D. 293
Schimmack, U. 376
Schimmelmann, B. G. 286
Schindler, I. 146
Schlaff, C. 20
Schlosser, D. A. 290
Schlösser, S. 286
Schmader, T. 67, 70, 75
Schmid, K. 121
Schmitt, L. 107
Schmitt, M. M. 361
Schmitt, M. T. 52, 65–67, 70–73, 76–77, 82, 99,
    190, 219, 297, 302, 362
Schmitz, N. 315
Schneider, J. A. 138
Schneider, M. 323
Schnicke, M. K. 112, 117
Schnurr, P. P. 127
Schofield, D. 357
Schofield, P. E. 325–326
Scholliers, P. 224
Schomer, K. G. 232
Schönberger, M. 232
Schuh, S. C. 27, 96, 365
Schuler, R. S. 86, 364
Schwab, K. 236
Schwab, R. L. 86, 364
Schwartz, C. 184
Schwartz, J. 68
Schwarzer, R. 91, 97
Scoboria, A. 159

Scott, J. A. N. 161
Scott, J. G. 162
Scott, K. M. 316
Scrignaro, M. 46
Seal, B. 206
Sebastian, A. 211
Seddon, R. 55, 249
Sedgwick-Taylor, A. 316
Seeley, J. R. 162
Seeman, T. E. 131
Seifert, R. 122
Seifert, T. 211
Seligman, M. 160, 168
Selinger, E. 313
Sellers, R. M. 69
Sellwood, W. 287
Selten, J. P. 294
Seltzer, M. 111
Selye, H. M. D. 84–86, 102
Semenkovich, C. F. 134
Semmer, N. 87
Sempértegui, G. A. 168
Sentell, T. L. 67
Serdarevic, M. 136
Serfaty, M. 302
Sethi, N. 283
Seymour-Smith, M. 55, 352
Shackleton, E. H. 262
Shafran, R. 206
Shah, P. 327, 331
Shah, R. 161
Shahly, V. 204
Shalev, A. Y. 112
Shamah, D. 59
Shaner, J. L. 65, 141
Shankar, A. 137
Shankar, S. 268–269
Shapiro, K. J. 40
Sharman, L. 300, 302, 356
Sharpe, M. 311, 316
Shattock, L. 310
Shaver, P. R. 161
Shaw, R. 126
Shea, M. E. 206
Shea, M. T. 163
Shearer, J. 179
Sheasby, J. 317
Sheffield, D. 263
Sheikh, J. I. 110
Sheldon, A. M. 221
Shelton, J. N. 69, 80
Shelton, R. C. 157–159

Shen, W. W. 285
Shepherd, B. 108
Shepherd, C. 311
Shepherd, J. 236
Sherbourne, C. D. 158
Sherer, M. 236
Sherif, M. 14, 21, 141
Sherman, C. J. 255
Sherman, R. A. 255
Sherry, S. 206
Sherwood, A. 68
Shields, C. 231, 245
Shiell, A. 43–44
Shim, R. S. 36
Shin, L. M. 110, 123
Shipley, B. A. 135
Shirinyan, D. 263
Shively, C. A. 40, 49
Shorter, E. 158
Shoup, J. A. 315
Shubert, T. 134
Shull, W. H. 230
Shum, D. 233–234
Sibley, C. G. 27
Sidanius, J. 67, 69–70
Siegert, R. 234
Siegler, I. C. 133
Siegrist, J. 58
Sigal, R. J. 209
Silani, G. 268
Silove, D. 108, 162, 230
Silva, J. 245
Silver, J. 230
Silver, M. 14
Silverman, R. A. 48
Simon, B. 75
Simpson, G. M. 289
Simpson, T. L. 182
Sinclair, C. 325
Sinclair, S. 65
Singer, T. 268
Singh, M. K. 158
Singh-Manoux, A. 46
Sinitsyn, V. 239
Sintemaartensdijk, N. 41
Sirigu, A. 268
Sitko, K. 335
Sivilotti, M. L. A. 311
Skewes, J. 260, 265
Skinner, J. B. 181
Sklar, L. S. 86
Skoner, D. P. 162

Skyt, I. 258
Slade, M. D. 144
Slavich, G. M. 329
Sledge, W. H. 98
Sloan, D. M. 127
Sloan, F. A. 1
Slopen, N. 189
Slovic, P. 325
Smart Richman, L. 66–68
Smeets, R. J. E. M. 315
Smink, F. R. E. 204
Smit, H. J. 214
Smit, J. H. 168
Smith, J. R. 218
Smith, B. W. 370
Smith, B. 373
Smith, C. 46, 209
Smith, D. E. 136
Smith, D. H. 230
Smith, H. J. 46
Smith, L. G. E. 146
Smith, M. E. 110
Smith, M. T. 316
Smith, N. G. 361
Smith, T. B. 3
Smith, T. W. 135
Sniehotta, F. 209
Snow, D. A. 59
Soderhamn, O. 140
Sofsky, W. 122
Sohlberg, M. M. 231
Soininen, H. 135
Sokol, B. W. 60
Solnit, R. 123
Solomon, A. 135
Solomon, P. 92
Song, Y. S. 361
Sonis, J. 114
Sosa, R. 263
Sotsky, S. M. 158, 163
South, E. I. 201, 333
Southwick, S. M. 110
Sowden, A. J. 209
Spahlholz, J. 65
Spalding, T. W. 134
Sparer, J. 92
Sparks, L. 326
Spears, R. 7, 71–72, 75, 99, 166, 268, 346, 348, 362
Spector, A. 151
Spector, J. 236
Spellacy, F. 237

Spencer, M. 68
Spencer, R. L. 39
Spencer, S. J. 142
Spijker, J. 157
Spinhoven, P. 168
Spinnato, J. A. 263
Spiro III, A. 146
Spiro, A. 135
Spitz, G. 230
Srinivasan, N. 12, 29
St Claire, L. 80, 141, 155, 317, 321–322
Stacy, R. 17
Staerklé, C. 52–53, 56
Stagoll, B. 66
Staiger, P. K. 19, 27, 185, 189, 197–198
Stalker, K. L. 247
Stam, R. 110
Stang, P. E. 316
Stangor, C. 75
Stanton, A. L. 315
Staples, M. P. 325
Starchina, Y. 239
Stark, C. 17, 19, 55, 169, 199, 201, 302, 348
Starks, R. D. 292
Stathopoulou, G. 181–182
Steel, C. 67, 287–288
Steel, Z. 162
Steele, C. M. 142
Steele, J. 179
Stefanucci, J. K. 142
Steffen, P. R. 68
Steffens, N. K. 27, 96, 148, 150, 191–192, 201, 215, 218, 222, 331, 338, 350–351, 356, 361, 365, 379
Stein, M. B. 111, 316
Steinbrecher, N. 310
Stein-Morrow, E. A. 135
Steketee, G. 113
Steptoe, A. 137, 315
Sterling, P. 86
Stevens, M. 325
Stevens, S. 302
Stevenson, C. 29, 51, 73, 268
Stewart, E. 261
Stewart, J. J. 140
Stewart, N. A. J. 17
Stewart, T. L. 146
Stice, E. 162, 204, 213–214, 223
Stieger, S. 268
Stirling, E. 213
Stolbach, B. C. 115
Stone, L. 310

Stott, C. 117–120
Stout, R. L. 182, 186–187
Strahm, S. 65
Strang, J. 135, 316
Straus, R. 102
Strausser, K. S. 273
Strayer, D. L. 142
Strecher, V. J. 208
Stronge, S. 27
Struening, E. L. 244
Stuber, J. 189
Stucke, T. S. 273
Sturchen, M. A. 236
Styron, T. 161
Subasic, E. 7, 29
Subramanian, S. V. 8, 44
Suedfeld, P. 86, 92, 97–98
Sui, X. 325
Sullivan, M. J. 258–259, 263
Sullivan, P. F. 159
Suls, J. M. 5
Sundin, J. 112
Sung, C. Y. 329
Sunstein, C. R. 218, 313
Surgenorb, P. W. G. 357
Susser, E. 294
Sutker, P. B. 114
Suvisaari, J. 278
Suzuki, T. 157
Swaab, R. 333
Swartz, H. A. 288
Swift, H. J. 144
Swim, J. K. 75
Swinburn, B. 211, 225
Swinson, R. P. 367
Syme, S. L. 27, 36–37, 60, 137
Szreter, S. 7

Tabuteau-Harrison, S. 244
Taffe, J. R. 232
Tajfel, H. 12, 14–15, 18, 19, 43, 46, 48, 49, 58, 77, 78, 99, 223, 235, 240, 242, 245, 273
Takeuchi, D. 68
Talipski, L. A. 247
Tanaka, S. 161
Tandon, A. 315
Tang, Y. 138
Tangney, J. P. 206, 215
Tapper, K. 325
Tarrant, M. 7, 25, 65, 218, 325, 327
Tarrier, N. 114, 283, 287
Taşdemir, Ö. 127

Tate, R. L. 230
Tate, R. 232
Taylor, A. 316
Taylor, C. B. 223
Taylor, D. M. 48
Taylor, L. F. 140
Taylor, M. D. 91, 135
Taylor, M. 288
Taylor, S. E. 69, 71, 91, 135, 327
Tear, M. J. 162
Teasdale, J. D. 161
Tedeschi, R. G. 108
Teesson, M. 185
Teixeira, C. P. 70
Temerlin, J. W. 17
Temerlin, M. K. 17
Temkin, N. R. 231
Teng, F. 275
Tennant, C. 162
Tennen, H. 315
Terry, D. 219, 325
Terry, L. 98, 219, 325
Testa, M. 75
Tewari, S. 12, 31
Thaler, R. H. 218, 313
Thase, M. E. 288
Thatcher, G. W. 94
Thisted, R. A. 162
Thoburn, J. 114
Thoits, P. A. 55
Thoits, P. 88–89
Thomae, N. 76
Thomas, K. C. 157
Thomas, K. R. 244
Thomas, S. L. 224
Thompson, E. P. 69, 70
Thompson, J. K. 95, 211, 214
Thompson, K. 95
Thompson, P. D. 325
Thompson, S. 137
Thorn, B. E. 316
Thorndike, A. N. 325
Thornicroft, G. 157, 169, 281
Thurecht, L. 42
Tice, D. M. 273
Tidy, E. 316
Tiggemann, M. 213
Tillotson, K. M. 258
Timko, C. A. 213, 223
Todis, B. 231
Toga, A. 228
Tollefson, D. 181

Tolppanen, A-M. 135
Tomaka, J. 137
Tomita, H. 110
Tompson, M. C. 289, 290
Tones, B. K. 324
Tones, K. 311
Tonks, J. 31, 55, 248, 333, 349, 358
Toobert, D. J.
Tooley, E. 370
Topel, R. H. 3
Torgerson, C. 228
Toscani, L. 325
Toschke, A. M. 230
Toumbourou, J. T. 175
Toumbourou, J. W. 188
Touyz, S. 213
Tovin, M. M. 140
Trace, S. E. 206
Tracey, I. 261
Tracie, M. 158
Tran, K. 377
Tran, N. 288
Tranel, D. 230
Trapnell, P. D. 358
Tredoux, C. 76
Trench, B. 184
Trifiletti, E. 125
Trindall, N. 53
Tripp, D. A. 259
Tristan, J. 223
Truax, P. A. 161
Truong, M. 67
Trzesniewski, K. H. 375
Tsang, A. 292
Tsang, H. W. 292, 316
Tsivrikos, D. 26, 44, 55, 57, 237, 273, 335, 348, 349
Tsuang, M. T. 159
Tsuboi, K. 213
Tsui, P. W. 316
Tucker, J. L. 25
Tun, P. T. 131
Turecki, G. 159
Turner, A. P. 317
Turner, B. S. 162
Turner, C. W. 135
Turner, J. A. 316
Turner, J. C. 4, 10, 15, 17, 18, 19, 23, 24, 25, 27, 29, 30, 43, 46, 48, 49, 76, 78, 94, 99, 139, 142, 163, 164, 166, 172, 215, 216, 223, 235, 240, 242, 245, 247, 270, 273, 319, 325, 333
Turner, R. J. 108

Turner, R. 265
Tuval-Mashiach, R. 112
Twamley, E. W. 214
Twenge, J. M. 207, 273
Twomey, S. 227
Tybjærg-Hansen, A. 222
Tyerman, A. 231, 233
Tyler, T. R. 46
Tyrka, A. R. 206
Tyrovola, S. 170, 333

Uchida, H. 157
Uchino, B. N. 328
Ulijaszek, S. J. 211
Uller, C. 190
Ulman, R. B. 111
Underwood, P. W. 91, 95
United Nations Children's Fund 44
United Nations. 131–132
Unruh, A. M. 259
Uskul, A. K. 190
Ustun, B. 315
Ustyuzhanin, D. 239
Uysal, S. 230

Vaananen, A. 43
Vaes, J. 73
Vaglum, P. 186
Vahtera, J. 43
Vaillant, G. E. 131, 133
Väisänen, E. 323
Vallen, B. 222
Van Baak, M. A. 211, 215
Van Bavel, J. J. 220, 268
Van den Berg, P. 210, 213, 214
Van der Heijden, G. J. 316
Van der Wouden, J. C. 316
Van Dessel, N. 316
Van Dick, R. 27, 29, 94, 96, 365
Van Dyck, R. 168
Van Hoeken, D. 204
Van Horn, J. 228
Van Ittersum, K. 218
Van Kessel, K. 316
Van Knippenberg, A. 48, 77
Van Marwijk, H. 316
Van Praag, H. 134
Van Ree, J. M. 311
Van Rijswijk, W. 30, 48
Van Stralen, M. M. 136
Van Straten, A. 161
Van Tulder, M. 92

Van Zee, A. 311
Van Zomeren, M. 346
Vanable, P. A. 372
Varese, F. 335
Vargha-Khadem, F. 110
Varnes, L. 10, 19, 26, 30, 44, 51, 78, 80, 96, 99, 142, 169, 244, 245, 273, 303, 333, 346, 358, 364
Vartanian, L. R. 210, 214
Vase, L. 258
Vasterling, J. J. 114
Veale, D. 161
Vedel, E. 184
Vedsted, P. 323
Vega, E. 362
Veisani, Y. 340
Veith, R. C. 110
Velicer, W. F. 207
Veling, W. 294
Verdeli, H. 163
Verdes, E. 315
Vergouwe, Y. 286
Verkuyten, M. 122
Vermetten, E. 110
Versari, A. 125
Vervoort, T. 263
Vezzali, L. 125
Victor, C. 137
Visscher, B. R. 71, 283, 327
Visscher, P. M. 71, 283, 327
Vitousek, K. 206
Vlaeyen, J. W. S. 258, 315
Vliek, M. L. W. 346
Vogel, D. L. 362, 363
Vogt, T. M. 313
Von Dawans, B. 94
Von Frey, M. 255
Von Friederichs-Fitzwater, M. M. 317
Von Korff, M. 316
Von Ranson, K. M. 206
Vormedal, K. 54, 84, 326, 360, 375
Vos, T. 158, 307
Voss, M. W. 134
Voudouris, N. J. 94, 270, 271, 276, 327
Vowles, K. E. 316
Vredenburg, K. 165
Vries, H. D. 136
Vythilingam, M. 110

Wade, T. D. 206, 362, 363
Wadley, A. L. 219, 325
Wagner, T. H. 133
Wagner, T. 286
Wahl, O. F. 344

Wahler, E. A. 176
Wainwright, S. P. 265
Waite, L. J. 137, 374
Wakefield, J. R. H. 18, 163, 165, 190, 244, 275, 294, 297, 304, 323, 326–327, 335
Wakley, G. 308
Wakslak, C. J. 69
Walden, J. 286
Waldinger, R. J. 131, 133
Waldron, B. 232
Waldron, I. 206
Walker, A. 209
Walker, R. B. 131
Walklate, S. 95
Wall, P. D. 254
Wallace, R. B. 148
Waller, G. 161
Walsemann, K. M. 67
Walsh, E. M. 211, 218
Walsh, M. 110
Walsh, R. S. 232, 247
Walter, J. 236
Walter, Z. C. 44, 47, 49, 58, 59, 70, 169, 281, 291, 333
Walton, G. M. 144, 340
Walwyn, R. 311, 316
Wampold, B. E. 161, 170
Wang, C. C. 317
Wang, C. E. A. 168
Wang, H.-X. 138
Wang, J. 108
Wang, M. 146, 315
Wang, W. (2009) 268
Wann, D. L. 19, 48
Wansink, B. 218
Ward, C. 234
Ward, J. 178
Ward, L. C. 316
Ward, M. 28
Ward, N. 142
Ward, R. A. 139
Warden, D. L. 236
Wardle, J. 137, 215
Warmerdam, L. 161
Warner, R. 48
Waroquier, L. 211
Warren, J. T. 80
Watanabe, K. 157
Waterloo, K. 168
Waterreus, A. 281
Watkins, B. A. 211
Watkins, C. J. 317
Watkins, J. T. 163

Watson, A. C. 68, 169, 362
Watson, B. M. 28
Watson, J. M. 142
Watt, I. S. 209
Wearden, A. J. 283
Webb, H. 189
Wecking, C. 29
Wegge, J. 29
Wegner, D. M. 258
Weich, S. 302
Weil, A. 114
Weiner, B. 69
Weinman, J. 315
Weishaar, M. 168
Weiss, A. 110, 135, 136
Weiss, J. 39
Weiss, R. D. 179
Weiss, S. M. 39
Weiss, D. S. 110, 366
Weissman, M. M. 163, 288
Welch, J. 283
Wells, K. B. 158
Wells, Y. 140
Werthessen, N. 102
Wessely, S. 92, 115
West, L. A. 137
West, R. 209
Westgate, E. C. 184
Wetherell, M. S. 15, 46, 76
Wexler, D. 92
White, J. 316
White, K. M. 219
White, M. 138, 338
White, P. D. 311, 316
Whiteford, H. A. 157
Whitehouse, H. 261
Whiteley, P. F. 44
Whitely, R. 302
Whiteside, U. 207
Whitlock, E. P. 315
Whyte, K. P. 313
Wickham, S. 294, 335
Wicklund, R. A. 207
Wicksell, R. K. 316
Wiech, K. 261
Wiggins, K. 370
Wilcox, K. 222
Wilke, H. 48, 77
Wilkinson, R. 36, 172
Wilksch, S. M. 206
Willems, L. N. A. 315

Williams, A. C. 316
Williams, A. 263
Williams, D. R. 68, 71
Williams, E. 283
Williams, J. L. 325
Williams, J. 278, 294
Williams, K. D. 273
Williams, K. 273
Williams, R. 26, 123
Williams, V. S. L. 375
Williams, W. H. 232
Williamson, H. 310
Williamson, M. 289
Williamson, P. R. 340
Willinge, A. 213
Willingham, J. 28
Willison, K. 278
Wills, T. A. 91, 95, 97, 162
Wilson, A. 352
Wilson, B. A. 227, 235–236, 240
Wilson, G. 146
Wilson, J. P. 111
Wilson, M. E. 40
Wilson, R. S. 138
Wimo, A. 131
Winblad, B. 138
Windle, M. 181
Windsor, T. D. 148
Winegardner, J. 230
Winehouse, A. 189–190
Wines, C. 114
Wingfield, J. C. 40, 329
Winstanley, J. B. 230
Winter, G. 127
Wiseman, C. V. 211
Wiseman, E. 332
Wisniewski, S. R. 288–289
Witkiewitz, K. 182
Wittrock-Staar, M. 214
Wiuf, C. 284
Wohl, M. J. A. 220
Wolfe, C. D. A. 230
Wolfe, R. 293
Wolff, B. B. 258
Wong, D. K. 232
Wong, V. 135
Wong, W. 289
Wood, S. 323
Woodall, J. 311
Woods, A. 278
Woods, B. 151

Woods, R. T. 152
Woodward, S. H. 110
Woolcock, M. 7
Woong Yun, G. 213
Work Group on Substance Use Disorders 179
World Bank 65
World Health Organization 44, 62, 204, 236, 307, 344
Wormington, S. V. 184
Worrell, M. 161
Woyshville, M. J. 286
Wray, N. R. 159, 283
Wright, C. C. 317
Wright, C. J. 235
Wright, C. L. 58
Wright, K. L. 280
Wright, R. 31, 297
Wright, S. C. 48, 220
Wurm, M. 102
Wuthnow, R. 53
Wyatt, G. 363
Wyatt, H. 211, 215
Wykes, T. 287–288

Xavier, M. 204
Xie, H. 289
Xu, K. 58
Xu, X. 268
Xygalatas, D. 260, 265

Yamagishi, T. 28, 294
Yamamoto, K. 367
Yang, J. 222
Yarasheski, K. E. 134
Yates, P. J. 237
Yehuda, R. 108

Yeomans, M. R. 206
Yildiz, A. A. 122
Yip, B. H. 283
Yip, T. 68
Ylvisaker, M. 232–235
Yoder, N. 25, 219, 325, 331
Young, B. M. 57
Young, H. 75
Young, J. E. 168
Young, R. M. 182
Ysseldyk, R. 19, 27, 364, 375–376
Yzerbyt, V. Y. 70

Zaccardo, M. 213
Zadro, L. 273
Zahniser, J. H. 292
Zajecka, J. 157–158
Zarate, R. 289
Zastowny, T. R. 283
Zautra, A. J. 97, 126
Zebel, S. 346
Zeeman, H. 235
Zeybek, A. 294
Zhang, A. 57–58, 74, 78, 82, 379
Zhao, C. 134
Zheng, L. 247
Zhou, X. 263
Zijdenbos, I. L. 316
Zimmerman, J. B. 134
Zimmerman, R. S. 319
Zink, T. 20
Zlati, A. 169
Zoellner, L. A. 115
Zuo, Z. 268
Zywiak, W. H. 182, 188

Subject index

Aboriginal 116
abuse 17, 27, 55, 80, 84, 108–110, 115–116, 120,
    123, 128, 161, 175–176, 179–182, 184, 189,
    191, 200, 292, 302, 327, 329; physical 123, 302;
    see also substance abuse
acceptance and commitment therapy (ACT) 316
acceptance coping 93
acquired brain injury (ABI) 11, 55, 227–251;
    adjustment and social identity change 236–240;
    cognitive impairment 230–232, 234–235,
    247–248, 250–251; costs and benefits of
    disclosure 250; disclosure decisions 243–244,
    250; injury severity and life satisfaction 247;
    nature and impact 227–231; post-traumatic
    growth 242, 244–247, 250; stigma 232–233,
    236, 240, 243–244, 250
acute pain 11, 252–277; appraisal 254, 258–260,
    263, 268–270, 272, 275–276; benefits and costs
    260–261; coping 263, 272, 275–276; definition
    252–254; gate control theory 257–258; meaning
    making 254; psychological benefits 260; rituals
    253, 260, 265–266; social pain 254, 263,
    272–274
adaptive pacing therapy 311
addiction 11, 55, 63, 116, 123, 175–202; multiple
    group memberships 190–193; residential
    and community treatment 185–186; social
    dislocation theory 188; social identity approach
    to 176, 187–200; social identity model of
    cessation maintenance 195–197; social identity
    model of recovery 197–198, 200–201; stigma
    188–190, 193; support groups 176, 184,
    186–187, 189, 191–192, 200; therapeutic
    community 191–195, 197, 199, 201
African Americans 49, 52, 67, 69–70, 72, 82
ageing 11, 55, 131–156, 166; age discrimination
    146; aged-based self-categorization 139–146;
    collective action 146–147; group intervention
    138, 153–155; health concerns 141; loneliness
    137; memory 137, 141–146, 151; mobility
    strategies 145; retirement 139, 146, 148, 150;
    social identity approach to 133, 136, 138–154;
    stereotypes 139–147, 154–155; symptom
    perception 139, 141, 155

achondroplasia 83
Alcoholics Anonymous (AA) 176, 186–187,
    191–193, 195–197; *see also* support groups
allostatic dysregulation 109
Alzheimer's disease 144, 229; *see also* dementia
anhedonia 157, 280
anorexia nervosa 204–206
antidepressant medication 158–159
anxiety 30, 36, 46, 66–68, 80, 94, 111, 114, 122,
    152, 154, 161, 169–171, 174, 182, 230, 232,
    256, 283, 287–288, 291, 300, 310, 316, 320,
    340–342, 347, 367–369
appraisal 74, 89–93, 95, 98, 116, 258, 269–270,
    272, 275, 316; primary 90–91, 93, 98, 269, 275,
    316; secondary 90–93, 95, 98, 269–270, 272,
    275
arthritis 4, 133, 307, 311, 316–317
asthma 133, 307–308, 317, 320, 329–330
attachment theory 161, 168
attitudes 89, 92, 140, 183, 189, 191, 200, 207–210,
    218, 221, 320, 325
attribution 69, 167–169, 173, 265
Australia 12, 18, 31, 36, 42, 59, 140, 179, 187–189,
    243, 281, 290–292, 303–304, 345, 349–351,
    356, 359, 361, 364, 369, 372, 375, 379
autism 30, 247
autobiographical memory 114, 116

BBC Prison Study 49–50, 52, 62, 99, 101–103,
    294–295, 297
Behavioural Couples Therapy (BCT) 184
binge eating disorder 204–205, 207
biochemical models 158–160, 165, 172
biological approaches 178
biomedical approaches 4–5, 7, 9, 283–286,
    309–311, 322–323, 329
bipolar disorders 278–281, 288–289
bio-psychosocial model of challenge and threat
    (BPM-CT) 41
brain injury *see* acquired brain injury (ABI);
    identity change after brain injury; traumatic brain
    injury (TBI)
breast cancer 68
buffering model of social support 53, 173, 273, 306

bulimia nervosa 205, 207, 323
bullying 99, 101, 297
burnout, measures 86, 99; *see also* stress, burnout

cardiovascular disease 4, 42, 66, 68, 133, 307, 325
Canada 59, 82, 116, 376
cancer 36, 45, 56, 68, 86, 133, 203, 307–311, 313, 325–326, 328–329
Cantril Self-Anchoring Striving Scale (Cantril Ladder) 376–377
capabilities 232–233
care 1, 27, 29, 36, 61, 64, 67, 69, 77, 79–81, 97, 125, 131, 133–134, 140–142, 145–146, 151–152, 155, 157, 172, 179, 185, 210, 221–222, 226, 235, 245, 248, 260, 278, 288–289–291, 309–311, 313, 316–319, 321–324, 329, 331, 334, 348–349, 358, 365; *see also* older adults in residential care
carers 27, 237, 333; motivation 323; well-being 327
catastrophising 258–259, 315–316
cerebral palsy 322
Chile 104, 125, 249
China 58, 78, 149, 239, 377, 379
choirs 7, 291, 300, 324
chronic fatigue syndrome 307, 310, 312, 316
chronic mental health conditions (CMHC) 11, 278–306; acquisition of identity 300; and recovery 280, 286, 289–290, 292–293, 297–305; community approaches 290–293; family-focused therapy 289–290; illness identity 297, 303; managing mental health stigma 302–303; mental health service reforms 287, 290, 293; social identity approach to 278, 290, 293–303; social and vocational activities 293; social marginalization 283, 293–294; social support 290, 292, 300, 302–306; stereotype rejection 303, 306
chronic fatigue syndrome 307, 310, 312, 316
chronic pain 133, 252, 277, 307, 311, 316
chronic physical health conditions (CPHC) 11, 252, 307–331; appraisal 316, 321, 329; essentialism 320, 330; expression of symptoms 309–313, 315–317, 319–321; health promotion strategies 325; health risk behaviours 324–326; illness identities 320–321, 327, 330; medically unexplained symptoms 310, 316, 320, 323; normative influence 325–326; nudge policies 313, 325; provision of healthcare services 321–324; self-management programs 316, 327; social identity approach to 309, 319–329; treatment adherence 323, 330
civility 125

Civil Rights Movement 78
cohesion *see* social cohesion
cognitive alternatives 58, 74, 78–79, 81, 98–99
cognitive behavioural therapy (CBT) 114, 161, 163, 168, 170, 172, 181, 183, 196, 231, 248, 287–289, 297, 311, 316, 335; and trauma 114; and depression 161, 163, 168, 170, 172; and eating disorders 203, 204–207, 213, 333, 359, 372; and addiction 181, 183, 196; and acquired brain injury 231, 248; and chronic mental health conditions 287–289, 297; and chronic physical health conditions 311, 316
cognitive-behavioural models 161–162
cognitive dissonance theory 265
cognitive restructuring 114
collective action 7, 73–74, 125, 146–147, 190
collective coping strategies 99
collective protest 75–76
collective resilience *see* resilience
collective response to stressors 51, 74, 76
collective self-regulation 120
common fate 124–125
communication 25, 28, 236, 289–290, 333
community 1–2, 7, 12, 27, 31, 36, 43–44, 51–52, 59–60, 69, 92, 101–102, 116, 122–123, 148, 150, 166–168, 170, 173, 176, 178, 180, 184–185, 187, 190–195, 197, 199–201, 216, 235–237, 259, 286–287, 290–293, 297–301, 304–305, 314, 324, 329, 331, 348–353, 358, 361, 364–365, 367, 369, 371–375
comorbidity 284, 289
concealment 71, 73–74, 243, 250, 347, 363–364; of health condition 320, 327; of stigma 70–71, 73–74
conditioning 113, 181
conflict 14, 18, 89, 100–101, 106, 112, 116–117, 121–123, 126, 129, 157, 183, 290, 327, 329, 335; family 122; interpersonal 183; intergroup; *see also* intergroup relations
connection *see* social connection
consumer perspectives 424
contingency reinforcement treatment 181
control 30–33, 37, 39–43, 45, 52, 56, 60, 69–70, 77, 80, 87, 90, 110, 114–115, 120, 127, 134, 136, 148, 151–152, 163–166, 181–182, 184–185, 191, 193, 196–197, 203, 206–209, 211, 216, 218–220, 225, 248, 257–258, 261–262, 270, 273, 288, 296–297, 317, 323, 327–328, 336, 343, 347, 364, 375
coping 52, 67, 71, 73, 77–78, 84, 90–91, 93, 97, 99–100, 108, 114, 121, 176, 182, 200, 232–233, 241, 245, 263, 272, 275–276, 287,

315–317, 327, 329–330; acceptance (*see* acceptance coping); appraisal 74; biological and psychosocial responses 72–73; strategies 72–73
core beliefs 161, 167–168
cortisol responses to stress 39–40, 67–68, 94, 101, 110, 328
critical incident stress debriefing 115, 128
critical health psychology 317–318
crowds 27, 118–120, 129, 230, 269, 347, 357; common fate 124–125; conflict 121; self-policing 120; physical crowds 120; psychological crowds 120; shared social identity 13, 27, 118–119

dementia 30, 131, 133–135, 142–144, 150, 152, 229, 240, 247–248, 349, 358, *see also* Alzheimer's disease
depersonalisation 21–22, 86
depression 157–174, 367; after traumatic brain injury 162; antidepressant mediations 158–159; and concealable group membership 169; and social relationships 161–165; cognitive approaches to 157, 160–163, 167–168, 170, 172; discrimination 169; interpersonal psychotherapy 163; loneliness 162; measures 165, 168; relapse 158, 163–164; social identity approach to 163–172; social withdrawal 160, 162
diabetes 1, 4, 7, 36, 66, 133, 203, 248, 286, 307–308, 311, 316–317, 323
diagnostic categories 207
diagnostic testing 309
dieting 203–205, 210, 213, 221, 223, 347, 371–372
disadvantage *see* socio-economic status (SES)
disasters 91, 108, 117, 123, 126, 129; *see also* collective resilience
disclosure 243, 250, 303, 347, 363–364; measures 347
discrimination 15, 18–20, 36, 57, 63–79, 81–82, 99, 116, 146, 169, 190, 210–211, 215, 222, 224–226, 243–244, 254, 281, 294, 302, 304, 320, 347, 362 (*see also* age discrimination; gender; prejudice; racial discrimination; religious groups; stigma; weight stigma); age (*see* age discrimination); ambiguity *vs.* uncertainty 89; appraisal and coping 74–76, 263, 276; biological and psychosocial responses 66–67, 72; buffers against pathological outcomes 72, 78, 206; collective strategies 78, 146; dwarfism (*see* dwarfism); gender (*see* gender discrimination); perceived control 77; pervasiveness 64, 74, 76,

81; racial (*see* racial discrimination); religious (*see* religious groups discrimination); support 63, 69, 71–74, 76; stress 67–68, 99; gender (*see* gender discrimination); individualistic strategies 76; pervasiveness 64, 74, 76; social mobility 72, 74–75, 77, 247
disability 36, 65–66, 131, 134, 158, 227, 229–231, 236, 240, 243, 291, 300, 307–308, 316–318, 320
driving cessation 148
dwarfism 19, 77, 83

eating 11, 78, 134, 136, 183, 188, 203–226, 252–253, 261, 267, 313, 315, 323, 325, 332–333, 359, 371–372; disorders 203–226; group-based stigma 222–224; social identity approach to 203, 215–216, 218, 221; norms 207, 215–222, 224; prejudice 210; situated identity-enactment model (SIE) 203, 217–219, 220, 224; social cognitive models, 207–211; socio-economic status 216; social and cultural influences 204, 211–214; thin ideal 211, 213–214, 221–222
education 8, 36–37, 42, 45–46, 56–58, 60–61, 67, 78, 140, 179, 187, 190, 195, 210, 216, 236, 281, 292, 303, 324; *see also* students
effervescence 29
efficacy *see* self-efficacy
emotional support 91, 191, 354, 360
empowerment 52, 60, 129
English Longitudinal Study of Ageing (ELSA) 148, 150
epigenetics 214, 327, 329
ethnic minorities 25, 169, 176; discrimination 169; social support 176
eustress 85, 97–98, 102
exclusion *see* discrimination
exercise 1–2, 8, 36, 68, 86, 94, 134, 136, 148, 150, 188, 190, 193, 213, 216, 223, 233, 307, 311, 315, 317, 336, 345; *see also* sport, benefits of 134
exhaustion 85–86, 102, 364–365
extreme events 129; *see also* war crimes

family 4–5, 8, 17, 20, 29, 42, 57, 84, 88, 91, 96, 104, 116, 122, 144, 150, 161, 165, 168, 175–176, 178, 180, 182, 184, 188, 190–195, 200, 215–216, 219, 231–233, 235, 237–238, 240, 250, 281, 283–284, 289–290, 293–294, 297, 301, 304–305, 354–355, 360–361, 373; identification 294; support 175–176, 191–196, 232–233; therapies 184
Fatboy Slim beach party in Brighton 117–119

fat talk 221
frequent attendance 323

Gallup World Poll 377
gate control theory 257–258
gender 20, 24–25, 36, 65–66, 70–71, 75–76, 80,
    93–94, 146, 161–162, 164, 190, 204, 259, 267,
    292, 319, 329–330, 341; discrimination 20, 65,
    76; *see also* sexuality, women
general adaptation syndrome (GAS) 84, 86
general practitioners (GPs) 313, 323;
    communication skills training 311, 317; health
    promotion 313; normative health beliefs 316,
    325
graded exercise therapy 311
group identification *see* social identification
groups 47–48, 51, 186, 195, 197, 353, 355;
    as mechanism in treatment 72, 78, 306; as
    psychological resources 52, 191
GROUPS 4 HEALTH 332–345; effectiveness 332,
    334, 339–342; program 332, 335–343; social
    disconnection 332–333, 334–335, 344; social
    identity mapping 338; theoretical underpinnings
    334–335
group identification 10, 51–53, 72–73, 77, 82,
    139, 149, 152, 155, 169, 173, 188, 295, 300,
    305–306, 326, 352; and health and well-being
    51–53, 72–73, 305; positive effects on health 52
group norms *see* norms
group psychotherapy 114, 163, 168, 170, 173, 233,
    288–289, 316

Hajj at Mecca 28, 357
happiness scales 31, 276
Headway UK 243
health and well-being measures 347, 364;
    affect 347, 370; burnout (chronic stress) 347,
    364–365; job satisfaction 347; life satisfaction
    347, 376–377; personal self-esteem 347, 375;
    post-traumatic stress 347, 366–367; traumatic
    experiences 366, 369
health belief model 207–208, 210
health beliefs 207–208, 210
health gradient 36–37, 41–46, 56, 60–61
health promotion 138, 209, 309, 313–314,
    324–326, 331; approach 309, 311–315, 329;
    social identity approach to 313, 324–325
health promotion approach 309, 311–315, 329
health-related behaviour 17, 75, 165, 170; and
    health-related outcomes 139; psychosocial
    models 41; social identity and health promotion
    17, 32, 34

health services 8, 37, 79–80, 141, 287, 290, 293,
    309, 321, 323
hearing loss 141, 155, 307, 320–322
hedonic model of pain 260–263
helping 15, 25, 44, 53, 55, 59, 66, 79, 88, 103,
    111, 119, 125, 134, 179, 184, 213, 232, 234,
    236, 274–275, 277, 288, 297, 303, 330, *see also*
    social support
Hillsborough disaster (1989) 118
HIV/AIDS 308
holistic approach (to ABI) 235–236, 240
homelessness 47–48, 56, 58–59, 168, 170, 291,
    300
horizontal epidemiology 308
housing 8, 36, 45, 48, 56, 58–59, 64, 67, 126,
    179, 187, 281–283, 292, 301; *see also*
    homelessness
humiliation 99
Hurricane Andrew (1992) 91
Hurricane Hugo (1989) 91
hysteria 111

identity-affirming behaviours 122
identity change 39, 53–56, 58, 61–62, 126,
    146, 148–149, 162, 188, 193, 195–197,
    199–202, 233–234, 236–240, 245, 249–250,
    260–261, 294, 335; social identity model of
    identity change (SIMIC); after brain injury
    235, 239, 250; and ageing 55, 146, 148–149;
    bio-psychosocial perspective 41; implications
    for rehabilitation 195, 200, 233–236, 240;
    neuropsychological contributions 230, 250;
    personal and social processes 246; self-
    discrepancy in long-term adjustment 233–234;
    social neuropsychological cure 230; stress and
    adjustment 53–55, 239; Y-shaped model of
    rehabilitation change processes 234; *see also*
    driving cessation
identity measures 346–347; crowd identification
    347, 357; multiple identities 347–350; personal
    identity strength 347, 358; social identification
    346–348, 364; social identity continuity 347,
    351–352
identity restoration 19, 47, 71, 78, 196, 240, 320,
    453
identity salience *see* social identity salience
Illness Perception Questionnaire (IPQ) 436
Impact of Events Scale (IES-R) 366–367
immigrants 52, 219, 294
immune system 86, 327–329
inclusive victimhood 122
India 12, 266, 268

individual differences 9, 68–70, 86, 109, 135, 206, 209, 218, 258–260, 315

individual mobility 48–49, 51, 57, 72, 74–75, 77, 223, 243–245, 250, 320

ingroups 47, 80, 270, 361; social support 49, 80, 270, 361; and solidarity 49, 89; support for outgroups 80, 270, 361

instrumental support 91, 360

integrated social identity model of stress (ISIS) 99–100, 103

intention 74, 188–189, 207–210, 221, 258, 288, 310, 347, 371–372

interaction *see* social interaction

intergroup conflict *see* intergroup relations

intergroup relations 18, 21, 41, 67, 70, 141

interpersonal and social rhythm therapy (ISRT) 288–289

interpersonal conflicts 183

interpersonal stress models 161–163, 172

interpersonal psychotherapy (IPT) 163, 165, 288, 335

isolation *see* social isolation

Jewish identity 269

job satisfaction scales 89

Kosovo war 121

language 6, 22, 24, 278; *see also* communication

Latino Americans 67

leadership 25, 27, 65, 89, 123, 222–223, 290, 314

learning 113, 152, 181, 232–233, 236, 260, 336; difficulties 113, 232

life events 53, 84, 87, 89, 108, 161–163, 283, 294, 332, 361, 366

life satisfaction 18, 31, 46, 52, 55, 66, 96, 148, 169, 199, 239, 246, 292, 300, 340–342, 347, 376–377; Cantril Self-Anchoring Striving Scale 376–377; measures 340–342; Satisfaction with Life Scale (SWLS) 341, 376; social capital 7–8, 293; social connections 55, 59, 138, 149–150, 249, 337; trust 97, 294

life thread model 234

life transitions 39, 52–56, 58, 61, 139, 148, 155, 194, 335

Little People of American (LPA) 83

London terrorist bombings (2005) 104, 124

long-term medical conditions *see* chronic physical health conditions

loneliness 5, 74, 137, 162, 294, 327, 332–333, 336, 340–342, 347, 373–374

Magh Mela 12–13, 31, 268–269, 272

mass emergencies 117, 129; *see also* resilience

mass panic *see* panic

medically unexplained symptoms (MUS) 310, 316, 320, 323

medication 5, 111, 133, 158–159, 176, 178–179, 256, 263, 275, 278, 284–286, 288–290, 292, 304, 311, 317, 320, 329; antidepressant 158–159; multiple 311; side effects 133, 158, 278, 286, 311

meaning 15, 17–18, 21, 26, 29, 32, 53, 56–57, 87, 93–94, 96, 100, 102, 110, 115, 121, 124, 128, 144, 165–167, 173, 191, 218, 241, 245, 247, 251–252, 254, 256, 258, 263, 267, 269–270, 275, 289, 293, 297, 319, 334

measures of identity, health, and well-being 346–379; health and well-being measures 347, 364–378; identity measures 346–358; psychological measures 358–364

memory 110, 113–114, 116, 123, 137, 141–146, 151, 230–232, 234–236, 248, 366; autobiographical (*see* autobiographical memory); older adults 142–146

mental illness identity 303

metacognitive contextual training 451

metaphoric identity mapping (MIM) 233

mindfulness 183, 257, 316

Mindfulness-Based Relapse Prevention (MBRP) 182

minimal group studies 14–15, 18

mood 5, 18, 47, 107, 133, 152, 157, 160, 167–168, 172, 230–231, 233, 235–236, 278, 280–281, 286–288, 290, 299–301

morbidity 149, 284, 289; *see also* disability

mortality 2–3, 36, 42, 55, 69, 135, 148–149, 307, 311, 378; and social relationships 135–136, 148–149; and stress 55, 69, 135

motivational interviewing 136, 178–180, 187, 209

multiple group memberships 48, 55, 61, 190–193, 239, 271–273, 327, 340; in addiction 55, 190–193

multiple identities 26, 44, 190–191, 270–271, 273, 323, 333, 347–349; in life transitions 191, 194; measures 270, 347–349; in the workplace 29–30, 89–90, 108

multiple sclerosis, 229, 244, 320, 326–327

Muslims 27, 75

Narcotics Anonymous (NA) 186, 192, 195–197, 370–371; *see also* support groups

national identity 97, 121, 166, 325

Nazis 64, 122

needs hierarchy 36, 39, 42, 46, 49
Nepal 42, 126
normalisation 93
norms 7–8, 21, 24–25, 33, 43, 117, 122, 129, 166,
169, 175, 183, 186–189, 191–193, 195–197,
200–201, 207, 215–222, 224, 325–326, 329,
347, 350, 359, 368; eating 217–222
nudges 218, 313, 331

obesity 2, 5, 36, 42, 68, 133, 203–206, 209, 211,
215–216, 219, 222–225, 327, 331
older adults 55, 64, 73, 133–146, 148, 150,
152–155, 322, 333–334, 344, 348, 358, 379;
discrimination (*see* ageing, age discrimination);
and hearing loss 141; self-categorization
139–146; driving cessation, 148; in residential
care 134, 145; social interventions 133–137
opponent process theory 261
Organization for Economic Co-operation and
Development (OECD) 43
organizational citizenship 30, 36, 94
organizational identification 400

panic 92, 118, 123, 230, 368; attacks 122; mass 92
paranoia 294–297, 306, 347, 372–373
perceived behavioural control 207
perceiver readiness 23, 25, 139, 168, 196
permeability of group boundaries 19, 74, 77–78,
81, 100
personal control 31, 317, 347, 364
personal identity 15, 17, 21, 31, 46, 72, 92–94,
125, 127, 246, 248, 347, 358
personal identity reconstruction 233–234, 248
personal identity strength 17, 246, 347, 358
personal mobility strategies 145
personality 5, 7, 34, 68, 82, 86–87, 102–103,
135–137, 166, 173, 206–207, 215, 230, 276,
278, 306, 331; disorder 206–207
phantom limb pain 255
pharmacotherapy 178–179, 181, 185
physical activity 1, 42, 133–134, 136, 138, 148,
150, 313, 334, *see also* exercise
physiological models 39–41, 123, 254–258
pilgrims 27–28, 31, 33, 267–269, 272, 357
political groups; and group identification 10,
51–53, 72–73, 77, 82, 139, 149–154, 169,
188, 295, 300, 305–306; and suicide 12, 29, 35,
59–60, 280, 288, 303, 357
Positive and Negative Affect Scale (PANAS)
370–371
post-traumatic growth 108, 123–126, 128, 242,
244–247, 250–251

post-traumatic stress disorder (PTSD) 104–105,
107–111, 113–114, 117, 120–123, 126–127,
129–130, 366–367
power 7, 11–12, 30–33, 36, 44, 46, 51, 129, 158,
165, 201, 207, 219, 221, 263, 275, 313, 317, 340,
343–344
prejudice 14–15, 18, 65, 71, 99, 146, 210, 281,
297, 303; *see also* discrimination
primary care 125, 310, 311, 322; *see also* general
practitioner
prison 29, 46, 49–52, 62, 91, 99, 101–103, 182,
294–295, 297, 364–365, 372, 376; *see also* BBC
prison study
productivity 236
protection–motivation theory 18, 30, 125, 136
prototypicality 24, 26, 325
psychoanalytic approach 111–112
psychological measures 358–364; disclosure/
concealment 363–364; social isolation 374;
social support 360–361
psychological needs 166
psychosis 92, 278, 280, 284, 286–287, 290,
294–297, 306
psychotherapy 114, 163, 168, 170, 173, 233,
288–289, 316
psychosocial models of health-related behaviour 5,
7, 41, 209, 235
PTSD *see* post-traumatic stress disorder

racial discrimination 52, 63–64, 73, 80; biopsychosocial responses 52; coping strategies 77,
90, 182; social support 52, 73, 80
racism *see* racial discrimination
Rat Park studies 188
RE-AIM model of health promotion 314
Reclink 291–292, 297–298, 305–306
recovery 26–27, 41, 55, 81, 115–116, 122–123,
128, 158, 176, 182, 184–189, 191–198, 201,
251, 277, 280, 286, 289–290, 292–293, 297,
302–305, 307, 315, 320
recovery model of mental health 293, 297, 304
rehabilitation 82, 122, 175–176, 182, 185, 187,
195, 200, 231, 233–236, 240, 248, 251, 292,
300, 370; *see also* acquired brain injury (ABI);
identity change after brain injury; older adults in
residential care; traumatic brain injury (TBI)
refugees 121–122
religious groups 192, 269; discrimination 190; and
group identification 188; and suicide 280
rejection-identification model 71–72, 82, 99, 302
relapse prevention model 182
residential care *see* older adults in residential care

resilience 104–130, 369; communication and trust 117, 120, 124–125; consequences of shared social identity 119, 124–126, 128; crowds 120, 129; empowerment 129; "resilience" vs "vulnerability", 131, 134; politics of 104, 109, 121, 127–129; preventing/minimizing risk 114, 126; relational transformation 124–125; social bonds 122; solidarity 118–119, 122, 124–125

retirement 53, 61, 63, 88, 139, 146, 148, 150, 162, 376

risk-taking 283, 324; *see also* social identity risk assessment

rites of passage 261

salutogenesis *see* eustress

Satisfaction with Life Scale (SWLS) 341, 376

schadenfreude 268

schemas 167, 169, 319

schizoaffective disorder 278–280, 291

schizophrenia 36, 278–289, 291, 293–294, 300, 306

School of Hard Knocks 299–301, 305–306, 356

selective serotonin reuptake inhibitors (SSRIs) 158

self-categorization 18, 21–26, 30, 34, 46–48, 71, 93, 95, 98, 139–146, 154–155, 163, 169, 196, 217, 247–248, 250, 276, 305, 319, 321–322, 325, 357

self-categorization theory (SCT) 18, 21–26, 139, 142, 196, 276, 319, 325; accessibility 26, 196, 321 (*see also* perceiver readiness); and older adults 26, 139–146; and social identity context 21–26; and social support 21–26; comparative and normative context/fit 23–25; in the workplace 89, 108; principles 23–24

self-concept 160, 163–165, 169, 197, 214, 232–235, 240, 248, 250, 319

self-continuity 54, 61–62, 113–115, 235, 237; *see also* social identity, continuity

self-determination theory 214

self-efficacy 52, 78–79, 87, 136, 148, 181–182, 186, 196–197, 199–200, 281, 317

self-esteem 14, 18–19, 26, 46–49, 52, 56–58, 66, 68–70, 77–78, 87, 115, 166, 184, 195–196, 206–207, 233, 244–245, 280–281, 300, 302–303, 305–306, 340–342, 347, 363, 375, 379

self-management programs (SMPs) 316

self-stereotyping 21–22

sex 45, 65, 164, 188

sexism *see* gender discrimination

sexuality 69

shame 68, 109, 122, 203, 225, 280, 328

Situated Identity-Enactment model (SIE) 217–219, 220

skeletal dysplasias 19–20, 77–78

sleep disturbance 107

smoking 1–2, 36, 42, 77–78, 87, 133–134, 138, 175, 178–179, 181, 189–190, 199, 313, 315, 324, 326–327, 329

social bonds 250

social capital 7–8, 37, 43–44, 126, 157, 293, 314; definition 7; life satisfaction 44, 46

social cognitive theory 7

social cohesion 44

social competition 20, 30, 99–100, 223, 241–242, 245; *see also* collective action

social connection 1, 27, 103, 150, 191, 260, 302

social creativity 20, 30, 99–100, 223, 241–242, 244–247, 250

social cure 10–11, 17, 34, 44, 103, 129, 166, 172, 185, 250, 254, 263, 268, 332–345; increase in research 173, 260–261, 263; *see also* social identity approach to health and well-being

social curse 129

social exclusion 8, 36, 190, 244, 276, 283, 327

social determinants of health 8–9, 37, 43–45, 57, 62, 138, 172, 331, 343

social disadvantage *see* Socio-Economic Status (SES)

social dislocation theory of addiction 188

social identification 17–18, 20, 24–25, 27, 29, 32–33, 45, 51, 59, 73, 81, 95–97, 99–102, 116, 118, 120–121, 139, 150, 152–153, 155, 165–167, 170, 188–189, 199, 219–220, 222, 241, 244, 247–248, 268, 294, 296, 302–304, 324, 326, 333, 340–341, 343–344, 346–348, 364, 379; measures 17, 150, 152, 341, 346, 348

social identity 12–35, 45, 52–53, 56, 71, 74, 79, 92, 95, 97, 115, 120, 123, 139, 163, 188, 193, 195, 215, 219, 236, 263, 267–269, 293–294, 297, 319, 321, 334, 346, 351–352; capital 9, 157, 293, 314; compatibility 349–350; continuity 351–352; definition 12–15; gain 54–56, 237–238, 240, 300, 338; and health promotion 313; loss 53, 149, 162, 201; measures 346–358; networks 55; resources 52–56, 238, 274, 336; and social context 218; trajectories 20

social identity approach 12–35, 45, 71, 92, 115, 139, 163, 188, 215, 236, 263, 293, 319, 334; to acquired brain injury 55, 227, 232, 236–248; to acute pain 252, 254, 263–274; to addiction 176, 187–200; to ageing 133, 138–154; to chronic mental health conditions 278, 290, 293–304; to chronic physical health conditions 309,

319–329; to depression 163–172; to eating 203, 215–224; to health and well-being 13, 17–19, 21, 27, 29, 31–34, 346, 351–353, 355–357; policy implications 44; practical implications 17; to social status and health 45–60; to stigma and health 19–20, 32; to stress 92–101; theoretical underpinnings 116, 334–335; to trauma and resilience 115–126

social identity continuity 54–57, 60, 237–238, 240, 338, 347, 351–352; *see also* identity change

social identity mapping 191–192, 201, 338, 347, 352–353, 356–357, 379

social identity model 39, 53–56, 62, 99–100, 103, 125–126, 162, 195–198, 216, 237, 294, 296, 306, 335; of cessation maintenance (SIMCM) 195–197; of collective resilience 125; of crowd psychology 129; of emergent paranoia 296, 306; of identity change (SIMIC) 39, 53–56, 62, 126, 237, 335; of impact of extreme events 129; of recovery (SIMOR) 197–198; of stress (ISIS) 99–100, 103

social identity reconstruction 233–234, 248

social identity salience 22–24, 93; and coping strategies 77, 90, 182, 287, 329; and disaster relief 30; and health behaviour 22–24; and organizational stressors 39, 94; and social support 29–30; and stress 93

social identity theory (SIT) 18–21, 23, 26, 30, 34, 46–47, 49, 51, 77–78, 82, 98–100, 245; principles 23, 51, 98

social inclusion 181, 299

social influence 24–26, 36, 92, 94, 188, 196–197, 214–216, 219, 221, 225, 232, 270, 276, 319

social interaction 7, 17, 29, 92, 114, 134, 161, 232, 244, 275, 333, 361

social isolation 135, 137–138, 162–163, 168, 194, 250, 280–281, 283, 292, 297, 304, 323, 329, 332–333, 340–342, 346; schema 168

social learning 260 *see also* learning

social mobility 247

social neuropsychological cure 230

social neuropsychology 230, 408

social relationships and health 52, 59, 98, 131, 137–138, 150, 155, 161–164, 181, 184, 231, 235, 246, 249–250, 275, 288, 331–332, 335; causal effects 137–138, 162–164; experimental studies 150, 158, 166, 263; family identification 294; group identification 139, 149–154, 295; multiple group memberships 48, 55, 61, 190–193; mortality 148–149; negative outcomes 332; positive effects 49, 52, 152, 237, 302

social support 2–3, 8, 29–30, 32, 39–41, 49, 51–52, 54, 59, 71–74, 80–83, 85, 91, 95–98, 102–103, 117, 122, 128, 137, 149, 152, 162–163, 165–166, 237, 243–244, 246, 250, 257, 260, 263, 270–271, 275, 277, 290, 292, 300, 302–306, 327, 346–347, 360–361; buffering hypothesis 162; cognitive 53, 58, 74, 162–163; definition 2–3, 8, 29–30; emotional 384; expectations of 125, 145; impact 39, 82; interpretation 123, 154; measures 39; material 31, 97–98; unsupportive interactions 347, 361

social solidarity *see* solidarity

socio-economic status (SES) 5, 36, 80, 162, 164, 216, 323; in community contexts 36, 216; disadvantaged groups 47–48, 51–52, 56, 59, 61; in education contexts 56–58; and health care 36, 80, 323; and health gradient 36; homelessness 168; in housing contexts 58–59; and identification with disadvantaged groups 47–48; mobility strategies 57, 145, 250; social identification 81, 165–166; sociological and epidemiological models 42–45

solidarity 15, 31, 41, 49, 89, 118–119, 122, 124–125, 166, 260, 265

sport 1–2, 7, 19, 93, 114, 118, 293; *see also* exercise, clubs 7

stages of change model *see* transtheoretical model

stereotype lift 144

stereotype threat 142

stereotypes 19–20, 80, 139–147, 154–155, 189, 302; of people with CMHC 302–303, 306; of older adults 139, 141

stigma 63–83, 189, 222, 302, 362; appraisal 70, 74–76; coping with 71–74; engagement with and health 63–67, 71–80; health services 79–80; and intention to quit addiction 189–190; sensitivity 68–69; *see also* discrimination; prejudice

stress 84–103; appraisal 89–92; buffering hypothesis 162; burnout 86; collective response 84, 89–95; epidemics 92; process 87, 92, 102; social identity approach to 92–101; transactional model 89–92, 94; *see also* workplace stress

stroke *see* acquired brain injury (ABI)

students 19, 26, 53, 55–58, 78, 93–94, 111, 140, 167–168, 184, 188–189, 219, 227, 299, 340, 346, 348–349, 356, 359, 361, 363–364, 370, 372–374, 376–377; *see also* education, health

subjective norms 208

substance abuse 27, 55, 175–176, 179–180, 182, 189, 191, 200, 292

support *see* social support

support groups 19, 53, 176, 184, 186–187, 191–192, 200, 243, 293, 302, 305–306, 311, 328
suicide 12, 29, 35, 59–60, 280, 288, 303, 357; and social relationships 59, 288; and stress 288
sun protection 325
SWLS (Satisfaction with Life Scale) 341, 376
sympathetic nervous system 109–110, 328
symptom 5, 10, 46, 66, 69, 88, 104–105, 107, 123, 139, 141, 154–155, 162, 170, 230, 278, 280, 286–287, 294, 311, 316, 320–323, 341; appraisal 316, 321; diagnosis 104–105, 107, 170

TBI *see* traumatic brain injury
theory of planned behavior (TPB) 207, 210
therapeutic alliance 25, 33, 96, 97, 161, 170, 188
therapeutic communities (TCs) 123, 176, 185, 187, 191–195, 197, 199–201, 348
thin ideal 211, 213–214, 221, 222
top 10 tips for better health 343; medical tips 343; alternative tips 44–45; social identity tips 343
tranquillisers 278
transactional model of stress and coping *see* stress, transactional model
transtheoretical model 209
trauma 104–130; appraisal 117, 123; coping 108, 114, 121; experience 108–114, 116, 122, 162, 230; mass emergencies 117, 129; post-traumatic growth 108, 123–126; post-traumatic stress 104–105, 107, 117, 120–121, 129; psychoanalytic models 111–112; resilience 104–130; social identity approach to 115–126; social identity model of collective resilience 125; *see also* collective resilience; traumatic brain injury; war crimes; war crimes: Kosovo
traumatic brain injury (TBI) 230, 233, 235, 238; associated problems 230–231; depression 230, 232; emotional well-being and social linkage 232; self-conceptualisation 232–235; *see also* acquired brain injury (ABI); identity change after brain injury
Trier Social Stress Test 94

trust 7–8, 15, 27–29, 33, 43–44, 80, 117, 120, 124–125, 161, 166, 267, 294, 302, 323, 331, 373
Type A behaviour pattern (TABP) 86–87
Type B behaviour pattern (TBBP) 86

university *see* students
Unsupportive Social Interactions Inventory 361
United Kingdom (UK) 1, 30, 61, 103, 118, 129–130, 153, 179, 190, 197, 202, 243, 290, 293, 327, 348–349, 352, 357–358, 360, 365, 369, 371, 373
United Nations (UN) 44, 108, 131–132
United States (US) 1, 20–21, 25, 31, 49, 59, 65, 70, 77–78, 91, 108, 133, 137, 146, 159, 184, 188, 219, 225–226, 242–243, 286, 290, 311, 328, 379
US Civil Rights Movement *see* Civil Rights Movement

vaccination 325
validation 124–125, 369, 371, 378
vulnerability 54, 68, 71, 142, 149, 158, 168, 175, 206, 214, 238, 335

war crimes 122; humiliation 122; Kosovo 121–122; Nazi 122
weight stigma 65, 75
weight loss 136, 206, 209, 213, 220, 223–225, 317, 327, 331; *see also* dieting
women 21, 23–25, 37, 55, 59, 65, 69, 73, 75–76, 80, 89, 93, 110, 115–116, 122, 132, 136, 149–150, 157, 161, 203, 204, 211, 213–214, 221–223, 225, 259, 265, 359, 371–372; *see also* gender; in abusive relationships 20, 116; coping style 99, 233, 327; discrimination 36, 75–76, 116, 215, 222
workplace stress 89–90, 92
World Health Organization 44, 62, 146, 156, 204, 236, 307, 344

Y-shaped model of rehabilitation change processes 233–236

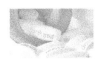

Hypotheses associated with the social identity approach to health

H1   (*the social identity hypothesis*): Because it is the basis for meaningful group life, social identity is central to both good and ill health.

H2   (*the identification hypothesis*): A person will generally experience the health-related benefits or costs of a given group membership only to the extent that they identify with that group.

H3   (*the group circumstance hypothesis*): When and to the extent that a person defines themselves in terms of a given social identity, their well-being will be affected by the state and circumstances of the group with which that identity is associated.

    H3a. When the group that defines a person's social identity is enhanced in some way (e.g., by success, high status, or advancement), social identity becomes a beneficial psychological resource and tends to have positive consequences for their well-being.

    H3b. When the group that defines a person's social identity is compromised in some way (e.g., by stigma, low status, or failure), the capacity for social identity to function as a beneficial psychological resource is reduced, and this will tend to have negative consequences for their well-being.

H4   (*the identity restoration hypothesis*): People will be motivated to restore positive identity when this is compromised by events that threaten or undermine their social identities (e.g., group failure, stigma, low status, or loss of group membership).

H5   (*the mobility hypothesis*): When circumstances threaten, undermine, or preclude positive social identity, if people perceive group boundaries to be permeable, they are likely to respond to the threat to positive identity through strategies of personal mobility.

H6   (*the creativity hypothesis*): When circumstances threaten, undermine, or preclude positive social identity, if people perceive group boundaries to be impermeable but group relations to be secure, they are likely to respond to the threat to positive identity through strategies of social creativity.

H7   (*the competition hypothesis*): When circumstances threaten, undermine, or preclude positive social identity, if people perceive group boundaries to be impermeable and group relations to be insecure, they are likely to respond to the threat to positive identity through strategies of social competition.

H8   (*the norm enactment hypothesis*): When, and to the extent that, a person defines themselves in terms of a given social identity, they will enact – or at least strive to enact – the norms and values associated with that identity.

H9   (*the influence hypothesis*): When, and to the extent that, people define themselves in terms of shared social identity, they will be more likely to influence each other.

H10 (*the prototypicality hypothesis*): People will have more influence in defining the meaning of a given social identity to the extent that they are seen to be representative of that identity.

H11 (*the multiple identities hypothesis*): Providing they are compatible with each other, important to them, and positive, the more social identities a person has access to, the more psychological resources they can draw upon and the more beneficial this will be for their health.

H12 (*the connection hypothesis*): When, and to the extent that, people define themselves in terms of shared social identity, they will be more likely to perceive themselves as similar and connected and to be positively oriented towards (e.g., trusting of) each other.

H13 (*the meaning hypothesis*): When, and to the extent that, people define themselves in terms of shared social identity, that identity will focus their energies and imbue them with a sense of meaning, purpose, and worth.

H14 (*the support hypothesis*): When, and to the extent that, people define themselves in terms of shared social identity, they will (1) expect to give each other support, (2) actually give each other support, and (3) construe the support they receive more positively.

H15 (*the agency hypothesis*): When, and to the extent that, people define themselves in terms of shared social identity, they will develop a sense of efficacy, agency, and power.

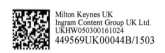